Condition-Specific Massage Therapy

Celia Bucci, MA, LMT

Wolters Kluwer
Health

Lippincott Williams & Wilkins

Philadelphia • Baltimore • New York • London
Buenos Aires • Hong Kong • Sydney • Tokyo

Acquisitions Editor: Kelley Squazzo
Product Manager: Linda G. Francis
Development Editor: Tom Lochhaas
Design Coordinator: Teresa Mallon
Marketing Manager: Shauna Kelley
Photography: Katrina Wittkamp
Art: Imagineering
Compositor: Aptara, Inc.

351 West Camden Street
Baltimore, MD 21201

Two Commerce Square
2001 Market Street
Philadelphia, PA 19103

Library of Congress Cataloging-in-Publication Data
Bucci, Celia, author.
    Condition-specific massage therapy/Celia Bucci.
      p. ; cm.
    Includes bibliographical references and index.
    ISBN 978-1-58255-807-3 (alk. paper)
    1. Massage therapy—Handbooks, manuals, etc.   I. Title.
[DNLM: 1. Massage—methods—Handbooks.   2. Musculoskeletal
Diseases—therapy—Handbooks.   WB 39]
    RM721.B882 2012
    615.8′22—dc22

                                        2010045790

For my father Vincenzo and my brother Jim. I wish I could give you a massage.

Reviewers

Rene Adams, MA
Pima Medical Institute
Santa Fe, New Mexico

Yves Charette, RMT
Collège Boreal
Sudbury, Ontario, Canada

Lloyd Mills, CMT
Massage Therapy Institute of Colorado
Denver, Colorado

Becky SanGregorio, LMT
Laurel Highlands Therapeutic Academy
Ebensburg, Pennsylvania

Antonella Sena, DC
Academy of Massage Therapy
Hackensack, New Jersey

Ljubisa Terzic, MD
Canadian College of Naturopathic Medicine
Toronto, Ontario, Canada

Barbara Uniatowski, LMT
Harris School of Business
Wilmington, Delaware

Foreword

Therapeutic massage has made incredible advances in the last few decades. While it is still used extensively as a method of general relaxation and stress reduction, the recognition of medical and healthcare benefits of massage therapy is now unquestioned. As a society we have spiraling healthcare costs and in many cases a decrease in positive outcomes from those invested costs. This situation has led to a renewed interest in complementary and alternative (CAM) health care approaches.

As the profession grows and matures we must clearly raise the bar of our educational standards. That can only happen in our schools and training programs when there are adequate educational resources to support the teachers and students in the classroom. We are gradually seeing an increase in quality educational resources for schools, but we still need enhancements to our collection of professional literature.

In addition to a shortage of books and resources for the classroom, there is also a lack of peer-reviewed medical literature about massage therapy. Continued advancements in the use of massage as a legitimate health care intervention is highly dependent on a growing body of peer-reviewed literature. Enhancing educational standards and encouraging research interest in massage therapy follows the emergence of textbooks emphasizing the clinical applications of massage.

Condition-Specific Massage Therapy is a valuable addition to the professional literature which will help move our profession forward and make the beneficial treatments of soft-tissue therapy available to a patient population greatly in need. In this text, author Celia Bucci brings detailed and specific clinical information to a level that will be accessible for many massage educators in their training programs. Her vision for making this information available to help the many clients in need is an inspiring call for all practitioners to improve their knowledge, skills, and understanding of various clinical conditions which clients may present.

There is an increasing degree of discussion about the importance of evidence-based practice in all health care fields. Bucci highlights that need for a strong evidence base to support the scientific understanding of our work. But more than simply giving the concept lip service she integrates these concepts into each chapter of the text. She states that this book is more of a *"what is"* than a *"how to"* approach. Her perspective and orientation for the text will help develop more *thinking practitioners*, not just those who are performing rote massage routines.

In our field there is no shortage of workshops, programs, books, or DVDs that are designed to teach a practitioner how to do a particular technique. What we are in greater need of are resources that help teach the practitioner how to think. Without essential clinical reasoning skills, those massage practitioners attempting to address complicated pain and injury complaints are simply acting as technicians. Because no person presents with the exact same pathology as another, massage practitioners must take advantage of their unique ability to individually tailor treatments to each person's needs. The essential clinical reasoning and critical thinking skills that Bucci emphasizes with her approach in this text are a great way to move in that direction.

The format she has chosen for this book is well suited to develop these essential critical thinking skills. Foundational principles of biomechanics, kinesiology, anatomy, assessment, and treatment are provided in the early chapters of the text. In the later chapters specific pathological conditions are addressed in extensive detail. Concepts applied to specific pathologies in the later chapters are built on the foundational knowledge established in these early chapters. Inclusion of critical thinking exercises and individual case studies is an excellent way to help the practitioner understand how to use this material in a realistic clinical context.

I was also impressed with the way in which information is presented visually throughout the book. The illustrations within the text highlight principles and greatly enhance the reader's understanding of concepts that are presented. Layered graphics help the reader understand anatomical relationships and better understand the pathological information presented about each condition.

This book can be a valuable resource both at entry-level educational programs and for practitioners already in professional practice. Having a highly readable resource like *Condition-Specific Massage Therapy* will help practitioners begin their career with a solid foundation. For those already in practice it is a valuable aid to enhance their understanding of situations they face each day in the clinic. I am very pleased to see a text like this available to support and enhance our professional literature and raise our educational discourse to a higher level.

Whitney Lowe
Sisters, OR

Preface

Massage therapy as a profession is in the midst of great, progressive change. Evidence-based practice and clinical applications are common topics in massage publications and education today. Our recognition as health care providers continues to grow as more consumers of massage use it for the relief of chronic pain and injury, and to improve athletic performance. At the same time, many new graduates entering practice begin their professional journey working in environments that the general public often perceives as indulgent, where general wellness and relaxation are the focus of treatment. Though my initial training focused on clinical massage, I began my professional journey working in a spa. I found during that time that regardless of the environments clients choose to receive massage, they often present with specific pain patterns, with or without a diagnosis, for which they seek at least temporary relief. Until they book a massage with a therapist familiar with their signs and symptoms, who can explain the possible causes and plan treatment that achieves the goal of long term improvement of symptoms, clients remain unaware of the health care benefits of massage therapy, or that the spa could be the perfect environment for the treatment of common chronic pain conditions.

Wellness massage is indeed therapeutic, and the massage therapist who can explain a pain pattern to their clients and incorporate specific treatments and self-care into general relaxation massage empowers clients with knowledge about their health while promoting the value of massage therapy as a treatment option for injuries, recurring pain, and athletic enhancement. As the profession evolves and becomes a more competitive and essential dimension of health care, the massage therapist has an advantage when they can assess clients' signs and symptoms and treat their probable causes of pain. These therapists are also more likely to develop a loyal clientele and gain extensive referrals because of the success they achieve in improving the client's symptoms.

Audience and Approach

In a typical massage therapy program it is difficult to teach a detailed, clinical approach to specific conditions because of time constraints. Moreover, students in a basic program may not yet know if, or how they want to specialize. In my opinion, the basic program is not the place for advanced clinical training. This is best taught in longer, specialized programs or through continuing education, and there are several marvelous books offering more detailed information than presented here. *Condition-Specific Massage Therapy* is a textbook intended for massage therapy students enrolled in a basic program and practicing therapists who want to hone their critical thinking and basic massage skills to target the structures involved in common chronic pain conditions.

Condition-Specific Massage Therapy is more of a "what is...?" than a "how to..." textbook. Signs, symptoms, anatomy, physiology, assessment, indications, contraindications, and treatment goals provide the critical thinking tools necessary to develop a treatment protocol that can be adapted to the practitioner's preferred therapeutic method, at their level of training. This also gives the practitioner who integrates energy therapies into massage a guide for using energy techniques that address the treatment goals for these conditions.

To use this book most efficiently, massage therapy students and practitioners should have:

■ The ability to find and palpate the origin, insertion, and belly of the major muscles
■ The ability to distinguish muscles, tendons and ligaments
■ The knowledge of endangerment sites and how to avoid them
■ The ability to perform a basic postural assessment

- The skills for applying basic strokes
- The knowledge of contraindications and cautions for massage
- The skill to find and use other texts as references for more specific questions.

Organization

The first chapter focuses on basic tools and concepts used throughout the text, including:

- Basic biomechanics
- The essential elements of a health history
- General interpretations of common signs and symptoms
- Atypical textures in tissues and how to address them
- The basics of ROM for assessment, treatment, and self care
- The general principles of massage and how to apply them
- The physiological effects of basic strokes
- Basic applications of hydrotherapy, mobilizations, and postisometric relaxation
- Planning and achieving treatment goals
- The basics of self care

The second and third chapters describe fascia and trigger points, their role in chronic pain, and guidelines for treatment. Research continues to show that resolving trigger points and fascial restrictions are fundamental in reducing spasm, lengthening shortened muscles, normalizing posture, and resolving chronic pain. Each chapter describing a specific condition includes the assessment and treatment of fascial restrictions and trigger points commonly found in those conditions.

The remaining chapters cover specific conditions independently. Chapters 4–11 describe conditions affecting specific locations, organized from superior body location (tension headaches) to inferior (plantar fasciitis). Because the structures involved in tension headaches, for example, are similar to those involved in hyperkyphosis, this arrangement gives the readers consecutive opportunities to study these structures, encouraging proficiency by repetition. Chapters 12–14 describe conditions that can affect structures throughout the body (muscle strain, ligament sprain, tendinopathy). Once the reader reaches these chapters, they will studied most of the muscles and joints of the body specifically, making it easier for them to adapt to conditions that can occur nearly anywhere.

Each condition chapter includes the following:

UNDERSTANDING [THE CONDITION]

- Explanation of the condition and the anatomical structures involved
- Common signs and symptoms
- Possible causes and contributing factors
- Conditions commonly confused with or contributing to the condition described
- Contraindications and special considerations for treatment
- Current research on the benefits of massage for the condition

WORKING WITH THE CLIENT

- Important questions for the client's health history
- Postural assessment
- Standard ROM for joints involved and common outcomes from ROM testing
- Simple orthopedic tests
- Origin, insertion, action, and innervation of muscles commonly involved
- Photograph showing trigger points and referral areas common to the condition
- Treatment goals
- Client self-care and suggestions for further treatments

PROFESSIONAL GROWTH

- Case study with SOAP notes
- Critical thinking exercises

Features

Condition-Specific Massage Therapy has been designed to encourage students to use critical thinking skills when addressing clients' needs. Elements to help reach that goal include:

- **Icons**

  Icons representing treatment goals are repeated throughout the text to encourage students to focus on outcomes instead of simply trying to memorize treatment steps. These will help students incorporate the techniques of their preferred massage modality to achieve the client's treatment goals.

- **Treatment Overview Diagram**

  This diagram provides a visual overview of the treatment goals for each condition. It is organized according to four general principles of massage sequencing:
  - general → specific → general
  - superficial → deep → superficial
  - proximal → distal → proximal
  - peripheral → central → peripheral

  The diagram focuses on treatment goals and the general principles of massage rather than rigidly specifying step-by-step procedures, allowing the therapist to incorporate their preferred techniques to achieve those goals.

- **Artwork**

  Photographs with the referenced muscles illustrated over the model's skin to show precise location of the structures to be addressed are included in each of the chapters that refer to the treatment of specific muscles. To help students recognize the condition, Chapters 4-11 also includes a photograph of a client in anatomical position alongside a photograph of a client whose posture shows postural deviations common to the condition described. To aid in developing the treatment plan, these photographs highlight muscles that are shortened or lengthened in the deviated posture.

- **Massage Therapy Research**

  This section summarizes some of the current research into the benefits of massage for treating the condition. In some cases, research is not yet available, and students should feel encouraged to embark on their own research projects.

- **Case Study and SOAP Note**

  Each condition chapter includes a case study with SOAP notes.

- **Critical Thinking Exercises**

  In each condition chapter, a list of critical thinking exercises is included for classroom discussion or homework to encourage students to consider unique situations when planning treatment.

Online Resources

Instructor resources available for *Condition-Specific Massage Therapy* include:

- Image bank of all art in the text
- A syllabus, and lesson plans for each chapter.
- PowerPoint slide presentations

All readers have access to an e-book, which can be accessed by visiting the website at http://thePoint.lww.com/Buccile (use the access code on the inside front cover of this book). Also on thePoint you will find links to relevant clips from *Acland's Video Atlas of Human Anatomy!*

Achieve Your Goals

As you read these chapters you'll surely notice some repetition. In many cases this repetition is verbatim. This is intentional, and while it may be tempting to pass over these repeated phrases, I strongly recommend reading them each time. There are many common elements to these conditions, their assessment and their treatment, and many of these repeated phrases are applicable beyond the conditions described in this text. While I could have phrased these elements slightly differently to avoid the tedium of repetition, I chose to repeat them exactly to help the reader commit these core concepts to memory. By the time you've read these phrases several times, my hope is that the concepts will be very clear and that their application will flow naturally.

Condition-Specific Massage Therapy will prepare you to contextualize the complaints you're most likely to hear in your practice. Without going deeply into clinical detail, this book explains how to use your basic skills to educate and treat clients with common musculoskeletal conditions. The features of this book were designed with consideration for diverse learning styles and to accommodate the wide variety of techniques known as massage therapy. I hope that above all this book demonstrates that basic skills provide a strong foundation for reaching clinical therapeutic goals in any massage therapy environment.

Your comments, questions, corrections, and other suggestions are sincerely welcomed. You can reach me at celia@preventchronicpain.com.

Celia Bucci, LMT

About the Author

Celia Bucci graduated from the Soma Institute, National School of Clinical Massage Therapy. She has practiced clinical massage in environments ranging from spas and resorts to sports clinics and currently runs a private practice at Illinois Masonic Hospital. Celia served as Secretary and Communications Liaison for the Illinois Chapter of the American Massage Therapy Association, and Editor of its newsletter *Keeping In Touch*. She was awarded the chapter's 2010 Distinguished Service Award.

Before embarking on her career in massage therapy, Celia earned a B.A. in Communications Studies from DePaul University, and an M.A. in Cultural Studies from the University of Iowa. Celia became a producer of theater, film, and cultural festivals, and a sound designer and sound engineer for performing artists. After visiting Trinidad and Tobago and experiencing a culture that reveres nature and living at a leisurely pace, she decided to put the phone down, step away from the computer, and slow it all down.

Acknowledgments

My mom Elisa taught me many practical skills—not the least of which is kneading pasta and bread dough. This, I believe, was my first and most fundamental lesson in palpating texture, tone, and temperature. Grazie, mamma! I'm pretty sure my sister Mary taught me to speak English, and I know she nurtured me as I was growing up. My brother Domenic showed me how much cool stuff happens outside the box. Thanks forever to both of you.

One day, Teresa Sieg Hajdu visited the school where I was teaching to talk about the books LWW had to offer. We chatted about the future of massage therapy education, and she asked me whether I'd ever considered writing a book, which I hadn't. Now my book is written and it's largely thanks to you, Teresa. That day changed my professional journey profoundly. You opened the door for me, and I am truly grateful.

After that, John Goucher read my proposal, passed it around, and told me that the project was accepted. I think I stopped breathing for a few seconds. Thanks for getting this ball rolling John, and thanks to Linda Francis and Tom Lochhaas for helping me keep the ball out of the middle of the road. Kelley Squazzo and Shauna Kelley got this book off my computer and into your hands. Thanks Kelleys! Though I still don't know your names, thanks to the reviewers of this text. Your comments and suggestions are much appreciated. Special thanks to James Clay and David Pounds for your innovative style of illustrating the musculature.

I might not have had the idea for this book if Emmanuel Bistas hadn't trusted me to design and teach the course that inspired it, or if my students hadn't asked so many great and complicated questions. And I might not have had the idea to teach a course on condition-specific massage if the Soma Institute hadn't provided me with a fantastic education that delved deeply into anatomy, physiology, kinesiology, and pathology, and encouraged me to apply critical thinking instead of memorizing techniques. Thank you Emmanuel, Soma, and all of my former students.

Mightiest thanks to my clients who, one session at a time, help me learn how all of this works, and whose confidence in me is a gift I cherish.

Many, many thanks to Geoff Greenberg and Steve Switzer for being my personal librarians. As many thanks to Jeanne Kim, Allison Ishman, Joe Muscolino, and Laura Allen for indulging me in conversations about what happens in the human body, and how to be an author. Cheers to Angie Palmier for regularly reminding me what I'm capable of. I hope you won't regret that!

Christopher Maceyak, Mary Brogger, Cyndi Elliot, Patti Renda, Judy Cohn, David Borreguero, and Karen Stanczykiewicz let me pull them away from fun and relaxation to pose for the photos I needed for the first draft of these chapters. That was really cool of you. Thanks to Josh Hudson, Xochitl Vinaja, Nestor Battung, and Caitlin Bauler for striking the poses that appear in this book, and to Katrina Wittkamp for capturing them. You're all beautiful.

Daliah Saper very generously provided legal counsel in the early stages of this project. I've never even met her. She's the friend of a friend who helped a complete stranger. How often does that happen? Susan Salvo, Jennifer Watrous, and Kelly Milford liked my work. That helped me pay the rent. I wouldn't have been able to focus so intently on this project without the opportunities you provided. Thanks y'all.

Fiona Rattray, Linda Ludwig, Janet Travell, David Simons, Thomas Myers, Ruth Werner, Bruno Chikly, Whitney Lowe, Andrew Biel, Leon Chaitow, Sandy Fritz, Erik Dalton, and Jean Pierre Barral taught me most of what I've learned about manual therapy so far. I encourage every reader of this book to delve more deeply into studying massage therapy as health care from these scholars and their protégés.

Ultimately, thanks to Freak Nation. You know who you are. I hope you also know how grateful I am to have you in my life. You listened to me and supported me throughout this long process. Now, finally, we can talk about something else.

Contents

PART III Conditions Affecting Locations Throughout the Body   285

CHAPTER

1

The Basic Tools for Specific Treatment

WHAT IS CONDITION-SPECIFIC MASSAGE?

Simply put, condition-specific massage refers to the application of massage techniques to treat the common contributing factors of a specific condition. Therapists may choose to supplement their basic education with advanced studies in massage techniques such as clinical, orthopedic, sports, and Thai massage; disciplines such as reflexology; and spa therapies. Regardless of the style of massage one chooses to practice or the environment in which one works, the clients we treat often suffer pain related to an injury or chronic postural imbalance. While the techniques we use to treat pain may differ, many of the treatment goals remain consistent.

Massage practitioners bring varying levels of expertise to their treatment of specific conditions. All massage therapists have expert knowledge of the musculoskeletal system. Advanced education and specialization is important for the therapist who plans to develop a practice treating complicated chronic pain and injuries. However, for uncomplicated cases of the common conditions explained in this book, basic massage therapy skills are often sufficient to minimize pain and facilitate postural balance.

This book focuses on using the basic skills learned in a core massage therapy program to treat the contributing factors involved in conditions most often seen in massage therapy environments ranging from medical facilities to spas. The emphasis on treatment goals allows you, the therapist, to apply the techniques of any modality you pursue. With an understanding of the physiological effects of techniques, you can match techniques with the treatment goals for specific conditions, as outlined in the following chapters, to develop treatment plans.

This chapter reviews the basic tools massage therapists use to design an effective treatment plan based on therapeutic goals. Each of the subjects covered in this book can be studied in much greater detail than presented here, and each tool can be used with greater specificity and for purposes beyond those learned in a basic massage curriculum. What is offered here is a way to integrate the treatment of specific signs and symptoms into general relaxation massage as well as a stepping stone toward the study of a more focused approach to treating specific conditions.

In some cases, clients with the conditions described in this book may have issues or complications that require advanced skills and training to treat them adequately. If you are unsure of whether your skills are adequate to properly treat a client with a complicated condition, discuss it with a mentor or therapist with advanced training. It may turn out that your assessment of the client is correct and your treatment plan is perfectly appropriate. If you are still unsure after discussing the case with a more experienced practitioner, refer the client to another massage therapist or health care provider who has the training and experience necessary to manage a complicated case. Attempting to treat a client whose case is beyond your experience may hinder the client's recovery and could turn the client away from massage therapy altogether. With the client's legal consent, ask the referred provider to discuss their assessment and treatment goals with you; this is a great way to learn by experience.

BASICS OF BIOMECHANICS

In general, biomechanics is the study of how mechanical models apply to living organisms. For massage therapists, biomechanics describes the relationship between the bones and joints and the internal and external forces that act upon them to either make us move or stabilize static postures. Muscle tension is the mediator in the push and pull between anatomical structures and the forces that act upon them. Knowing the basics of musculoskeletal biomechanics can reveal how typical biomechanical functioning is stressed by a client's posture and activities and helps you plan treatment. Understanding the relationship between anatomy and force is a valuable tool for assessing pain and injury.

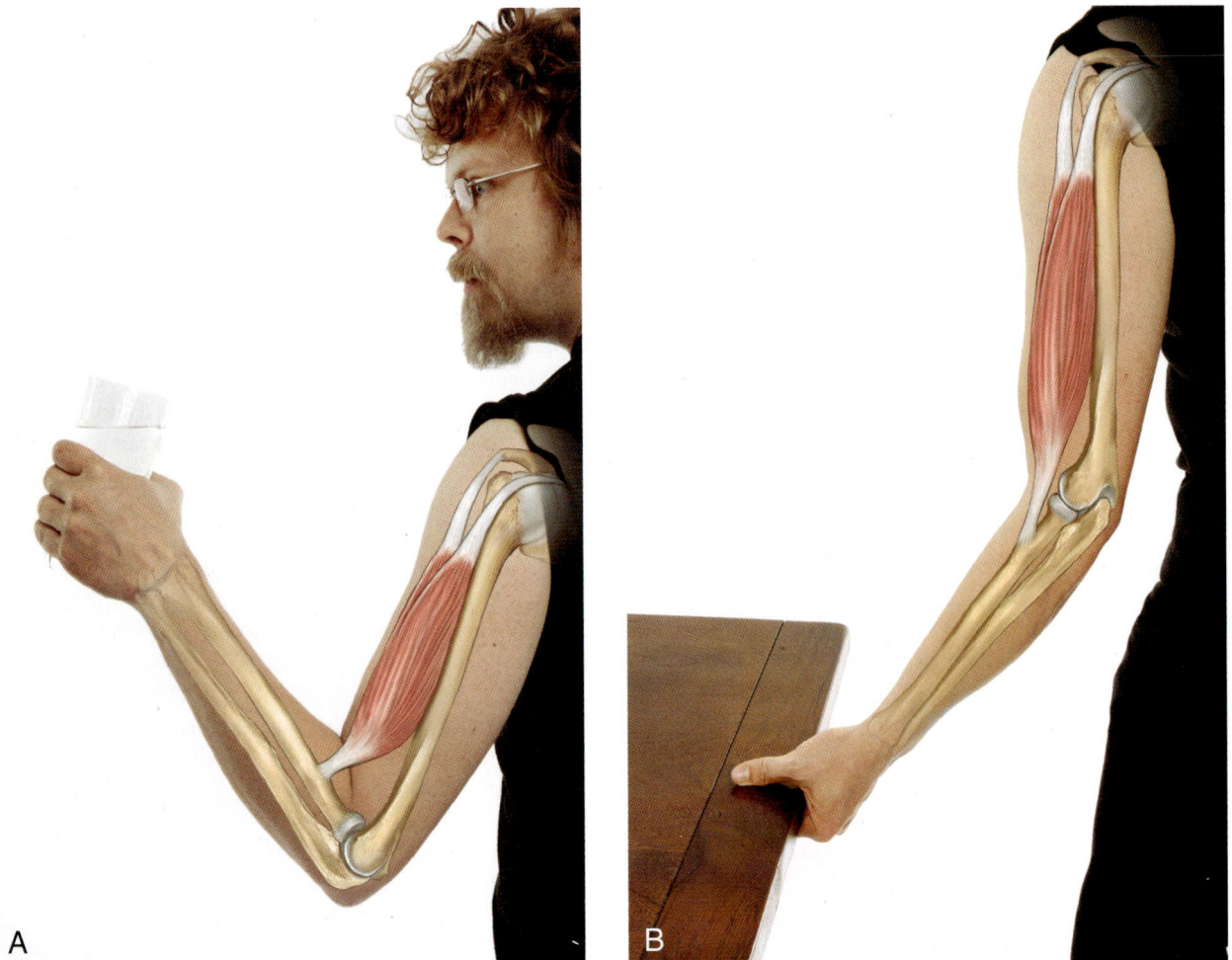

A   B

Figure 1-1 **Isotonic and isometric contractions.** An isotonic contraction produces the movement of a joint (A), while an isometric contraction does not (B).

When muscle tension is greater than the resistance against it, the length of the muscles responsible for the given action change to produce movement. This is an isotonic contraction (Fig. 1-1). Isotonic contractions are either concentric (muscle shortens) or eccentric (muscle lengthens). Concentric and eccentric contractions are described in more detail below. When we are healthy, muscle contractions are easily greater than the resistance of gravity and the weight of our own bodies, making them sufficient to produce fluid movement. The swing phase of the gait cycle, for example, is composed of isotonic contractions. The stronger the muscle is, the more resistance it can overpower.

When resistance is greater than muscle tension, the length of the muscle does not change and no movement occurs. This is an isometric contraction. The stance phase of gait involves isometric contractions. No matter how healthy we are, our muscle contractions will never be strong enough to move the planet Earth, but they contract isometrically to keep us standing.

When muscle fibers are recruited to perform an action, each myofibril contracts either completely or not at all. This is referred to as the "all or nothing" principle. The force of a contraction is generated not by the degree of contraction in each muscle fiber but by the number of fibers recruited that contract fully to produce the necessary force. For example, if gravity is the only source of resistance against a movement, such as when you flex your elbow to scratch your nose, few fibers that produce that movement need to be recruited. However, when the source of resistance to elbow flexion is a 40-pound child, many more fibers must contract. This can help explain why a specific portion of a muscle shows more signs of strain than other areas of the same muscle.

Agonists and Antagonists

Each of the movements described above require the coordination of muscles that function either as agonists, which produce the movement, or as antagonists, which oppose the movement (Fig. 1-2). All muscles can be either agonists or antagonists depending on the action being

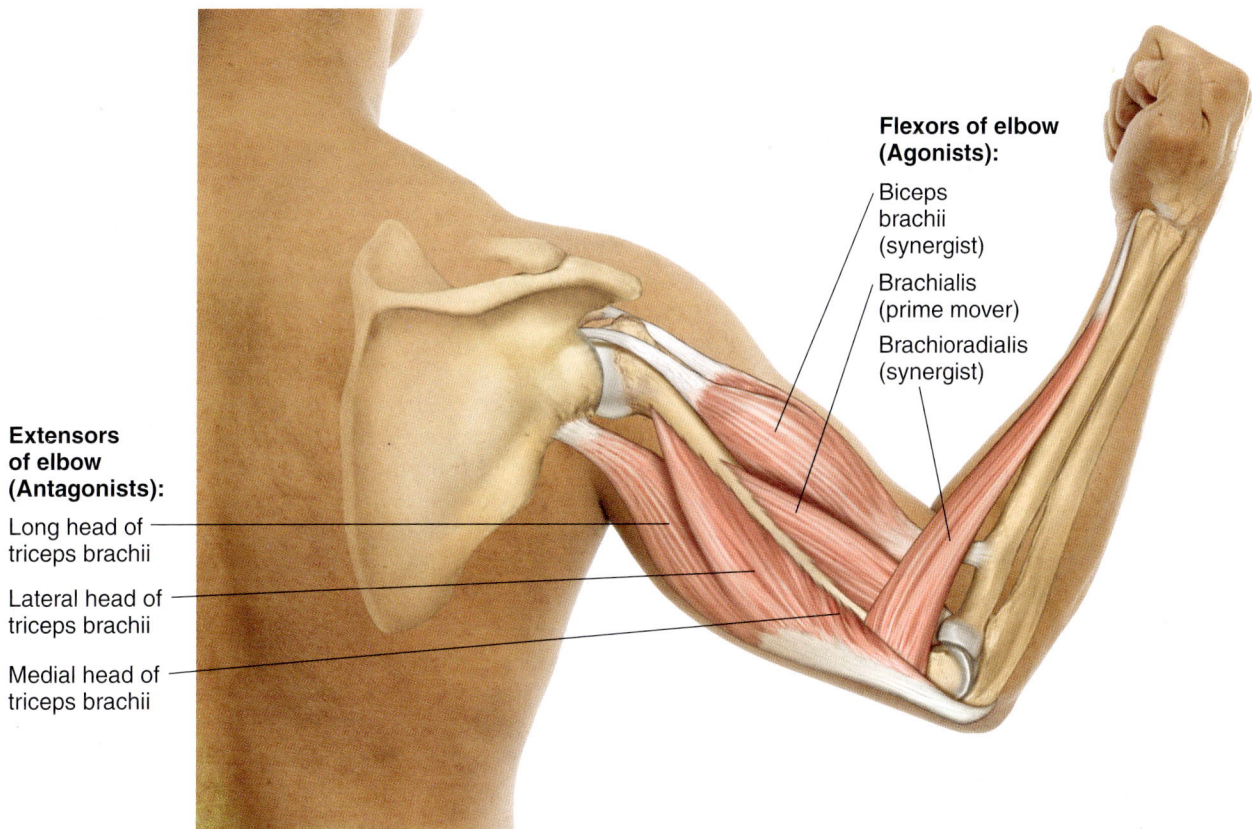

Flexors of elbow (Agonists):
Biceps brachii (synergist)
Brachialis (prime mover)
Brachioradialis (synergist)

Extensors of elbow (Antagonists):
Long head of triceps brachii
Lateral head of triceps brachii
Medial head of triceps brachii

Figure 1-2   **Agonist and antagonist during during flexion of the elbow.** The agonist produces movement by contracting concentrically, while the antagonist controls the rate and speed of that movement by contracting eccentrically.

performed. Both agonists' and antagonists' fibers are recruited according to the "all or nothing" principle described above.

The agonists of a movement, which include the prime mover and its synergist(s), are the muscles that contract concentrically to produce movement. A concentric contraction is one in which fibers shorten to produce the force needed for action. The prime mover is the main muscle responsible for a given movement and is usually the biggest or strongest of the muscles responsible for that particular action. In flexing the elbow, for example, the brachialis muscle is the prime mover; it contracts concentrically.

Synergists are muscles that assist the prime mover when the force needed requires the concentric contraction of several muscles. Synergists are the smaller muscles capable of performing the same action as the prime mover. Frequent synergists to the brachialis for flexing the elbow include the biceps brachii and brachioradialis, although any muscle that flexes the elbow may become involved. The number of muscles and the strength required to assist the prime mover in its action depend largely on the amount of resistance involved. Lifting a pen may not require the contraction of many fibers of the prime mover for elbow flexion nor the recruitment of synergists. However, lifting a heavy box of books may require the contraction of all of the fibers of the prime mover for elbow flexion and the recruitment of all of its synergists. When the prime mover for a particular action is injured, its synergists (among other structures) often help to compensate for the dysfunction. These can become prone to hypertonicity and injury when called upon to carry out actions normally performed by the bigger, stronger, prime mover.

Antagonists are muscles that oppose agonists to ensure that movement is fluid. The antagonist lengthens against the shortening of the agonists to control the speed and rate of contraction, resulting in smooth movement. Without antagonists to control the speed and rate of contraction, a strong impulse to flex your elbow to scratch your nose could result in a black eye! The antagonists during flexion of the elbow are the triceps brachii; they contract eccentrically. An eccentric contraction is one in which fibers lengthen to keep movement fluid. The number of fibers recruited to antagonize an action depends on the amount of force needed to control the speed and rate of a concentric contraction. Flexing your elbow while picking up a pen may require the recruitment of a few fibers of the antagonists to elbow flexion, while lifting a box of books may require the recruitment of all of the antagonists' fibers. Conversely, the triceps are agonists for extending the elbow and are antagonized by the elbow flexors.

Understanding these differences is important for planning treatment because the prime mover and synergists involved in an action that contributed to an injury are prone to shortening and are likely to need lengthening, while the antagonists of that action are more prone to overstretching or microtearing and are likely to need strengthening. Once you treat the shortened muscles involved in a dysfunction, it is essential to assess their antagonists for injury and instruct the client to strengthen them when appropriate so that they become strong enough to help keep the shortening of the agonists from recurring.

Often, the coordination of agonists and antagonists is compromised not by an action that caused an injury but by a static posture that holds agonists in a shortened position and antagonists in a lengthened position. For example, a truck driver or data entry clerk is prone to developing hyperkyphosis because they spend hours with the pectorals shortened and the rhomboids lengthened. Because this client often feels pain between the shoulder blades, we rush to treat those muscles, and we should. However, if we do not also lengthen the pectorals and instruct the client on how to strengthen their antagonists, the rhomboids have little chance of performing optimally against the resistance of the chronically shortened pectorals.

Most activities are performed by a variety of muscular movements that occur in phases. For example, when we flex our elbows, we may also be pronating or supinating the forearm, flexing or internally or externally rotating the shoulder, and so on. Therefore, it is necessary to consider the agonists, synergists, and antagonists in each of the actions or postural deviations that contribute to dysfunction. In addition, while agonists and antagonists oppose each other in an isotonic contraction, such as when walking, isometric contractions affect the muscles on either side of the joint involved nearly equally. When you are standing still, both the hamstrings and quadriceps are contracting isometrically to maintain balance.

RANGE OF MOTION

Range of motion (ROM) is a general term that describes all of the possibilities of movement of a joint. ROM does not describe the functionality of muscles, although the results of ROM testing, which indicate the functionality of a joint, may lead to your examination of the muscles responsible for that movement and of other soft tissues involved. The ROM of each joint depends on the shape of the joint as well as the muscles and other tissues surrounding that joint. When referring to ROM, it is important to name the joint involved, the action involved, and whether the action is passive, active, or resisted (e.g., active flexion of the elbow). If the client feels pain during ROM testing, ask where the pain is felt so that you can begin to pinpoint the source and determine whether the agonist or antagonist, muscle or tendon, ligaments, joint capsule, or bones of the joint are primarily responsible. While a visual estimate is often sufficient to recognize dysfunction, ROM can be measured more precisely with a goniometer (Fig. 1-3).

In active ROM, the client moves the joint through its range by consciously contracting muscles (Fig. 1-4). Active ROM can be free (AF ROM: active free range of motion) when the client moves without any help, or it can be assisted (AA ROM: active assisted range of motion) if weakness makes it difficult for the client to move the joint unassisted. Since it allows the client to control the amount of movement and stay within a pain-free range, only active ROM testing should be used during the acute stage of injury to prevent undue pain or re-injury.

Passive ROM (P ROM) describes action at a joint that is produced by a force other than muscle contraction across that joint (Fig. 1-5). Gravity, a wall or other surface, another part of the client's body, and the massage therapist are external forces that can produce P ROM. To test P ROM, move the relaxed client's joint through its range without their assistance. You may choose

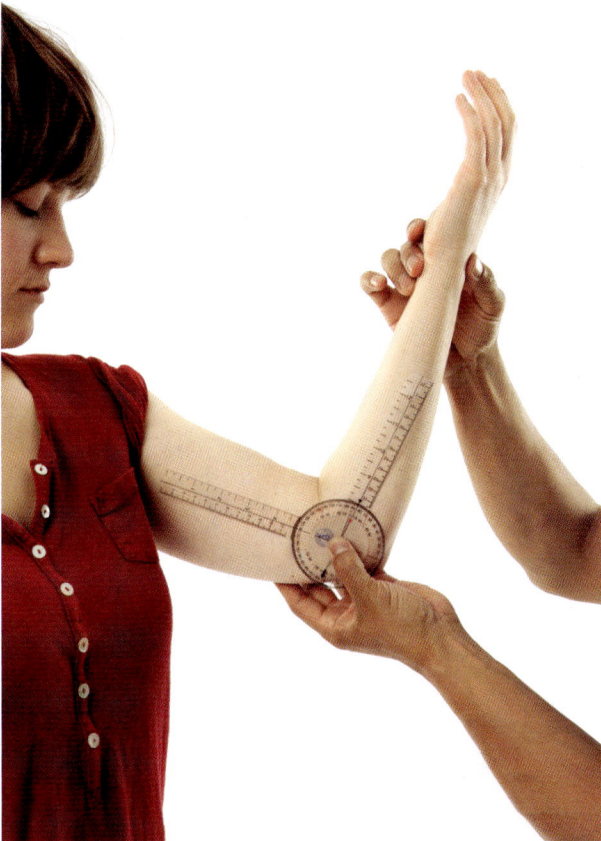

Figure 1-3   Goniometer. ROM can be measured precisely with a goniometer.

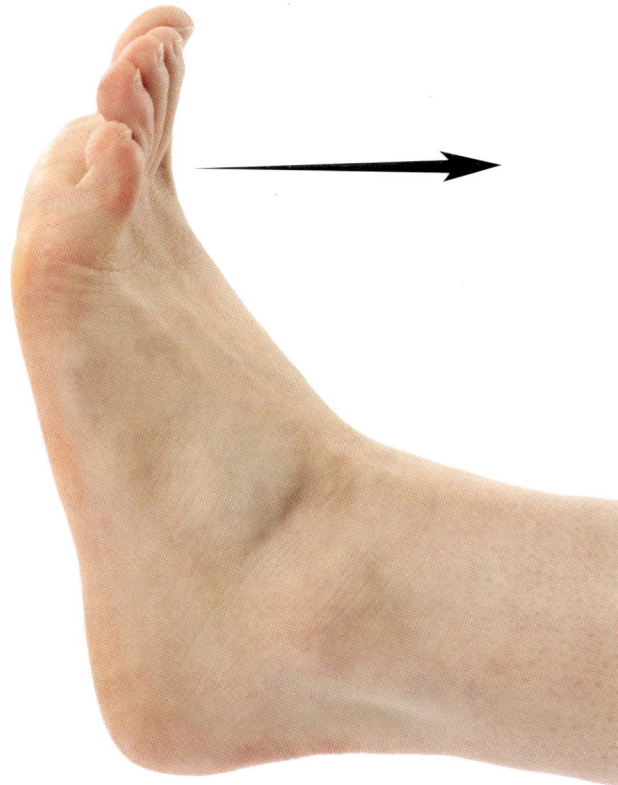

Figure 1-4   Active dorsiflexion of the ankle. In AF ROM, the client moves the joint through its range by actively contracting muscles without assistance or external resistance.

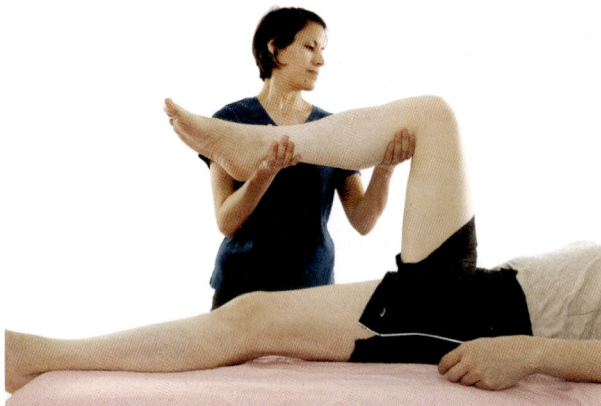

Figure 1-5   Passive flexion of the hip. In P ROM, the therapist moves the relaxed client's joint through its range.

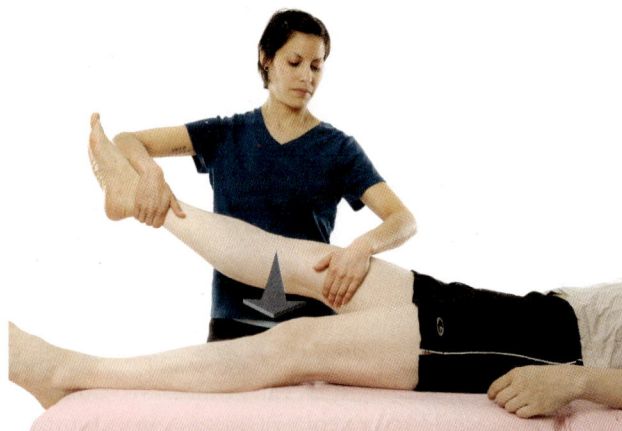

Figure 1-6   Resisted adduction of the hip. In R ROM, the client actively moves a joint through its range while the therapist applies resistance. In this image, the client is moving his leg straight toward the camera, resisted by the therapist's pressure.

this option if the client is too weak to move the joint or if you want to test the joint for structural abnormalities or for the dysfunction of noncontractile tissues.

Resisted ROM (R ROM) is an active contraction by the client that is resisted by an external force such as a weight, a wall or other surface, or the massage therapist (Fig. 1-6). To test R ROM, instruct the client to move the joint actively while you resist their effort just distal to the joint being tested. You do not need to resist the action to the point of immobility or trembling, which would obscure the results. Minimal resistance is enough to engage structures and recruit receptors that are not engaged in AF or AA ROM. R ROM should not be used in the acute stage of injury.

CLIENT ASSESSMENT

It is always essential to learn as much as you can about the client's health history before proceeding with condition-specific massage. Many conditions may have underlying contributing factors—such as systemic conditions, past trauma, side effects from medication, and personal stress—that involve contraindications or require special consideration in a treatment plan. It is important to get as much detail as you can and use critical thinking to see the big picture.

Health History

OLDRFICARA (read: "Ol' Dr. Ficara") is a mnemonic to help you remember important questions to ask the client when collecting the basic, subjective information you need to make an accurate assessment and plan treatment. The answers to these questions may have different implications depending on the client's condition. These are discussed in greater detail in the chapters on specific conditions.

   Onset—When did the symptoms begin?
   Location—Where are the symptoms felt?
   Duration—How long do the symptoms last when they occur?
   Radiation—Do the symptoms radiate to another part of the body?
   Frequency—How often do the symptoms occur?
   Intensity—Using a pain scale, what is the level of pain with these symptoms?
   Character—Describe what the symptoms feel like.

Aggravating factors—What makes the symptoms worse?

Relieving factors—What makes the symptoms diminish?

Associated factors—This includes more specific questions based on the information you have collected so far and questions about any medical diagnoses, medications, other treatments, past injuries, and any other detail that may help you plan treatment. (The following chapters list questions that are important for specific conditions.)

What do Signs and Symptoms Tell You?

A client's signs and symptoms can tell you much of what you need to know to assess a mild or moderate condition. Signs are objective and measurable by the therapist. These include postural deviations, ROM assessment, tone, temperature, and texture of soft tissues. Symptoms are subjective and are measured by the client. These include level of pain, fatigue, and quality of life. Knowing what a client feels before beginning a postural assessment or special tests helps you focus your assessment and save time. While each client's case and subjective description may vary, some general interpretations of signs and symptoms listed in Table 1-1 can be helpful.

Use a pain scale when assessing the client's symptoms. Research some of the many methods used to assess pain, and choose one that helps you make the best connections between the client's subjective description and treatment goals (Fig. 1-7). Always remember that pain is subjective and that clients' pain tolerance may vary widely. In your verbal assessment, ask the client about their level of pain during activities of daily living. A scale of 1-10 is commonly used where 10 represents a level of pain that significantly hinders or even prevents activities of daily living. A level 9 or 10 pain during activities of daily living may indicate a serious condition or a severe or acute injury. Refer these clients to their health care provider if you suspect a systemic condition or if the injury requires medical attention. In the case of a severe or acute injury that is not contraindicated for massage, even if you have received clearance from a health care provider to perform massage therapy, you may not be able to work locally, and you should not work deeply. You may opt to reschedule treatment of this client until the injury has reached the subacute or chronic stage, or refer the client to a massage therapist with advanced training. Note that all pain matters; do not underestimate the importance of even a level 2 or 3 pain, especially if it is chronic. A healthy neuromusculoskeletal system should produce no pain at all.

You also need to assess any pain a client experiences during treatment. Using a 1-10 scale again, 10 represents pain that would cause the client to pull away from your touch. Ask the client to let you know when you approach level 6 or 7, because once pain reaches a level 8, the client may not be able to remain fully relaxed. If you are going to use a technique that produces pain above a level 8, such as some trigger point techniques, explain this to the client in advance to try to keep him or her from tensing the muscles. Many clients believe that treatment is most beneficial when it is deep and painful. Explain to your clients that treatment is most effective when it is delivered slowly and deliberately, one layer at a time, with the client as relaxed as possible. The treatments described in this text should not be painful. Keeping the client calm and relaxed is crucial. Reminding the client to breathe during deep techniques may help ease pain and prevent him or her from tensing the muscles.

Range of Motion Assessment

When testing ROM to assess a dysfunction, it is best to test active ROM of the joint first. The client will likely restrict AF ROM to a range within their comfort zone. Use the client's active range as a guide when performing P ROM and R ROM testing to avoid causing the client unnecessary pain or further injury by moving beyond their comfort range. Moreover, forcing joint movement through its full range can affect the accuracy of your assessment. You want to assess what the client can achieve only up to the point of discomfort. This will give you the information you need to assess what may be keeping the client from reaching the full range. When using ROM as part of your treatment or recommending it for self-care, be careful to stay within a comfortable range and to limit resistance or repetition that may reproduce symptoms.

Table 1-1	General Interpretations of Subjective Descriptions	
Subjective Description	**During Activities of Daily Living**	**During Palpation or Treatment**
Sharp pain	Recent trauma to soft tissue.	Compression of or friction to torn fibers.
	Acute stage of an injury, such as torn muscle fibers, tendon, or ligament, felt particularly with movement, often relieved at rest.	Compression of a bone spur, cyst, or other abnormal growth.
	A condition involving an internal organ (local, deep pain).	An internal organ condition, when working on the abdomen.
	Compression or impingement of a nerve, in particular if accompanied by burning or tingling, felt at rest or with activity.	
Dull, aching pain, or stiffness or tightness	Trauma to the muscle in the nonacute stage.	Ischemia due to the client's posture during treatment or to the technique applied.
	Hypertonicity.	Area of accumulated metabolites.
	Swelling.	Hypertonic or fatigued muscles.
	Myofascial or joint restriction.	
	Active trigger point.	
	Syndrome such as fibromyalgia.	
Burning pain or sensation	Compression of a nerve.	Compression of a nerve due to the client's posture during treatment or to the technique applied.
	Cutaneous trigger point.	
	Damage to periosteum (local sensation).	
Tingling or numbness	Nerve compression, impingement, or lesion.	Ischemia or compression of a nerve due to the client's posture during treatment or to the technique applied.
	Holding the same posture for a long period.	
	Ischemia.	
	Systemic medical conditions involving nerve damage or ischemia (e.g., diabetes).	
	Vitamin or mineral imbalance.	
	Toxic exposure.	
	Side effect of radiation.	
Throbbing pain	Inflammation.	Prolonged compression of blood vessels.
	Acute injury.	
	Sluggish venous or lymphatic flow.	
Increasing pain on movement	Active trigger point.	Active trigger point.
	Spasm.	Spasm.
	Torn fibers.	Torn fibers.
	With radiating pain, irritation of a nerve.	With radiating pain, irritation of a nerve.
Decreasing pain on movement	Edema or decreased circulation relieved by increasing circulation.	Edema or decreased circulation relieved by increasing circulation.
	Latent trigger point.	Latent trigger point.
Pain unaffected by movement	Cutaneous trigger point.	Cutaneous trigger point.
	Pain is referred.	Pain is referred.
Weakness	Injury or condition affecting nerves, muscles, or neuromuscular junction.	Compression of a nerve or blood vessel due to the client's posture or the therapist's technique.

Table 1-1	General Interpretations of Subjective Descriptions (Continued)	
Subjective Description	**During Activities of Daily Living**	**During Palpation or Treatment**
Paresthesia (prickling, itching, pins and needles sensation on skin)	Nerve involvement ranging from simple compression to tumors. Compromised circulation. Diabetes. Hypothyroid condition. Vitamin deficiency. Rheumatoid arthritis. Lupus.	Compression of a nerve. Stimulation of cutaneous reflex zone.
Hyperesthesia (abnormally high sensitivity to stimulus)	Chemical stimulants (e.g., caffeine). Trauma to head or spinal cord. Anxiety.	Stimulation of the central nervous system. Anxiety.
Heat	Inflammation.	Increased circulation resulting from repetitive stroking. Technique initiates inflammatory process.
Cold	Ischemia.	Compression of blood vessels.

As an assessment tool, AF ROM gives you information about both contractile and noncontractile tissues in and surrounding the joint. If the AF ROM of the affected joint causes pain or is reduced compared to the same, healthy joint on the other side of the body, this could indicate trigger points, adhesions, scarring, or injuries to the agonist, synergist, or antagonist for that movement as well as possible abnormalities in bone, ligaments, bursa, menisci, or other tissues. If the client feels no pain but is unable to move the joint through its full range, this could indicate weakness in the agonist or synergists of that motion and may indicate neurological involvement. Such results should lead you to test those muscles more specifically either with R ROM to test strength or with palpation to test texture, tone, temperature, and tenderness (see Palpation section below).

As an assessment tool, P ROM may reveal information about joint dysfunction that is unrelated to muscle contraction. By eliminating muscle contraction as a factor in this assessment, you may be able to deduce that pain or restriction is caused by injury or inflammation that is not wholly muscular in nature. Bursitis, meniscal tears, bone spurs, ligament instability, dislocations, fascial restrictions, or other problems may then become evident.

End feel is the term for the sensation the therapist feels when applying overpressure, that is, adding just a bit of pressure at the end of the client's comfortable passive range of motion. You add only enough pressure to feel if and how the joint springs back. You do not want to add enough pressure to push the joint beyond the client's comfortable ROM. A healthy end feel is one that occurs when overpressure is added to the P ROM of a joint that has full ROM and results in a gentle spring back with no discomfort. This is the normal response to overpressure when the shape of the joint and functional soft tissue surrounding the joint are the only things that limit its range. A pathological end feel, in contrast, is the sensation you feel when overpressure is added to the P ROM of a joint that cannot reach full ROM or results in discomfort because an unhealthy structure stops it short. Table 1-2 summarizes healthy and pathological end feels.

As an assessment tool, R ROM can give you information about the client's strength and the health of the nerves that send impulses to the muscles that move the joint being tested. If R ROM tests elicit pain, it is likely that there is a trigger point or a strain to the muscle or tendon crossing the joint. Depending on the degree of strain, the results may be similar to AF ROM. If R ROM reveals weakness without pain, nerves may be involved.

Visual Analogue Scale

Choose a Number from 0 to 10 That Best Describes Your Pain

No Pain					Distressing Pain					Unbearable Pain
0	1	2	3	4	5	6	7	8	9	10

ASK PATIENTS ABOUT THEIR PAIN
INTENSITY–LOCATION–ONSET–DURATION–VARIATION–QUALITY

"Faces" Pain Rating Scale

0 NO HURT	1 HURTS LITTLE BIT	2 HURTS LITTLE MORE	3 HURTS EVEN MORE	4 HURTS WHOLE LOT	5 HURTS WORST

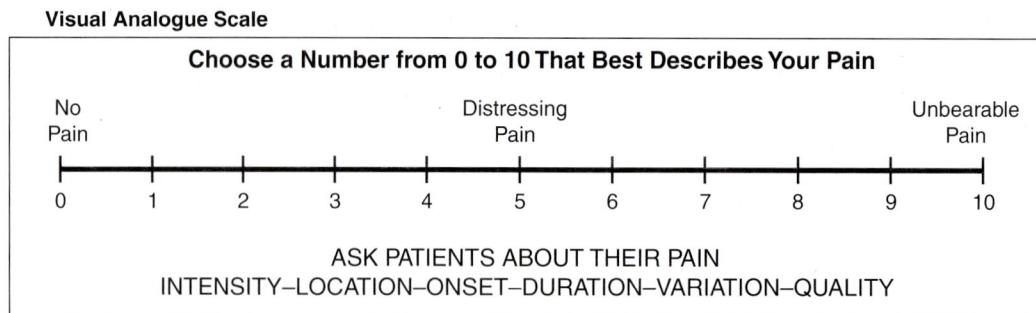

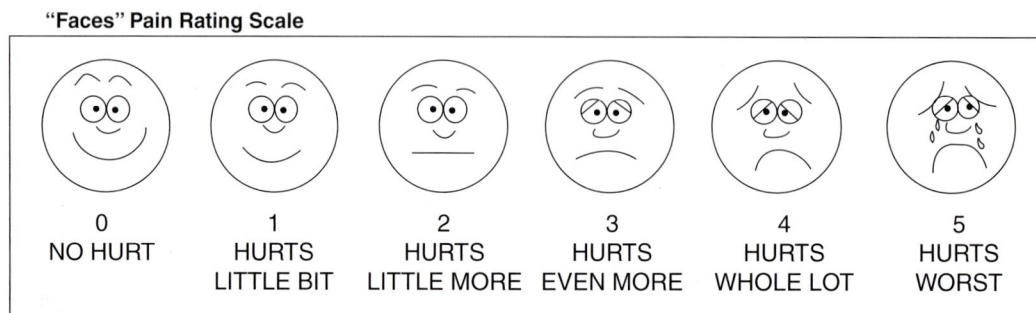

Behavioral Observation Pain Rating Scale

Categories	Scoring		
	0	1	2
Face	No particular expression or smile; disinterested	Occasional grimace or frown, withdrawn	Frequent to constant frown, clenched jaw, quivering chin
Legs	No position or relaxed	Uneasy, restless, tense	Kicking, or legs drawn up
Activity	Lying quietly, normal position, moves easily	Squirming, shifting back and forth, tense	Arched, rigid, or jerking
Cry	No crying (awake or asleep)	Moans or whimpers, occasional complaint	Crying steadily, screams or sobs, frequent complaints
Consolability	Content, relaxed	Reassured by occasional touching, hugging, or talking to. Distractable	Difficult to console or comfort

Each of the five categories (F) Face; (L) Legs; (A) Activity; (C) Cry; (C) Consolability is scored from 0 to 2, which results in a total score between 0 and 10.

Figure 1-7 **Pain scales.** Many methods are used to assess pain. Research a few, and choose one that best suits your needs and the needs of your clients. From Yeznach Wick J. Pain in a special population: the cognitively impaired. Pharmacy Times 2007. Available at http://www.pharmacytimes.com/issue/pharmacy/2007/2007-01/2007-01-6171.

Palpation

Your fingers have many sensory receptors that give you the ability to detect even the most minor inconsistencies in tissues. While developing palpation skills, be patient with yourself. You may not yet be fully able to quickly make the connections between what you read here and what you feel with your hands. It takes time and practice with many different bodies to develop accurate palpation skills.

Many of the strokes used at the beginning of treatments are excellent palpation tools that can reveal atypical properties, such as hypertonicity, in a general way. With the more local tissues involved

| Table 1-2 | Joint End Feel | | |

Type of End Feel	Cause of Limitation	Healthy End Feel	Pathological End Feel
Soft tissue approximation	Normal mass of soft tissue at end of range (e.g., elbow flexion is limited by meeting of biceps and anterior forearm muscles).	Painless for client. Therapist feels soft compression of one muscle against another with spring back following overpressure.	N/A
Muscle end feel	Full length of muscle reached (e.g., dorsiflexion is limited by the length of plantar flexors).	Client feels stretch. Therapist feels tension and spring back following overpressure.	Client may feel pain if adhesions or scarring are present. Therapist feels abrupt end of range.
Capsular end feel	Joint capsule reaches full stretch (e.g., external rotation of shoulder).	Painless for client. Therapist feels firm sensation with little give as if stretching leather, with spring back following overpressure.	Soft capsular end feel is similar to healthy end feel, but client feels pain and muscle guarding. Common with sprains, acute inflammation, and stiffness, and felt throughout range.

Hard capsular end feel ends in resistance and no give. |
Ligamentous end feel	Ligaments surrounding joint (e.g., abduction of extended knee).	Client feels no pain. Therapist feels firm end with no give, and spring back following overpressure.	Referred to as loose ligamentous end feel. Client may feel pain. Therapist is able to move joint beyond normal range.
Bony end feel	Bony structures of joint (e.g., full extension of knee).	Client feels no pain. Therapist feels abrupt end of range with spring back following overpressure.	Client may feel pain. Therapist feels abrupt, hard stop before full range due to callus, fracture, or myositis ossificans. An end feel that is rough or gravelly may indicate chondromalacia or crepitus.
Muscle spasm	Reflexive muscle spasm to prevent further movement.	—	Client feels pain and stops movement suddenly with possible rebound due to spasm.
Boggy end feel	Joint effusion or edema (common with sprains and capsular restrictions).	—	Client may feel pain. Therapist feels soft, mushy end.
Empty end feel	Severe pain.

Rare except with grade 3 sprain, impingement, dislocation, acute bursitis, or tumor. | — | Client feels severe pain. Therapist feels no restriction or no appreciable end to range, but movement is protectively stopped by client, without spasm, as contraction would cause compression and increase pain. |

in specific conditions, it is important to take your time with palpation for your assessment to be comprehensive and accurate. When palpating locally for specific irregularities like scar tissue or strains, your movement should cover only 1 inch of tissue in 5-10 seconds. Slow, deliberate palpation in an area solid with adhesions and hypertonicity may also release superficial tissues and reveal deeper, more specific causes of dysfunction. Focus intently when you palpate to avoid missing subtle details. Begin superficially and work toward deeper palpation. Even when palpating deep tissues, avoid heavy pressure that may change the texture of the surrounding tissues, transfer too much information to the receptors in your fingers, and obscure your results. Ease your way into the deeper layers.

Focused palpation reveals inconsistencies in the texture, tone, temperature, and tenderness of tissues that might help explain the causes of dysfunction and pain. The norms for these characteristics may differ slightly from client to client, so you need to palpate bilaterally to make a comparison between tissues that you suspect are contributing to poor posture or pain and the tissue of the same structure on the unaffected side. Table 1-3 is a general guide to some of the characteristics you may discover.

MASSAGE THERAPY

General Principles of Massage

Once you have collected information to help you understand the client's particular situation, you can plan treatment with specific goals. A wide variety of techniques are at our disposal to achieve these goals, and we plan the sequence of these techniques to best address the factors involved in the client's dysfunction. By choosing techniques with physiological effects that match the treatment goals and by following the general principles of massage, you can plan effective treatment for the client's specific condition no matter what modality you practice. The general principles described below complement each other so well that applying one will often satisfy the others. For example, in many cases, when you begin treating generally, you will very likely also be working superficially and proximally. When treating specific structures, you are often also working deeply and distally.

GENERAL-SPECIFIC-GENERAL

The general-specific-general principle applies with all techniques for general relaxation or to treat specific conditions and is elemental for a full body massage or more localized treatment. This principle involves applying techniques generally both before and after applying them specifically. The intent is to accomplish general goals before focusing on specific goals and to work systemically before treating locally. General goals include acclimating the client to your touch, reducing sympathetic firing and engaging parasympathetic mechanisms of the nervous system, and increasing circulation. Once you have applied general techniques, you are ready to work more specifically. This could mean using a technique with a targeted physiological effect (e.g., reducing adhesions after you have increased circulation) or applying a variety of techniques to the specific tissues involved in the condition (e.g., treating the wrist to reduce adhesions, lengthen shortened tissues, and mobilize the joint after treating the body generally to open channels of circulation and attend to compensating structures). Following the specific treatment, work generally again to clear the area, move fluids and metabolites toward the heart or lymph nodes, and relax the nervous system, which may have been excited by your specific treatment.

An example of the general-specific-general principle is to apply superficial effleurage to the whole body before applying petrissage and deep effleurage to the quadratus lumborum; then follow this local treatment with clearing strokes to move the contents you have released through the proper channels toward the nearest lymph nodes. This sequence applies the principle in a general Swedish massage that incorporates specific focus on the low back. Another example is applying warming strokes and superficial myofascial release to the neck and shoulders before stripping individual neck muscles and treating trigger points, then following with clearing strokes toward the trunk. This sequence applies the principle in a treatment for tension headaches.

SUPERFICIAL-DEEP-SUPERFICIAL

The superficial-deep-superficial principle also applies with all techniques for general relaxation or to treat a specific condition and is elemental when planning a full body massage or a more localized treatment. This principle involves applying techniques to superficial tissues both before and

Table 1-3	Common Characteristics of Injured Tissue

Characteristics	How it Feels to the Therapist	Therapeutic Goals
Adhesions—tissues stick together	Superficially, it may feel as if the skin does not move freely over superficial muscles. Deeper structures may feel as if they are one. You may be unable to differentiate individual muscles or fiber directions if adhesions are present.	Release adhesion to allow tissues to move freely and independently.
Hypertonicity—increased tone in muscle belly, often accompanied by dehydration, and may be neurological in nature.	Tissue feels resistant and harder than healthy tissue. Shape is distorted. Fiber direction may be obscured. Often accompanied by adhesions and may contain trigger points.	Reduce tone—release tension with heat, massage, and lengthening.
Hypotonicity—reduced tone in muscle belly, often accompanied by fluid retention, and may be neurological in nature.	Tissue feels spongy and softer than healthy tissue. Fibers may feel inflated. Contractile strength may be reduced but functional.	When indicated, increase tone with cold, stimulating strokes, and isolated concentric contractions.
Atrophy—muscle wasting, often the result of a systemic condition or lack of use.	Tissue feels spongy and softer than healthy tissue. Contractile strength is minimal to nonexistent.	Treatment depends on the cause. If systemic, discuss with health care professional. If disuse is the cause, perform isolated contractions with gradual introduction of resistance.
Taut—overstretched or pulled tightly.	Tissues feel like tightly pulled strings, as on a guitar. Fibers are easily isolated and may strum when applying cross-fiber strokes. Often accompanied by adhesions and may contain trigger points.	Reduce adhesions and trigger points if found. Encourage activities and postures that do not add length to the muscle.
Myofascial trigger points—hyperirritable spot in a taut band of skeletal muscle.	When palpable, feels like a knot or a bump. Trigger points are often obscured by adhesions and hypertonicity and are revealed only when superficial layers are treated first.	Reduce tone, metabolites, ischemia, or other factors contributing to trigger points, followed by stretching to restore normal muscle length.
Scar tissue	An interruption in fiber direction or an uncharacteristic, immovable bump or divot in tissue with accompanying adhesions.	Break up scar tissue, and realign with healthy fiber direction.
Fibrosis—formation of tough, fibrous tissue; often part of the healing process but can become chronic.	Thick, often lumpy, moveable tissue. Sometimes feels as if fibers are inflated or swollen.	Halt fibrous formation by increasing circulation and restoring muscle function. In chronic cases, use friction to reduce nodules when not contraindicated (e.g., with rheumatoid arthritis) followed by stretching the affected fibers.
Panniculosis—fibrosis or increased viscosity of subcutaneous fascia.	Superficial. Feels coarse and granular. Skin may look dimpled.	Skin rolling or other myofascial technique to reduce viscosity.
Crepitus—crackling sound made when two rough surfaces in the body make contact.	Feels similar to adhesion but with audible and palpable crackling.	Reduce adhesions and release gasses or metabolites that contribute to crepitus. Increase circulation to flush tissues.
Inflammation—local response to injured cells characterized by dilation of capillaries, heat, and swelling.	Local, sometimes visible swelling that is often red and warm or hot to the touch.	Massage is locally contraindicated when inflammation is acute. Increase venous flow proximally to encourage removal of metabolites.
Edema—accumulation of interstitial fluid.	Skin may look swollen, stretched, or shiny. Texture may feel boggy or gelatinous.	Massage is locally contraindicated. Increase venous and lymphatic flow proximally to encourage reabsorption.

(continued)

Table 1-3	Common Characteristics of Injured Tissue (Continued)	
Characteristics	**How it Feels to the Therapist**	**Therapeutic Goals**
Heat—dilation of blood vessels, often red, and a sign of inflammation.	Warm or hot to the touch.	Heat may be a sign of infection, which is a contraindication. If no infection is suspected, encourage venous return and lymphatic flow.
Cold—constriction of blood vessels, often pale and dry, and may result in reduced hair growth.	Cool or cold to the touch.	Cold may be a sign of ischemia and may result from a systemic condition. If no contraindications exist, increase circulation to warm the area.

after applying them to deeper tissues. Working superficially first ensures that you treat tissues layer by layer, reducing the possibility of shocking the client's tissues and causing kick-back pain (i.e., pain that occurs in the hours or days following treatment, especially when treatment progresses too deeply too quickly).

An example of the superficial-deep-superficial principle is to apply light effleurage to the whole back before applying deeper effleurage and petrissage to the erector spinae; then end with superficial clearing strokes toward the heart. Using the same sequence next with the extremities would apply all of the general principles for a full body, general relaxation massage. Another example of the superficial-deep-superficial principle is warming the tissues of the forearm, releasing superficial fascial restrictions, breaking deeper adhesions with cross-fiber friction, stripping individual muscles that cross the wrist, treating the flexor retinaculum, stretching the tissues, and ending first with deep and then with superficial clearing strokes toward the axilla. This sequence applies the principles in the treatment of carpal tunnel syndrome.

PROXIMAL-DISTAL-PROXIMAL

The proximal-distal-proximal principle also applies with all techniques for general relaxation or to treat a specific condition and is elemental for a full body massage or more localized treatment. This principle involves applying techniques closest to the trunk before applying them to the extremities, finishing with strokes back toward the trunk. By beginning treatment proximally, you open the channels of circulation so that whatever fluids you move when working distally have a clear, open path back to the lymph nodes and heart. After treating distally, it is essential to encourage circulation back toward the trunk so that metabolites and edema do not reaccumulate distally or at the site of the injury.

An example of the proximal-distal-proximal principle is beginning treatment on the back, working next on the extremities, and finishing with clearing strokes back toward the trunk. This applies the principle in a full body relaxation massage. Another example is to treat the thigh and leg before frictioning scar tissue around the malleoli, and then use clearing strokes to encourage venous return proximally. This applies the principle in the treatment of a sprained ankle in the chronic stage.

PERIPHERAL-CENTRAL-PERIPHERAL

The peripheral-central-peripheral principle applies when treating specific injuries and is elemental for planning localized treatments. This principle involves applying techniques around the periphery of an injury before working directly on it. The proximity of your treatment to the central area of an injury depends on the stage of the injury and the client's tolerance. You may not be able to treat the area of injury directly in your initial sessions but may be able to approach it gradually in subsequent sessions.

By treating peripherally, you can move metabolites that have accumulated in low concentrations around the injury to clear the area for moving metabolites in higher concentrations closer to the specific site. Likewise, adhesions and scar tissue are likely to be less dense in the periphery of an injury than directly on it, and treating the periphery first may make it easier to approach the center. Finally, the client probably feels less pain in the periphery than at the site, so as long as working locally is not contraindicated, you can slowly approach the area and gradually ease any anxiety about having the injury touched. Ending with treatment at the periphery aids in venous return and reduces kick-back pain, possibly because the focus moves away from the injury toward tissues with more integrity.

An example of applying the peripheral-central-peripheral principle is to reduce adhesions and hypertonicity in the hamstrings on either side of torn fibers before breaking up scar tissue and realigning fibers at the site of injury; follow this with clearing strokes over the whole leg working toward the trunk to increase venous return. This applies the principle in the treatment of a hamstring strain in the subacute or chronic stage.

Physiological Effects of the Basic Strokes

Each of the strokes used in massage therapy has physiological effects that may vary depending on the depth and speed of their application. The Arndt-Shultz law explains that weaker stimuli activate physiological effects while stronger stimuli inhibit them. For example, beginning your work superficially and then gently and slowly working into deeper tissues will have a more positive physiological effect than quickly applying force. The most effective treatment includes a combination of strokes chosen and applied in a sequence specifically intended to produce a desired effect. This is especially important when using massage to treat specific conditions that have overt contributing factors. Because of its physiological effects, a massage stroke may also be contraindicated by your treatment goals or may not be appropriate for clients with certain local or systemic conditions. For example, if one of your treatment goals is to reduce local inflammation, applying friction on or near the area would be contraindicated by your goal. See Table 1-4 for more general contraindications.

The three basic effects of massage strokes are mechanical, reflexive, and chemical. A mechanical effect changes the shape or tone of the tissue and often results from force. Lengthening a shortened muscle by using deep gliding strokes is an example of a mechanical effect. A reflexive effect occurs when the stroke applied accelerates or decelerates a response, often in the nervous system, and is generally intended to restore homeostasis. Dilation of blood vessels following the release of a compressive force to a previously ischemic area is an example of a reflexive effect. A chemical effect occurs when a stroke encourages the release or absorption of chemicals in the body. Massage resulting in an increase in serotonin—a neurotransmitter that regulates mood and reduces irritability—is an example of a chemical effect.

It may not be possible to precisely identify a single effect with each use of massage strokes largely because practitioners do not always apply them in exactly the same way and because each client's physiological response may be slightly different. In addition, it may not be possible to isolate one effect from another when a stroke produces more than one effect. There is currently great interest in investigating the physiological effects of massage strokes in more detail. Organizations like the National Institutes of Health are soliciting research to help explain exactly why these techniques work. We do, however, have a fundamental understanding of how the techniques generally affect the systems of the body. Table 1-4 summarizes the basic strokes used in massage and many of their physiological effects. Consider the following general principles when choosing strokes and determining what depth and speed to use when applying them:

- If the stroke increases circulation or lymph flow, it is best to apply it in the direction of venous return (toward the heart) or lymphatic flow (toward the nearest lymph nodes).
- The depth of strokes influences the therapeutic effect. Using a stroke superficially will affect the superficial tissues, while applying it deeply will affect the deeper tissues. It is best to work the superficial tissues thoroughly before accessing the deeper tissues, to prevent kick-back pain.
- The speed of strokes influences the therapeutic effect. Applying a stroke slowly is more likely to be relaxing and may enhance the mechanical effects intended. Applying a stroke quickly is more likely to stimulate the tissues resulting in shorter reflexive effects.

Table 1-4	Physiological Effects, Therapeutic Goals, and Contraindications to the Basic Massage Strokes		
Stroke	**Physiological Effects**	**Therapeutic Goals**	**Cautions and Contraindications**
Effleurage or gliding	Increases venous circulation. Stimulates lymph flow. Increases mobility of tissues. Dilates arterioles. Stimulates mechanoreceptors.	Mobilize fluid. Increase circulation. Increase lymph flow. Reduce edema. Increase absorption of metabolites into lymph. Reduce pain. Reduce tension. Reduce spasm. Lengthen tissue. Soften scar tissue.	Open wounds. Local or systemic infection. Varicosities (if significant enough to damage vessel). Edema (if significant enough to tear skin). Bruises. Dermatitis. Local cortisone injection. Following radiation therapy. Fever. Any diagnosis that suggests impaired cardiovascular function.
Petrissage or kneading	Softens and increases pliability of tissues. Creates space around fibers. Warms tissues. Affects muscle spindles and Golgi tendon organs to reflexively relax muscle. Increases superficial and deep circulation. Stretches scar tissue.	Increase circulation. Mobilize fluid. Mobilize tissues. Mobilize metabolites for removal. Reduce tension. Reduce spasm.	Open wounds. Local cancer. Local infections. Chronic inflammation. Gross edema. Circulatory condition (particularly local, such as thrombosis). Acute injury. Reduced tone or atrophy. Local cortisone injection. Large varicose veins.
Compression	Softens tissue. Flattens tissue. Stimulates muscle spindles to initiate reflexive muscle relaxation. Stimulates nerves. Arterioles dilate following release.	Increase circulation. Relieve trigger points. Reduce tension. Reduce spasm.	Open wounds. Local cancer. Local infections. Chronic inflammation. Gross edema. Local cortisone injection. Circulatory condition (particularly local, such as thrombosis). Nerve impairment. Acute injury.

Table 1-4	Physiological Effects, Therapeutic Goals, and Contraindications to the Basic Massage Strokes (Continued)		
Stroke	**Physiological Effects**	**Therapeutic Goals**	**Cautions and Contraindications**
Vibration	Stimulates nerves.	Loosen mucus in lungs.	Open wounds.
	Stimulates mechanoreceptors.	Reduce spasm.	Acute injury.
	Initiates reciprocal inhibition.	Reduce edema.	Local cortisone injection.
	Reduces pain.	Aid in resetting muscle function.	On thorax: heart failure, thrombosis, or severe hypertension.
			Local cancer.
			Infections.
			Gross edema.
			Circulatory insufficiency.
			Following radiation therapy.
			Hyperesthesia.
			Varicosities.
Tapotement or percussion	Stimulates nerves.	Increase circulation and lymph flow.	Open wounds.
	Stretches tendons, resulting in contraction of muscle and inhibiting its antagonist.	Pain relief.	Acute injury.
	Stimulates weak muscles.	Aid in resetting muscle function.	Local cortisone injection.
	Contracts superficial blood vessels when applied superficially.	Loosen and move mucus in lungs.	On thorax: heart failure, thrombosis, or severe hypertension.
	Dilates vessels by releasing histamine.		Local cancer.
			Infections.
			Gross edema.
			Circulatory insufficiency.
			Following radiation therapy.
			Hyperesthesia.
			Hypertonicity.
			Fresh scars.
			Varicosities.
Friction	Breaks up adhesions.	Increase inflammation to reduce adhesions and initiate tissue repair.	Acute injuries.
	Initiates inflammatory process.	Reduce adhesions.	Fresh scars.
	Provides pain relief.	Break down scar tissue before realignment.	Local inflammation or edema.
	Helps tissue repair.		Use of NSAIDs within 4 hours of treatment.
			Local cortisone injection.

Hydrotherapy

Hydrotherapy, or water therapy, can be a useful therapeutic tool in massage treatments. Hydrotherapy can also be a great self-care tool when clients apply it correctly. There are numerous methods for applying hydrotherapy including baths, steam, and heat or ice packs. Study these in detail if you choose to use them or recommend them for self-care. This book focuses on moist heat and ice packs used during therapy as well as simple hydrotherapy options for self-care.

The temperature of the hydrotherapy source must be higher or lower than body temperature to have an effect. The greater the difference in temperature is, the more profound the effect will be. Hydrotherapy must be adjusted to the client's tolerance as well as for the particular condition. When using hydrotherapy during treatment, be sure to check in with the client frequently to ensure that the temperature is not extreme. If it is, add an additional layer of wrap around the source of hydrotherapy, or otherwise adjust the temperature of the source to suit the client's tolerance.

The application of heat should always be moist. Dry, electric heat can dehydrate soft tissue locally, which may result in thicker adhesions and the accumulation of metabolites. This condition could hinder the outcome of your treatment and may be painful for the client. Regardless of your source of heat—hydrocollator, thermal water pack, or other supply—be sure that the wrap you use is clean and moist.

The source of cold should also always be covered by a clean wrap, though applications of cold hydrotherapy in these chapters do not require external moisture. In some cases, as described in the following chapters, it is recommended that ice applications be maintained until the area is numb. Before reaching that point, the client may briefly experience pain from the extreme cold. Explain this to the client in advance and ask him or her to let you know if the pain becomes too much to endure the entire process. Add an additional layer of wrap if this occurs. Once the discomfort has ceased and numbness occurs, remove the source of cold to avoid frostbite.

In all cases, be sure that the weight of your hot or cold source is not so heavy that it would compress injured structures, nerves, or vessels. Table 1-5 lists the effects, goals, and contraindications for simple hot and cold hydrotherapy applications.

Contrast hydrotherapy involves alternating hot and cold applications. Contrast is best used to reduce congestion in tissues because it causes vasodilation followed by vasoconstriction, which increases local circulation and creates a flushing effect. This effect partly depends on the difference in temperature of the hot and cold applications; hot and cold applications have a greater effect than warm and cool ones. In general, the heat application should last two to three times longer than the cold application, and the contrast should be repeated two or three times. Because vasoconstriction occurs in 20–30 seconds, 60–90 seconds of heat followed by 20–30 seconds of cold, repeated two or three times, is sufficient. End contrast therapy with cold to reduce prolonged fluid accumulation.

In some cases, adding salt to a bath may improve the therapeutic outcome. By the process of osmosis, water crosses a permeable or semi-permeable membrane, such as the skin, in an attempt to balance the concentration of sodium on either side of the membrane. If the water used in hydrotherapy has a higher concentration of sodium than the body, such as when salts are added to a bath or when one is in the ocean, water exits from the body through the skin into the salted water. This effect is best used therapeutically to reduce inflammation. When the water used in hydrotherapy contains no salt, the concentration of sodium is higher in the body, so water from the bath will pass through the skin into the body. This is best used when tissues are dehydrated or to dilute a high concentration of metabolites.

Drinking water is also an application of hydrotherapy. We encourage our clients to drink water after a treatment to help flush metabolites and to rehydrate tissues. In general, we should all drink water everyday to replace lost fluids and to keep tissues well-hydrated. If you wait until you feel thirsty, dehydration has already begun. Drinking water throughout the day is key to good health.

Table 1-5	Hydrotherapy		
Hydrotherapy Application	**Physiological Effects**	**Therapeutic Goals**	**Local and Systemic Cautions and Contraindications**
Heat	Elicit parasympathetic response.	Increase circulation.	Local or systemic inflammation or edema.
	Dilate vessels locally.	Soften tissues.	Infection.
	Increase metabolism.	Rehydrate tissues.	Open wounds.
	Increase local nutrient flow.	Flush metabolites.	Cardiovascular disease.
	Increase inflammation.		Overstretched or atrophied tissues.
	Diminish muscle tone.		Injury in acute phase.
	Diminish muscle spasm.		Hyper- or hyposensitivity.
	Diminish velocity of nerve conduction.		Extremities of diabetics.
	Decrease pain perception.		
Cold	Elicit sympathetic response.	Decrease inflammation and edema.	Insufficient circulation (e.g., Raynaud's).
	Constrict vessels locally (primary effect in first 30 seconds or so—the body responds to this by increasing circulation in an attempt to balance temperature. With longer application, vasoconstriction returns).	Slow the inflammatory process induced by friction.	Cardiovascular disease.
			Hyper- and hyposensitivity.
			Client feels cold.
	Decrease circulation (with long applications).		Open wounds.
	Decrease inflammation.		Tissues with increased tone.
	Decrease metabolism.		
	Increase muscle tone.		
	Decrease pain perception.		

Mobilization

As a therapeutic tool, active free ROM can reduce adhesions, restore mobility, increase circulation of blood and lymph, and reset neuromuscular function and proprioception. AF ROM can be used during massage treatment or as self-care. When using AF ROM during treatment, be sure to limit movement to the client's tolerance and use repetition only as long as the action remains comfortable. When instructing the client in self-care, it is essential to demonstrate the activity you are recommending and to tell the client to stay within a range of motion and repetition that does not reproduce symptoms. Ask the client to perform the activity in your presence and recommend adjustments to ensure that he or she will not harm himself or herself when practicing alone.

As a therapeutic tool, passive ROM has many of the same effects as active ROM: reduces adhesions, restores joint mobility, increases circulation of blood and lymph, and resets neuromuscular function and proprioception. When using P ROM during treatment, be sure to respect the client's tolerance and to use repetition only as long as the action remains comfortable. When instructing the client in self-care, it is essential to demonstrate the activity you are recommending and to tell the client to stay within a range of motion and repetition that does not reproduce symptoms. P ROM is suggested for self-care using an external force (e.g., by passively extending the wrist against a desk to lengthen shortened wrist flexors).

As a therapeutic tool, resisted ROM can be used to strengthen weak or lengthened muscles and to reset the nervous system by using resisted, voluntary contractions followed by stretching, which may encourage the lengthening of a shortened muscle. Unlike R ROM for testing, when using resistance therapeutically, the intention is to apply enough resistance to motivate the client to produce a strong contraction. Use these techniques only if the client is strong enough and willing. Some clients may feel anxious about performing resisted exercise in the early stages of healing. Be certain to stay within the client's comfort zone, and use repetition only as long as the action remains comfortable.

Post-Isometric Relaxation

Proprioceptors are nervous system receptors that detect the position and action of body parts, the relationship of one body part to the others, muscle tension and stretch, joint position, and the speed and direction of movement (Fig. 1-8). In short, proprioceptors process information that is internal to the body and convey it to the brain to help you know that you are, for example, sitting rather than standing or walking rather than running. They help you know where your arm is in relation to the rest of your body when you raise it. The main proprioceptors involved in musculoskeletal function are muscle spindles, Golgi tendon organs, and joint kinesthetic receptors. Muscle spindles are located in the muscle belly and detect the amount of stretch in the muscle fibers. Golgi tendon organs are found in tendons and in the musculotendinous junctions; they

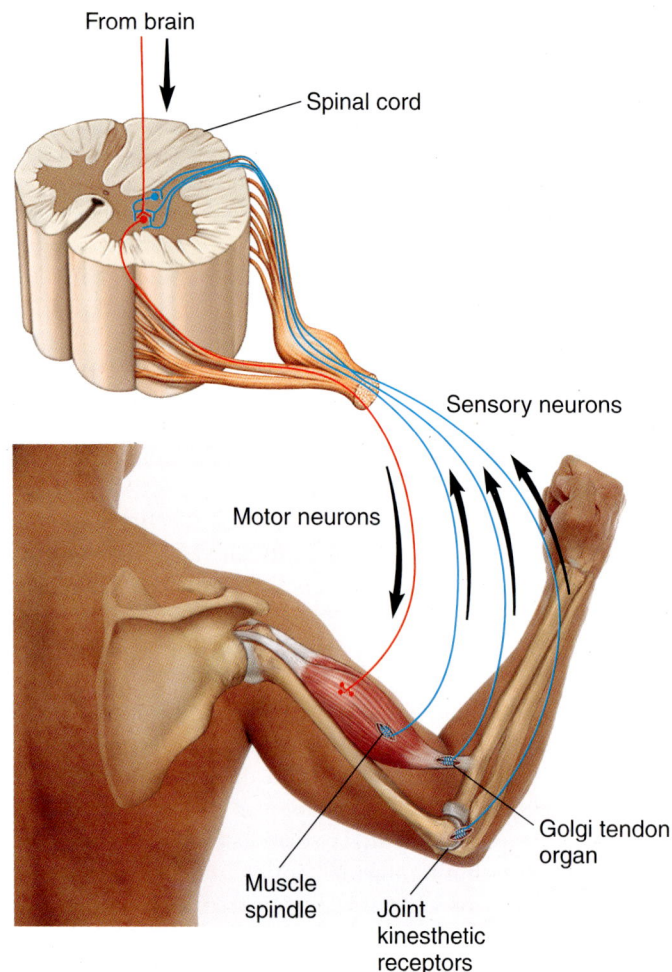

Figure 1-8 Proprioceptors. Proprioceptors process information that is internal to the body and convey it to the brain.

detect tension in those structures. Joint kinesthetic receptors are found in joint capsules; they detect pressure and movement of the joint.

When dysfunction occurs, especially if it is chronic, proprioceptors may adapt to the imbalance, compromising proper function. When muscle spindles and Golgi tendon organs misfire, resting muscle tone is set too high, which results in hypertonicity (atrophy is less likely to be associated with proprioceptor dysfunction and more likely to be associated with dysfunction of the central nervous system or the spinal roots of the peripheral nervous system). When joint kinesthetic receptors misfire, sensitivity to pressure and movement of the joint is reduced and may result in reduced ROM or chronic postural deviations. Proprioceptive neuromuscular facilitation and muscle energy technique are therapeutic methods that alternate periods of contraction and relaxation with the goal of resetting the nervous system so that a shortened muscle can lengthen more fully, the joint can move more freely, and proprioceptors can then return to normal function. For a few seconds following the contraction in these exercises, nerve impulses are repressed, which allows the muscle to be passively lengthened further. Never use these techniques with a fracture, severe or acute injury, or if the client is not receptive to or capable of resisted contractions.

There are many such exercises within each method that have slightly varying therapeutic goals. This book focuses on post-isometric relaxation (PIR) to encourage proper proprioception. Once you have studied this and other such techniques closely, you will have a variety of options better suited to the client's particular needs. All of these techniques are most effective following strokes that increase circulation, soften tissues, and initiate the lengthening of shortened tissues. You should notice the client's shortened muscle lengthen with each repetition of the steps outlined below. You may be able to reach normal resting length of the muscle with a few repetitions of PIR in a single session. If not, the client may not be ready to reach full ROM. As long as the exercise is comfortable for the client, you can repeat it in subsequent visits until normal resting length and tone is achieved. The following sequence describes PIR. It is best to explain these steps to your client before beginning so that you can coordinate movement together.

1. Position the muscle in a comfortably lengthened position. The muscle should not be lengthened to the point of a stretch.
2. Ask the client to contract the muscle against your resistance for 10 seconds. Your resistance should not require the client to use full strength but should be enough to resist full ROM. If you feel the client begin to shake or the client feels discomfort, decrease your resistance.
3. Be sure that the proximal end of the joint is securely supported in your hands as you ask the client to relax the contraction and breathe slowly and deeply. If the joint were not supported, the client would maintain a contraction to keep the structure from falling or moving too quickly.
4. Slowly lengthen the muscle as fully as you can without causing discomfort, and hold this position for approximately 15 seconds.
5. Repeat—two to four times or as indicated.

The following exercise demonstrates proprioceptive dysfunction and the benefit of massage and post-isometric relaxation in correcting it. Work with a partner. If your partner has an area of tension or pain, or if your assessment reveals a postural imbalance, apply this exercise to the affected joint. Ask your partner to close his or her eyes and adjust his or her posture unaided until he or she believes that the joint you are assessing is in anatomical position. For example, if your partner walks or stands with the hips in external rotation, ask him or her to close the eyes and adjust the hips until he or she believes that the toes are pointing forward and both hips are in anatomical position. If his or her neck is laterally flexed and rotated, ask him or her to close the eyes and point the nose straight ahead with the eyes level. If a chronic postural imbalance has affected proprioception, it is likely that his or her perception of anatomical position is skewed in the direction of the imbalance (i.e., the hips remain laterally rotated to some degree, or the neck is still somewhat laterally flexed and rotated even though your partner perceives it as balanced). Now, treat the muscles responsible for the ROM in question. In the example above, lengthen the lateral rotators of the hip or the lateral flexors and rotators of the neck, and end with a few rounds of PIR. Reassess your partner's posture, asking him or her to close the eyes and stand in anatomical position. Has the imbalance improved? If your partner has had a long history of postural imbalance, the improvement after one treatment may be minimal. However, in some cases, a single application of massage followed by PIR can make a profound difference.

CLIENT SELF-CARE

Client self-care is important for achieving treatment goals. Massage therapy can usually help to alleviate signs and symptoms, but the client must take an active role in reducing contributing factors and prolonging the effects of treatment. Stretching, strengthening, and becoming more aware of posture and activity are some of the suggestions that may improve the treatment outcome. When educating clients about self-care, you must consider their whole situation and make suggestions appropriate for their level of strength, general health, and stage of healing. It is best to begin slowly with simple exercises and few repetitions to be certain that the client can perform self-care activities without causing further injury, fatigue, or distress. It is also essential that you demonstrate all suggested activities to ensure that the client understands them clearly, reducing the possibility of injury. If you have legal access to pictures or can create precise descriptions of self-care exercises, give them to your clients as these can be excellent guides.

The most common reason clients give for skipping self-care is lack of time. One way to encourage clients to perform self-care is to make recommendations that they can incorporate into their activities of daily living rather than having to schedule a separate time for a specific regimen. Simple, effective self-care exercises can be performed while talking on the phone, reading e-mail, watching television, or taking a shower. Some of these are described in the following chapters, and you can suggest additional self-care activities that fit nicely into your clients' lifestyles.

A client who diligently complies with self-care recommendations usually heals more quickly and remains symptom free longer than one who does not. However, as much as we want to heal clients, we cannot force them to follow our recommendations. Ask your clients if they have performed the self-care exercises you suggested. If they hesitate or admit that they have not, explain that self-care may expedite healing, but do not insist or judge. Encourage clients to perform self-care, but it is not appropriate to criticize or reprimand those who do not comply.

Stretching

A stretch is a procedure in which the distance between the bony attachment sites of a muscle is increased. Stretching is recommended after the client's mobility has increased and pain has decreased enough for you to perform ROM exercises without the client feeling intense symptoms. The target tissues for stretching exercises are those involved in the condition which have shortened due to injury, repetitive activity, or static postures. They should include compensating structures such as fascia, muscles, tendons, and ligaments unless the injury is acute and those structures have shortened or are in spasm as a protective measure to splint the joint.

Stretches should never be forced. The client should stretch to lengthen the tissue within their comfort zone. When possible, encourage the client to remain relaxed and to minimize muscle contractions once in the posture that produces the stretch. Watch the client performing the stretch. If you notice, for example, that when stretching the neck the client contracts the levator scapulae, help him or her to recognize this by using your own body to demonstrate what it looks like when he or she stretches compared to how you recommend the stretch, or by gently resting your hand on the structure that you want the client to relax while performing the stretch. One way to minimize muscle contractions during a stretch is to perform it passively with the assistance of gravity or a surface like a wall or desk.

A stretch should be steady, without force or bouncing. It takes time for soft tissues and proprioceptors to accommodate the muscle's new length. Ask the client to hold each stretch steadily for at least 15 seconds, taking deep breaths throughout. On exhalation of a deep breath, the client may be able to reach a deeper stretch without pain.

Strengthening

Strengthening is achieved by actively contracting the targeted muscles. An active contraction occurs when one deliberately brings the bony attachment sites of a muscle closer together. Strengthening exercises are recommended only when the client is strong enough and the pain is reduced enough for the client to perform exercises without causing further injury or distress. The target tissues for strengthening exercises are those involved in the condition, which have lengthened or weakened due to injury, repetitive activity, or static postures. These should include all compensating structures unless the injury is still in an acute stage or where strengthening a muscle would adversely affect its antagonist. For example, if you were unable to reduce adhesions or spasm in the biceps brachii, attempting to strengthen the triceps could cause a reaction in the biceps or its synergists, intensifying the spasm or tearing the tissues. The client may be more capable of strengthening the muscle safely after subsequent visits when spasm has subsided.

Strengthening exercises should be performed slowly and fluidly. The client should exercise within their comfort zone. When possible, encourage the client to target very specific tissues without contracting muscles that do not need strengthening. This may not always be possible, but it is most effective when it is possible. Watch the client perform the active contraction. If you notice, for example, that when strengthening the middle trapezius and rhomboids, the client elevates the scapula or rotates the glenohumeral joint, help him or her to recognize this by demonstrating what it looks like when he or she performs the exercise compared to how you recommend doing it or by gently resting your hand on the structure that you want the client to relax.

Resisted ROM can be used to strengthen the antagonists of shortened muscles and, when followed by a passive stretch to a shortened muscle, to reorient a nervous system that has become accustomed to a postural imbalance. When instructing the client in self-care, it is essential to demonstrate the activity you are recommending and to tell the client to stay within a range of motion, resistance, and repetition that does not reproduce symptoms. Ask the client to perform this activity before leaving the clinic so you can see that he or she understands how to perform it correctly.

In all strengthening exercises, resistance and repetition should be limited to the client's comfort zone. Strengthening exercises should not cause undue fatigue or pain. One or two slow repetitions free of external resistance performed a few times a day may be most appropriate in the early stages of healing. As the condition improves, the client may become better able to perform more repetitions with greater resistance.

Hydrotherapy

Hydrotherapy can be a relaxing, effective form of self-care when the client applies it correctly. When recommending hydrotherapy for self-care, follow the guidelines in the earlier Hydrotherapy section. Explain these guidelines so that clients understand why they should use salt or not, why the application time is important, why moisture is essential, when hydrotherapy is contraindicated, and why drinking water is important. You can create written explanations for your clients to ensure that they use hydrotherapy correctly.

Breathing

Deep, diaphragmatic breathing is an essential element of overall good health. Many of us take breathing for granted. We are often so busy that we rush through our breaths as we rush through our lives. Shallow breathing contributes to anxiety, emotional distress, and pain. Helping our clients recognize their breathing pattern and teaching them to adjust to a more relaxed diaphragmatic breathing can have a profound effect on healing. Slow, diaphragmatic breathing calms the sympathetic nervous system and delivers more oxygen through the circulatory system. When used in treatment or during self-care, deep breathing can enhance muscle relaxation and reduce the client's anxiety about their pain or about the massage techniques being used to help relieve their pain. Moreover, instructing the client to recognize their breathing can help him or her to focus on the moment instead of being distracted by where he or she has been or is going next.

Assess your client's breathing at the beginning of treatment by placing one hand on the abdomen and one hand on the sternum and observe movement in these areas as the client breathes. The abdomen should expand first and more forcefully than the sternum. If you notice that the client breathes primarily in the chest or primarily in the abdomen, help him or her to become aware of this by asking him or her to place one hand on the abdomen and the other on the chest to feel the imbalance. Explain that the abdomen should expand first, the ribs expand next, and the sternum elevate last. If this does not help the client to adjust his or her breathing pattern, add gentle pressure to the sternum to minimize the movement of the chest and encourage him or her to breathe into the abdomen, or add gentle pressure to the abdomen to minimize its movement and encourage expansion of the chest. Encourage the client to use this technique to assess and adjust breathing by practicing for 3-5 minutes each day. The goal is to adapt this pattern for normal breathing. You can instruct the client to use this exercise while he or she is being treated, particularly when you approach an area that is tender or during trigger point therapy, and while performing self-care exercises.

When assessing a client's breathing or while recommending breathing exercises, consider the health of his or her respiratory system. Not all clients are capable of practicing deep, diaphragmatic breathing. In addition, ensure clients do not hyperventilate or become dizzy; emphasize that the exercise should be slow and relaxed. Following is an example of a breathing exercise used to focus the mind, relax the nervous system, and reduce generalized pain; it can also be directed to the area you are treating and during self-care exercises:

1. The client can be seated, supine, or prone, using bolsters as desired.
2. Instruct the client to inhale gently while imagining that the breath is white like a clean coffee filter. Ask the client to send this breath (filter) to the toes.
3. As he or she exhales, ask the client to imagine that the pure white breath filters out any impurities in the toes and feet leaving the tissues pink or red with clean, oxygenated blood. The client can also imagine that the breath exhaled is grey or tinted by the impurities filtered out. If the client cannot imagine fresh pink tissue after one breath, have him or her send another breath to the area until the tissues feel clean and oxygenated.
4. The next inhalation is sent to the calves, filtering impurities there with the exhalation, leaving behind fresh, clean tissues.
5. Continue this exercise superiorly, including the upper extremities, until all tissues feel cleaned by the pure, deep breaths.

RANGE OF MOTION ASSESSMENT

Treatment Goals

Planning treatment includes assessing signs and symptoms related to a client's complaint(s) and assessing the client's general health history to determine the best course of therapy in order to achieve treatment goals within the scope of practice for massage therapy. The client and therapist work together to determine appropriate, individual treatment goals. Planning treatment sometimes requires working with a health care team to ensure that all health care providers for a particular client understand each other's treatment goals and to ensure that those goals are complementary. The primary principle in planning treatment is to "do no harm."

With your assessment of the client's signs and symptoms, health history, posture, and ROM, you are ready to put the pieces together and determine treatment goals. While each client's case requires individualized planning, there are several treatment goals common to most moderate cases of the conditions in the chapters that follow: reducing adhesions, increasing circulation, reducing tension, treating trigger points, manually lengthening shortened tissues, passively stretching shortened tissues, and clearing the area treated.

REDUCE ADHESIONS

Because adhesions are often superficial and myofascial release is best performed without emollient, reducing adhesions is a good place to begin. Fascia tends to be thick and dense around muscles that are short, while it is thin and taut around muscles that are stretched. Kneading, cross-fiber friction, and the specific myofascial release strokes explained in Chapter 2 reduce adhesions. Heat, stretching, and mobilizations may also reduce adhesions.

INCREASE CIRCULATION

Venous and lymphatic circulation may be compromised in areas where tissues are adhered, hypertonic, or frequently held in a flexed position. When circulation is reduced, fewer nutrients get in and fewer metabolites get out of the tissues. Areas in which circulation is reduced can become dehydrated and adhered. Gliding, kneading, and percussion increase circulation. Although compression may temporarily reduce circulation, the release of compression temporarily increases circulation. When repeated, compression and release may increase the flow of circulation through the affected area. Heat, mobilizations, and stretching also increase circulation.

REDUCE TENSION

Muscle tension increases during sustained concentric or eccentric contractions. While it is tempting to assume that short, tight muscles are more likely to develop tension than long, weak muscles, this is not always the case. For example, the long, weak erector spinae, stretched over an increased thoracic curve, contract for long periods in an attempt to balance the spine over a stable center of gravity. Although stretched and taut, they may also be tense and hypertonic. Gliding, kneading, and broad compressions help reduce tension and restore normal resting tone. Heat, mobilizations, stretching, and post-isometric relaxation may also reduce tension.

LENGTHEN TISSUE

Short, tight muscles cause and perpetuate postural imbalance and contribute to keeping opposing muscles long and weak. In addition to reducing the tension that has accumulated in these tissues, it is important to lengthen them to encourage the restoration of normal resting length. Firm and deep gliding strokes along with pin and stretch techniques are ideal for manually lengthening tissues.

TREAT TRIGGER POINTS

Trigger points perpetuate the sustained contraction of isolated muscle fibers. As long as trigger points remain activated, it is unlikely that normal resting tone or neuromuscular function can be fully restored. In general, deep gliding, cross-fiber strokes, compression, heat, and stretching help to deactivate trigger points. Chapter 3 explains trigger points and describes treatment options in more detail.

Treatment icons: Increase circulation; Reduce adhesions; Reduce tension; Lengthen tissue; Treat trigger points; Passive stretch; Clear area

PASSIVE STRETCH

After applying techniques that reduce adhesions, increase circulation, and relax contracted muscles, a full passive stretch held for 15–30 seconds helps to elongate the crimped collagen fibers found in noncontractile tissues such as tendons and ligaments (see Chapters 13 and 14). This is an important part of restoring proper posture. The full passive stretch, particularly as part of post-isometric relaxation, also helps to restore proprioception and proper neuromuscular function. A full passive stretch is achieved by increasing the distance between the attachment sites of the affected muscle while the client remains relaxed.

CLEAR AREA

Most massage therapy techniques release and mobilize metabolites that have accumulated as a result of dysfunction. Clearing strokes help move fluids containing metabolites through the circulatory and lymphatic systems where the fluids are cleansed and the metabolites are neutralized or excreted. Broad gliding strokes, both superficial and deep, are ideal for clearing locally and systemically. Mobilizations may also help increase circulation and clear the local area.

STRENGTHENING WEAKENED MUSCLES

Strengthening weakened muscles is also an important part of restoring proper posture and neuromuscular function. It is not included in the treatment goals above because even though percussion, vibration, and cold hydrotherapy may contribute to increasing muscle tone strengthening is a goal best achieved by self-care. Each of the following condition-specific chapters include recommendations for strengthening structures that are commonly weak. Recommend strengthening exercises, explain why the strengthening of weak muscles is important, and ask the client if he or she is performing self-care exercises between appointments. Remember, however, that these are recommendations that the client may or may not follow.

BIBLIOGRAPHY AND SUGGESTED READINGS

Biel A. *Trail Guide to the Body: How to Locate Muscles, Bones and More*, 3rd ed. Boulder, CO: Books of Discovery, 2005.

DeDomenico G. *Beard's Massage: Principles and Practice of Soft Tissue Manipulation*, 5th ed. St. Louis, MO: Elsevier, 2007.

Donoghue P, Doran P, Dowling P, et al. Differential expression of the fast skeletal muscle proteome following chronic low-frequency stimulation. Biochim et Biophysica Acta—Proteins & Proteomics. 2005;1752:166–167.

Fritz S. *Mosby's Fundamentals of Therapeutic Massage*, 4th ed. St. Louis, MO: Elsevier, 2009.

Fritz S, Chaitow L, Hymel GM. *Clinical Massage in the Healthcare Setting*. St. Louis, MO: Mosby/Elsevier, 2008.

Hendrickson T. *Massage for Orthopedic Conditions*. Baltimore, MD: Lippincott Williams and Wilkins, 2003.

Hertling D, Kessler RM. *Management of Common Musculoskeletal Disorders: Physical Therapy Principles and Methods*, 4th ed. Philadelphia, PA: Lippincott Williams and Wilkins, 2005.

Ingalls CP. Nature vs. nurture: Can exercise really alter fiber type composition in human skeletal muscle? Journal of Applied Physiology. 2004;97(5):1591–1592.

Petty NJ, Moore AP. *Neuromusculoskeletal Examination and Assessment: A Handbook for Therapists*, 2nd ed. Edinburgh, UK: Churchill Livingstone, 2001.

Rattray F, Ludwig L. *Clinical Massage Therapy: Understanding, Assessing and Treating over 70 Conditions*. Toronto, ON: Talus Incorporated, 2000.

Simons DG, Travell JG, Simons LS. *Myofascial Pain and Dysfunction: The Trigger Point Manual* Vol. 1, 2nd ed. Baltimore, MD: Lippincott Williams & Wilkins, 1999.

Turchaninov R. *Medical Massage*, 2nd ed. Phoenix, AZ: Aesculapius Books, 2006.

U.S. National Library of Medicine and the National Institutes of Health (ADAM). Numbness and tingling. Available at http://www.nlm.nih.gov/medlineplus/ency/article/003206.htm. Accessed Summer 2008.

Yeznach Wick J. Pain in a special population: The cognitively impaired. Available at http://www.pharmacytimes.com/issue/pharmacy/2007/2007-01/2007-01-6171. Accessed Winter 2010.

Fascia

UNDERSTANDING FASCIA

Fascia is one of the most studied tissues in the human body today. It became so significant in scientific literature worldwide that in 2007 the International Fascia Research Congress (http://www.fasciacongress.org/) was established to explore the importance of fascia for both conventional and complementary health care. Previously thought to be a passive connective tissue, research has established biomechanical and adaptive properties of fascia that are becoming widely recognized as an integral part of homeostasis and an essential element in the long-term resolution of many chronic conditions.

Fascia is soft but dense, fibrous connective tissue forming a continuous, three-dimensional matrix that provides support and shock absorption for the structures of the body; communicates vital information about tension and compression throughout the body; and facilitates the absorption of nutrients and removal of toxins and metabolites (Fig. 2-1). Fascial fibers form dense, irregular connective tissue with a multidirectional arrangement (Fig. 2-2). Fascia covers all of our organs, nerves, muscles, and bones, and while it separates one structure from another, its continuous matrix also connects the structures of the body.

There are three types of fasciae. Superficial fascia, or subcutaneous fascia, is just beneath the skin. It is composed largely of connective and adipose tissues. It connects the skin to the superficial muscles and supports the superficial nerves and blood vessels. Superficial fascia stores water and fat, which help insulate the body. Deep fascia, also called myofascia, is denser than superficial fascia and covers the muscles. It binds the individual fibers that form single muscles and connects individual muscles into groups. The types of collagen and concentrations of elastin change as myofascia reorganizes within the continuous matrix to form the denser tendons, which attach muscle to bone, and ligaments, which support the bones that form a joint. Healthy myofascia allows muscles to move independently and holds nerves and blood vessels that supply structures deep to the skin. Visceral fasciae form the sacs that hold our organs within their cavities and are named according to the organ they support: pericardia (heart), pleura (lungs), and peritonea (abdomen).

While fascia has different forms and functions depending on its location, it is all integrated into a single, continuous, three-dimensional matrix. Massage therapy often focuses on the actions of individual muscles or muscle groups for the purpose of assessing dysfunction and planning treatment. However, because they are bound together, when we assess and treat muscles, we are also necessarily assessing and treating fascia. Every muscle functions within the fascial web (Fig. 2-3). Thus, when we are successful in relaxing a muscle in spasm, the restoration of its normal resting length is unlikely if the fascia surrounding it is bound and shortened. For this reason, understanding the structure and function of fascia can have profound implications for treatment outcomes.

Fascia primarily comprises ground substance, collagen, and elastin. Ground substance—resembling a thin or diluted gel—gives fascia a fluid character. Ground substance holds cells together and allows for the exchange of substances between cells and the interstitial fluid that

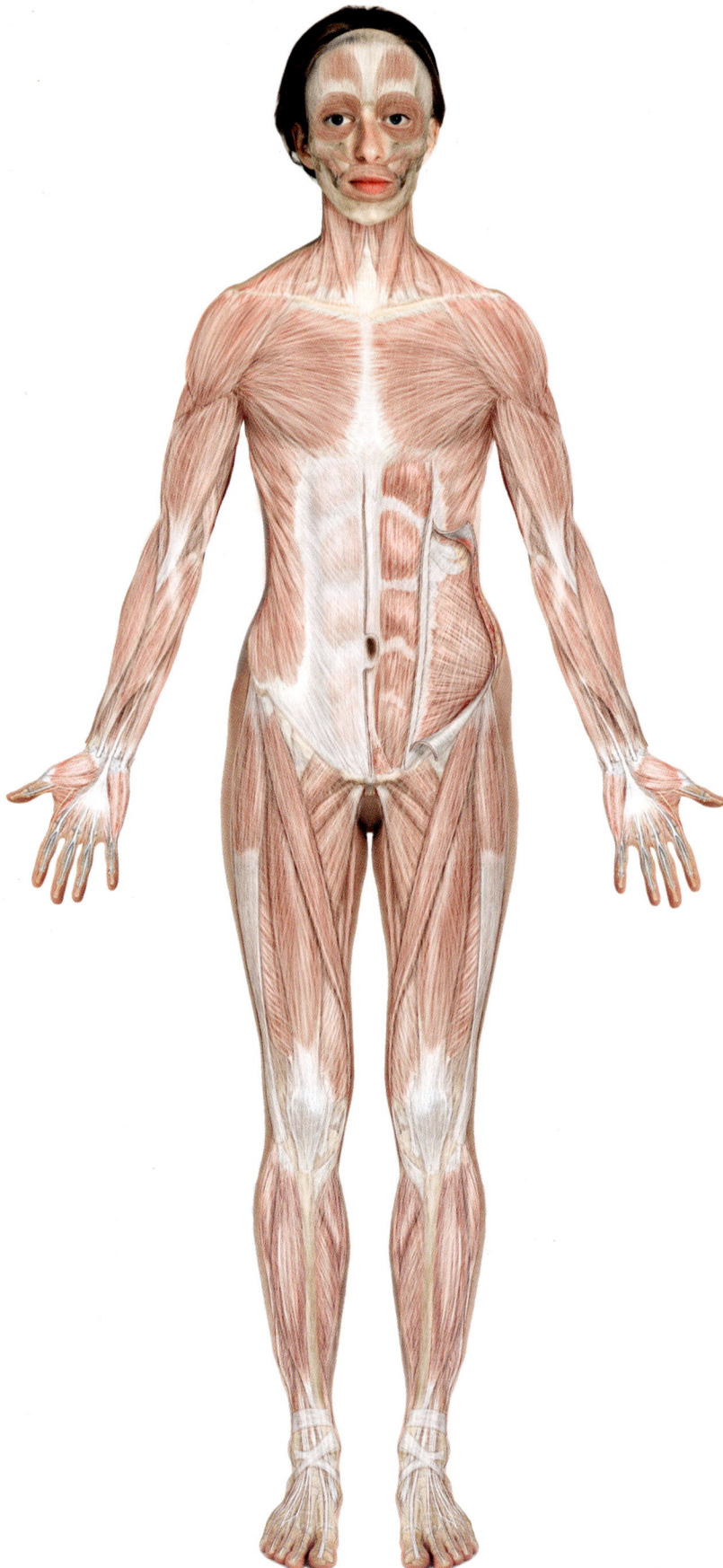

Figure 2-1 **Human fascia.** Fascia is a three-dimensional matrix of connective tissue that provides support and shock absorption for the structures of the body. Fascia surrounds our organs, nerves, muscles, and bones. The areas in white represent regions of thick fascia. (*continued*)

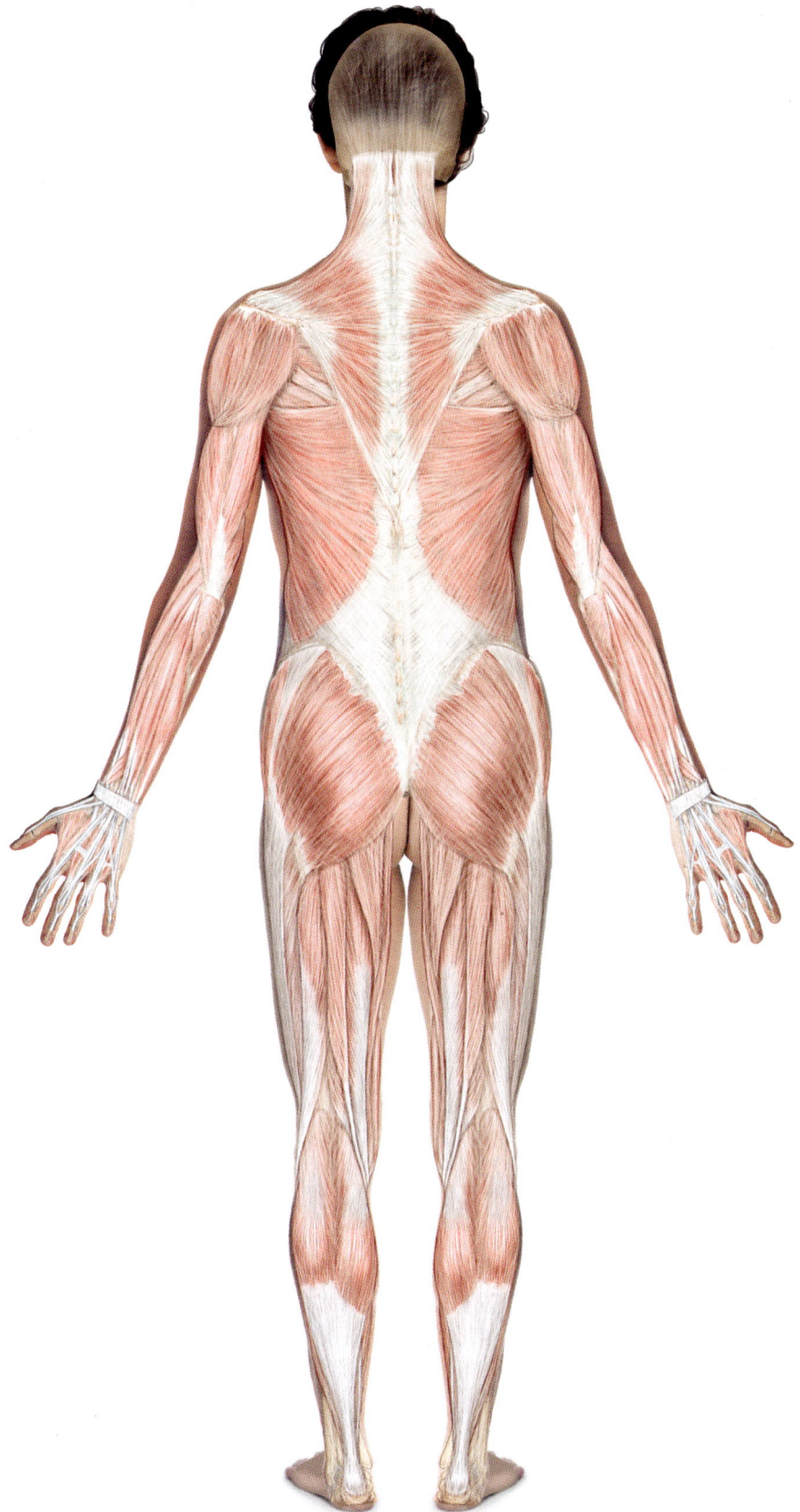

Figure 2-1   (*Continued*)

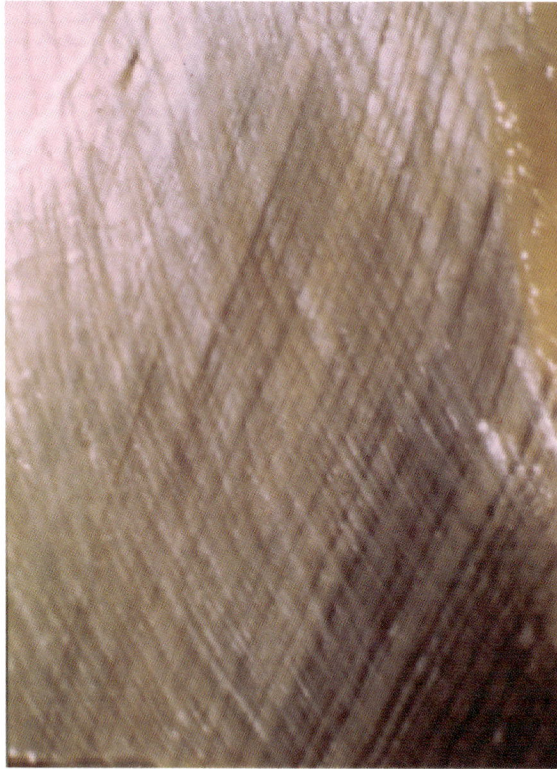

Figure 2-2 **Dense irregular connective tissue.** The multidirectional fiber arrangement of fascia allows for a wide range of movement. Photo copyright Ronald A. Thompson, Ida P. Rolf Research Foundation; used by permission.

bathes them, letting nutrients in and metabolites and toxins out. Ground substance can change in density according to the tissue's needs—a characteristic referred to as thixotropy. Movement, heat, and hydration keep it fluid, and this fluidity in muscles allows for freer movement. Lack of movement, cold, and dehydration cause it to thicken, and thickening inhibits free movement. This is much like what happens to a can of paint. When left alone, particularly in a cool environment, the paint becomes thicker and less mobile. Stir it up, and it begins to liquefy. During the initial healing stage of an acute injury, restricted movement may help prevent re-injury. However, in the subacute and chronic stages, or when a chronic dysfunctional pattern results from postural imbalance, fascia becomes tight and bound, and the thicker, more viscous ground substance is less effective in exchanging substances. Fewer nutrients make it into the cells, and metabolites and toxins are more likely to accumulate locally. Reducing the viscosity of ground substance is one of the goals of myofascial release. Shearing forces, as applied in many massage strokes, reduce viscosity.

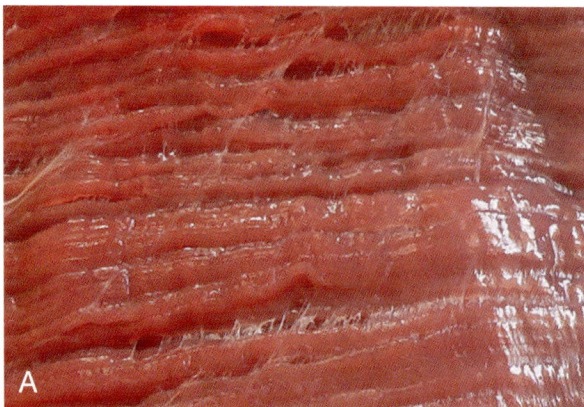

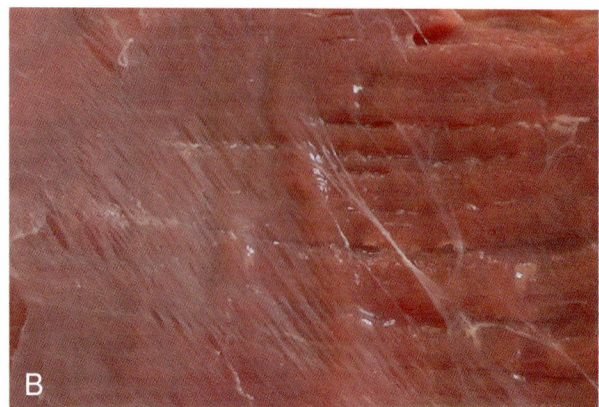

Figure 2-3 **Fascial web.** The fascial web weaves between muscle fibers (A) and surrounds groups of fibers (B). Photos provided courtesy of www.terrarosa.com.au.

Collagen, a protein that easily binds and forms fibers or threads, gives fascia its strength and resilience. Many different types of collagen are found in the human body, each contributing slightly differently to the capabilities of the tissues it forms. The combinations and concentrations of these different collagen fibers allow for the wide variation of connective structures in the body. Collagen makes fascia highly resistant to overstretching and tearing. However, because collagen fibers are so prone to binding, when dysfunction begins, collagen plays a key role in the development of adhesions and is the main component of scars. Elastin—another protein—makes fascia flexible and stretchy, allowing it to reshape as the body moves in every possible direction. When movement allows fascia to stretch slowly, these changes are gradual and fluid. However, when dysfunction puts fascia in a constant stretch, it lengthens and cannot recoil as muscles do. As it stretches, it loses fluid and becomes rigid, dehydrated, and adhered. In time, with proper healing that includes reducing adhesions, restoring the fluidity of ground substance, and removing the offending action or posture, new fibers can form to reestablish the fascia's strength and elasticity.

Fascia is also packed with integrins—receptors that detect tension and compression outside the cells they surround and then communicate this information directly into those cells. This gives fascia the remarkable ability to adapt and instruct the cells it covers to adapt to the body's needs at any given time. Under strain, the primary cells of fascia, called fibroblasts, secrete cytokines, which are immune-responsive substances that encourage inflammation. This suggests that fascia has immunological properties. Cytokines are also communicative. When functioning optimally, these communicative properties of fascia encourage adaptation and healing of the injured structures it is connected to. However, when integrins are overloaded and fibroblasts become hyperactive, the once adaptive response can become chronic and pathological. Recent studies have explored the hyperactive inflammatory response as a factor contributing to fibromyalgia.

It was recently discovered that fascia is also embedded with smooth muscle cells that aid in its adaptation to tension and the demands of the structures it surrounds. When stretched abruptly or for an extended period, fascia increases resistance, actively contracting against the stretch. This may explain the increased tone and fibrotic texture of stretched fascial tissue. Fascia is thoroughly innervated by mechanoreceptors such as Golgi receptors, Ruffini and Pacini corpuscles, and miniscule nerve endings, providing both sensory and motor functions that serve as receptors for pain as well as tension and pressure. Deliberate pressure, whether slow and steady or fast and variable, stimulates these individual receptors. This initiates a cascade of changes in autonomic functions that range from local changes in viscosity and metabolism to more systemic adaptations such as muscle relaxation and emotional calming, depending on the receptor's functions. This may explain why myofascial release to one area of the body can have profound healing effects in distant areas and why treating dysfunctional fascia can be an effective way of restoring healthy muscle tone.

Myofascial dysfunctions tend to follow patterns along what are referred to as myofascial lines (also called myofascial meridians), described in detail in Thomas Myers' (2008) *Anatomy Trains*. These lines are tracks of myofascia within the matrix, which support the common lines of pull (muscle actions) along which strain and tension are transmitted through the body to move the skeleton. These lines of fascia continue past the insertion of a single muscle, linking it to structures that experience tensile stress in similar directions. For example, a myofascial line links the plantar muscles to the calf muscles, hamstrings, gluteals, erector spinae, and suboccipitals all the way up to the galea aponeurotica (Fig. 2-4). Local strain at any point along that line may be transmitted along the whole line, often producing symptoms and dysfunction somewhere other than at the original site of strain.

To understand myofascial lines and the tendency of dysfunctional patterns to develop along them, we must first understand the concept of tensegrity. Tensegrity (tensional integrity) describes the character of a structure, the integrity of which depends on balanced tension across its rigid parts (Fig. 2-5). Tension in one part of the structure must be balanced by tension in another. In the human body, the rigid parts are our bones. By themselves, the bones would simply stack upon each other, compressed by gravity, eventually collapsing under their own weight. The skeleton is stabilized by the constant tension of muscles, tendons, and ligaments—our tensile structures. And fascia, which binds these structures, distributes tensile stress throughout its

Myofascial chain	Bone attachments		Myofascial chain	Bone attachments

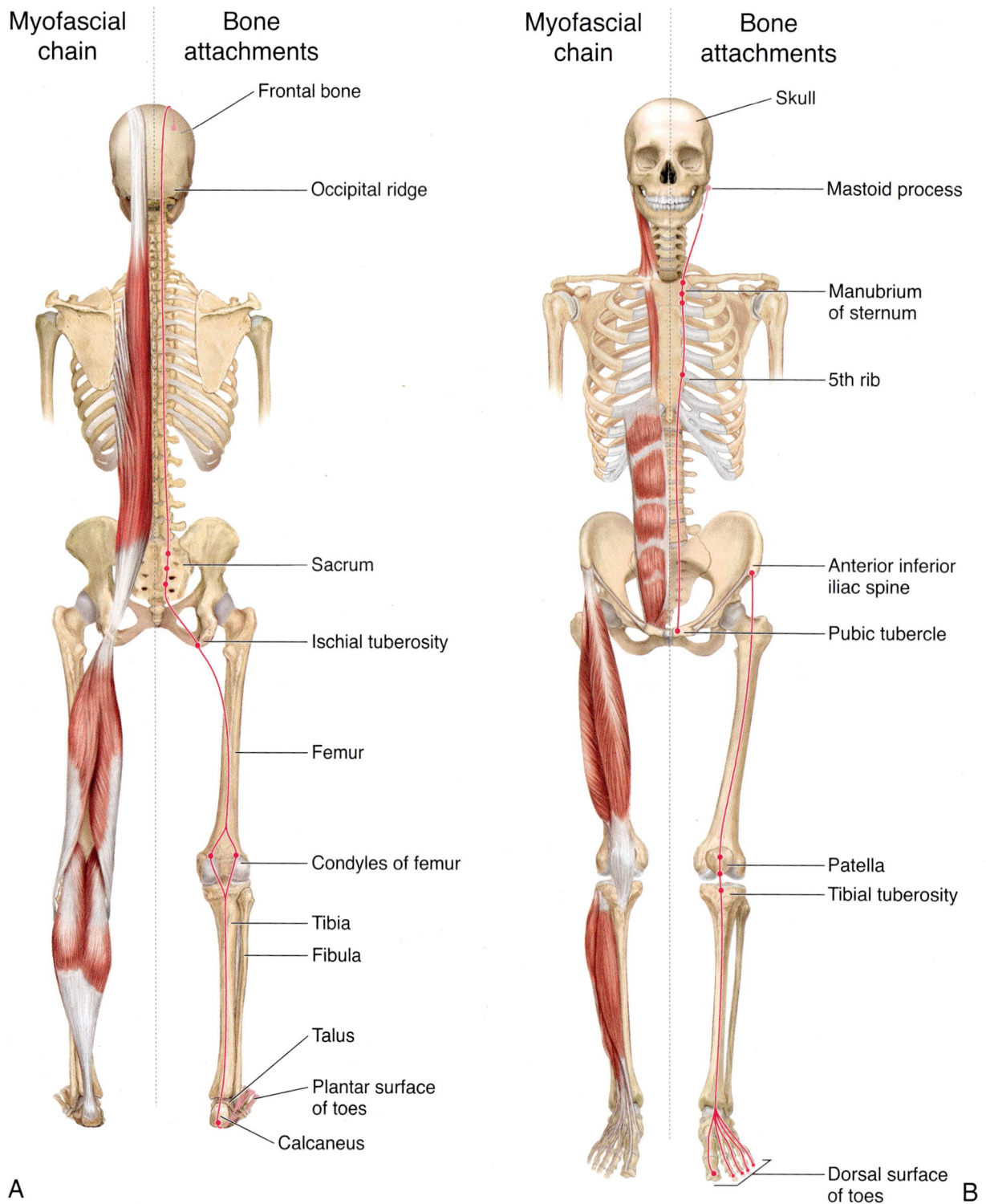

Figure 2-4 **Myofascial lines.** The superficial back line (A) and the superficial front line (B) connect the head to the feet through the body.

webbing to prevent any single, localized area from being subject to the full force of a movement or gravity.

When stress to one part of a structure is increased, especially when the stress is repetitive, myofascial fibers reorganize and stiffen along the direction of applied stress (Fig. 2-6). Under maximum strain, as when chronically lengthened, this alignment of fibers can become virtually linear, losing the multidirectional character that allows for remarkable freedom of movement

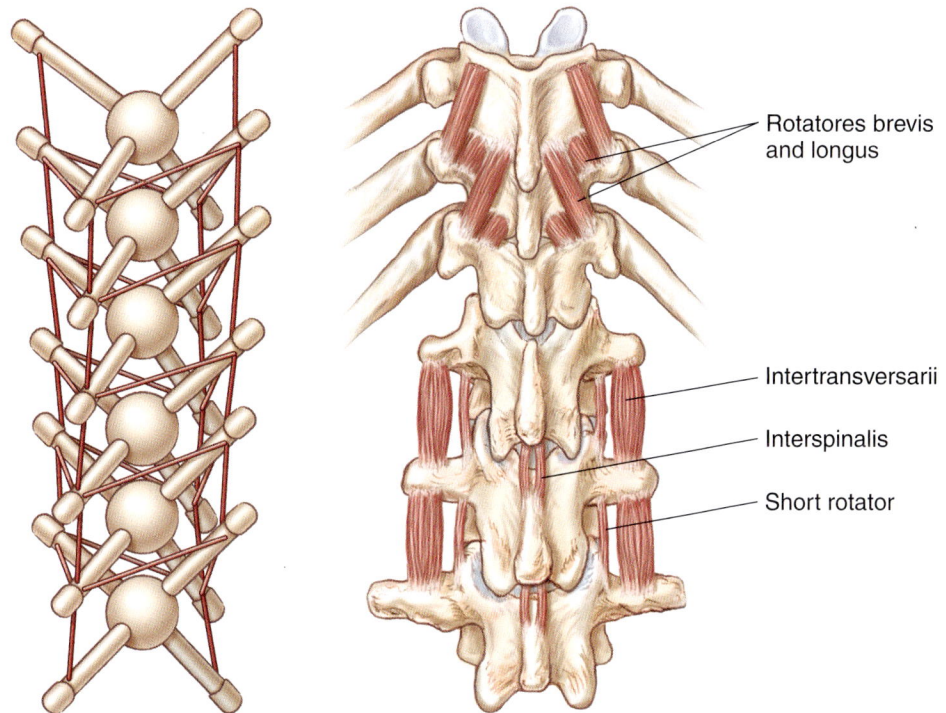

Figure 2-5   Tensegrity. A tensegrity structure depends on balanced tension across its rigid parts. The stellated tetrahedron on the left and the spine on the right are flexible yet stable structures. They can move in multiple directions and bear a load in any position. In the spine, tension is balanced across the rigid bones by muscles and fascia.

and resilience against stressors. This is much like what happens when you pull the ends of a cotton ball. In a relaxed state, the fibers of a cotton ball are arranged in multiple directions, like a loosely knit mesh. When you slowly pull the ends, you can see the fibers straighten and reorganize along the line of the stress (stretch) you are applying. As you continue to pull, most of the fibers reorganize into this longitudinal alignment. The rigidity of those aligned fibers provides protection against the stress you are applying (you have to pull with more force to lengthen them fur-

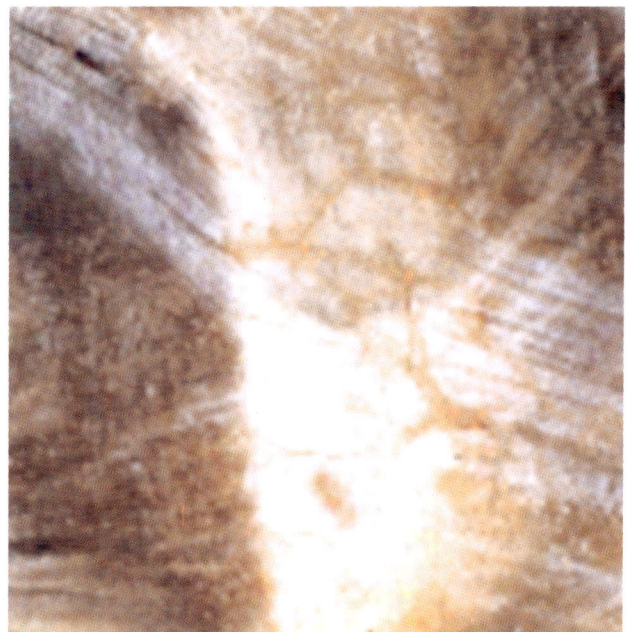

Figure 2-6   Pectoral fascia under stress. Myofascial fibers of this pectoralis major have reorganized diagonally, from upper left to lower right, stiffening along the direction of applied stress. Photo copyright Ronald A. Thompson, Ida P. Rolf Research Foundation; used by permission.

ther), and makes the fibers more efficient against stress aligned in that direction (as when cotton is spun into yarn or thread). However, when aligned to accommodate stress in a single direction, the fibers also lose the freedom of random movement. Conversely, if you squeeze a cotton ball tightly, its fibers become compressed, changing the density of the once fluffy ball. To restore its fluff, you would loosen the fibers slowly and gently, uncrimping the densely packed fibers and increasing the spaces between them.

When one area of the body is repeatedly subject to a pattern of tension or stress in the same direction, the muscles that contract in that direction often shorten and their antagonists lengthen. The fascial webbing surrounding those structures follows, becoming short, thick, and compressed or long, narrow, and stretched. In either case, function is compromised, restricting movement and reducing pliability. If the local fascia loses function within the tensegrity model, stress is distributed along the fascial line that contains that structure to compensate for the weakness. Left untreated, tensegrity along that line falls out of balance. Ultimately, adhesions, hypertonicity, trigger points, and chronic pain syndromes may develop.

For example, a client with hyperlordosis (see Chapter 8) often presents with shortened hip flexors and lumbar extensors and lengthened hamstrings and abdominal muscles. The fascia surrounding the shortened soft tissues bunches up and becomes dense and bound to the shortened muscles and other local structures. This fascia needs to be released and lengthened to restore free movement of each structure individually and to allow the muscles to regain a normal resting length and tone. The fascia surrounding the lengthened structures stretches, with fibers aligning virtually linearly in the direction of tension, and creates a belt-like band that binds to the surrounding soft tissues. That band of virtually unidirectional fibers initially serves to prevent tearing and to protect the structure from more dramatic misalignment, but in doing so, it restricts free and random movement, ultimately weakening the structure. In both cases, adhesions and compromised function affect the circulation of fluids that feed the soft tissues and remove toxins and metabolites. Toxins accumulate; nutrition is diminished; function is compromised; and trigger points, pain, and weakness develop. Since a tensegrity structure distributes stress along the direction of tension, such dysfunction can occur anywhere distant from the site of strain along the line of tension.

The remainder of this chapter focuses on myofascia, with particular attention to its superficial layers, its contribution to chronic pain, and the role massage therapy can play in restoring proper function. However, untreated fascial restrictions can have a profound effect not only on the function of the musculoskeletal system but also on any organ within all systems of the body. Applying myofascial release to treat structures other than the musculoskeletal anatomy requires advanced training in myofascial release. The References and Selected Readings section at the end of this chapter includes articles with more clinical detail than presented here, and many continuing education offerings focus on the finer details of fascial health and homeostasis.

Possible Causes and Contributing Factors

Mechanical overload, whether caused by an acute incident, repetitive misuse, or postural imbalance, is a primary contributing factor in the development of myofascial restrictions. Immobility following an injury or as a result of static postures held for long periods may also cause the thickening of ground substance, which contributes to myofascial adhesions and compromises the exchange of nutrients and waste products. Daily exercise reduces the risk of developing broad myofascial restrictions, and studies have shown that injuries heal better when activity is reintroduced as soon as possible. Chilling the fascia, whether directly—such as with prolonged use of an ice pack—or indirectly—such as when sitting near an air conditioning vent, may also cause a thickening of ground substance, reducing fascial mobility and its ability to transfer nutrients and metabolites. Prolonged compression of myofascia by external sources, such as the straps of a bag or a utility belt, may reduce fluid content and contribute to adhesions.

Scar formation binds fibers together and increases adhesions. In the initial 24–48 hours following injury, the inflammatory process aids in providing nutrients and clearing the area to promote healing. Fibroblasts become very active, producing ground substance and collagen to reestablish integrity in the injured structure. These fibers are laid down more randomly than when fibroblasts actively restore and reinforce healthy tissue. As the scar matures, the collagen fibers bind tightly and harden to prevent further damage from tensile stress. Untreated, scar tissue shrinks and tightens, ground substance diminishes, adhesions solidify, and both the structure and function of the injured tissue are compromised. The period of scar tissue maturation is an ideal time to apply myofascial techniques to soften and reorient fibers, reduce local adhesions, and minimize the risk of spreading dysfunction throughout the matrix.

Pathologies including chronic inflammation, infection, hormonal imbalance, and nutritional deficiencies can also affect the normal functioning of fascia, though dysfunction may not be apparent until weeks, months, or even years later. Trauma, fatigue, and physical or emotional stress can perpetuate myofascial dysfunction. Congenital conditions such as bone length discrepancies may encourage compensatory patterns that include myofascial restrictions.

Each of the conditions described in this book will likely involve myofascial restrictions because the postures or traumas that contribute to these conditions can also contribute to tensile stress and adhesions. Releasing myofascial restrictions that contribute to these conditions is necessary to fully resolve the signs and symptoms associated with them.

Contraindications and Special Considerations

First, it is essential to understand the cause of the client's pain. Refer the client to his or her health care provider if symptoms are severe or significantly reduce his or her activities of daily living. These are a few general cautions:

- **Infection.** Fascial restrictions can be associated with chronic infections that cause inflammation. Massage is systemically contraindicated until the infection is resolved.
- **Acute injury.** Do not treat local to an acute injury. Performed without advanced training, myofascial release may be too aggressive for newly injured tissues. Wait until the subacute or chronic stage, when the tissues are more stable.
- **Producing symptoms.** Take care to keep the level of pain within the client's tolerance. Explain the process of treatment and the sensations your client may experience before you begin so that the client is aware and prepared. Understanding may keep the client from tensing up.
- **Hypermobile joints and overstretched muscles.** It is best not to fully stretch a muscle or fascia that is already lengthened or crosses a hypermobile joint. Fascial restrictions found in such areas should be treated with strokes that bring the joints on either end of the stretched fascia closer together, releasing only the affected fibers.
- **Treatment duration and pressure.** If the client is elderly, has degenerative disease, or has been diagnosed with a condition that diminishes activities of daily living, you may need to adjust your pressure as well as the treatment duration. More frequent, half-hour sessions may suit the client better.
- **Friction.** Do not use deep friction if the underlying tissue is at risk for rupture. To avoid re-injury, allow time for scarring and tissue regeneration before applying friction. Do not use deep friction if the client is taking anti-inflammatory medication or anticoagulants. Friction initiates an inflammatory process, which may interfere with the intended action of anti-inflammatory medication. Recommend that the client refrain from taking such medication for several hours before treatment if his or her health care provider is in agreement. Because anticoagulants reduce clotting, avoid techniques that may cause tearing and bleeding.

Assessing and Treating Myofascia

Pain and reduced ROM resulting from musculoskeletal injury or postural imbalances will almost certainly involve some degree of myofascial dysfunction. A client will not likely complain specifically about fascial restrictions but will likely refer to a general or specific area of pain or tension. If your client has been evaluated by a health care professional to rule out more serious contributing factors and has had a variety of treatments targeting muscles but continues to experience pain, fascial restrictions may be preventing the return of normal resting length and tone. In general, where muscles are short and tight, the myofascia is likely to be bulky, fluid filled, and adhered to the affected muscles and surrounding tissues in the shortened position. Where muscles are lengthened and weak, the myofascia will likely be stretched, flat, narrow, dehydrated, and adhered in the long, strap-like form.

As a general rule, you want to move fascia in the direction that you want the affected structure to move. For example, if the pectoral fascia is bound in the shortened position due to internal rotation of the shoulder, lengthen the pectoral fascia from the clavicle and sternum toward the humerus to encourage external rotation. If the fascia of the upper back is stretched along with the erector spinae due to an increased curve of the thoracic spine, move the fascia inferiorly to help reduce the kyphosis (Fig. 2-7). Take care not to use techniques that stretch fascia that is already lengthened due to injury or postural imbalance.

Once you have completed a postural assessment that helps indicate which structures may be contributing to the client's symptoms, palpation will give you the most direct and accurate picture of the client's myofascial health. One key to accurate palpatory assessment is distinguishing between muscle fibers and fascia and recognizing the musculotendinous junctions where fascia tends to be thickest. Density and mobility will provide clues. Hypertonic muscle fibers feel broadly dense, knotty, or crunchy but can usually be identified individually. Apply pressure to a hypertonic muscle until you feel resistance, and as it releases, you can palpate more deeply before you feel the next level of resistance. Fascial restrictions require more focused assessment. A hand that is too heavy may push past the superficial fascia, and you might miss those restrictions. Moreover, myofascial restrictions can be small and localized and easily passed by if you are not focused. A myofascial restriction will slow or even stop your stroke if you move along it slowly and intently.

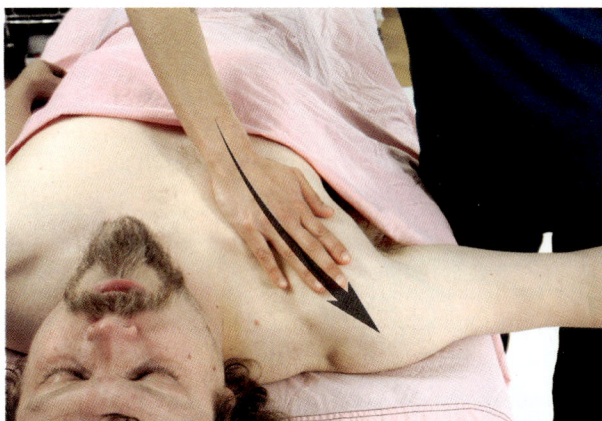

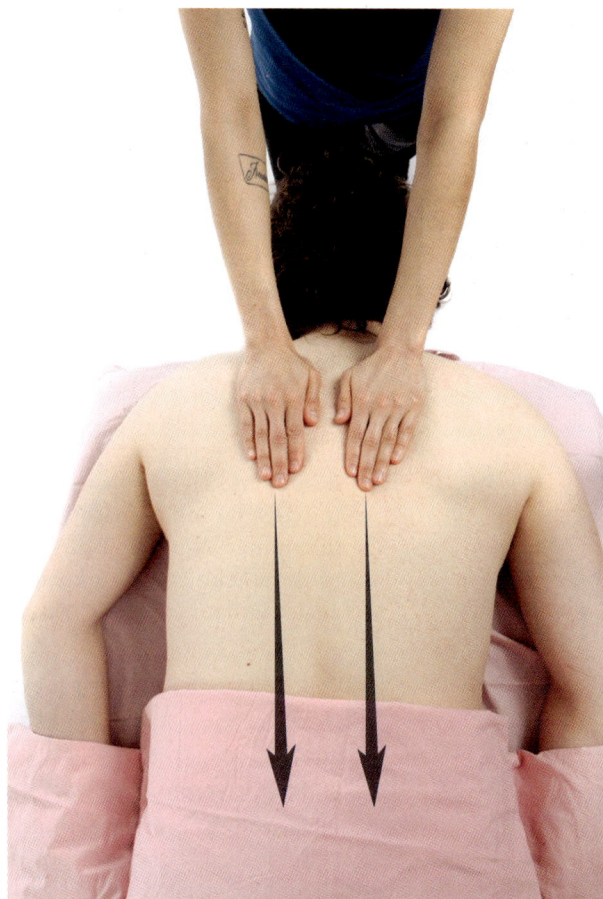

Figure 2-7   Myofascial release. Treat myofascial tissues in the direction that you want the structure to move. For example, if the pectoral fascia is shortened due to internal rotation of the shoulder, lengthen the tissues from the clavicle and sternum toward the humerus to encourage lateral rotation of the shoulder. If the fascia of the upper back is stretched along with the erector spinae due to an increased curve of the thoracic spine, move the fascia inferiorly to help reduce the kyphosis.

It is best to assess and treat myofascial restrictions before applying emollient to prevent gliding over the restrictions. Check the skin, muscles, attachment sites, and any ligaments in the area for immobility and adhesions. Assess the texture, temperature, tone, and tenderness of the tissues in the affected areas as well as distant structures known to contribute to pain in those areas. Restriction is indicated by an inability of a superficial structure, such as skin, to glide smoothly over a deeper structure, such as muscle. Cross fiber strokes are an effective way of initially breaking up adhesions and increasing space between structures or fibers. Skin rolling is an excellent technique for both assessing and treating superficial myofascia (Fig. 2-8). Using both hands, grasp a piece of skin between your thumbs and the index and middle fingers, and gently push the skin away from you with your thumbs while your fingers walk across the skin to gather and roll it. Begin your roll in an area where tissue is easy to grasp, and move toward the area you suspect to be adhered. Rolling a wad of tissue between your fingers will become more difficult and tender over myofascia that is dense or adhered. The texture of the affected tissue may feel gritty or fibrotic. When gripping the affected superficial tissues, you may see dimpling similar to the texture of orange peel (Fig. 2-9). Repeating skin rolling several times over the affected area may be sufficient to release restrictions.

Restrictions may also be recognized as tissues that do not spring back after compression or stretching. Gently compress and hook into the tissue and, without gliding, try to move it in all directions. Tissues that do not move freely or do not spring back when released are likely adhered. For a large area of restriction, a broad stretch is a good beginning (Fig. 2-10A). Place the flat palms and fingers of both hands over the restricted area. It is helpful to begin with your hands close to, or even touching each other so you can monitor the stretch by watching the space between you hands increase. Without gliding over the skin, move your hands away from each other in the direction you intend to stretch the fascia until you feel movement. For example,

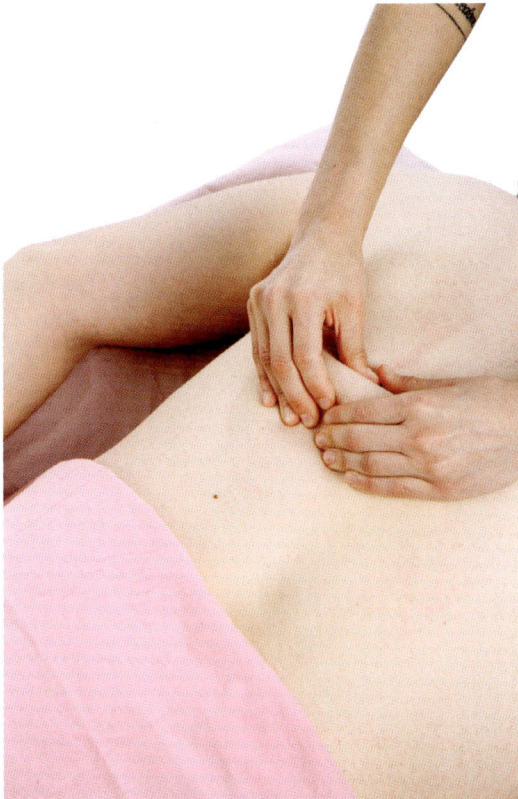

Figure 2-8 **Skin rolling.** Skin rolling is an effective technique for both assessing and treating myofascial restrictions. Notice the red streaks superior to the therapist's hands indicating vasodilation and increased circulation as a result of skin rolling.

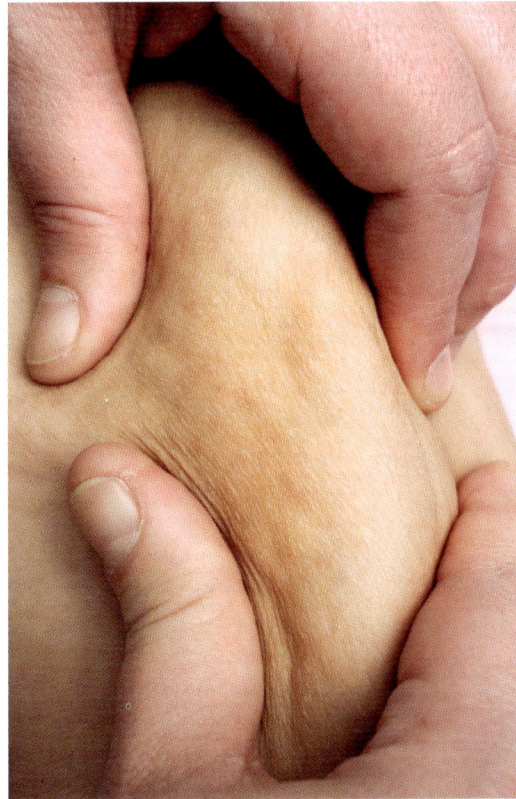

Figure 2-9 **Orange peel texture.** Dimpling of the skin suggests superficial fascial restrictions.

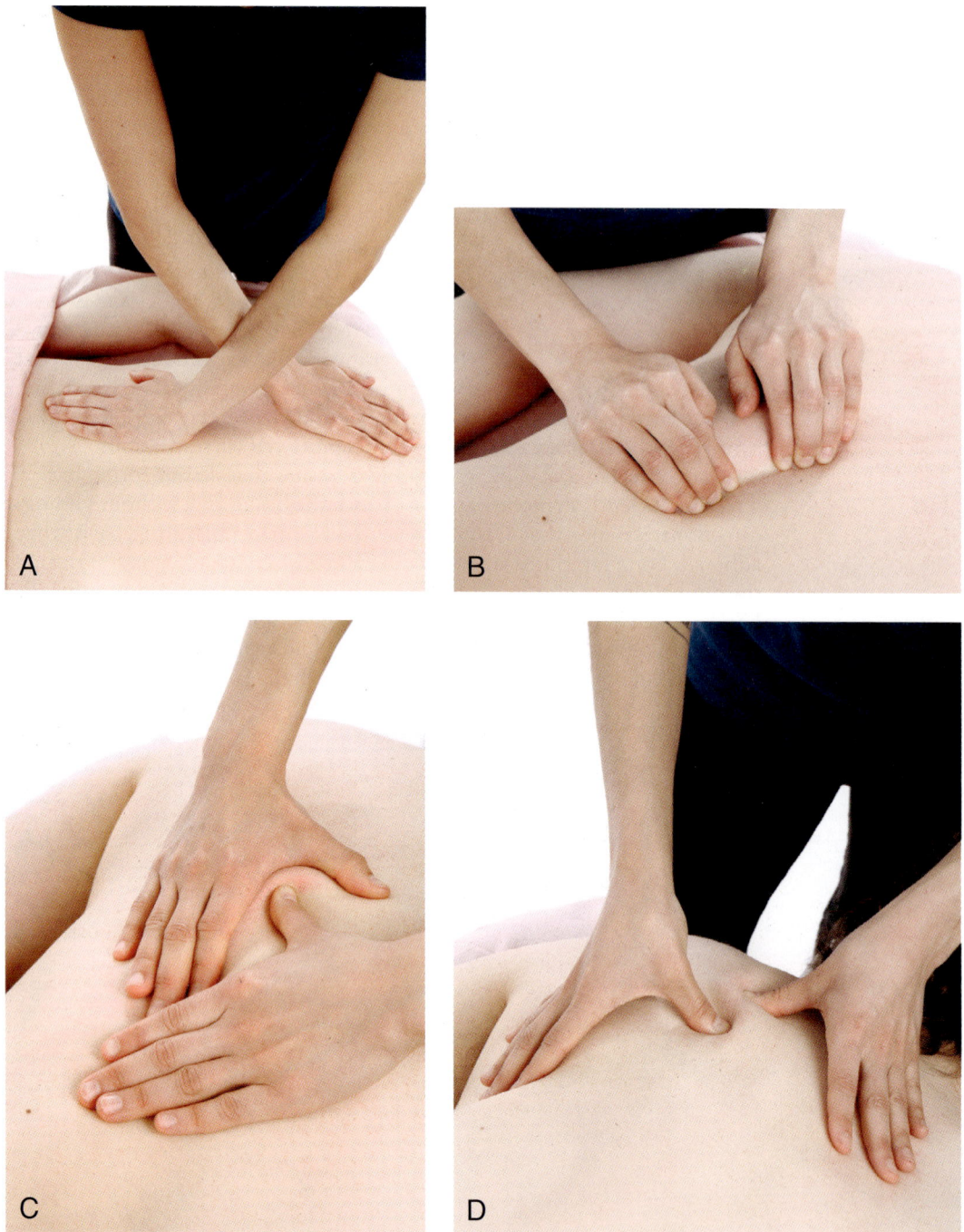

Figure 2-10 **Myofascial release.** Broad release (A), focused release (B), C strokes (C), and S strokes (D) are all effective methods of releasing myofascial restrictions.

if you are reducing restrictions along the latissimus dorsi, begin with your hands over the area of restriction, and move them so that one is moving toward the ilium and the other is moving toward the axilla. Use only enough pressure to make contact with the fascia and move it, without compressing the underlying structures.

If the restriction is more localized, a more focused technique is recommended (Fig 2-10B). The number of fingers you use depends on the size of the area of the local restriction. Begin with the fingers close to or touching each other so you can monitor the amount of stretch achieved. If you are working deeply, treat the superficial tissues first to ease access to the deeper structures. Use only enough pressure to access and maintain contact with the affected tissues. Without gliding, move your fingers away from each other in the direction you intended to stretch the fascia until

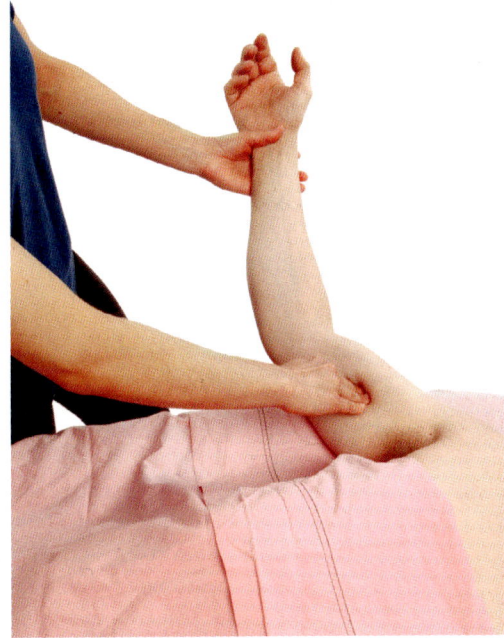

Figure 2-11 **Assessing and treating deep myofascia.** Press gently into the tissue at an angle and use short strokes to assess deeper myofascia. Once you have entered the area, if you need to work more deeply, adjust the angle of your compression vertically, perpendicular to the target tissue.

you feel movement. For example, if you are releasing an adhesion along the superior fibers of the pectoralis major, place a finger or two of each hand along those fibers. Move the fingers of one hand toward the clavicle, while the others move toward the humerus.

Superficial and deep fascial restrictions can also be released by distorting the shape of the tissue. Use only enough pressure to access the affected tissues. A C-stroke is performed by placing one hand in the area of restriction with the thumb and index finger creating the C shape, while one or two fingers of the other hand push the tissues into the curve of the (Fig. 2-10C). An S-stroke is performed by placing the thumbs or fingers of one hand parallel to those of the other, and then moving the hands in opposite directions to form the S shape (Fig. 2-10D).

Assessing deeper tissues requires even more focused palpation. Begin by gently pressing your fingertips at an angle toward the tissues to be assessed (Fig. 2-11). Once you have entered the area, if you need to work more deeply, adjust the angle of your compression vertically, perpendicular to the target tissue. For example, to access the fibers of the brachialis that are deep to the biceps brachii, enter the area at an angle via the edge of the distal biceps until you make contact with the brachialis. Once you feel it, if you need to gain even more direct access, adjust your angle, approaching perpendicular contact, moving the biceps further out of the way, allowing you to treat the deeper fibers of the brachialis. Move your fingers across a small area of the fibers to release adhesions and along the fibers to lengthen them as necessary.

When assessing the deeper myofascia, feel for independent mobility of each affected muscle, and note the texture of the connective tissues around it. Myofascial restrictions will reduce independent mobility. For example, when you find a taut band of fibers that indicates the possible presence of a trigger point (see Chapter 3), palpate around the edges of the taut band. You will likely feel a thread of dense connective tissue that not only encapsulates the taut band but also adheres it to the surrounding tissues, preventing these tissues from moving freely and independently. Slow, cross-fiber strokes are a good assessment tool for deeper myofascial restrictions and an excellent tool for releasing them. If you find a deep restriction, maintain contact with it through the superficial layers, and hook and stretch it until you feel release. Follow this with slow, firm longitudinal strokes to lengthen shortened fascia.

During your assessment and treatment, the client may report sensations such as burning, itching, scratching, or pinpricks. These sensations indicate the presence of myofascial restrictions during assessment and the release of myofascial restrictions during treatment. Instruct your client to breathe deeply while you are treating areas that are painful, and take care not to cause a level of pain that keeps the client from relaxing. As the tissues release, the level of discomfort should decrease. The client may report a calming sensation in an area distant from where you are working, which is likely the result of stress being released along the affected fascial lines.

To get the best results, hold a myofascial stretch until you feel the tissue release. This can take up to a minute or longer. Be patient and take care to use only as much pressure as you need to access the affected tissue. These strokes may leave a dent or other distortion in the tissue when you release it. In most cases, this will last for only a few seconds, but in extreme cases, the distorted shape caused by your compression may last longer due to pitting edema. Chronic edema and large areas of pitting edema should be assessed by a medical professional.

Massage Therapy Research

What follows is a small sampling of the research describing the effects of massage therapy techniques for the treatment of myofascial dysfunction. The references at the end of this chapter include additional studies, and even those represent only a small sample of the literature on massage treatment for myofascial dysfunction. Several of the following chapters also include references to research in which myofascial release is central to positive outcomes.

In a study titled "Tensegrity Principle in Massage Demonstrated by Electro- and Mechanomyography," Kassolik et al. (2009) tested the electrical and mechanical activities of muscles that are distant from but indirectly connected to the muscles being massaged. Thirty-three men received either a massage to the brachioradialis while the middle deltoid was tested for activity or a massage to the peroneals while the tensor fasciae latae was tested. Although no significant electrical activity was noted in the middle deltoid during the massage of the brachioradialis, electrical activity in the tensor fasciae latae increased with the massage to the peroneals. Mechanical activity increased in both scenarios. The authors conclude that the tensegrity principle applies during the use of massage techniques, an observation that has great implications for the treatment of muscle tension.

LeBauer et al. (2008) produced a case report titled "The Effect of Myofascial Release (MFR) on an Adult with Idiopathic Scoliosis," describing the treatment of an 18-year-old female with significant curves in the thoracic and lumbar spine. Her complaints included low back pain and bilateral hip pain. The subject had worn a brace for approximately 6 months when she was 12 years old and reported that before using the brace she had no pain related to her scoliosis. Posture and gait were assessed, pain was measured using a Visual Analog Scale (VAS), and the subject completed questionnaires assessing her self-reported pulmonary function as well as her quality of life, both before and after MFR. She received 6 weeks of treatment consisting of 45-minute sessions twice per week. Comparison of pre- and post-treatment data revealed improvements in pain, thoracic and lumbar rotation, and posture. VAS, pulmonary function, and quality of life all had significant improvements following MFR. The authors concluded that a single case study cannot confirm that such results are typical and encouraged further investigation of MFR for the treatment of idiopathic scoliosis.

In the case report titled "Efficacy of Myofascial Release Techniques in the Treatment of Primary Raynaud's Phenomenon," Walton (2008) describes the results of the treatment of a 35-year-old female who had been suffering symptoms including pallor and decreased temperature in the extremities due to vasoconstriction, followed by numbness and throbbing pain as blood returned to the extremities for 12 years. Baseline information was collected for 3 weeks before treatment and 3 weeks following treatment. The subject kept a log describing the frequency, duration, and severity of symptoms and the number of digits affected. Five 45-minute myofascial treatments were administered to the upper back, neck, and arms, along the myofascial meridian, over a 3-week period. The duration and severity of symptoms improved over the course of treatment, although the frequency of symptoms and number of digits affected varied little compared to pretreatment measurements. The author notes that while these findings are encouraging, further study including a larger sample size, longer observation period, and a control group is necessary.

PROFESSIONAL GROWTH

CASE STUDY

Maria is a 28-year-old horticulturalist. She is very fit and very flexible. She maintains an active lifestyle, participating in sports and martial arts. She has pain in her right heel.

Subjective

Maria reported feeling intense pain in her right heel, which was constant when she was using the foot. She felt less pain at rest, but it returned with each step throughout the day. She stated that her foot sometimes felt "full" or swollen. She pointed to a spot on the medial, anterior, inferior calcaneus, explaining that at its worst she felt severe pain in that spot, and at times she felt a "buzzing" around the area and up the ankle, a few times reaching the middle of her calf. The pain does not decrease after walking or other activities of the foot. She has no pain in the left foot or elsewhere on the body. Maria stated that until approximately 2 years ago, she had walked primarily on the balls of her feet. After developing chronic low back pain, she had begun a regular, intensive stretching program and began practicing yoga regularly to get her heels to touch the floor, and to reduce the low back pain. She was successful in both, walking flat on her feet without back pain, but had developed a gradually increasing pain in her heel beginning approximately 6 months ago. She has seen her primary care provider and was referred to an orthopedist who then referred her to a podiatrist. X-rays showed no bone spurs or fractures to the bone. All three health care providers diagnosed plantar fasciitis and recommended wearing a boot to prevent plantar flexion when she sleeps. She was unsatisfied with the diagnosis because when she researched plantar fasciitis, she did not think her symptoms matched those in the literature. After practicing all of the recommended self-treatments and exercises, her symptoms were not relieved, and on some days, felt worse. It has become so intense that she has had to discontinue practicing yoga, Hapkido, and working out. She is terribly concerned about being sedentary and is eager to get back to these activities.

Objective

Maria appears healthy and vibrant. When talking about her heel pain, she looks stressed.

A postural assessment revealed head slightly forward, elevated right shoulder, severe hyperlordosis with anterior pelvic tilt, elevated left ilium with slight rotation of the pelvis toward the left. She has a slight valgus of the calcaneus bilaterally. When she lies supine, her non-weight-bearing posture reveals extension of the toes, pes cavus, and significant plantar flexion. The right ankle joint is very flexible; she feels a stretch but no pain with passive dorsiflexion. Palpation produced pain only at the anterior inferior, medial calcaneus, near the attachment of the abductor hallucis, and along the inferior tendons of the tibialis posterior, flexor digitorum longus, and flexor hallucis longus. The fascia of the entire right lower leg is extremely dense and adhered. Compressing the tissues in any area of the leg created significant dimpling, particularly along the superior, medial aspect of the calcaneal tendon. Further palpation revealed fascial restrictions along the whole superficial back line. The fascia is dense and strap-like along the thorax, and slightly tender with skin rolling. The fascia is thick and bound in the thoracolumbar area, surrounding the anterior iliac crest, tensor fasciae latae, and into the iliotibial band. There was a trigger point in the medial, inferior aspect of the soleus, which referred into the heel, reproducing the pain she feels when walking.

Action

Began supine, releasing fascia of the anterior hip and lengthening hip flexors. Maria was able to tolerate only minimal to moderate stretching of this fascia in the beginning. I applied cross-fiber strokes followed by lengthening the hip flexors. I did not treat iliopsoas today because of the time restriction and to avoid combining the intensity of iliopsoas treatment with intense myofascial release. Turning the client prone, I stretched the hip flexors. I performed myofascial release to the full superficial back line. Treatment of the thorax was pleasant for the client, but minimal to moderate stretching of the thoracolumbar fascia caused intense burning and itching. Fascia of the lateral thigh is thick and adhered bilaterally, and myofascial techniques produced intense burning and itching near the iliotibial band. Fascia of the lower leg is particularly thick with much dimpling upon even minimal compression. I focused the majority of my time on broadly loosening the super-

ficial fascia of the legs, progressing to deeper, more specific fascial stretches to the deep tissues of the posterior leg where accessible. Maria felt extreme burning and pinching with a moderate myofascial stretch along the right medial calcaneal fascia. Deeper palpation along the tibia was extremely painful, which raised concerns of medial plantar and tibial nerve involvement, so I worked only superficially in those areas, gently stretching it, and will revisit the area as layers of fascia release. I applied muscle stripping and lengthening strokes to the gastrocnemius and soleus, treating a trigger point in the right soleus. In the initial seconds of compression, Maria stated that the pain intensity had increased from level 6 to 8 and the pressure felt deeper, although I had not increased the pressure I was applying. Over the course of approximately 30 seconds, the pain reduced from level 8 to 4. I applied broad lengthening strokes to the plantar fascia of the right foot, taking care not to reproduce pain in the heel, followed by a deep stretch and post-isometric relaxation to the plantar flexors.

Maria reported feeling looser and freer in movement, although she still feels moderate pain in the heel.

Plan

I demonstrated deep stretches to the hip flexors. If these do not begin to reduce the resting length of the hip flexors, I will treat iliopsoas in subsequent visits. I also demonstrated deep stretches to the plantar flexors and superficial kneading of the iliotibial band. I suggested treatments twice per week with a focus on releasing thoracolumbar fascia, hip flexors, and plantar flexors. I will reassess for trigger points in the quadratus lumborum, lumbar erector spinae, hip flexors, and deep plantar flexors as superficial tissues release.

CRITICAL THINKING EXERCISES

1. Become more familiar with the texture of muscle compared to fascia by slowly and gently palpating a few of the large muscles (gastrocnemius, biceps brachii, and rectus femoris) in your partner, with the goal of finding their musculotendinous junctions. Look at photos while you palpate if it helps you locate the junction. When you find it, move an inch toward the muscle belly, then an inch toward the tendon, and identify the differences in tone and texture. Try this on both healthy tissues and those you think may be contributing to your partner's postural deviations or pain. The more sensitive your fingers become to these differences, the more success you will have with identifying fascial restrictions.

2. Begin by finding an area of superficial myofascial restriction on a partner. Place your two index fingers over the restricted area with the fingers as close together as possible. Slowly pull them in opposite directions without gliding on the skin. Watch and feel as the space between your fingers increases and the tissue releases.

3. The area surrounding the superior angle of the scapula is often dense, painful, and adhered. Muscles with a wide variety of fiber directions emanate from that general area. How should you proceed in releasing the layers of tissue? Describe the order of tissues that you will treat, the techniques you will use, and the direction of force that you will apply to reduce restrictions and adhesions.

4. Conduct a short literature review to learn about the relationship between myofascial dysfunction and one or more of the following:
   - Neurotransmitter imbalance
   - Chronic infections
   - Thyroid dysfunction
   - Diabetes
   - Stress

BIBLIOGRAPHY AND SUGGESTED READINGS

Arroyo-Morales M, Olea N, Martinez M, et al. Effects of myofascial release after high-intensity exercise: A randomized clinical trial. Journal of Manipulative and Physiological Therapeutics. 2008;31:217–223.

Biel A. *Trail Guide to the Body: How to Locate Muscles, Bones and More,* 3rd ed. Boulder, CO: Books of Discovery, 2005.

Chaudhry H, Huang C-Y, Schleip R, et al. Viscoelastic behavior of human fasciae under extension in manual therapy. Journal of Bodywork and Movement Therapies. 2007;11:159-167.

Fascia Research Congress. About Fascia. Available at http://www.fasciacongress.org/about.htm. Accessed Fall 2009.

Hertling D, Kessler RM. *Management of Common Musculoskeletal Disorders: Physical Therapy Principles and Methods*, 4th ed. Philadelphia, PA: Lippincott Williams & Wilkins, 2006.

Ishman A. Ishman Bodycare Center and Institute. Fascial Link Therapy. Available at http://www.ibodycare. com/FascialLinkTherapyTMCourseDescriptions08_06.pdf. Accessed Summer 2010.

Kassolik K, Jaskolska A, Kisiel-Sajewicz K, et al. Tensegrity principle in massage demonstrated by electro- and mechanomyography. Journal of Bodywork and Movement Therapies. 2009;13(2):164–170.

Kirilova M, Stoytchev S, Pashkouleva D, et al. Visco-elastic mechanical properties of human abdominal fascia. Journal of Bodywork and Movement Therapies. 2009;13(4):336–337.

Langevin HM. Connective tissue: A body-wide signaling network? Med Hypotheses. 2006;66(6):1074–1077.

LeBauer A, Brtalik R, Stowe K. The effect of myofascial release (MFR) on an adult with idiopathic scoliosis. Journal of Bodywork and Movement Therapies. 2008;12(4):356–363.

Liptan GL. Fascia: A missing link in our understanding of the pathology of fibromyalgia. Journal of Bodywork and Movement Therapies. 2010;14:3–12.

Manheim C. *The Myofascial Release Manual*, 3rd ed. Thorofare, NJ: Slack Inc., 2001.

Mayo Foundation for Medical Education and Research. Fibromyalgia. Available at http://www.mayoclinic. com/health/fibromyalgia/DS00079. Accessed Fall 2009.

Myers TW. *Anatomy Trains: Myofascial Meridians for Manual and Movement Therapists*, 2nd ed. London, UK: Churchill Livingstone, 2008.

Rattray F, Ludwig L. *Clinical Massage Therapy: Understanding, Assessing and Treating over 70 Conditions*. Toronto, ON: Talus Incorporated, 2000.

Scheumann DW. *The Balanced Body: A Guide to Deep Tissue and Neuromuscular Therapy*, 3rd ed. Philadelphia, PA: Lippincott Williams and Wilkins, 2007.

Schleip R. Fascial plasticity –a new neurobiological explanation: Part 1. Journal of Bodywork and Movement Therapies. 2003;7(1):11–19.

Schleip R. Fascial plasticity—a new neurobiological explanation: Part 2. Journal of Bodywork and Movement Therapies. 2003;7(2):104–116.

Schleip R, Klingler W, Lehmann-Horn F. Fascia is able to contract in a smooth muscle-like manner and thereby influence musculoskeletal mechanics. Proceedings of the 5th World Congress of Biomechanics, Munich, Germany 2006, 51–54.

Simons DG, Travell JG, Simons LS. *Travell & Simons Myofascial Pain and Dysfunction: The Trigger Point Manual*, 2nd ed. Baltimore, MD: Lippincott Williams and Wilkins, 1999.

Stanborough M. *Direct Release Myofascial Technique: An Illustrated Guide for Practitioners*. London, UK: Churchill Livingstone, 2004.

Walton A. Efficacy of myofascial release techniques in the treatment of primary Raynaud's phenomenon. Journal of Bodywork and Movement Therapies. 2008;12(3):274–280.

Werner R. *A Massage Therapist's Guide to Pathology*, 4th ed. Philadelphia, PA: Lippincott Williams and Wilkins, 2008.

Myofascial Trigger Points

UNDERSTANDING MYOFASCIAL TRIGGER POINTS

There has been much recent research into myofascial trigger points. While this research continues to investigate theories about them, to date, there is no single agreed-upon explanation for the pathophysiology of trigger points and no universally accepted diagnostic criteria. *Myofascial Pain and Dysfunction: The Trigger Point Manual* by Simons and Travell (1999) is a seminal resource for the study of trigger points and is a primary source of information in this book. This chapter presents an overview of myofascial trigger points, their contribution to chronic pain, and the role massage therapy can play in relieving the symptoms they cause. Many continuing education offerings focus on the finer details of trigger point therapy for those interested in advanced training.

Trigger points may be found in epithelial tissue, connective tissue, nerves and muscles. Trigger points in muscles and fascia are called myofascial trigger points, and these will be the focus of this chapter. The term *trigger point* is used throughout this text to refer to myofascial trigger points.

A myofascial trigger point is a spot in a skeletal muscle that shows evidence of an excessive, prolonged response to stimuli. The spot is palpated as a nodule within a taut band of muscle fibers (Fig. 3-1). Trigger points refer pain to a location distant from the nodule in predictable patterns. When chronic pain is not relieved by manual manipulation of the symptomatic area, it is possible that the pain is referred from a trigger point in another area. For example, a trigger point in the upper trapezius often causes headache pain (Fig. 3-2). Several of these referral patterns are shown in Chapters 4 to 11. Trigger points can also cause other referred reactions including spasm; dilation or contraction of blood vessels; or secretion of fluids, such as tears or saliva, and can cause the referred inhibition of another muscle.

Trigger points are frequently found at the neuromuscular junction. The neuromuscular junction is the site of synaptic contact between the motor neuron and muscle fibers, where an action potential spreads from nerve to muscle to initiate a contraction (Fig. 3-3). In most human muscles, the neuromuscular junction occurs in the middle of the muscle fiber. At the neuromuscular junction, a synapse depends on the presence of the neurotransmitter acetylcholine (ACh), which is released locally to activate only those fibers recruited to produce a contraction. In a normal muscle contraction, the production, use, and breakdown of ACh happens quickly, limiting the duration of the contraction as well as the energy required for this process. The contracted muscle fibers are quickly released and are ready to respond to another action potential.

Circumstances including injuries, overuse, misuse, or systemic conditions can cause dysfunction at the neuromuscular junction, which results in a sustained contraction of the affected muscle fibers, creating the contraction knot we call a trigger point. The sustained contraction ini-

Taut band

Trigger point

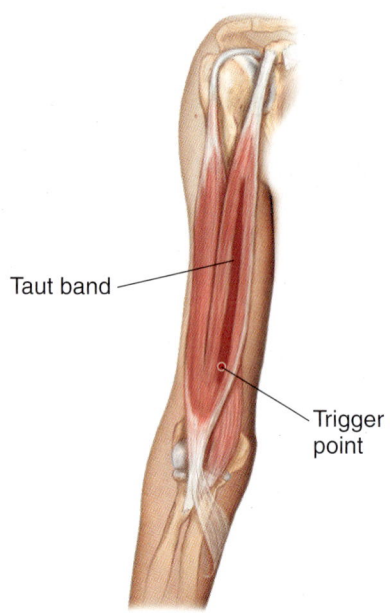

Figure 3-1 **Myofascial trigger point.** A myofascial trigger point is a hyperirritable spot in a skeletal muscle palpated as a nodule within a taut band of muscle fibers.

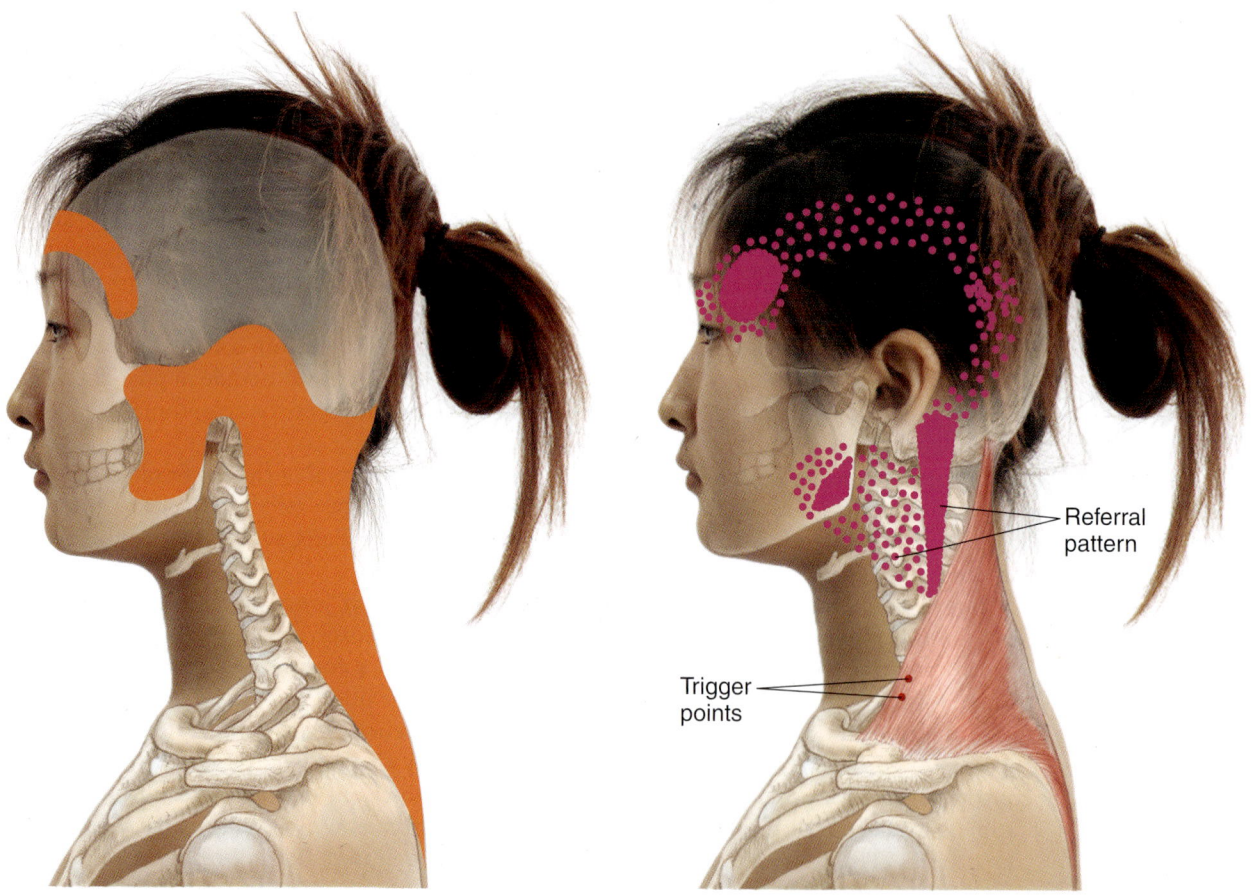

Common areas of tension headache pain

Common referral pattern for upper trapezius trigger points

Referral pattern

Trigger points

Figure 3-2 **Referred pain.** Trigger points refer pain into areas distant from the nodule.

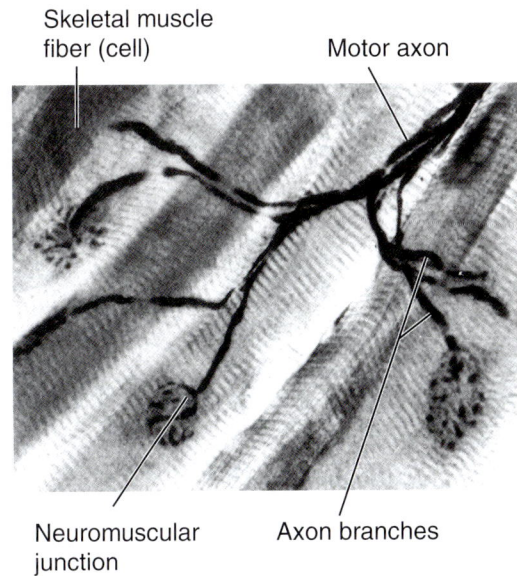

Figure 3-3   **Neuromuscular junction.** Nerves meet the muscle at the motor endplate to form a neuromuscular junction. From Cormack DH. *Essential Histology,* 2nd ed. Philadelphia, PA: Lippincott Williams & Wilkins, 2001.

tiates a cycle that perpetuates the contraction through a number of actions that may occur in variable order:

- Metabolic demand is increased because the sustained contraction requires energy.
- The contraction knot reduces circulation and the supply of oxygen and nutrients needed to meet the metabolic demand while promoting the accumulation of metabolic waste products that disturb local nociceptors and cause pain.
- Reduced circulation and increased metabolic demand depletes adenosine triphosphate (ATP) locally, which prevents the inhibition of ACh release and impairs the function of the pump that returns calcium to the sarcoplasmic reticulum.
- The continual imbalance of calcium, ACh, and ATP sustains the contraction.

The sustained contraction shortens muscle fibers and reduces their action potential, both of which affect the function of the muscle as a whole.

Studies suggest that a trigger point is actually a mass containing many dysfunctional motor endplates. Biopsies from cadavers have revealed that the diameter of the shortened muscle fibers containing trigger points is considerably greater than the diameter of healthy muscle fibers. This makes the knot feel bigger and denser than the healthy tissue around it. A taut band may occur because the contraction pulls fibers toward the knot, leaving them taut on either side of the knot (Fig. 3-4). The degree of dysfunction and irritability in the trigger point influences the intensity of pain more than the size of the muscle does. Active trigger points in small, minor muscles are just as likely to cause severe pain as trigger points in big, major muscles.

Trigger points are categorized as active, latent, or satellite. An *active trigger point* causes symptoms with normal activities of daily living and at rest. The referred sensation elicited by compressing an active trigger point will likely replicate the client's pain during daily life (i.e., the client will be familiar with this sensation). A *latent trigger point* is painful only on compression. While it is also found within a taut band of muscle and produces referred sensation that is characteristic for that trigger point, a latent trigger point does not cause pain during activities of daily living or rest, and the referral elicited by compression may not be familiar to the client. A latent trigger point can become active with overuse or other irritating factors. A *satellite trigger point* is one that develops within the referral area of an active trigger point, in an overloaded synergist, or in the antagonist of the muscle containing a trigger point. Satellite trigger points are often deactivated when the primary trigger point that induced it is deactivated.

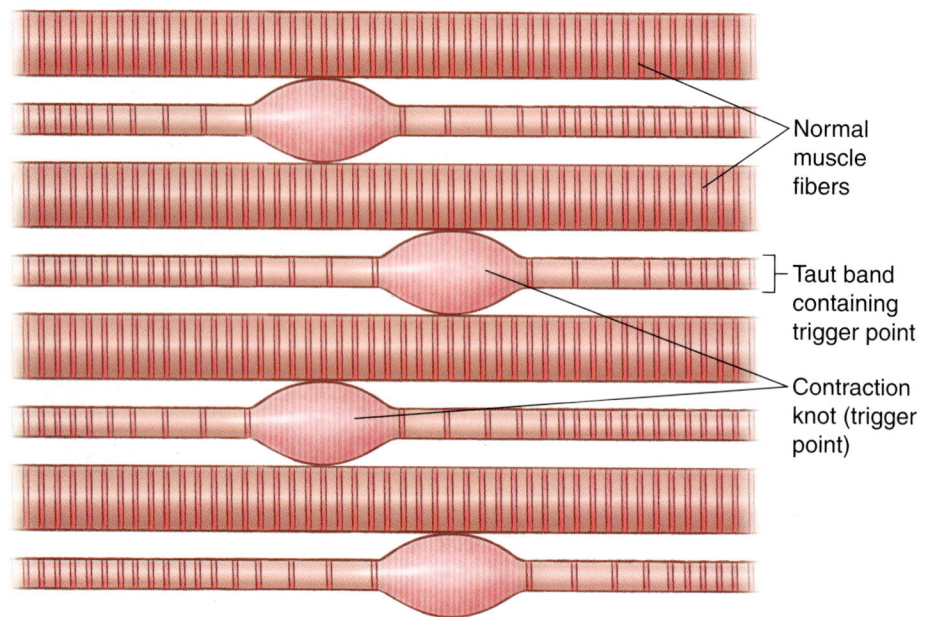

Figure 3-4   Taut band of muscle. Note how the contraction knot increases tension on either side of the knot, pulling the affected fibers taut and making them thinner.

Common Signs and Symptoms

Clients with trigger points often initially report pain in a general area. For example, a trigger point in the scalenes may refer pain around the medial aspect of the scapula, which the client will often call neck or shoulder pain. Trigger points rarely produce sharp or easily localized pain unless the point is directly compressed. Symptoms such as numbness, tingling, or prickling are sometimes reported. Compression of a trigger point causes predictable, referred pain or tenderness in an area either surrounding or distant from the trigger point. Active trigger points produce pain with activity, while at rest, and when compressed. The pain may be felt at the site of the trigger point or in its referral zone. Reducing the factors that contribute to an active trigger point can cause it to become latent, but it can become active again when improper use of the affected muscle or involvement of another factor aggravates it. Referred pain can become chronic unless the active trigger point is deactivated. Chronic, painful trigger points can disturb sleep. Lack of sleep can consequently increase sensitivity to pain, exacerbating symptoms. A break in this cycle is necessary to relieve the chronic condition.

It may be difficult for the client to relax a muscle containing a trigger point. Muscle tension, hypertonicity, and spasm may develop in muscles containing active or latent trigger points. This may cause the client to perform actions clumsily. Affected muscles may be short and tense, may fatigue quickly, and may not lengthen fully without pain. Pain may be worse with passive lengthening than with an active contraction because the client will limit active motions to avoid pain. Limiting the function of the prime mover containing a trigger point can lead to overloading of its synergists and antagonists, which may in turn cause trigger points to develop in those muscles. Reflex inhibition caused by trigger points may lead to weakness in muscles that show no sign of atrophy. Clients may be less aware of the dysfunction caused by trigger points than they are of pain.

Referred autonomic phenomena including dilation or constriction of blood vessels, changes in local temperature, sweating, goose bumps, and production of tears or saliva may be caused by trigger points. Proprioceptive irregularities including dizziness, ringing in the ears, and problems maintaining balance may also result from trigger points in some muscles. Strumming a taut band at the site of a trigger point may shorten the affected fibers, eliciting a local twitch response (Fig. 3-5). This twitch response, which feels like a quick flutter of the muscle fibers, is often used as a diagnostic criterion for assessing trigger points.

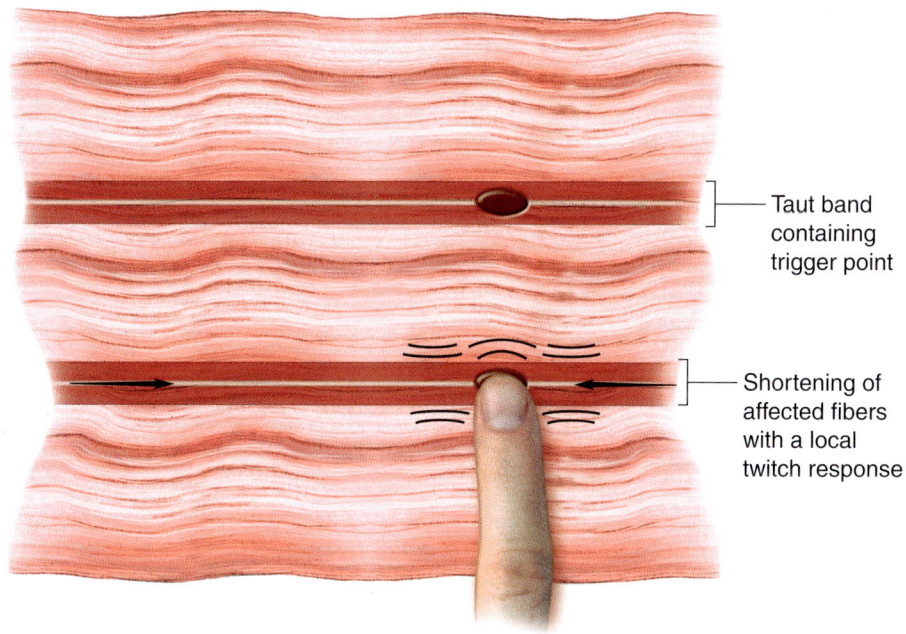

Figure 3-5 **Local twitch response.** Strumming a taut band at the site of a trigger point may shorten the affected fibers, eliciting a local twitch response. Adapted from Simons et al. (1999).

Possible Causes and Contributing Factors

Mechanical overload of a muscle, whether by acute incident or repetitive misuse, is a primary contributing factor to the development of trigger points. Active trigger points in muscles that are held in a shortened position will cause pain in the area of the trigger point or its referral zone. Latent trigger points in muscles that are regularly held in a shortened position may become active. Muscle contraction, particularly from the shortened position or against resistance, aggravates trigger points.

Muscles that are shortened due to postural imbalance are prone to developing trigger points. Postures that hold affected muscles in a shortened position, such as during sleep, sitting at a desk or in a car, or holding other inactive postures, may exacerbate pain. Actively lengthening a muscle containing a trigger point shortens its antagonist. Performing this stretch too quickly or forcefully can activate a trigger point in the antagonist. People who exercise their muscles daily are less likely to develop trigger points than those who are generally sedentary but occasionally participate in short bouts of intense activity.

Chilling a muscle, whether directly when using an ice pack or indirectly, such as when sitting near an air conditioning vent, may activate a trigger point. Compression of muscles by external forces, such as the strap of a bag or a utility belt, may contribute to the development or activation of trigger points. Nerve compression may encourage the development of trigger points in the muscles it innervates. Pathologies including organ insufficiency and inflammatory conditions such as arthritis can activate trigger points. Trauma, fatigue, and physical or emotional stress can also activate and perpetuate the symptoms of trigger points.

Conditions that affect metabolic, endocrine, or chemical homeostasis including thyroid conditions, diabetes, gout, and clinical depression can be perpetuating factors. Deficiency in vitamins or minerals including B, C, folic acid, magnesium, calcium, and iron can contribute to or delay the healing process of trigger points. Chronic bacterial or viral infections and some allergies may lead to chronic trigger points. Regular exposure to toxic chemicals, such as those in environmental pollution and pesticides, or heavy metals, such as mercury, may also play a role.

Most of the conditions described in this book will likely involve trigger points because the postures or traumas that contribute to these conditions can also contribute to the development of trigger points. Deactivating trigger points that contribute to these conditions is often necessary to fully resolve the signs and symptoms associated with them.

Because trigger points can occur in any muscle and are perpetuated by factors that include chronic infections and visceral disease, they can contribute to and be confused with many other conditions throughout the body. For example, pain in the pectoral area may result from a trigger point but can also be a symptom of cardiac disease, while trigger points in the abdominal muscles can mimic as well as contribute to digestive distress. Travell and Simons suggest that trigger points may contribute to a wide variety of chronic conditions to a much greater degree than is currently recognized by health care professionals. Table 3-1 lists some of the general conditions commonly confused with or contributing to trigger points. Because it may be difficult to distinguish pain referred by a trigger point from pain that results from a more serious condition, it is particularly important to understand the client's health history, precipitating events, and other possible causes for pain before initiating treatment. Consult your pathology book for more detailed information. If you are unsure and the client's signs and symptoms resemble those of a more serious condition, particularly if the client has other risk factors, refer him or her to a health care provider for a medical assessment.

Contraindications and Special Considerations

First, it is essential to understand the cause of the client's pain. Because trigger points refer pain and other autonomic symptoms that may also result from serious conditions, refer the client to his or her health care provider if symptoms are severe or significantly reduce activities of daily living. These are a few general cautions:

- **Infection.** Trigger point pain can be associated with or may mimic pain related to local or systemic infections. Massage is systemically contraindicated until the infection is resolved.
- **Acute injury.** Do not treat trigger points local to an acute injury such as a strain or sprain. Trigger point therapy may be too aggressive for recently injured tissues. Wait until the subacute or chronic stage, when the tissues become more stable.
- **Producing symptoms.** Compressing a trigger point will produce local or referred pain. Take care to keep the level of pain within the client's tolerance. Explain the process of treatment before beginning so that the client is aware and prepared to experience this pain during treatment. Knowing what to expect may keep the client from tensing up. Instructing the client to breathe through the technique may help reduce pain.
- **Kick-back pain.** Treating a taut band or trigger point too vigorously may cause the client to experience symptoms within hours or days following treatment. Work slowly, one layer at a time, to prepare the deeper tissues for treatment. Avoid treating one area too intensely, and avoid treating several trigger points in the same area in one session. Always follow frictions and compressions with a full, passive stretch within the client's tolerance. Heat may also help to release the trigger point and reduce the possibility of kick-back pain.
- **Hypermobile joints and overstretched muscles.** It is best not to fully stretch a muscle that crosses a hypermobile joint or one that is already overstretched. When treating a trigger point in these circumstances, use a localized pin and stretch or muscle stripping to lengthen only the affected fibers.
- **Treatment duration and pressure.** If the client is elderly, has a degenerative disease, or has been diagnosed with a condition that diminishes his or her activities of daily living, you may need to adjust your pressure as well as the treatment duration. Frequent half-hour sessions may suit the client better.
- **Friction.** Do not use deep frictions if the health of the underlying tissues is at risk for rupture. Allow time for scarring and tissue regeneration to avoid re-injury. Do not use deep frictions if the client is taking antiinflammatory medication or anticoagulants. Friction initiates an inflammatory process, which may interfere with the intended action of antiinflammatory medication. Recommend that the client refrain from taking such medication for several hours before treatment if his or her health care provider agrees. Because anticoagulants reduce clotting, avoid techniques such as friction that may cause tearing and bleeding.

Table 3-1	Differentiating Conditions Commonly Confused with or Contributing to Myofascial Trigger Points		
Condition	**Typical Signs and Symptoms**	**Testing**	**Massage Therapy**
Myofascial pain syndrome	Persistent muscle aches or pain Muscle or joint stiffness Muscle tension Trigger points Pain interrupts sleep	Physical exam Palpate for trigger points Referred pain or twitch response Other tests may be performed to rule out other sources of pain	Massage therapy is indicated.
Fibromyalgia	Constant, dull, widespread aching or pain Tender points Fatigue Sleep disturbances Signs and symptoms of possible coexisting conditions including chronic fatigue syndrome, depression, headaches, irritable bowel syndrome, and post-traumatic stress disorder	Physical exam Pain lasting at least 3 months 11 of 18 points positive for tenderness Blood tests to rule out other conditions	Massage is indicated. It is important to distinguish the tender points of fibromyalgia from trigger points that refer pain elsewhere. Fibromyalgia is often exacerbated by deep pressure and may require a soft touch.
Angina Pectoris	Chest pain Pain in arms, neck, jaw, shoulder, or back Nausea Fatigue Shortness of breath Anxiety Sweating	Physical exam Risk factors Blood test Electrocardiogram Stress test Chest x-ray Echocardiogram CT scan	Trigger points in pectoralis major may mimic some symptoms of angina pectoris. If the client presents with risk factors or the symptoms listed here, refer him or her to a health care provider prior to treatment. When risk factors are present, massage is indicated only if cleared by a primary health care provider and if the client is able to perform normal activities of daily living.
Migraine	Episodic or chronic Moderate or severe Often unilateral Pulsating or throbbing Aggravated by physical activity Aura, nausea, vomiting, sensitivity to light and sound	Diagnosed by signs and symptoms, familial history, and response to treatment MRI or CT to rule out other causes EEG to rule out seizures	Trigger points in SCM, temporalis, and the posterior cervical muscles may mimic the symptoms of migraines. Massage may not be appropriate during a migraine but may reduce intensity and frequency when performed regularly between headaches.
Tension headache	Dull, aching, vice-like pain Pain in neck and shoulders Scalp tenderness Loss of appetite Fatigue Insomnia Mood changes Trouble concentrating	Often self-assessed Physical exam Blood tests, CT, or MRI to rule out other conditions	Massage is indicated. See Ch. 5. Trigger points in the SCM, muscles of mastication, posterior cervical muscles, suboccipitals, and upper trapezius may contribute to tension headaches.

(continued)

Condition	Typical Signs and Symptoms	Testing	Massage Therapy
Dysmenorrhea (severe menstrual cramps)	Throbbing or cramping in low abdomen Pain radiating to back and thighs Nausea Dizziness	Assessed only when cramps are severe enough to disrupt activities of daily living, suggesting other contributing factors Ultrasound CT or MRI Laparoscopy	Trigger points in the lower rectus abdominis can mimic the pain of dysmenorrhea. It is best to wait until the menstrual cycle is over and swelling and tenderness in the abdomen have subsided before assessing and treating trigger points.
Earache and tinnitus	Ear pain Ringing in ears Hearing loss Fever Irritability	Physical exam of ear, mastoid, nose, and throat	Pain in or around the ear and mastoid may indicate infection. Massage is contraindicated until infection is resolved. Trigger points in the deep masseter can cause earache or tinnitus. Trigger points in the lateral pterygoid and SCM may also cause tinnitus.
Temporomandibular joint disorder (TMJD)	Pain in the jaw, face, ears, or neck Stiffness in jaw Difficulty chewing Reduced ROM Locking of jaw Clicking in jaw Uneven bite Headaches	Physical exam X-ray of teeth CT scan of bones MRI of joint's disc	Massage therapy is indicated for TMJD. Advanced training is necessary. Some states have restrictions against working intra-orally. Trigger points in the masseter or lateral pterygoid may cause TMJD pain.
Infant colic	Predictable bouts of crying Inconsolable crying Changes in posture including flexed hip, clenched fists, and tense abdominal muscles	Physical exam Diagnostic test to rule out other causes	Massage is indicated to relieve the symptoms of colic. Training in infant massage is advised. Trigger points in the abdominal muscles may contribute to the pain of colic.
Spasm/cramp (contracture)	Sudden, often sharp pain in affected voluntary muscle Palpable and often visible mass of hypertonic muscle tissue	Often self-assessed X-ray or MRI may be used to assess extent of damage	Massage is indicated. Discuss with health care provider if repeated spasm may be related to an underlying condition or side effects of medication.
Bursitis	Pain, especially with activity or palpation Heat, redness, swelling, or tenderness	Physical exam ROM tests X-ray or MRI if conservative treatment is not successful	Massage is systemically contraindicated if bursitis is due to infection and is locally contraindicated in the acute stage to avoid increased swelling. In the subacute stage, massage to structures surrounding the joint is indicated.
Diabetes	Frequent urination, frequent thirst, increased appetite, fatigue, nausea	Physical exam Fasting blood sugar test	Massage is indicated when tissues are not compromised, and circulation and nerve conduction are healthy.
Gout	Redness, heat, and swelling Sudden, intense pain—often at night—that diminishes gradually over a couple of weeks	Physical exam Blood and urine uric acid concentration tests Synovial fluid test	Massage is contraindicated during acute attacks. Gout may indicate other systemic conditions. Work with the health care team.

Massage Therapy Research

What follows is just a small sampling of the research describing the effects of massage therapy techniques commonly used for the treatment of trigger points. Trigger points have been studied in great detail by practitioners in fields ranging from massage therapy, physical therapy, and chiropractic care to anesthesia, cardiology, and neurology. Each of the condition chapters in this book also includes references to research in which trigger point therapy is central to the positive outcomes described.

For the studies described here, the pressure pain threshold (PPT) represents the least amount of pressure that causes the subject to perceive pain, which is measured using an external instrument called an algometer. The visual analog scale (VAS) represents the results of a questionnaire answered by each subject.

The study "Effectiveness of a Home Program of Ischemic Pressure Followed by Sustained Stretch for Treatment of Myofascial Trigger Points" (Hanten et al., 2000) tested the possibility that a home care program designed, demonstrated, and monitored by a trained practitioner could help alleviate the pain associated with trigger points. Forty subjects diagnosed with one or more trigger points in the neck or upper back were randomly divided into two groups. One group was instructed to apply gradually increasing pressure to their trigger point using a Thera Cane® until they felt release, followed by a 30–60 second stretch, at least twice a day for 5 days. The control group was assigned a 5-day home program of active ROM exercises to be performed 10 times each, at least twice a day, for 5 days. Both groups were instructed not to perform any treatment on days 6 and 7. PPT and VAS were reported before treatment and on the third day after treatment. Subjects also reported the duration of their pain over a 24-hour period. The subjects performing compressions reported greater improvement in PPT and VAS. Functionality was not studied in this trial. The authors concluded that a home program of compression and stretching, occasionally monitored by a trained clinician, reduces pain and the number of visits to a clinic, although it is not clear whether this provides any improvement in function.

In 2006, Fernández-de-las-Peñas et al. published "The Immediate Effect of Ischemic Compression Technique and Transverse Friction Massage on Tenderness of Active and Latent Myofascial Trigger Points: A Pilot Study." Forty subjects with neck pain for at least 2 consecutive weeks, who had received a diagnosis of either latent or active trigger points in the upper trapezius, were randomly divided into two groups. Subjects in Group A received a single treatment in which the therapist applied gradually increasing pressure to the trigger point in the lengthened upper trapezius fibers until the subject felt pressure and pain. This amount of pressure was maintained until the subject reported a 50% decrease in pain. The pressure was then increased until the subject felt pain again, and the process was repeated for 90 seconds. The subjects in Group B received 3 minutes of continuous transverse friction to the relaxed upper trapezius fibers, applied slowly, using pressure that approached the PPT. Both PPT and VAS were assessed before treatment and 2 minutes after treatment. In both groups, there was a significant improvement in the PPT and VAS. There was no remarkable difference in outcomes between the two groups, nor was there any remarkable difference in results after treatment for a latent trigger point versus an active trigger point. The authors noted that positive results are obtained when the therapist applies only enough pressure to feel an increase in tissue resistance, and that there may be no clear reason to use pressure that causes pain or ischemia. They suggested that while ischemic compression and friction reduce pain resulting from trigger points, further study is needed to determine whether the amount of pressure applied to a trigger point during treatment affects the results.

In 2009, Ibáñez-García et al. published a comparative study titled "Changes in Masseter Muscle Trigger Points Following Strain-Counterstrain or Neuro-muscular technique." Seventy-one subjects, aged 20 to 65 years, who had received a diagnosis of latent trigger points in the masseter muscle, were divided into three groups. Group A was treated with neuromuscular therapy. The therapist used the thumb to apply six to eight muscle stripping strokes to the masseter. Each stroke lasted 4–5 seconds. Group B was treated with strain-counterstrain. The therapist located the trigger point in the masseter muscle, then applied gradually increasing pressure until the subject felt pain. The subject's position was then changed until pain was reduced by approximately 75%, and the new position was held for 90 seconds. The subject was then passively moved into the neutral position. Group C, the control group, received neither treatment nor a sham procedure. Each participant lay supine in a neutral position for 5 minutes and was assessed after treatment. Each group participated in one session per week for 3 consecutive weeks. PPT, VAS, and ROM for active opening of the mouth were measured prior to and 1 week after treatment. Both the neuromuscular and strain-counterstrain groups showed significant improvement compared to the control group. Differences between the neuromuscular and strain-counterstrain groups were insignificant. The authors noted limitations in their study, which reported only the immediate effects of treatment. Studies analyzing long-term effects are needed. In addition, while the subjects had received a diagnosis of masseter trigger points, all were asymptomatic and their results may be different from subjects who are presenting with pain. However, latent trigger points are clinically relevant and can become active. Finally, because the control group received no treatment, the study cannot rule out a placebo effect in the other groups that showed improvement. The authors recommend a trial that includes a sham technique to validate the improvements shown with neuromuscular therapy and strain-counterstrain.

WORKING WITH THE CLIENT

Client Assessment

Assessment begins at your first contact with a client. In some cases, this may be on the telephone when an appointment is requested. Ask in advance if the client is seeking treatment for specific pain so that you can prepare yourself.

Table 3-2 lists questions that may aid your assessment.

POSTURAL ASSESSMENT

The client's description of the location of his or her pain will help you to determine which muscles may harbor the trigger point(s) that refer pain to that location. This will also help you to determine which muscles are short, weak, or otherwise inhibited. Allow the client to enter the room ahead of you while you assess his or her posture and movement. Clients may avoid postures or movements that lengthen or overload a muscle containing a trigger point. Look for imbalances in movement or patterns of compensation that may give additional clues about the location of trigger points. For example, a client with low back or leg pain may have a trigger point that shortens the piriformis, which may cause the client to stand with the hip laterally rotated. A client with shoulder pain may have a trigger point that shortens the scalenes on one side, which could cause the client to hold the head in slight lateral flexion to the same side and slight rotation to the opposite side to avoid lengthening the shortened scalenes. Look for reduced mobility or a favoring of one side. If the lower body is affected, watch as the client walks, climbs steps, sits, and stands from sitting. If the upper body is affected, watch as the client opens the door, takes off his or her coat, or picks up a pen. Notice if the client rotates the trunk to avoid rotating the head when turning to talk to you. Notice if he or she is able to perform these activities without assistance or if he or she avoids lengthening or loading certain muscles.

When assessing standing posture, be sure that the client stands comfortably. If he or she deliberately tries to stand in the anatomic position, you may not get an accurate assessment of his or her posture in daily life. When trigger points affect the lower body, the client may stand in a position that keeps resistance off the affected muscles. This, in turn, may initiate imbalances in posture from the feet up to the spine. Check for irregularities in the ankles, knees, hips, and low back. When the upper body is affected, the client may hold the joint in a position that keeps the injured muscle from stretching. This may initiate compensating patterns that protect the affected muscle. Look for imbalance in the shoulders and rotations in the arm, forearm, and cervical or thoracic

Table 3-2	Health History

Questions for the Client	Importance for the Treatment Plan
When did the symptoms begin?	Onset of symptoms may help you determine whether trigger points are the result of a recent injury or recent episode of misuse or if the condition is chronic or recurrent.
Did you receive an injury or surgery to this area?	An explanation of prior injury to the area may help you determine the contributing factors. Surgery and resulting scar tissue may increase the risk of developing trigger points.
Do you have a history of chronic infection, metabolic disorders, or other chronic health conditions?	Chronic health conditions may be a contributing factor in the client's pain or may be a predisposing factor in the development of trigger points.
Have you seen a health care provider for this condition? What was the diagnosis? What tests were performed?	Medical tests may reveal the condition contributing to trigger points. If no tests were performed to make a diagnosis, use the tests described in this text for your assessment. If your assessment is inconsistent with a diagnosis, ask the client to discuss your findings with his or her health care provider or ask for permission to contact the provider directly.
Where do you feel symptoms?	The pain reported by a client may either indicate the site of the trigger point or its referral zone or may result from restricted ROM because a muscle crossing the joint contains a trigger point.
Describe what your symptoms feel like.	Active trigger points usually cause steady, aching pain that is somewhat diffuse. Trigger points rarely produce sharp, pinpointed pain. Remember that clients are not likely to realize that a spot in one part of the body can refer symptoms to another part of the body, so it is important for you to make that connection.
Describe your posture during sleep, work, or other activities of daily living.	Holding a muscle in a shortened position may contribute to trigger points.
Do any movements make your symptoms worse or better?	This may help you locate weakness in structures producing such movements. Resisted activity or activities that lengthen the muscle containing a trigger point are likely to increase symptoms. Adding slack or reducing tension in the muscle may decrease symptoms.
Are you taking any prescribed or over-the-counter medications or any herbal or other supplements?	Medications of all types may contribute to symptoms or have contraindications or cautions.
Have you had a corticosteroid or analgesic injection in the past 2 weeks? Where?	Local massage is contraindicated. A history of repeated corticosteroid injections may affect the integrity of muscle and tendons, increasing the risk of injury. Use caution when applying pressure or cross-fiber strokes. Analgesics reduce sensation and may cause the client to allow you to work too aggressively.
Have you taken a pain reliever or muscle relaxant within the past 4 hours?	The client may not be able to judge your pressure and may allow you to work too aggressively.
Have you taken anti-inflammatory medication such as NSAIDs (e.g., aspirin or ibuprofen) within the past 4 hours?	Deep friction causes inflammation and should not be performed if the client has recently taken an anti-inflammatory medication. Regular use of anti-inflammatories may also contribute to collagen degeneration.

spine. You may not be able to attend to all of the compensating patterns in the early treatments, but may be able to return to them once the primary trigger point(s) are deactivated.

ROM ASSESSMENT

ROM assessment may reveal limitations that the client was unaware of. Clients with trigger points are often more conscious of pain than they are of limitations. Because the pain of trigger points is often referred, ROM assessment, particularly against resistance or in a full passive stretch, will help you pinpoint the muscle containing a trigger point that is referring pain. Since it allows the client to control the amount of movement and stay within a pain-free range, only active ROM should be used during the acute stage of injury to prevent undue pain or re-injury.

Active ROM

Compare your assessment of the client's active ROM in the affected joints to the values listed in the Average ROM boxes in Chapters 4 to 11.

- **Active ROM of the affected joint** may be limited but may not cause pain if the movement is slow and steady, whereas a quick or forceful active contraction of a muscle containing a trigger point will be limited and likely painful. The client may limit movement to the pain-free range.

Passive ROM

Compare the client's P ROM on one side to the other when applicable. Note and compare the end feel for each range (see Chapter 1 for an explanation of end feel).

- **P ROM of the affected joint** may produce no symptoms or restriction when that movement shortens the muscle, but is often restricted and produces pain on a full passive stretch. The location of pain during a full passive stretch of the affected joint may reveal the referral pattern for that trigger point and help to determine the location of the trigger point.

Resisted ROM

Use resisted tests to assess the strength of the affected muscle. Compare the strength of the affected side to the unaffected side when possible.

- **R ROM of the affected joint** may reveal weakness in the affected muscle and will likely produce pain local to the trigger point or in its referral zone. Pain is most likely when the resisted contraction is initiated with the muscle in a shortened position.

SPECIAL TESTS

Numerous orthopedic tests are specific for trigger points in individual muscles. These specific, named tests largely comprise combinations of compression, passive lengthening, and resisted contractions of the affected muscles. It is important to learn these tests in advanced training that is focused on clinically oriented treatments or research. For now, length and strength assessment, a full passive stretch of the affected muscle, and palpation are sufficient tools for assessing trigger points. Use ROM testing as described above, and refer to Chapters 4 to 11 for special tests of the muscles affected by those conditions.

PALPATION ASSESSMENT

Place the muscle in a fully relaxed and comfortably lengthened position when palpating for trigger points. If a muscle can be grasped between the fingers, a pincer grip may be a good option for palpating trigger points (Fig. 3-6). For muscles that cannot be gripped, compress the area between your finger and the muscle or bone deep to the affected muscle. When palpating for trigger points, it is essential to work slowly, with full concentration. They can easily be missed when working broadly or quickly. Locate the taut band first. A taut band feels something like a guitar string, pulled tight, that rolls under your finger when you strum across it using pressure. Palpation along the length of the taut band may reveal a nodule—the trigger point. Compression of this nodule causes more local or referred pain than pressure to any other part of the taut band. This spot can be very small—even the size of a pinhead—so it is important to palpate slowly and to stay focused. If the nodule is mobile and does not seem to be embedded in a muscle or fascia, it may be a lipoma. Lipomas are fatty nodules that should not be directly compressed or treated with friction.

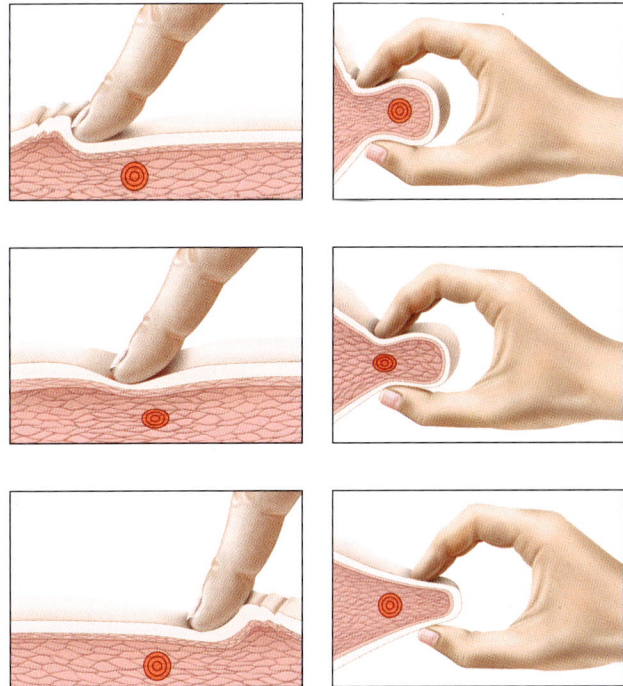

Figure 3-6   Palpating trigger points.
Begin your flat finger (left images) or pincer grip (right images) palpation on one side of the suspected trigger point, moving slowly and deliberately over it to the other side of the trigger point. The client will likely feel a higher level of pain when you make direct contact with the trigger point than when palpating the fibers that surround it. Adapted from Simons et al.

Applying direct pressure to the trigger point often elicits pain or other referred sensations. This sensation may occur immediately upon pressure or 10 or more seconds later. If the trigger point is active, this sensation will be familiar to the client, resembling the pain he or she experiences during activities of daily living. Strumming the taut band or applying pressure to the precise trigger point may cause a local twitch response, which feels like a brief flutter of the muscle and is likely due to a spinal reflex. The local twitch response supports an assessment of the presence of a trigger point. The local twitch response may be momentarily painful for the client. It may also reduce tension in the muscle. The tissue surrounding the trigger point may be dense and adhered and have the rough, granular texture of panniculosis.

It is essential to adequately warm the tissues and reduce adhesions and hypertonicity in order to palpate a small or deep trigger point. The area around the affected trigger point may be cool due to ischemia. Repeated rubbing or scratching of the area containing trigger points may cause the skin to become red and itchy, possibly due to overly sensitive mast cells releasing histamine, which causes the blood vessels to dilate upon minor trauma. It is unclear why this condition, called dermographia, occurs or if it is directly related to trigger points.

Some trigger points cause symptoms other than pain or weakness. For example, trigger points in the sternocleidomastoid (SCM) may cause dizziness, ringing in the ears, or the production of tears. Several books, including *Travell and Simons' Trigger Point Manual*, and much continuing education are dedicated to detailed explanations of these individual responses. In this book, each condition chapter contains an illustration of the relevant trigger points and their referral patterns.

Condition-Specific Massage

Trigger points often contribute to musculoskeletal injuries or chronic pain conditions. For example, plantar fasciitis may have origins in a trigger point that shortens the gastrocnemius. Trigger points should always be considered when assessing chronic pain conditions. When trigger points contribute to the symptoms of musculoskeletal conditions, the following recommendations are incorporated into treatment to aid healing and reduce the risk of further injury. Releasing the contraction knot of a trigger point, restoring proper circulation through the muscle, and restoring normal muscle length and neuromuscular function are the basic goals of treating trigger points.

Because trigger points can occur in any muscle, the descriptions of techniques here do not specify locations since they are described more fully in later chapters. Use the resources in the following chapters when needed to determine the muscle fibers' direction, joints that have been crossed, tissues that are superficial versus deep, and so on. In some cases, such as with myofascial pain syndrome, trigger points can cause systemic symptoms and significantly reduce the client's activities of daily living. In addition, trigger points may be complicated by other conditions such as infection, metabolic insufficiency, or complex nerve lesions. A complicated case involving trigger points should be supervised by a professional with advanced training or referred to a primary health care provider.

It is essential for the treatment to be as relaxing as possible. Strumming or compressing a trigger point may cause pain at the upper end of the client's tolerance. Explain this to your client, asking him or her to let you know when your pressure approaches the upper end of his or her tolerance. Ask the client to breathe deeply during the application of the technique to help relax the muscle and nervous system, which may allow you to use more pressure when necessary. As the trigger point is deactivated, the referral pain will also diminish. Because treatment to the affected muscle can be uncomfortable, it is best to alternate treatment directly to the trigger point with more general treatment, stretches, and joint mobilizations. In addition, treating aggressively or attempting to resolve several trigger points in one session may cause kick-back pain. You may not be able to fully resolve chronic symptoms related to trigger points in one session. Do not try to do so by treating aggressively. Remember that you are working on tissue that is compromised. Ask the client to let you know if any part of your treatment reproduces symptoms, and always work within his or her tolerance.

There are many methods for treating trigger points including vapocoolant spray, moist heat, stretching, and muscle energy techniques. The following suggestions for treating pain, weakness, and limited ROM caused by trigger points are easily incorporated into the treatments suggested for the specific conditions described in other chapters of this book. The following description is generalized for any affected muscle. Refer to Chapters 4 to 11 for images and treatment suggestions pertaining to specific muscles.

- The area of pain reported by the client will give you clues about the possible location of an active trigger point. Use the illustrations of trigger point referrals in the following chapters or a more detailed trigger point chart, such as Travell & Simons' Trigger Point Flip Charts, to match the client's complaint with the referral area of a trigger point.
- Positioning and bolstering depends on the area to be treated. The muscle containing a trigger point should be comfortably lengthened, but not stretched.
- If you find edema, apply superficial clearing strokes toward the nearest lymph nodes and, when possible, bolster the area to allow gravity to draw fluid toward the thorax.

- If swelling is minor or absent, apply brief moist heat to the affected area to soften adhesions and increase circulation. If inflammation is present, do not use heat.

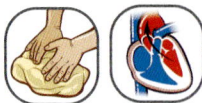

- Use your initial warming strokes to increase superficial circulation, soften tissues, and assess the tissues broadly surrounding the suspected trigger point and those that may be compensating. You should be able to initially assess tissues for adhesions, hypertonicity, protective muscle spasm, and tensile stress, all of which will help you to determine how to focus your treatment.

- Before applying emollient, assess and treat fascial restrictions around the affected muscle(s).

Treatment icons: Increase circulation; Reduce adhesions; Reduce tension; Lengthen tissue; Treat trigger points; Passive stretch; Clear area

- Soften the tissues peripheral to the trigger point, beginning proximally (closest to the trunk). Pay special attention to the affected muscle and its synergists. If the antagonists are accessible, treat these now, or return to this step when the client changes position. Circular kneading and cross-fiber strokes are effective for both softening tissues and reducing adhesions.

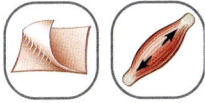

- Once the superficial tissues are pliable enough to allow for deeper work, apply friction strokes to reduce the remaining adhesions and apply lengthening strokes to peripheral tissues that are short and tight, beginning proximally. Muscles with fiber direction and actions in common with the injured muscle may have shortened to protect the injured muscle from further injury. If you find taut bands within these peripheral muscles, assess for additional trigger points.

The following steps describe treatment options for trigger points. In the following chapters, this treatment is represented by the icon to the left.

- Locate the taut band. It is easiest to find the taut band when the muscle is relaxed in a comfortably lengthened position. Shortening the muscle adds slack, which reduces tension, and makes the taut band more difficult to palpate. Feeling a twitch in the muscle as you palpate is a good indicator that you have found a taut band and possibly a trigger point.
- Begin with slow lengthening strokes along the taut band. Muscle stripping is sometimes sufficient to release a trigger point. If this happens, the taut band may also release and become slack.
- If muscle stripping is sufficient to resolve a trigger point, apply a full stretch to the muscle.
- If lengthening strokes do not release the taut band, slowly palpate along it to find the trigger point. This will be the most tender spot within the taut band. You may feel a nodule. Because a trigger point can be very small and obscured by adhesions and hypertonicity, this step requires slow and deliberate palpation. A good general rule is to take 6 seconds to palpate 1 inch of muscle.
- Once you have found the trigger point, compress it slowly. Your pressure may cause discomfort but should not cause pain. Remind the client to use the pain scale you described at the beginning of treatment to let you know when your pressure approaches a level of pain that keeps him or her from relaxing. Slow, deep breathing may make the treatment more comfortable and may improve the outcome of trigger point therapy.
- While compressing the trigger point, ask the client to let you know if the level of pain decreases. In addition, ask the client to describe any referred sensations.
- The compression can be held for as little as 10 seconds or as long as 1 minute. As you apply pressure, the fibers may begin to lengthen and become slack. Increase your pressure slightly to take up that slack so that you can maintain direct contact with the nodule. If you feel the resistance in the tissue decrease during compression, increase your pressure slightly until you feel the resistance again. If you feel the nodule move, do your best to follow it. This may require using one hand to stabilize the taut band while the other compresses the trigger point.
- While applying pressure to the trigger point, it may help to change the direction of your pressure slightly by making tiny movements around the nodule. This may give you more direct access to the contracted fibers.
- If you hold the compression for 10–20 seconds and the trigger point does not release, follow with lengthening strokes and Swedish techniques to the surrounding area. You can return to the trigger point, applying a few short rounds of compression followed by lengthening. The client's pain level may reduce with each application.
- If you apply compression for 20–60 seconds and the trigger point does not release, do not apply another round. Prolonged compression is an aggressive form of treatment that causes ischemia, and repeated applications may result in kick-back pain. You can return to this spot in a subsequent session.
- If you did not feel the trigger point or taut band release sufficiently, perform postisometric relaxation to the affected muscle. Assess muscle length and the taut band following postisometric relaxation.
- Follow any of the above methods with a slow, passive stretch of the affected muscle. Ask the client to remain as relaxed as possible. Hold the stretch for 15–30 seconds.
- Heat may be applied directly to a trigger point or taut band that did not fully relax. Heat increases circulation, softens adhesions, and may allow the muscle to lengthen more fully.

TREATMENT GOAL

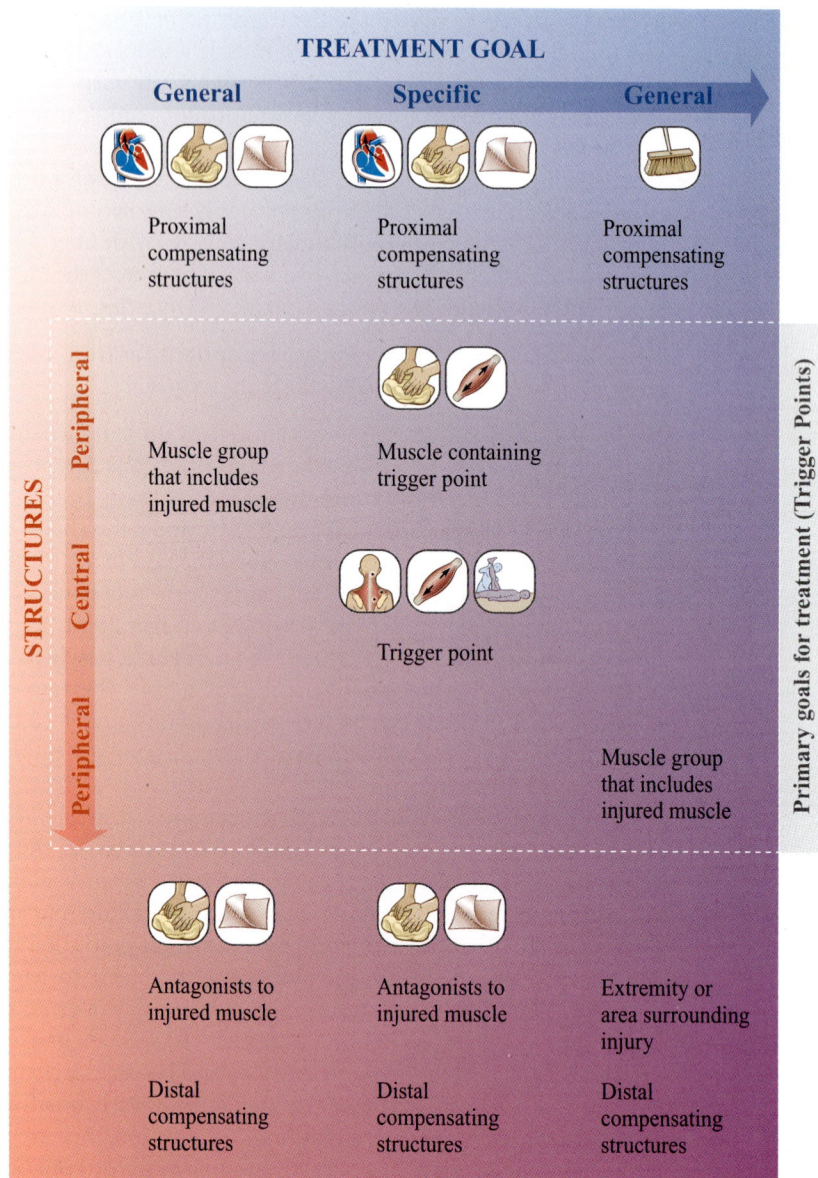

Figure 3-7   Trigger points treatment overview diagram. Follow the general principles from left to right, or top to bottom, when treating trigger points.

- If you were unable to address the antagonists of the injured muscle, reposition the client and address them now.

- Clear the areas treated.

The Treatment Overview diagram summarizes the flow of treatment (Fig. 3-7).

CLIENT SELF-CARE

Avoiding further injury is a primary concern when recommending self-care. Reducing or eliminating habitual offending activities and other perpetuating factors is crucial for long-term relief from trigger points. The client must learn to recognize when he or she is holding the affected muscle in a shortened position and which of his or her activities of daily living are putting undue stress on muscles that have developed trigger points. You can help clients learn how to modify such activities to avoid overstressing the muscle. In many cases, the most important modification is simply slowing down to avoid the reflex responses that shorten muscles. The following are intended as general recommendations for stretching and strengthening muscles involved in the client's condition. The objective is to create distance between the attachment sites of muscles that have shortened, and to perform repetitions of movements that decrease the distance between the attachments of muscles which have weakened. If you have had no training in remedial exercises and do not feel that you have a functional understanding of stretching and strengthening, refer the client to a professional with training in this area.

Clients often neglect self-care due to time constraints. Encourage them to follow these guidelines:

- Instruct the client to perform self-care throughout the day, such as while talking on the phone, reading e-mail, washing dishes, or watching television instead of setting aside extra time.
- Encourage the client to take regular breaks from stationary postures or repetitive actions. If the client's daily activities include hours of inactivity, suggest moving for at least a few minutes every hour to prevent adhesions and reduced circulation. If the client's daily activities require repetitive actions that contribute to trigger points, suggest resting for at least a few minutes every hour or reducing the offending activity as much as possible.
- Demonstrate gentle self-massage of the muscles containing trigger points to keep adhesions and hypertonicity at bay between treatments. Applying moist heat may also help alleviate symptoms of trigger points. Instruct the client to follow self-massage and moist heat with a full passive stretch.
- Demonstrate all strengthening exercises and stretches to your client and have him or her perform these in your presence before leaving to ensure that he or she is performing them correctly and will not harm himself or herself when practicing alone. Stretches should be held for 15–30 seconds and performed frequently throughout the day within the client's limits. The client should not force the stretch or bounce. A stretch should be slow, gentle, and steady, keeping every other joint as relaxed as possible.
- Recommend stretching and strengthening exercises according to your findings in ROM testing and palpation.

Stretching

Maintaining proper length and tone of the affected muscle, its synergists, and its antagonists is essential to resolving trigger points and reducing the risk of further injury. For the contraction knot of a trigger point to be released, the affected fibers must be fully lengthened. Each stretch should be relaxed while reaching the full range possible within the client's tolerance. Stretches should be performed throughout the day, particularly before and after intense activity. Take care to instruct the client to begin slowly, gradually increasing the stretch as symptoms diminish and ROM improves. Stretching an injured muscle too quickly or too deeply may initiate a reflex response, which may result in spasm. In addition, when the affected muscle is lengthened, its antagonists are shortened. If the antagonists are involved in protective splinting, contracting them too quickly or too deeply may also result in spasm.

The results of ROM testing and palpation will determine which muscles have shortened and need to be stretched. In general, stretching occurs when the distance between the attachment sites of the muscle is increased. Refer to Chapters 4 to 11 to find stretches for specific muscles or groups of muscles.

Strengthening

A muscle with trigger points may not function efficiently, which may affect the ROM of the joint it crosses. While it is important to lengthen the affected fibers to eliminate a trigger point and keep it from returning, the client may also need to restore strength to a muscle affected by trigger points. In addition, strengthening the antagonists of muscles harboring trigger points may help keep the affected muscle from reflexive shortening. Strengthening weakened muscles is equally important for restoring proper function to the affected joint. The results of ROM testing and palpation will determine which muscles have weakened and need to be strengthened. In general, active or resisted contractions strengthen muscles. As with stretching, a strengthening program should progress gradually. Pain-free, active ROM is effective for gradually restoring strength to weakened muscles. These exercises should be introduced slowly and increased in intensity only within the client's tolerance. As healing progresses and the risk of re-injury diminishes, add resistance to active ROM. Refer to Chapters 4 to 11 for exercises to strengthen specific muscles or muscle groups.

SUGGESTIONS FOR FURTHER TREATMENT

Treatment duration and frequency can vary widely when trigger points are a contributing factor in the client's condition. New trigger points resulting from a recent injury or newly developed pattern of activity or inactivity may be resolved in a single treatment. An acute trigger point that has been unrecognized or ignored may have become chronic. Chronic trigger points may lead to other factors, such as adhesions, hypertonicity, or weakness, that require more attention. When treating specific conditions such as those described in other chapters, it may be necessary to include assessment and treatment of trigger points in each session. As the client learns new postures and methods for performing pain-free activities, other muscles may respond to these changes. A trigger point treated in the last session may have resolved, while another one may become active.

There should be some improvement with each session. If this is not happening, consider the following possibilities:

- There is too much time between treatments. It is always best to give the newly treated tissues 24–48 hours to adapt, but if too much time passes between treatments in the beginning, the client's activities of daily living may reverse any progress.
- The client is not adjusting his or her activities of daily living or is not keeping up with self-care. As much as we want to fix the problem, we cannot force a client to make the adjustments we suggest. Explain the importance of his or her participation in the healing process and encourage the client to follow your recommendations, but be careful not to judge or reprimand a client who does not.
- The condition is advanced or involves other musculoskeletal complications that are beyond your basic training. Refer this client to a massage therapist with advanced training. Continuing to treat a client whose case is beyond your training could hinder his or her healing and turn the client away from massage therapy altogether.
- The client has an undiagnosed, underlying condition. Discontinue treatment until the client sees a health care provider for medical assessment.

If you are not treating the client in a clinical setting or private practice, you may not be the therapist who takes this client through the full program of healing. Still, if you can bring some relief in just one treatment, it may encourage the client to discuss this change with his or her primary health care provider and seek manual therapy rather than more aggressive treatment options. If the client agrees to return for regular treatments, the symptoms are likely to change each time, so it is important to perform an assessment before each session.

PROFESSIONAL GROWTH

CASE STUDY

Todd is a 58-year-old bank executive. He has pain in his left shoulder that was intermittent until about 6 weeks ago, when it became constant. Todd spends many hours working at a computer and talking on the telephone. He stays fit by rock climbing and playing basketball and other sports on the weekends and some evenings. Todd stated that he has been athletic since childhood and has been well trained to warm and stretch his muscles before and after strenuous activity.

Subjective

Todd reported feeling pain in his left shoulder that used to come and go but has become fairly constant over the past 6 weeks. He has also noticed that from time to time he feels pain radiating down his arm and into his thumb. When asked if he had any injuries, he replied "No" but quickly added that he had been in a side-impact car accident approximately 3 years ago. He had been taken to the hospital following the accident, but no injuries were found. Twenty-four hours later, he had told his health care provider that he felt a little stiffness in his neck, although it was not debilitating. His provider prescribed a neck brace, which Todd wore for approximately 3 days until the aching stopped. He has had no manual or physical therapy since the accident. Todd stated, with frustration, that he has been taking ibuprofen nearly every day for the past month, and while this helps him get through the workday, he is concerned that it will cause stomach problems. When asked, Todd stated that his shoulder does not hurt when he is playing basketball, but he has stopped climbing because the symptoms are intense when he bends his head back to look up. He feels the worst pain when he straightens his neck after holding the phone between his left ear and shoulder. He also feels pain when riding his bike. When asked, he described that he leans forward to reach his handlebars with his neck bent back to look forward while riding his bike. When asked, he stated that he feels no numbness, tingling, or weakness in his arm or hand.

Objective

Todd appears healthy and vibrant. He had no difficulty turning the doorknob or taking off his coat. I noticed that after filling out his form, he lifted his head very slowly and had a brief, pained expression on his face. I asked if he felt pain at that moment, and he said he did not notice anything.

Postural assessment revealed left lateral flexion of the neck and right rotation of the neck. The left shoulder is elevated. Trunk is slightly flexed toward the left. Rotating the neck to the left produced pain in the shoulder after 3 seconds. Todd stated that he felt like it was about to hurt in his arm too. Extension of the neck produced pain along the levator scapula after 5 seconds. Vertebral artery test was negative for circulation deficiency. Adson's test was negative for compression of neurovascular bundle.

Tissues of the neck, particularly the left anterior neck, are dense and adhered. Crepitus was both felt and heard with superficial cross-fiber strokes. Gentle pincer grip to the left SCM was instantly tender. No referred pain. Trigger points were found in the anterior scalene, approximately 1 inch superior to the clavicle. Pressure on the trigger point produced pain in the shoulder instantly, and into the arm within 5 seconds. Palpation of the area around the scapula and down the arm caused no pain; Todd stated that it felt good. Levator scapula and upper trapezius are hypertonic and tender. No trigger points were found here, although this may be because the tissues are dense and adhered. I will reassess in a follow-up treatment.

It is possible that the side-impact car accident resulted in whiplash that was not properly treated.

Action

We began in the supine position. I performed myofascial release from the skull toward the ribs anteriorly, toward the acromion process laterally, and toward the scapula posteriorly. I applied more specific superficial techniques to release fascia surrounding the left SCM and scalenes. The tissue is dense and adhered and may contain minor scar tissue. Crepitus was evident during cross-fiber strokes across scalenes. I applied emollient and general Swedish techniques to the neck and shoulders to warm and lengthen the superficial muscles. I applied pincer grip kneading to the full length of the SCM. This produced pain at level 5 initially. Pain reduced to 1 after three repetitions. With the SCM softened, I accessed the scalenes. I began with three rounds of slow muscle stripping to the full length of the anterior scalene. The client reported pain at a level 5 along the muscle, increasing to level 7 as the stroke approached a nodule in the muscle. No twitch response was felt. After the third round of muscle stripping, the pain remained at level 6 at the most tender spot. I applied direct pressure to the nodule for 10 seconds. The client reported familiar pain referred into the shoulder at level 4 and less so into the arm. I increased the length of the scalenes slightly by laterally flexing the neck toward the right before each round of compressions. By the third round, local pain in the anterior scalene reduced to 4 and referred pain was described as "a shadow of the pain I felt in the beginning." I felt what may have been a twitch response, although it was minor and could have been a movement of the muscle related to breathing. I continued muscle stripping to the middle and posterior scalene. I found nothing other than hypertonicity in the middle scalene. The posterior scalene was locally painful at level 4 but produced no referred pain. I applied a full passive stretch to the left scalenes by laterally flexing the neck toward the right with a slight rotation toward the left for 20 seconds.

I performed general deep tissue techniques to neck extensors and pectorals. I then turned the client prone and continued general deep tissue techniques to the upper back. I found taut bands between the scapula and spine. Due to hypertonicity and adhesions, it is unclear whether these are the rhomboid or serratus posterior superior. Deep forced breathing did not help to distinguish between the rhomboid and serratus. I focused on releasing adhesions between the scapula and spine and on reducing hypertonicity in the levator scapulae and upper trapezius.

Plan

Todd rescheduled for one week from today. I will assess the scalenes, the rhomboid/posterior serratus, the trapezius, and the levator scapula again during the next session.

I demonstrated a gentle massage to the neck to keep adhesions at bay until the next session. I suggested that he do this while lying down so that the neck and shoulder are cradled and the muscles do not need to actively contract. I demonstrated scalene stretches. I recommended that Todd perform a full, slow, gentle rotation of the neck for 20 seconds out of each hour that he sits at his computer, followed by a full stretch to the scalenes. I suggested using a speaker phone or ear buds to avoid holding the phone with his shoulder.

CRITICAL THINKING EXERCISES

1. Your client reports chronic pain in the gluteal area that has not been relieved by massage. You suspect that the pain may be referred by a trigger point in the quadratus lumborum. The area around the quadratus lumborum is dense and adhered, and it is difficult to distinguish the individual muscles in the area. Discuss methods for getting to the small trigger point in a deep muscle obscured by adhesions and hypertonicity. Create a self-care plan and a plan for future treatment.

2. Using books, Web sites, and other sources that describe trigger points in detail, find possible sources for pain in the following areas, keeping in mind that there may be more than one:
   - Around the eye
   - In the upper row of teeth
   - The thumb and index finger
   - The fourth and fifth fingers
   - The elbow
   - Across the iliac crests and sacrum
   - Near the greater trochanter
   - Down the posterior leg
   - At the patella
   - In the arch of the foot

3. Conduct a short literature review to learn about the relationship between trigger points and one or more of the following:
   - Vitamin deficiency
   - Chronic infections
   - Hypothyroidism
   - Hypoglycemia
   - Depression

BIBLIOGRAPHY AND SUGGESTED READINGS

Biel A. *Trail Guide to the Body: How to Locate Muscles, Bones and More*, 3rd ed. Boulder, CO: Books of Discovery, 2005.

Cormack DH. *Essential Histology*, 2nd ed. Philadelphia, PA: Lippincott Williams & Wilkins, 2001.

Fernández-de-las-Peñas C, Alonso-Blanco C, Fernández-Carnero J, et al. The immediate effect of ischemic compression technique and transverse friction massage on tenderness of active and latent myofascial trigger points: A pilot study. Journal of Bodywork and Movement Therapies. 2006;10(1):3–9.

Hanten WP, Olson SL, Butts NL, et al. Effectiveness of a home program of ischemic pressure followed by sustained stretch for treatment of myofascial trigger points. Physical Therapy. 2000;80(10):997–1003.

Hong CZ. Specific sequential myofascial trigger point therapy in the treatment of a patient with myofascial pain syndrome associated with reflex sympathetic dystrophy. Australasian Chiropractic & Osteopathy. 2000;9(1):7–11.

Ibáñez-García J, Alburquerque-Sendín F, Rodríguez-Blanco C, et al. Changes in masseter muscle trigger points following strain-counterstrain or neuro-muscular technique. Journal of Bodywork and Movement Therapies. 2009;13(1):2–10.

Mayo Foundation for Medical Education and Research. Bursitis. Available at http://www.mayoclinic.com/health/bursitis/DS00032. Accessed Spring 2009.

Mayo Foundation for Medical Education and Research. Diabetes. Available at http://www.mayoclinic.com/health/diabetes/DS01121. Accessed Summer 2009.

Mayo Foundation for Medical Education and Research. Fibromyalgia. Available at http://www.mayoclinic.com/health/fibromyalgia/DS00079. Accessed Summer 2009.

Mayo Foundation for Medical Education and Research. Menstrual Cramps. Available at http://www.mayoclinic.com/health/menstrual-cramps/DS00506. Accessed Summer 2009.

Mayo Foundation for Medical Education and Research. Myofascial Pain Syndrome. Available at http://www.mayoclinic.com/health/myofascial-pain-syndrome/DS01042. Accessed Spring 2009.

Mayo Foundation for Medical Education and Research. TMJ Disorders. Available at http://www.mayoclinic.com/health/tmj-disorders/DS00355. Accessed Summer 2009.

Rattray F, Ludwig L. *Clinical Massage Therapy: Understanding, Assessing and Treating over 70 Conditions*. Toronto, ON: Talus Incorporated, 2000.

Shah JP, Danoff JV, Desai MJ, et al. Biochemicals associated with pain and inflammation are elevated in sites near to and remote from active myofascial trigger points. Archives of Physical Medicine and Rehabilitation. 2008;89(1):16–23.

Shah JP, Gilliams EA. Uncovering the biochemical milieu of myofascial trigger points using in vivo microdialysis: An application of muscle pain concepts to myofascial pain syndrome. Journal of Bodywork and Movement Therapies. 2008;12(4):371–384.

Simons DG. New views of myofascial trigger points: Etiology and diagnosis. Archives of Physical Medicine and Rehabilitation. 2008;89(1):157–159.

Simons DG, Travell JG, Simons LS. *Travell & Simons' Myofascial Pain and Dysfunction: The Trigger Point Manual*, 2nd ed. Baltimore, MD: Lippincott Williams and Wilkins, 1999.

Simons DG. Understanding effective treatments of myofascial trigger points. Journal of Bodywork and Movement Therapies. 2002;6(2):81–88.

U.S. National Library of Medicine and the National Institutes of Health (ADAM). Gout. Available at http://www.nlm.nih.gov/medlineplus/ency/article/000424.htm#Symptoms. Accessed Winter 2009.

U.S. National Library of Medicine and the National Institutes of Health (ADAM). Migraine. Available at http://www.nlm.nih.gov/medlineplus/ency/article/000709.htm. Accessed Summer 2008.

U.S. National Library of Medicine and the National Institutes of Health (ADAM). Earache. Available at http://www.nlm.nih.gov/medlineplus/ency/article/003046.htm. Accessed Summer 2009.

Werner R. *A Massage Therapist's Guide to Pathology*, 4th ed. Philadelphia, PA: Lippincott Williams and Wilkins, 2008.

Hyperkyphosis

UNDERSTANDING HYPERKYPHOSIS

A healthy spine has four natural curves (Fig. 4-1). The two lordotic curves—cervical and lumbar—arc anteriorly. The two kyphotic curves—thoracic and pelvic—arc posteriorly. These curves are ideal in our species to maintain balance, absorb the impact of movement, and allow maximum flexibility for our particular types of activity.

Hyperkyphosis is an increased kyphotic curve. This chapter focuses on the more common thoracic hyperkyphosis: an increased thoracic curve most often accompanied by protracted scapulae, internally rotated shoulders, and a head-forward posture (Fig. 4-2). In a very short period relative to our evolution, human lifestyle has changed from one that was once considerably physical—hunting and gathering, walking, manual labor, and so on—to one that is becoming increasingly sedentary. Today, we spend a lot of time driving, sitting at a desk, working at a computer, watching television, and so on. These static postures put many of the body's joints in flexion. The hips, knees, thorax, and shoulders are often nearly immobile for hours at a time. Because of this, hyperkyphosis and hyperlordosis are two very common postural deviations that lead to chronic pain and reduced ROM in our modern lifestyle. Both of these postures may lead to other conditions, but you may find that normalizing the curves of the spine and leveling the ilia and scapulae will reduce pain and restriction and may facilitate your treatment of accompanying conditions.

Functional versus Structural Postural Imbalance

The hyperkyphosis described above is functional; its cause is primarily soft tissue dysfunction and postural deviations that result from an injury or activities of daily living. These deviations can be treated with manual therapy, self-care, and postural awareness. The therapeutic goal for functional hyperkyphosis is to lengthen the muscles that have shortened, have become hypertonic, and are pulling the bones out of alignment; to strengthen the muscles that have stretched and become weak; and to reset the neuromuscular system to recognize proper posture and diaphragmatic breathing as normal.

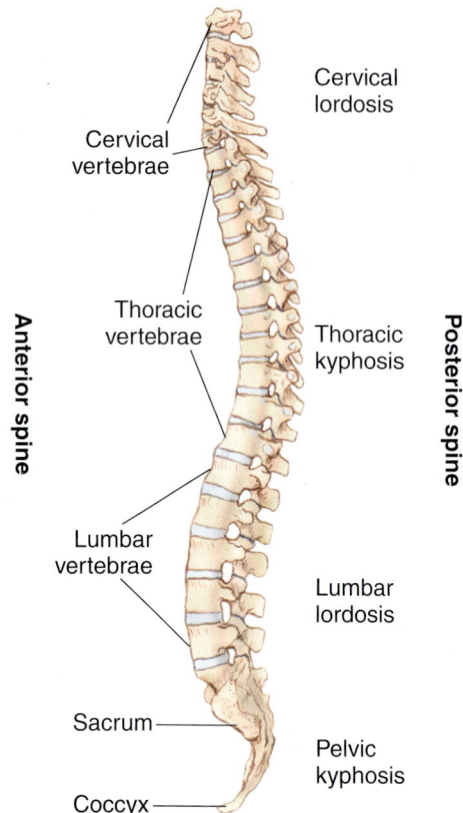

Figure 4-1 **Curves of the spine.** The cervical and lumbar lordotic curves arc anteriorly. The thoracic and pelvic kyphotic curves arc posteriorly.

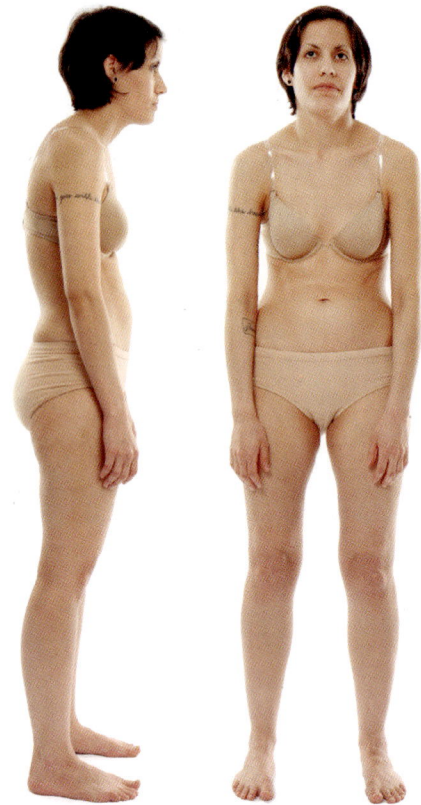

Figure 4-2 **Hyperkyphosis.** Hyperkyphosis involves an increased thoracic curve most often accompanied by protracted scapulae, internally rotated shoulders, and a head-forward posture.

A structural curve, in contrast, is primarily caused by changes in bones. Bone fusions, the development of spurs or new bony prominences, fractured bones that were not well set, osteoporosis, and degenerative disc disease are a few of the possible contributing factors. Manual therapy may offer pain relief, increase ROM, and slow the progression of postural imbalance but is unlikely to reverse the dysfunction. A client's health history may help you assess whether postural deviations are structural in nature, although a diagnosis of structural hyperkyphosis requires medical testing. When a client's hyperkyphosis is structural, it is best to discuss the condition with a health care provider to fully understand the causes. You may need to modify positioning, bolstering, length of treatment, and techniques to accommodate the client's particular needs.

Muscles of the Upper Cross

Thoracic hyperkyphosis is also referred to as upper cross syndrome. Coined by Vladimir Janda, MD, DSc, upper cross syndrome refers to an imbalance and dysfunction of the agonists and antagonists that move and support the thorax. The muscles that become short and tight and the muscles that become weak and overstretched form a cross through the upper thoracic spine (Fig. 4-3). You typically find the pectorals, anterior deltoid, and posterior neck muscles short and tight, while the muscles between the scapulae and those deep in the anterior neck are stretched and weak. The weakened muscles become less able to oppose the actions of the agonists that internally rotate the shoulders, protract the scapula, flex the thoracic spine, and pull the head forward. As this happens, the imbalance can become more profound and the body less able to reverse the process without intervention (Table 4-1).

Common Signs and Symptoms

The most common signs of hyperkyphosis are postural changes such as an increased thoracic curve, protracted scapulae, internally rotated shoulders, and a head-forward posture. The most common symptom of developing thoracic hyperkyphosis is pain between the scapulae and along the posterior neck. Overstretched muscles including the rhomboids, middle trapezius, and thoracic erector spinae form taut bands that may harbor trigger points. The primary function of the rhomboids and middle trapezius in a static posture is to keep the spine erect and the scapulae retracted. When the client's common posture stretches them, these muscles (and the nerves that innervate them) are working against the tight pectorals to try to bring the scapulae closer to the spine. If the pectorals are not lengthened, the rhomboids and middle trapezius are fighting a difficult battle, a form of overuse, and can become weak and easily fatigued. In addition, trigger points in the scalenes, levator scapula, trapezius, and latissimus dorsi all refer pain between the scapulae. With adhesions, trigger points, and spasm, the cervical and thoracic spine may become hypomobile if left untreated.

Internally rotated shoulders, protracted scapulae, and the head-forward position each involve muscles that, when hypertonic, may compress nerves and vessels, resulting in thoracic outlet syndrome (see Chapter 6), which is frequently mistaken for carpal tunnel syndrome (see Chapter 7) when the site of nerve compression is not correctly identified. When thoracic outlet syndrome develops, lymphatic structures may be compressed, causing insufficient drainage and edema; vasculature may be compressed, leading to insufficient circulation and ischemia; and nerves may be compressed, leading to pain, numbness, and tingling along their distribution and weakening or atrophy of muscles supplied by the compromised nerves.

With the thorax flexed, movement of the ribcage and the muscles of respiration are restricted, which may cause shallow breathing and can lead to chronic respiratory dysfunction. A client with prior respiratory disorders who develops hyperkyphosis may experience increased signs and symptoms of respiratory dysfunction. Protraction of the scapulae turns the glenohumeral joint

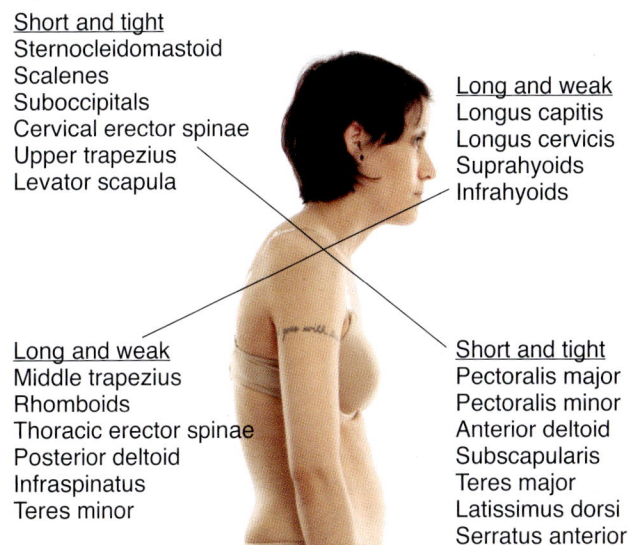

Short and tight
Sternocleidomastoid
Scalenes
Suboccipitals
Cervical erector spinae
Upper trapezius
Levator scapula

Long and weak
Longus capitis
Longus cervicis
Suprahyoids
Infrahyoids

Long and weak
Middle trapezius
Rhomboids
Thoracic erector spinae
Posterior deltoid
Infraspinatus
Teres minor

Short and tight
Pectoralis major
Pectoralis minor
Anterior deltoid
Subscapularis
Teres major
Latissimus dorsi
Serratus anterior

Figure 4-3 Muscles of the upper cross. Notice the relationship between the muscles that are short and tight and those that are long and weak.

Table 4-1	Muscles of the Upper Cross with Actions That Contribute to Hyperkyphosis
Muscles That are Short and Tight (with Agonist Action)	**Muscles That are Stretched and Weak (with Antagonist Opposition)**
Pectoralis major (internal rotation of shoulder)	Infraspinatus (internal rotation of shoulder)
Anterior deltoid (internal rotation of shoulder)	Posterior deltoid (internal rotation of shoulder)
Subscapularis (internal rotation of shoulder)	Teres minor (internal rotation of shoulder)
Teres major (internal rotation of shoulder)	
Latissimus dorsi (internal rotation of shoulder)	
Serratus anterior (protraction of scapula)	Middle trapezius (protraction of scapula)
Pectoralis minor (protraction of scapula)	Rhomboid major and minor (protraction of scapula)
SCM (head forward)	Longus capitis (head forward)
Scalenes (head forward)	Longus cervicis (head forward)
Upper trapezius (upper cervical extension)	Suprahyoids (upper cervical extension)
Levator scapulae (upper cervical extension)	Infrahyoids (upper cervical extension)
Suboccipitals (upper cervical extension)	Thoracic erector spinae (increased thoracic curve)
Cervical erector spinae (upper cervical extension)	

inferiorly, causing the rotator cuff muscles to compensate and become hypertonic. If left untreated, particularly if the client uses repetitive motions of the glenohumeral joint with resistance, frozen shoulder may develop. The head-forward posture and extension of the upper cervical vertebrae may stress the facet joints and lead to wearing of the intervertebral discs. When the head is in a forward position, the mandible is drawn posteriorly, which may contribute to dysfunction in the temporomandibular joint, often resulting in grinding of the teeth, called bruxism. Trigger points in the muscles of mastication refer pain into the teeth that can be mistaken for toothache. Trigger points in muscles including the SCM and upper trapezius may refer into the head, causing tension headaches. You may also find one or both shoulders elevated, or hyperlordosis (see Chapter 8). It is difficult to say which of these postural deviations begins the process, but as one develops, the others may follow as the body attempts to stay balanced on its center of gravity with the eyes level and looking forward.

Possible Causes and Contributing Factors

Pathologies that affect the integrity of bones are often the cause of structural hyperkyphosis. Porous bones (osteoporosis) become unable to bear weight and may cause the thoracic vertebrae to collapse upon each other, resulting in increased curvature. Nutritional deficiencies of calcium and vitamin D as well as increased consumption of calcium oxalate and carbonated beverages may play a role in the body's ability to rebuild bone. Ankylosing spondylitis—an autoimmune disease that causes arthritis or swelling in the spine—ultimately causes the vertebrae to fuse with the thorax in flexion. Tuberculosis that settles in the spine—an infection called Pott's disease—also results in deterioration of the vertebrae that can cause structural hyperkyphosis. Scheuermann's disease—an idiopathic condition that affects adolescents—occurs when the posterior aspects of the vertebrae grow faster than the anterior portion, causing the vertebrae to wedge and increase the thoracic curve. Congenital defects, such as spina bifida or muscular dystrophy, may also contribute.

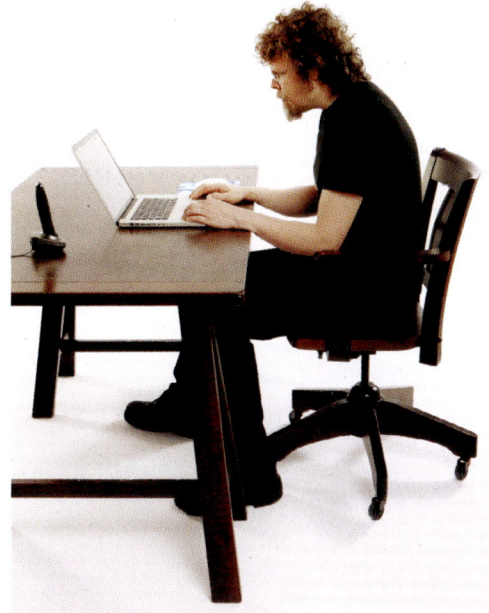

Figure 4-4 **Poor seated posture.** Poor seated posture that contributes to hyperkyphosis is common among desk workers.

The primary contributing factor to functional thoracic hyperkyphosis is poor posture. In some cases, as with muscular dystrophy or radiculopathy, poor posture results from muscle degeneration and interrupted innervation. More commonly, upper cross postural deviations result from voluntary poor posture. For example, if a client regularly performs activities that require the shoulders to be in flexion and internal rotation, the head is likely to jut forward, adding much weight to the anterior frontal plane (Fig. 4-4).

Try this yourself: Sit straight with your arms hanging comfortably at your sides. Slowly raise your shoulders into flexion and internal rotation as if to type on a keyboard, paying close attention to how your neck and head follow. Certainly, you can force your head to stay straight, but these movements often naturally cause the head to move slightly forward and the neck to flex slightly. Because we need to look straight ahead, the upper vertebrae of the neck extend to level the eyes. When this is a common, daily posture, the thoracic spine begins to curve posteriorly. Moreover, when a client regularly assumes this posture, the pectoral muscles are shortened and develop increased tone, while the middle trapezius and rhomboids become overstretched, making it difficult for them to resist the pull of the pectorals. Left untreated, the kyphotic curve will continue to increase, the scapulae will continue to protract, and the cervical and lumbar lordotic curves may continue to increase to compensate.

Exercise and sports involving resisted contraction in the pectoral muscles may contribute to hyperkyphosis. Professions that involve heavy lifting, repeated flexion and internal rotation of the shoulders, or a slouched posture may place the worker at risk. Age also plays a role as the bones become weaker over time, and the person performs less frequently those activities that keep the joints mobile. Poor eyesight or hearing, which may cause the client to thrust the head forward in order to see or hear better, may become a contributing factor if left unaddressed. Respiratory conditions affecting the tone of the muscles of respiration may also play a role.

Table 4-2 lists conditions that are commonly confused with or that contribute to hyperkyphosis.

Contraindications and Special Considerations

- **Underlying pathologies.** Ankylosing spondylitis, osteoarthritis, osteoporosis, degenerative disc disease, bone spurs, or fusions may be present. If you suspect one of these (consult Table 4-2 and your pathology book for signs and symptoms), refer the client to a health care

| Table 4-2 | Differentiating Conditions Commonly Confused with or Contributing to Hyperkyphosis |

Condition	Typical Signs and Symptoms	Testing	Massage Therapy
Osteoporosis	Bone or joint pain, tenderness, bone fractures, loss of height, slouching	Bone mineral density test CT, X-ray Urinary calcium test	Indicated in early stages and with health care provider approval in later stages. May reduce pain. Take care not to use force that may fracture a bone.
Spondylolisthesis (begins in lumbar, proceeds to thoracic spine)	Lumbar hyperlordosis Pain in low back, buttocks, and thighs Stiff back	X-ray	Massage is indicated. Use caution if bones are fragile. Stretching and strengthening encouraged.
Ankylosing spondylitis	Pain often begins in low back unilaterally and progresses bilaterally to upper back and throughout thorax Fatigue and anemia may develop	MRI Blood tests	Indicated to reduce pain, maintain mobility, and slow progress of spinal distortion Use caution if bones are fragile.
Scheuermann's disease (juvenile kyphosis)	Begins at puberty Pain, curved spine that worsens when bending, difficulty breathing, chest pain Signs and symptoms cease when child stops growing	X-ray Adam's forward bending test	Indicated to reduce pain
Pott's disease (tuberculous arthritis)	Slow onset Low-grade fever Excessive perspiration Loss of appetite Swollen, tender joints Spinal masses Numbness and tingling in extremities Reduced ROM	X-ray Tuberculin skin test (PPD) Aspiration of joint fluid Biopsy to test bacteria	Contraindicated until infection is resolved completely Work with health care provider in cases of abscesses or other contraindications. Massage may be helpful to reduce pain.
Muscular dystrophy	Many forms appear in childhood or adolescence, although a few may develop in adulthood Muscle weakness Loss of coordination Progressive, resulting in fixed contracture of muscles	Blood test for creatine level Electromyography Ultrasonography Muscle biopsy Genetic testing	Work with health care provider. Massage may reduce pain and delay contracture.
Paget's disease	Persistent bone pain Joint pain and stiffness Headache, neck pain Bowed legs Locally hot to touch Fractures Hearing loss Loss of height	X-ray Bone scan Blood test for serum alkaline phosphatase and serum calcium	Work with health care provider. Massage may help maintain flexibility. Use caution if bones are fragile.

Table 4-2	Differentiating Conditions Commonly Confused with or Contributing to Hyperkyphosis (Continued)		
Condition	**Typical Signs and Symptoms**	**Testing**	**Massage Therapy**
Nerve root compression (radiculopathy)	Muscle spasm, weakness, or atrophy Pain around scapula on affected side Neck pain Pain radiates to extremities Pain worsens with lateral flexion or rotation or when sneezing, coughing, laughing, or straining	Spurling's test Valsalva's test Neurological exam to test reflexes, sensation, and strength X-ray or MRI to assess for space occupying lesions	Indicated if cause and location are understood. Take care not to increase compression of nerve or reproduce symptoms.

provider for assessment before initiating treatment. If the client is diagnosed with an underlying pathology that is not contraindicated for massage, work with the health care provider to develop a treatment plan.

- **Endangerment sites.** Be cautious near the endangerment sites in the neck and axilla. Gently palpate for the pulse of the carotid artery before you begin working on the neck. Avoid this area; if you feel a pulse while working, back off slowly and avoid the area.
- **Treatment duration and pressure.** If the client is elderly, has degenerative bone disease, or has been diagnosed with a condition that diminishes activities of daily living, you may need to adjust your pressure as well as the treatment duration. Frequent half-hour sessions may suit the client better.
- **Positioning.** Use bolsters to position a client for comfort as well as to reduce postures that may contribute to hyperkyphosis. In the prone position, bolsters under the shoulders will reduce protraction of the scapulae. Adjust the face cradle to reduce extension in the neck. In the supine position, a bolster along the length of the spine and under the occiput will reduce protraction of the scapulae and extension of the neck. If hyperlordosis is present, a bolster across the anterior superior iliac spine in the prone position will reduce anterior pelvic tilt, and a bolster under the ankles may reduce tension in the low back. A bolster under the knees in the supine position may reduce tension on the low back.
- **Hydrotherapy.** Do not use moist heat on the neck or chest if the client has a cardiovascular condition that may be affected by the dilation of blood vessels. Severe hypertension and atherosclerosis are two examples of conditions where hydrotherapy is contraindicated. Consult your pathology book for recommendations.
- **Friction.** Do not use deep frictions if the client has a systemic inflammatory condition, such as rheumatoid arthritis or osteoarthritis, if the health of the underlying tissues is compromised or if the client is taking an anti-inflammatory medication. Friction may initiate an inflammatory process, which may interfere with the intended action of anti-inflammatory medication. Recommend that your client refrain from taking such medication for several hours before treatment if his or her health care provider agrees.
- **Tissue length.** It is important when treating myofascial tissues to not stretch tissues that are already overstretched. Assess for myofascial restrictions first and treat only those that are clearly present. Likewise, overstretched muscles should not be stretched from origin to insertion because their length should not be increased. If you treat trigger points, use heat or a localized pin and stretch technique instead of full ROM stretching. For example, because the rhomboids and middle trapezius tend to be overstretched, it is not advised to perform myofascial release or a full stretch from origin to insertion across the length of these muscles.
- **Hypermobile joints and unstable ligaments.** Be cautious with mobilizations if the client has hypermobile joints or if ligaments are unstable due to injury, pregnancy or a systemic condition.

Massage Therapy Research

Studies in journals covering subjects ranging from physical therapy to neuroscience report that hyperkyphosis results in structural changes or is caused by functional changes, such as the shortening or lengthening of muscles in the upper cross, and is often associated with neurological dysfunction. Although several articles describe exercise, yoga, chiropractic care, surgery, self-care, proprioceptive neuromuscular facilitation, and other methods of reducing the symptoms of hyperkyphosis, a thorough literature review reveals no research, case studies, or articles specifically showing the benefits of massage therapy for hyperkyphosis, kyphosis, or upper cross syndrome. Many of the studies addressing hyperkyphosis focus on increased thoracic curvature in the elderly as a result of osteoporosis. While much literature describes the phenomenon of increased thoracic flexion in a society prone to hunched, seated postures, research has not yet investigated massage as a specific treatment option for hyperkyphosis.

In 2008, Greig et al. conducted a study titled "Postural taping decreases thoracic kyphosis but does not influence trunk muscle electromyographic activity or balance in women with osteoporosis." As the title suggests, taping decreased the thoracic curve but had no effect on muscle tone associated with hyperkyphosis. Additional research is necessary to determine whether manual manipulation of the trunk muscles may have an effect on electromyographic activity and whether such an effect may suggest massage as a treatment option with longer-lasting effects.

Research into the benefits of massage for scoliosis, thoracic outlet syndrome, temporomandibular joint dysfunction, respiratory distress, and other syndromes commonly associated with hyperkyphosis is available. Although anecdotal evidence has suggested that manual therapy reduces pain and increases ROM when hyperkyphosis is present, additional research is needed to determine the benefits of massage therapy intended to lengthen shortened muscles, strengthen weakened muscles, and reset neuromuscular function for clients presenting with signs and symptoms of functional hyperkyphosis.

WORKING WITH THE CLIENT

Client Assessment

Hyperkyphosis is one of the most common postural deviations causing chronic pain and restricted ROM in the upper body. It involves many joints and nearly all of the muscles of the upper body. A wide variety of possible factors can contribute to the development of both structural and functional hyperkyphosis. All of these elements add up to many variations in how a client may present to you. For example, a client may hold the phone more frequently at his or her left ear with the left shoulder and present with left lateral flexion and right rotation of the neck, which suggests that the scalenes and SCM on the left side may be short and tight. Another client may frequently carry a heavy bag on the right shoulder and may present with an elevated right shoulder, which suggests that the upper trapezius and levator scapulae may be short and tight. Common presentations of hyperkyphosis are described below. However, it is essential to assess every joint to put together an accurate picture for each individual client. In addition, because treatment goals differ, it is important to know if the primary cause of hyperkyphosis is functional or structural.

Assessment begins at your very first contact with a client. In some cases, this may be on the telephone when an appointment is requested. Ask in advance if the client is seeking treatment for a specific area of pain so that you can prepare yourself.

Table 4-3	Health History

Questions for the Client	Importance for the Treatment Plan
Where do you feel symptoms?	The location of symptoms gives clues to the location of trigger points, injury, or other contributing factors.
Describe what your symptoms feel like.	Differentiate possible origins of symptoms and determine the involvement of nerves or blood vessels.
Do any movements make it worse or better?	Locate tension, weakness, or compression in structures producing such movements.
Have you seen a health care provider for this condition? What was the diagnosis? What tests were performed?	Bone density, blood, and respiratory function tests may indicate contributing factors. Medical tests may indicate that hyperkyphosis is structural in nature.
Have you been diagnosed with a conditionsuch as osteoporosis, rheumatoid arthritis or osteoarthritis, asthma, temporomandibular joint disorder, weakened vision or hearing?	Systemic and other conditions may contribute to signs and symptoms, may require adjustments to treatment, and may impact treatment outcomes.
Have you had an injury or surgery?	Injury or surgery and resulting scar tissue may cause adhesions, hyper- or hypotonicity, and atypical ROM.
What type of work, hobbies, or other regular activities do you do?	Repetitive motions and static postures that increase thoracic flexion, protracted scapulae, neck extension, or head-forward posture may contribute to the client's condition.
Are you taking any prescribed medications or herbal or other supplements?	Medications of all types may contribute to symptoms or have contraindications or cautions.
Have you had a cortisone shot in the past 2 weeks? Where?	Local massage is contraindicated.
Have you taken a pain reliever or muscle relaxant within the past 4 hours?	The client may not be able to judge your pressure.
Have you taken anti-inflammatory medication within the past 4 hours?	Deep friction may initiate an inflammatory process and should not be performed if the client has recently taken anti-inflammatory medication.

Table 4-3 lists questions to ask the client when taking a health history.

POSTURAL ASSESSMENT

Allow the client to walk and enter the room ahead of you while you assess posture and movements before the client is aware that the assessment has begun. Look for imbalances or patterns of compensation for deviations common with hyperkyphosis. Have the client sit at a desk or table to fill out the assessment form, and look for a slouching posture. If he or she is slouched, ask a question to draw his or her attention to you and away from the form. Notice whether he or she extends the thoracic spine or only the upper cervical spine when looking up at you. Extending only the upper cervical spine may indicate weakness in thoracic extension. Look for slight rotation of the neck when the client is looking straight ahead. This may indicate shortening of the contralateral upper trapezius, scalenes, or SCM or shortening of the ipsilateral levator scapulae, splenius, or cervical erector spinae. If the internal rotators of the shoulder are shortened, the client's elbow and forearm may not rest on the table while writing. Watch also as the client stands up to see whether he or she extends the thoracic spine or whether the momentum comes mostly from hip and knee extension. If hyperlordosis is also present, knee extension may be the primary force, and the client may use the table for assistance in standing. Supplement these findings with a standard assessment of the client's stationary, standing posture. Figure 4-5 compares the anatomic position to posture affected by hyperkyphosis.

ROM ASSESSMENT

Test the ROM of the neck, shoulders, and thoracic spine, assessing length and strength of both agonists and antagonists that cross the joints tested. If hyperkyphosis is structural in nature, do not perform ROM tests that move the affected joints into ranges that are inhibited by altered joint structure. For example, if thoracic vertebrae are fused into flexion, do not test extension of the thoracic spine. Since it allows the client to control the amount of movement and stay within a pain-free range, only active ROM should be used in the acute stage of injury to prevent undue pain or re-injury. Box 4-1 presents the average active ROM results for the joints involved in hyperkyphosis.

Active ROM

Compare your assessment of the client's active ROM to the values in Box 4-1. Pain and other symptoms may not be reproduced with active ROM assessment because the client may limit movement to a symptom-free range.

- **Active extension of the thoracic spine** may be reduced when muscle tension, adhesions, and trigger points in the extensors of the thoracic spine contribute to hyperkyphosis. The client may resist full active extension of the thoracic spine if this produces symptoms during activities of daily living.
- **Active flexion of the cervical spine** may be restricted due to weakened deep cervical flexors attempting movement against shortened upper cervical extensors.
- **Active rotation and lateral flexion** of the cervical spine may be reduced or cause pain due to hypertonicity or spasm in the rotators and lateral flexors of the cervical spine or the weakening of their antagonists.
- **Active external rotation of the shoulder** may be restricted due to adhesions, hypertonic internal rotators of the shoulder, and protraction of the scapula.

Passive ROM

Compare the client's passive ROM on one side to the other when applicable. Note and compare the end feel for each range (see Chapter 1 for an explanation of end feel).

- **Passive flexion of the cervical spine** may be restricted or cause discomfort due to shortened cervical extensors or dysfunction of the vertebrae.
- **Passive lateral flexion or rotation of the cervical spine** may be restricted unilaterally if the client's posture favors lateral flexion or rotation in the opposite direction.
- **Passive extension of the cervical spine** may be restricted by the head-forward posture due to tension in muscles such as the scalenes or SCM that also flex the cervical spine. If the head-forward posture is not present, passive extension of the cervical spine will likely occur with ease, although it may produce pain at the end point.
- **Passive external rotation of the shoulder** may be restricted if the scapula is protracted, causing the glenohumeral joint to be rotated inferiorly.

Resisted ROM

Use resisted tests to assess the strength of the muscles that cross the involved joints. Compare the strength of the affected side to that of the unaffected side.

- **Resisted extension of the thoracic spine** may reveal pain and weakness in the thoracic erector spinae.
- **Resisted retraction of the scapula** may reveal pain and weakness in the rhomboids and middle trapezius.
- **Resisted rotation or lateral flexion of the neck** may produce pain or a referral if the muscles responsible for that action are tight or contain trigger points, and may reveal weakness in their antagonists.
- **Resisted external rotation of the shoulder** may reveal weakness in the external rotators of the shoulder.

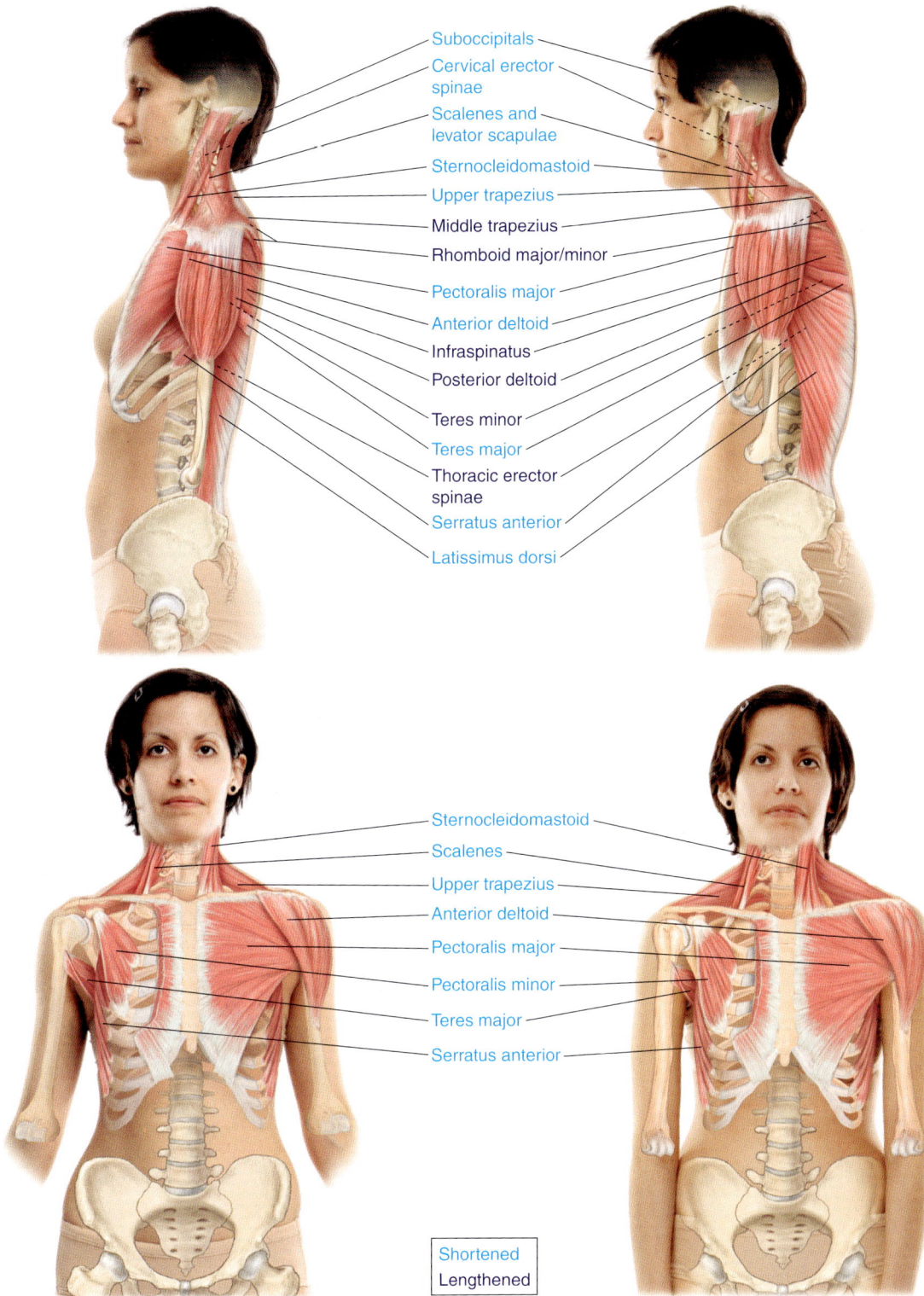

Suboccipitals
Cervical erector spinae
Scalenes and levator scapulae
Sternocleidomastoid
Upper trapezius
Middle trapezius
Rhomboid major/minor
Pectoralis major
Anterior deltoid
Infraspinatus
Posterior deltoid
Teres minor
Teres major
Thoracic erector spinae
Serratus anterior
Latissimus dorsi

Sternocleidomastoid
Scalenes
Upper trapezius
Anterior deltoid
Pectoralis major
Pectoralis minor
Teres major
Serratus anterior

Shortened
Lengthened

Figure 4-5 **Postural assessment comparison.** Compare the anatomical postures on the left to the hyperkyphotic postures on the right. Notice how the muscles of the upper cross react to the increased kyphotic curve and head-forward posture.

Box 4-1   AVERAGE ACTIVE ROM FOR JOINTS INVOLVED IN HYPERKYPHOSIS

Cervical Spine

Flexion 60°
SCM (bilateral)
Anterior scalenes (bilateral)
Longus capitis (bilateral)
Longus colli (bilateral)

Extension 55°
Upper trapezius (bilateral)
Levator scapulae (bilateral)
Splenius capitis (bilateral)
Splenius cervicis (bilateral)
Rectus capitis (bilateral)
Oblique capitis superior (bilateral)
Semispinalis capitis (bilateral)
Longissimus capitis (bilateral)
Longissimus cervicis (bilateral)
Iliocostalis cervicis (bilateral)

Lateral Flexion 20–45°
Upper trapezius (unilateral)
Levator scapulae (unilateral)
Splenius capitis (unilateral)
Splenius cervicis (unilateral)
SCM (unilateral)
Longus capitis (unilateral)
Longus colli (unilateral)
Anterior scalene (unilateral)
Middle scalene (unilateral)
Posterior scalene (unilateral)
Longissimus capitis (unilateral)
Longissimus cervicis (unilateral)
Iliocostalis cervicis (unilateral)

Ipsilateral Rotation 70–90°
Levator scapulae (unilateral)
Splenius capitis (unilateral)
Splenius cervicis (unilateral)
Rectus capitis (unilateral)
Oblique capitis (unilateral)
Longus colli (unilateral)
Longus capitis (unilateral)
Longissimus capitis (unilateral)
Longissimus cervicis (unilateral)
Iliocostalis cervicis (unilateral)

Contralateral Rotation 70–90°
Upper trapezius (unilateral)
SCM (unilateral)
Anterior scalene (unilateral)
Middle scalene (unilateral)
Posterior scalene (unilateral)

Shoulder

Flexion 180°
Anterior deltoid
Pectoralis major (upper fibers)

Biceps brachii
Coracobrachialis

Extension 50–60°
Posterior deltoid
Latissimus dorsi
Teres major & minor
Infraspinatus
Pectoralis major (lower fibers)
Triceps brachii

Internal Rotation 60–100°
Anterior deltoid
Latissimus dorsi
Teres major
Subscapularis
Pectoralis major

External Rotation 80–90°
Posterior deltoid
Infraspinatus
Teres minor

Abduction 180°
Deltoids
Supraspinatus

Adduction 50–75°
Latissimus dorsi
Teres major
Infraspinatus
Teres minor
Pectoralis major
Triceps brachii (long head)
Coracobrachialis

Horizontal Abduction 45°
Posterior deltoid
Infraspinatus
Teres minor

Horizontal Adduction 130°
Anterior deltoid
Pectoralis major (upper fibers)

Thoracic Spine

Flexion 30–40°
Rectus abdominis
External obliques
Internal obliques

Extension 20–30°
Spinalis
Longissimus
Iliocostalis
Multifidi
Rotatores
Semispinalis capitis
Latissimus dorsi
Quadratus lumborum

Lateral Flexion 20–25°
Spinalis (unilateral)
Longissimus (unilateral)
Iliocostalis (unilateral)
Quadratus lumborum (unilateral)
External oblique (unilateral)
Internal oblique (unilateral)
Latissimus dorsi (unilateral)

Ipsilateral Rotation 35°
Internal oblique (unilateral)

Contralateral Rotation 35°
Rotatores (unilateral)
Multifidi (unilateral)
External oblique (unilateral)

Mandible

Elevation (contact of teeth)
Masseter
Temporalis
Medial pterygoid

Depression 35–50 mm
Hyoids
Digastric
Platysma

Protraction 3–7 mm
Lateral pterygoid
Medial pterygoid

Retraction
Temporalis
Digastric

Contralateral Lateral Deviation 5–12 mm
Lateral pterygoid
Medial pterygoid

Respiration

Inhalation
Diaphragm
Scalenes
SCM
External intercostals
Serratus anterior
Serratus posterior superior

Exhalation
Internal intercostals
Serratus posterior inferior
Internal obliques
External obliques
Transversus abdominis

SPECIAL TESTS

The following special tests will help you determine when a client should be evaluated by his or her health care provider using X-ray or other tools, which may reveal conditions that are contraindicated or require special consideration when planning massage treatment.

The **vertebral artery test** may reveal insufficiency in the vertebral artery and is performed if the client experiences vertigo, blurred vision, or light-headedness during activities of daily living (Fig. 4-6).

1. Position the client seated in a chair facing you with the eyes open.
2. Instruct the client to fully rotate and extend the neck to one side for 30 seconds.
3. If, during this time, the client complains of nausea or dizziness or if you notice involuntary motion of the eyes, the test is positive for insufficient circulation through the vertebral artery, and the client should be referred to his or her health care provider.
4. If the test is negative on one side, test the other. Do not test the other side if the first side tests positive.

Spurling's test may reveal compression of a nerve or irritation to the facet joint in the cervical spine and is performed when the client has had an injury, complains of pain that radiates, or experiences numbness and tingling in the arm (Fig. 4-7). Although massage may not be contraindicated for a client with these conditions, refer the client to his or her health care provider for more detailed information or to a massage therapist with advanced training if you have not studied the client's condition in detail. If the client tests positive for vertebral artery insufficiency, do not perform Spurling's test.

1. If the client has recurring symptoms on one side only, begin with that side.
2. Stand behind the seated client and instruct him or her to extend, laterally flex, and rotate the head to the affected side.

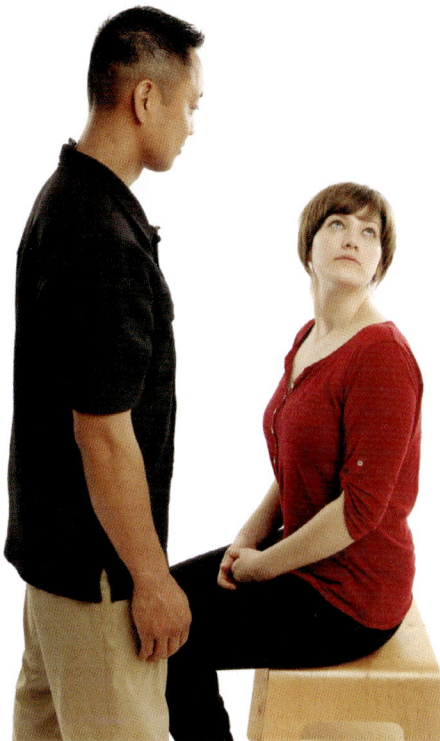

Figure 4-6 **Vertebral artery test.** Watch the client's eyes for any involuntary movement during this test.

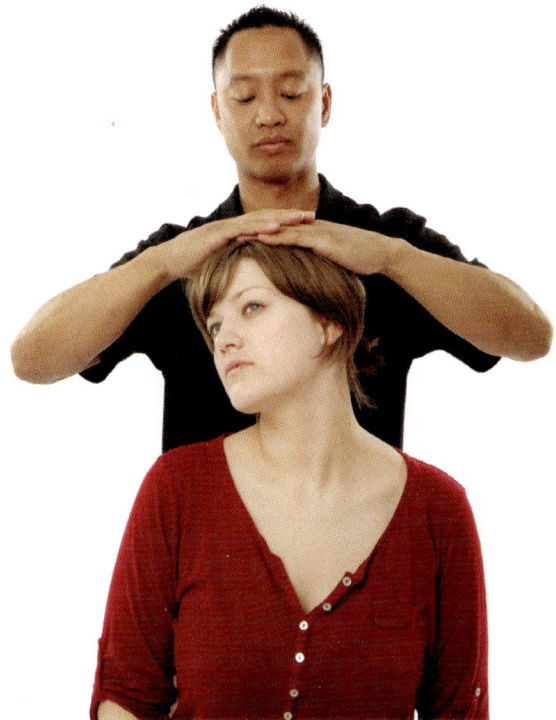

Figure 4-7 **Spurling's test.** Use gentle traction following this test to release pressure.

3. Gently and slowly press down on the client's head. If the client cannot extend, laterally flex, or rotate the neck, perform a simple compression test without these actions.
4. If the client experiences radiating pain, numbness, or tingling in the arm, the test is positive for nerve root compression.
5. Ask the client to describe the location of symptoms, because this may suggest which nerve is compressed.
6. If the client feels pain that does not move past the neck, the test is positive for irritation of the facet joint.
7. Applying gentle traction to the neck after the test may relieve symptoms. If traction does relieve symptoms, this is considered reinforcement that Spurling's test is positive for compression of a nerve or facet joint irritation.

The **Valsalva maneuver** may reveal a herniated disc, tumor, or other factor that increases pressure on the spinal nerves; it is used when the client complains of pain in a localized area along the spine, particularly when coughing or sneezing. A herniated disc does not contraindicate massage, but this test is not specific for the cause of increased pressure. For this reason, it is best to refer the client to his or her health care provider for further testing before performing a massage.

1. To avoid even a temporary reduction in circulation, do not perform this test if the client has tested positive for vertebral artery insufficiency or has cardiovascular disorders.
2. With the client seated and facing you, ask him or her to take a deep breath and then attempt to exhale against the closed throat (such as when moving the bowels).
3. The test is positive if the client feels pain in a localized spot along the spine.

PALPATION ASSESSMENT

Palpate the muscles of the upper cross to assess for hyper- and hypotonicity and myofascial restrictions. You are likely to find hypertonicity and myofascial restrictions in the pectorals, especially near the glenohumeral joint. The serratus anterior, subclavius, and anterior intercostals may also be adhered and hypertonic, particularly if the client slouches or has developed a pattern of shallow breathing. The SCM, upper trapezius, suboccipitals, cervical erector spinae, levator scapulae, and scalenes may be hypertonic, particularly if the client has developed the head-forward posture, elevated shoulders, or extension of the upper cervical spine. When internal rotation of the shoulder is present, you may also find adhesions and hypertonicity in the anterior deltoid, latissimus dorsi, subscapularis, and teres major.

Overstretched muscles may include the deep anterior neck muscles, rhomboids, middle trapezius, and thoracic erector spinae with the head-forward posture, protracted scapulae, and increased thoracic curve. With internally rotated shoulders, the posterior deltoid, infraspinatus, and teres minor may be lengthened.

Condition-Specific Massage

Because hyperkyphosis may be structural, it is essential to understand the client's health history. If a systemic condition or a degenerative bone or disc disease is present, discuss treatment with the client's health care provider and adjust the treatment accordingly. Treatment goals for structural hyperkyphosis may be limited to pain reduction. If thoracic outlet syndrome, chronic tension headaches, or hyperlordosis is present, refer to those chapters in this text for special testing and consideration of the neuromuscular characteristics. Temporomandibular joint dysfunction may also develop with hyperkyphosis. This disorder is not covered in this text, but you may treat the muscle of mastication generally to offer some relief; if you have not studied this condition in detail, refer the client to a massage therapist with training in this area.

It is essential for the treatment to be relaxing. You are not likely to eliminate the pain associated with hyperkyphosis or any of the associated conditions in one treatment. Do not try to do so by treating aggressively. Be sure to ask your client to let you know if the amount of pressure keeps him or her from relaxing. If the client responds by tensing muscles or has a facial expression that looks distressed, reduce your pressure. Remember that you are working on tissue that is compromised.

Ask the client to let you know if any part of your treatment reproduces symptoms. If deep palpation of a trigger point reproduces symptoms, explain this phenomenon to your client and ask him or her to breathe deeply during the application of the technique. As the trigger point is deactivated, the referral pain will also diminish. Common trigger points and their referral points are shown in Figure 4-8.

If any other symptoms are reproduced, adjust the client to a more neutral position, reduce your pressure, or move slightly off the area, and take note of this because it may help you understand more clearly exactly what is contributing to the client's symptoms. Instruct your client to use deep but relaxing breathing to assist in relaxation.

The following suggestions are for treatment that considers several factors involved in hyperkyphosis. Because several joints and many muscles are involved in this condition, your treatment will likely fill the entire session.

- Begin with the client in the supine position with a rolled towel along the length of the spine (Fig. 4-9). This bolster will retract the scapulae and lengthen the pectoral muscles. If the client's neck is in extension, fold a pillow case or hand towel into a bolster that is small enough to be placed under the occiput without obstructing your access to the posterior neck muscles.

- If the client has symptoms that suggest thoracic outlet syndrome, begin on the affected side. If both arms are affected, begin with the dominant side. See Chapter 6 on thoracic outlet syndrome for considerations concerning edema and reproduction of symptoms.

- Place moist heat on one pectoral if the client does not have a cardiovascular condition. After heating one pectoral, move the heat to the other side and begin treating the heated side. After heating the second pectoral, you can move the heat to the posterior neck if this is comfortable for the client.

- Before applying emollient, assess the tissues of the anterior upper cross for myofascial restrictions and release them if found. Adhesions are often found around the glenohumeral joint, along the anterior deltoid, along the lateral and posterior neck, and at the occiput.

- Reduce tension, then apply lengthening strokes to the full length of the pectoralis major to soften tissues to allow you to treat deeper structures (Fig. 4-10). Apply these strokes from sternum or clavicle toward the humerus to reduce internal rotation of the shoulder.

- Assess the pectoralis major for trigger points, and treat them if found. Common trigger points in the pectoralis major are found along the mid sternum, at the clavicular attachments, and along the inferior fibers, particularly near the axilla.

- Assess and treat the subclavius for hypertonicity and trigger points. The subclavius is a slight, thin muscle deep to the pectoralis major and may not be easily palpated (Fig. 4-11). Trust your knowledge of anatomy as you palpate along the inferior edge of the middle third of the clavicle toward the costal cartilage of the first rib. If you find and treat trigger points in the subclavius, use a pin and stretch technique to lengthen the muscle fibers.

- You can treat the pectoralis minor through the pectoralis major, but it is difficult to distinguish the two muscles when palpating both. You can access pectoralis minor more directly by pushing the lateral fibers of the pectoralis major medially as you palpate ribs 3, 4, and 5 (Fig. 4-12). This may be easiest by kneeling next to the client and placing his or her hand on

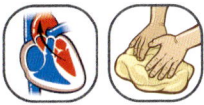

Treatment icons: Increase circulation; Reduce adhesions; Reduce tension; Lengthen tissue; Treat trigger points; Passive stretch; Clear area

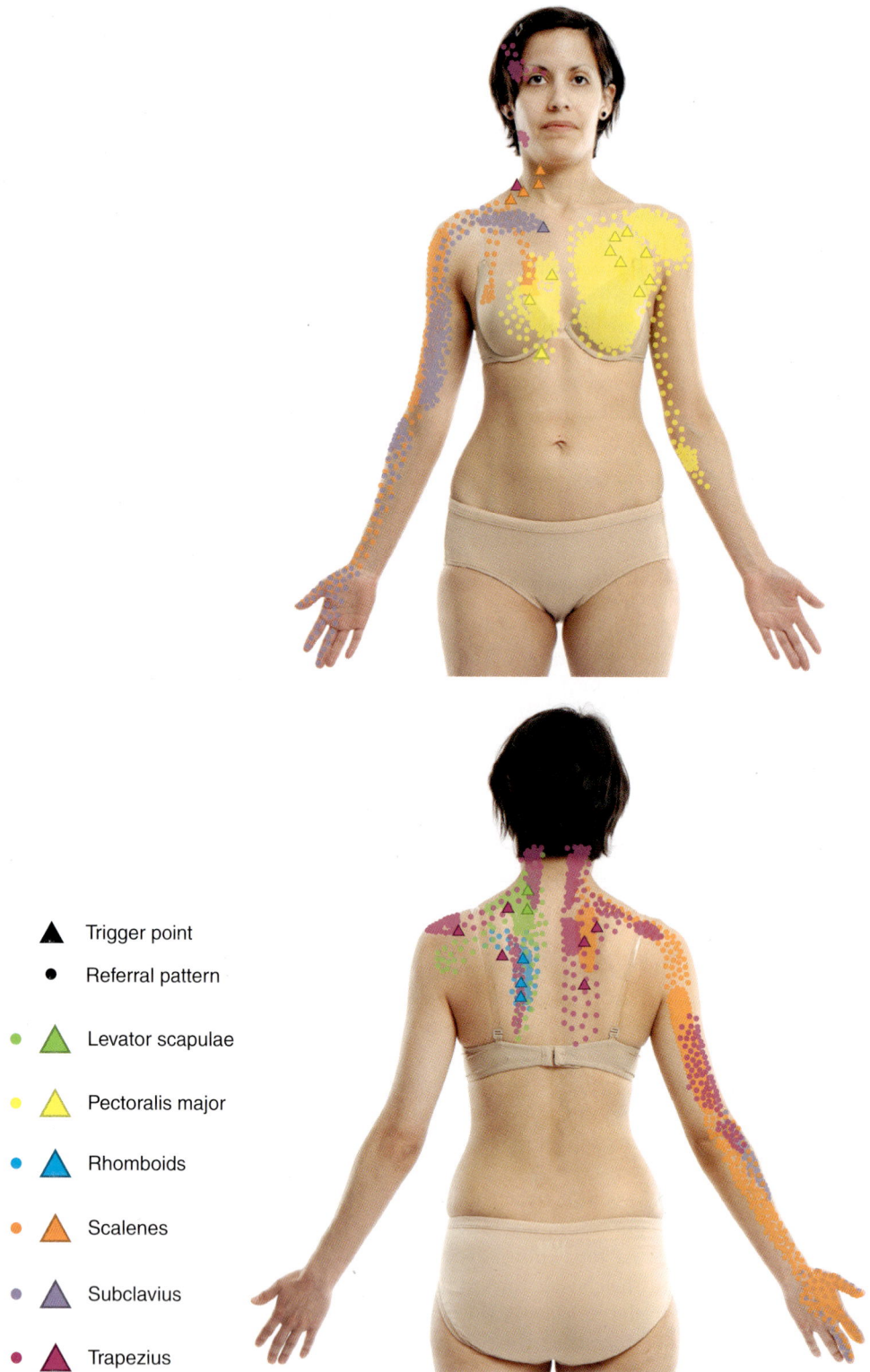

Trigger point

Referral pattern

Levator scapulae

Pectoralis major

Rhomboids

Scalenes

Subclavius

Trapezius

Figure 4-8   **Common trigger points associated with hyperkyphosis and their referral patterns.**

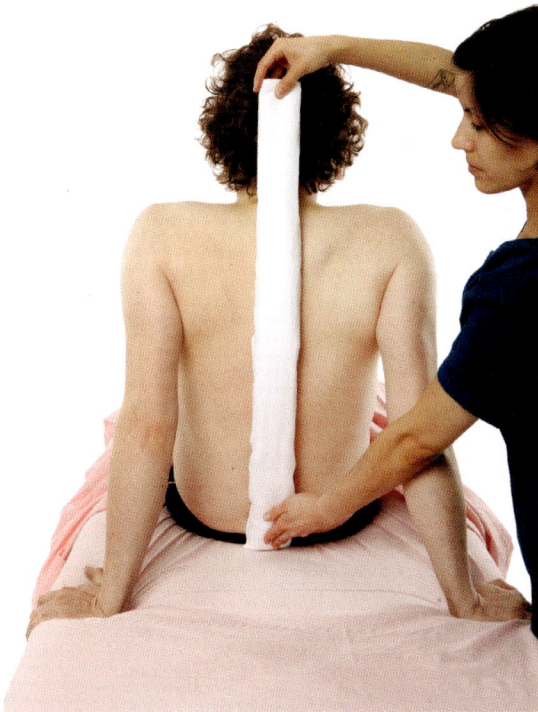

Figure 4-9   Bolster in supine position. Position the bolster along the spine before the client lays supine. Either use a bolster that is long enough to cradle the head, or use a small, folded towel or pillow case under the occiput so that the neck is not hyperextended.

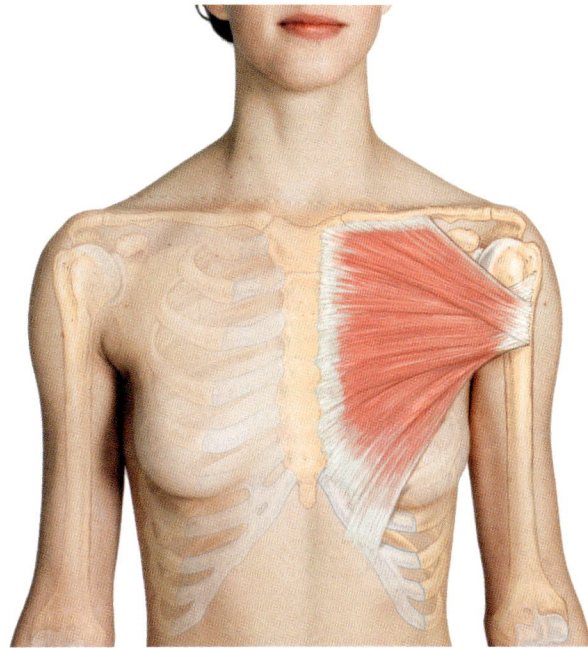

PECTORALIS MAJOR

Origin	Medial half of clavicle, sternum, and cartilage of ribs 1 to 6.
Insertion	Crest of greater tubercle of humerus.
Action	**All fibers** adduct shoulder, internally rotate shoulder, assist in elevating thorax in forced inspiration; **upper fibers** flex shoulder, horizontally adduct shoulder; **lower fibers** extend shoulder.
Nerve	Medial and lateral pectoral.

Figure 4-10   Pectoralis major. Short, tight pectorals contribute to the internal rotation of the shoulders. Adapted from Clay JH, Pounds DM. *Basic Clinical Massage Therapy: Integrating Anatomy and Treatment,* 2nd ed. Philadelphia: Lippincott Williams & Wilkins, 2008.

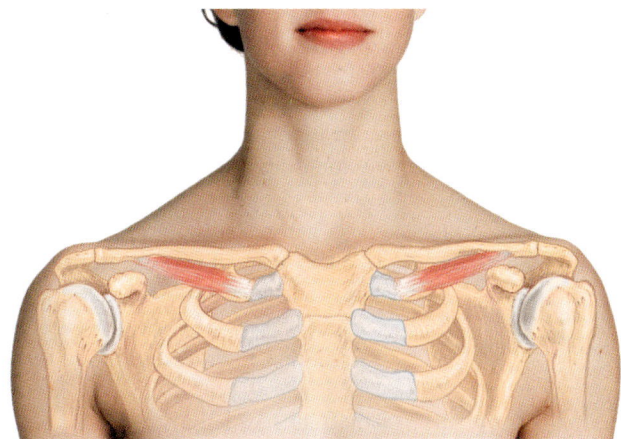

SUBCLAVIUS

Origin	First rib and costal cartilage.
Insertion	Inferior, lateral aspect of clavicle.
Action	Draws rib inferiorly and anteriorly, elevates first rib in inhalation.
Nerve	Subclavian.

Figure 4-11   Subclavius. The subclavius may be adhered and hypertonic when the thorax is flexed. Adapted from Clay JH, Pounds DM. *Basic Clinical Massage Therapy: Integrating Anatomy and Treatment,* 2nd ed. Philadelphia: Lippincott Williams & Wilkins, 2008.

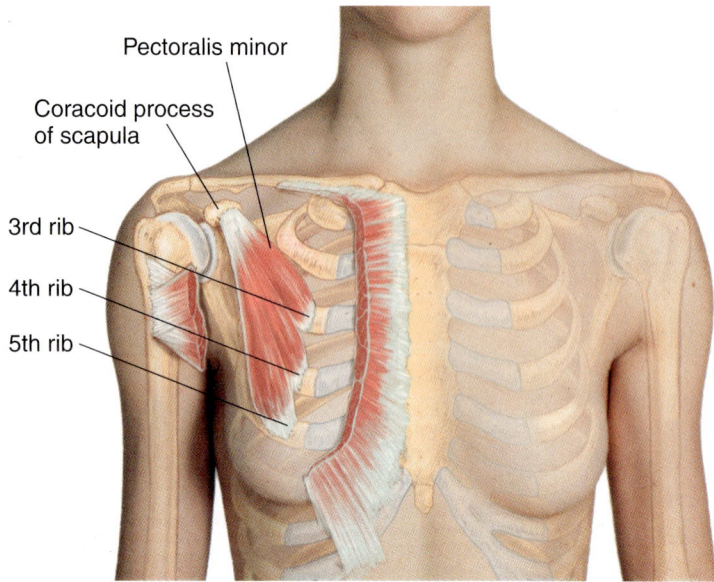

Pectoralis minor

Coracoid process
of scapula

3rd rib

4th rib

5th rib

PECTORALIS MINOR

Origin	*Third, fourth, and fifth ribs.*
Insertion	*Coracoid process.*
Action	*Depress scapula, protract scapula, tilt scapula anterior, assist in inhalation.*
Nerve	*Medial pectoral.*

Figure 4-12 **Pectoralis minor.** The pectoralis minor may be shortened if the scapulae are protracted. Figs. 4-12, 4-13, and 4-14 adapted from Clay JH, Pounds DM. *Basic Clinical Massage Therapy: Integrating Anatomy and Treatment,* 2nd ed. Philadelphia: Lippincott Williams & Wilkins, 2008.

your shoulder, which will gently lift the pectoralis major out of the way. This is also preferable to externally rotating the shoulder, which would put tension on a shortened pectoralis major. Once you have found the pectoralis minor, ask the client to depress his or her shoulder and feel for a contraction. If you are palpating through the pectoralis major, you may also feel it contract.

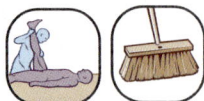

- If you treat myofascial restrictions, hypertonicity, and trigger points in the pectoral area, perform a full stretch to the pectorals, and close with clearing strokes. If you found the area to be only minimally affected, close with clearing strokes.

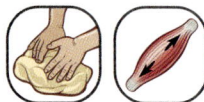

- Assess the anterior deltoid for hypertonicity (Fig. 4-13). Warm the tissues and lengthen them from the clavicle toward the deltoid tuberosity to reduce the internal rotation of the shoulder.

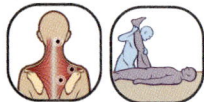

- Treat any trigger points found, and stretch the anterior deltoid using external rotation or by extending the shoulder off the edge of the table.

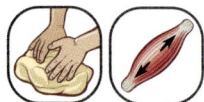

- With the head turned slightly away from the side you are treating, warm and lengthen the superficial neck muscles, particularly the upper trapezius, from the occiput to the acromion process (Fig. 4-14). Be very careful not to work in the endangerment areas. Avoid direct compression to nerves and blood vessels, and back away gently if you feel a pulse.

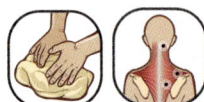

- Soften then lengthen the levator scapulae, splenius capitis, splenius cervicis, the suboccipitals, and the cervical erector spinae (Fig. 4-15). Treat any trigger points as necessary. Hooking your fingers under the occiput and gently rocking the head into minimal flexion and extension is an effective way of releasing the suboccipitals.

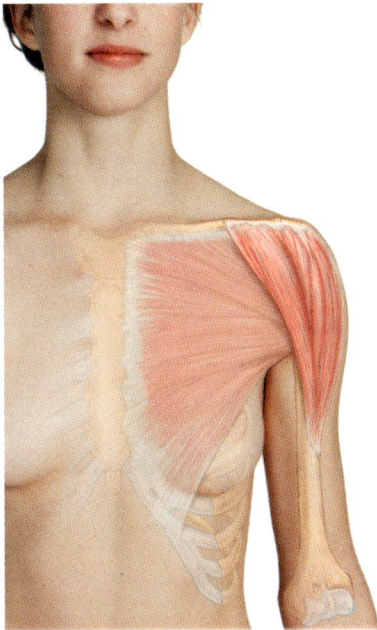

ANTERIOR DELTOID

Origin	Lateral third of clavicle, acromion process, spine of scapula.
Insertion	Deltoid tuberosity.
Action	**All fibers** abduct shoulder; **anterior fibers** flex shoulder, internally rotate shoulder, horizontally adduct shoulder; **posterior fibers** extend shoulder, externally rotate shoulder, horizontally adduct shoulder.
Nerve	Axillary nerve.

Figure 4-13 **Anterior deltoid.** The anterior deltoid may be short and tight if the shoulder is internally rotated.

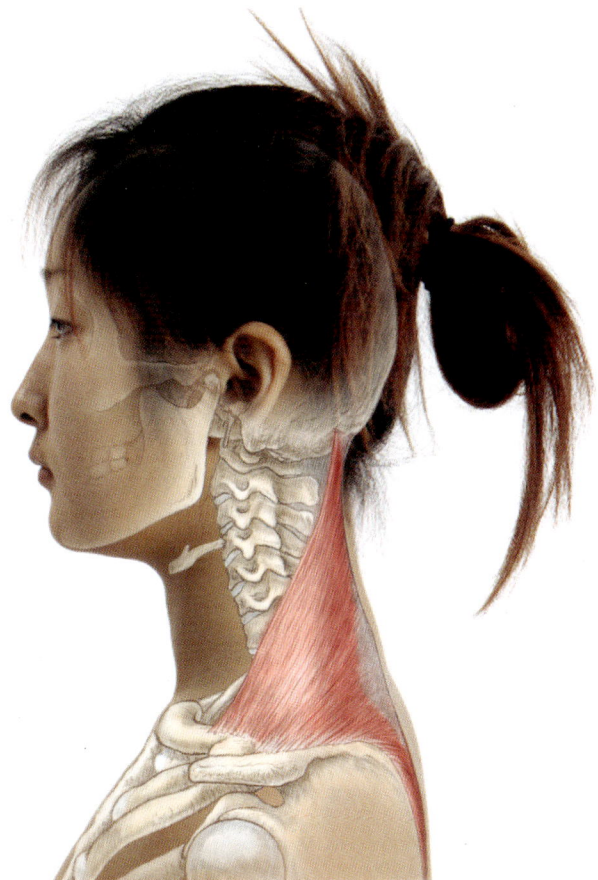

UPPER TRAPEZIUS

Origin	External occipital protuberance, medial superior nuchal line of occiput, ligamentum nuchae.
Insertion	Lateral third of clavicle, acromion process.
Action	**Bilaterally**: extend neck and head; **unilaterally**: ipsilateral lateral flexion of neck and head, contralateral rotation of neck and head, elevate scapula, upwardly rotate scapula.
Nerve	Spinal accessory and cervical plexus.

Figure 4-14 **Upper trapezius.** Treat the superficial upper trapezius before accessing the deeper neck muscles.

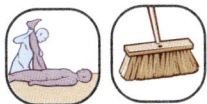

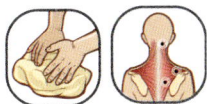

- If you treat hypertonicity and trigger points in the posterior neck muscles, perform a full stretch, and close with clearing strokes.

- Release the SCM; using pincer grip petrissage along its length is often effective. Treat trigger points if found. Trigger points in the SCM may cause vertigo, nausea, or ringing in the ears. Ask your client to let you know if any unusual sensations are felt, and reduce your pressure if necessary.

- Once you have softened the SCM and trapezius, you will have greater access to the scalenes (Fig. 4-16). To access the anterior scalene, gently push the SCM medially with one or two fingertips as you feel for the deeper scalenes. As you move the SCM medially, your fingers should be gently resting on the soft tissue covering the transverse processes of the cervical vertebrae. Use this as your guide for treating the anterior scalene. Once you have found it, ask the client to take a quick, forced breath into his or her chest, and feel for a contraction.

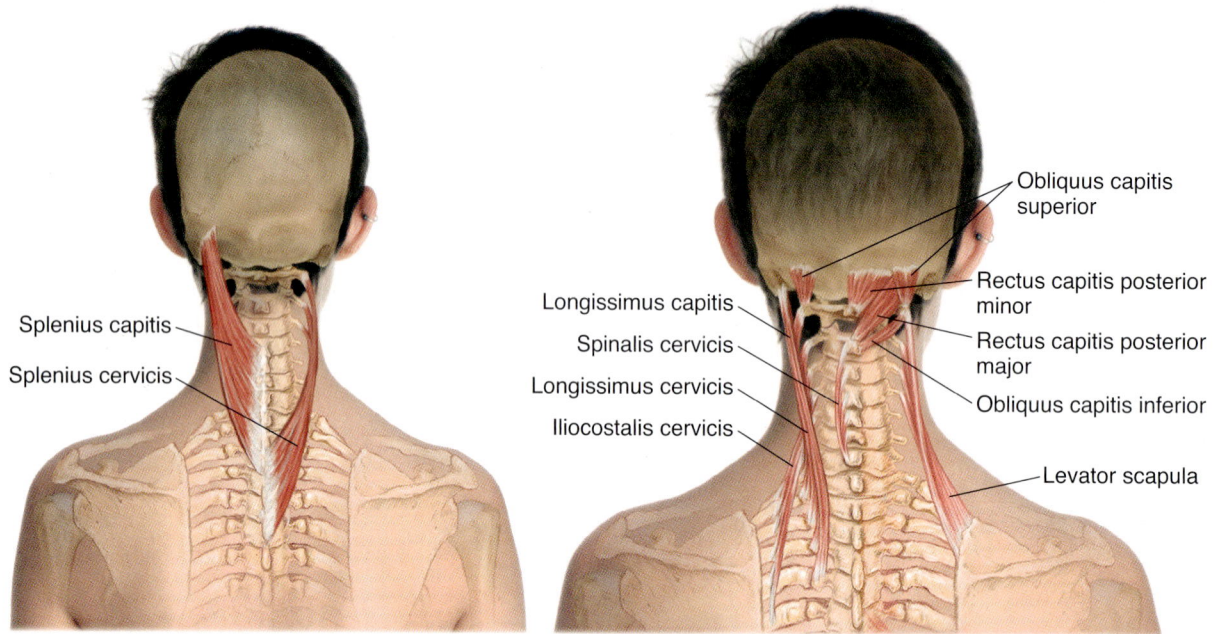

SPLENIUS CAPITIS

Origin	Ligamentum nuchae, SP of C7–T3.
Insertion	Mastoid process and lateral superior nuchal line of occiput.
Action	**Bilaterally:** extend neck and head; **unilaterally:** ipsilateral rotation and lateral flexion of head and neck.
Nerve	Branch of dorsal division of cervical nerves.

SPLENIUS CERVICIS

Origin	SP of T3–6.
Insertion	TVP of upper cervical vertibrae.
Action	**Bilaterally:** extend neck and head; **unilaterally:** ipsilateral rotation and lateral flexion of head and neck.
Nerve	Branch of dorsal division of cervical nerves.

LEVATOR SCAPULA

Origin	TVP of C1–4.
Insertion	Upper, medial border and superior angle of scapula.
Action	**Bilaterally:** extend neck and head; **unilaterally:** elevate scapula, downward rotation of scapula, lateral flexion of neck and head, ipsilateral rotation of neck and head.
Nerve	Dorsal scapular and cervical nerves.

SUBOCCIPITALS

Origin	SPs and TVPs of C1–2.
Insertion	Nuchal lines of occiput and TVP of C1.
Action	**Bilaterally:** tilt the head into extension, **unilaterally:** ipsilateral rotation of head.
Nerve	Suboccipital.

CERVICAL ERECTOR SPINAE: SPINALIS; LONGISSIMUS, ILIOCOSTALIS

Origins	Ligamentum nuchae, SP C7; TVPs T1–5; posterior ribs 1–12.
Insertion	SPs of C2–7; TVP C1–7, mastoid process; TVPs of lower cervicals.
Action	**Bilaterally:** extend vertebral column; **unilaterally:** ipsilateral lateral flexion.
Nerve	Dorsal primary divisions of spinal nerves.

Figure 4-15 Posterior neck muscles. Posterior neck muscles may be short and tight with an extension of the neck. Figs. 4-15 and 4-16, adapted from Clay JH, Pounds DM. *Basic Clinical Massage Therapy: Integrating Anatomy and Treatment,* 2nd ed. Philadelphia: Lippincott Williams & Wilkins, 2008.

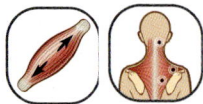

■ Lengthen the anterior scalene from the transverse processes to the first rib. Treat any trigger points found with muscle stripping and compression. It is often helpful once you have found a trigger point in the scalenes to compress it gently while slowly rotating the head ipsilaterally. Trigger points in the anterior scalene are often quite sensitive, and the client may feel cautious when you work deeply in the neck. Begin gently so as not to frighten the client or cause him or her to jerk the head. Remember that you are working in an area that is filled with nerves and vasculature. Trigger points in the scalenes may radiate across the top of the shoulder and into the arm, hand, and fingers. If the client also has thoracic outlet syndrome, symptoms may appear. Reduce your pressure, and realign the neck if necessary.

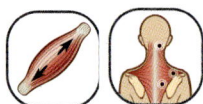

■ Find the middle and posterior scalenes by gently palpating the transverse processes and then moving slightly posterior. The middle scalene crosses the transverse processes as it heads toward the first rib. The posterior scalene is posterior to the middle scalene, and runs inferiorly toward the second rib. Once you have found them, ask the client to take a quick, forced breath into his or her chest, and feel for a contraction. Take the same cautions with the

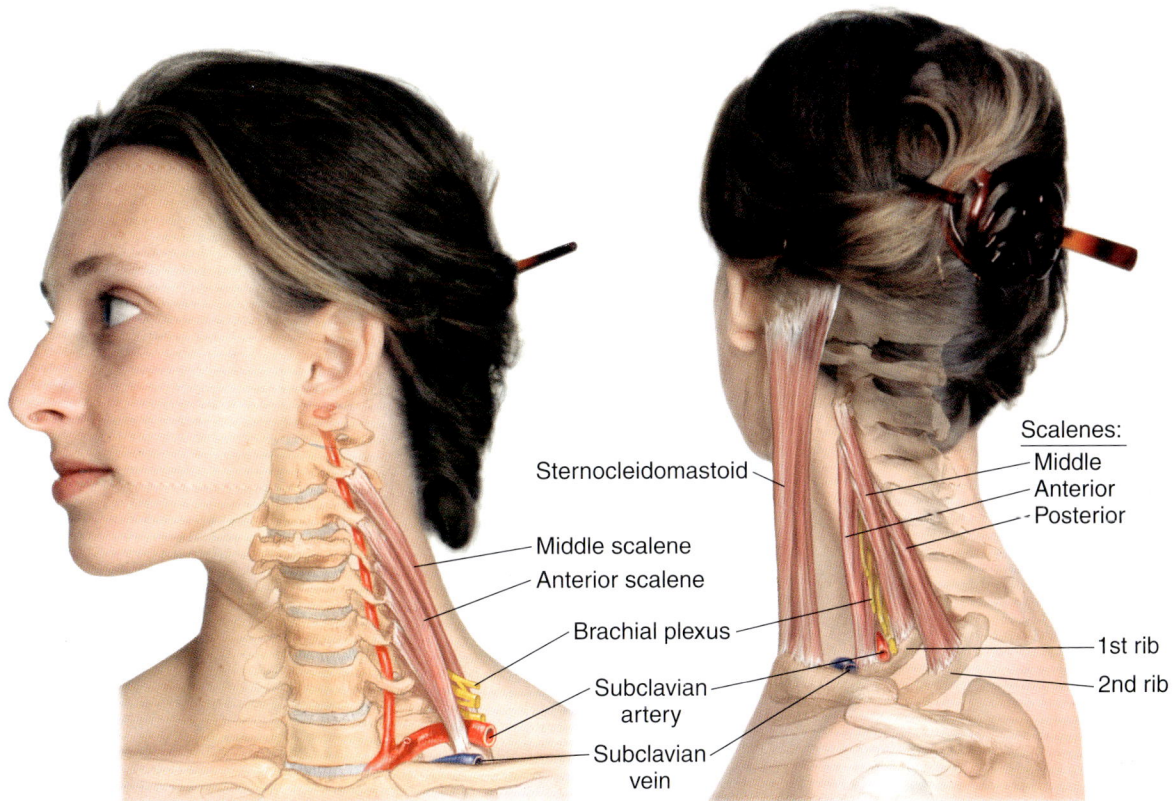

SCALENES

Origin	Anterior-TVP 3–6, middle-TVP 2–7, posterior-TVP 5–6.
Insertion	**Anterior**, 1st rib; **middle**, 1st rib; **posterior**, 2nd rib.
Action	**Unilateral**, ipsilateral lateral flexion and rotation of head and neck; **bilateral**, elevate ribs in inhalation and flex head and neck.
Nerve	Cervical.

STERNOCLEIDOMASTOID

Origin	Top of manubrium and medial third of clavicle.
Insertion	Mastoid process and superior nuchal line.
Action	**Unilateral**, ipsilateral lateral flexion and rotation of head and neck; **bilateral**, flexion of the neck, assist in inhalation.
Nerve	Spinal accessory XI.

Figure 4-16 **SCM and scalenes.** The SCM and scalenes may be short and tight with the head-forward posture.

middle and posterior scalenes as you did with the anterior scalene. Lengthen the muscles, and treat trigger points if found.

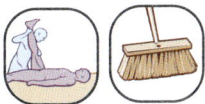

■ If you treat trigger points, stretch the scalenes by increasing the distance between their origins and insertions. Options for stretching include contralateral lateral flexion and ipsilateral rotation. If you found no trigger points, use clearing strokes, and turn the client into the prone position.

■ Turn the client to the prone position, and use rolled towels to bolster the shoulders. This will keep the pectorals lengthened, retract the scapulae, and reduce any stretch on the rhomboids and middle trapezius. The bolster should be placed under the shoulder and a few inches of the humerus to avoid adding tension to the joints.

■ Adjust the face cradle to reduce flexion in the cervical spine. If you see a crease in the skin on the back of the neck, lower the head rest slightly as long as this is comfortable for the client.

■ Reduce adhesions between the scapulae. These are commonly found around the superior angle of the scapula, at the vertebrae, and at the intersection of the lower trapezius and latissimus dorsi (Fig. 4-17).

■ When treating the middle trapezius and rhomboids, apply strokes from the scapula toward the spine. Remember that these muscles are often overstretched in hyperkyphosis. Stripping in the opposite direction may lengthen the already overstretched muscles.

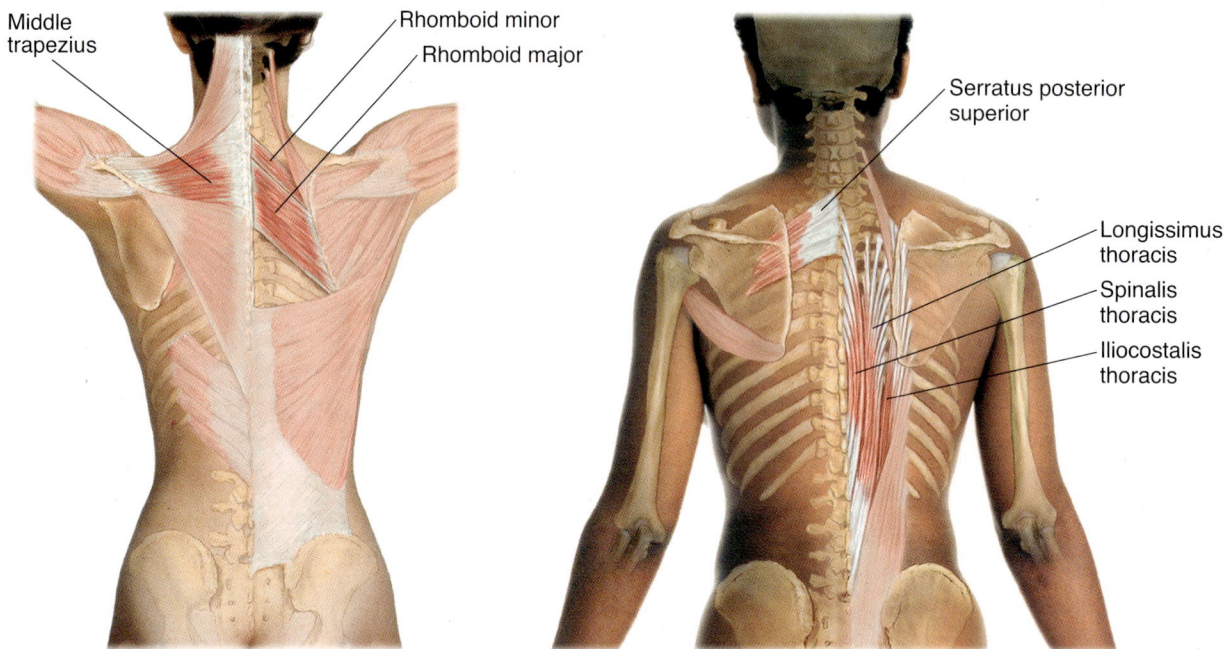

Middle trapezius

Rhomboid minor

Rhomboid major

Serratus posterior superior

Longissimus thoracis

Spinalis thoracis

Iliocostalis thoracis

MIDDLE TRAPEZIUS

Origin	SP of C6–T3.
Insertion	Acromion process and spine of scapula.
Action	Adduct and stabilize scapula.
Nerve	Spinal accessory and cervical plexus.

RHOMBOIDS

Origin	**Major**, SP T2–5; **minor**, SP C7–T1.
Insertion	**Major**, medial border of scapula between spine and inferior angle; **minor**, upper, medial border of scapula.
Action	Adduct, elevate, and downwardly rotate scapula.
Nerve	Dorsal scapular from brachial plexus.

SERRATUS POSTERIOR SUPERIOR

Origin	SP C7–T3.
Insertion	Posterior surface of ribs 2–5.
Action	Elevate ribs during inhalation.
Nerve	Spinal nerves I–IV.

THORACIC ERECTOR SPINAE

Origin	**Spinalis**, SP C7–L1; **longissimus**, common tendon; **iliocostalis**, ribs 1–12.
Insertion	**Spinalis**, SP thoracic vertebrae; **longissimus**, lower 9 ribs and TVP thoracic vertebrae; **iliocostalis**, ribs 1–6.
Action	**Unilateral**, ipsilateral lateral flexion of thorax; **bilateral**, extend thorax.
Nerve	Dorsal divisions of spinal nerves.

Figure 4-17 Middle trapezius, rhomboids, serratus posterior superior, and thoracic erector spinae. The middle trapezius, rhomboids, serratus posterior superior, and thoracic erector spinae may be overstretched and weak with protraction of the scapulae and thoracic flexion. Figs. 4-17, 4-18, and 4-19 adapted from Clay JH, Pounds DM. *Basic Clinical Massage Therapy: Integrating Anatomy and Treatment,* 2nd ed. Philadelphia: Lippincott Williams & Wilkins, 2008.

■ When treating the deeper thoracic erector spinae, cross fiber strokes may help separate adhered tissues. Apply strokes from superior to inferior to encourage thoracic extension.

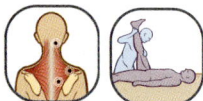

■ Assess the rhomboids, middle trapezius, and thoracic erector spinae for trigger points. It may be difficult to use compression on the erectors because of their rope-like texture. Try to isolate the trigger point and stabilize the tissue with one hand while you compress with the other to keep it from continually rolling away from your pressure. If you treat trigger points in these muscles, use a pin and stretch technique to lengthen only the affected area to avoid stretching the full muscle.

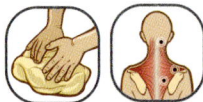

■ Assess the teres major, serratus anterior, and latissimus dorsi for hypertonicity and trigger points and treat if necessary (Fig. 4-18).

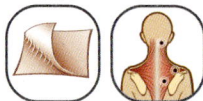

■ Assess the infraspinatus and teres minor for adhesions and trigger points and treat if necessary (Fig. 4-19).

■ If you have time, consider the other possible conditions that may develop with hyperkyphosis, and treat these areas. Tension headaches suggest additional treatment to the head, tem-

Anterior view of scapula
Attachment site of serratus anterior to anterior, medial edge of scapula

Attachment of latissimus dorsi to medial lip of bicipital groove of humerus

Serratus anterior

2
3
4
5
6
7
8
9

Latissimus dorsi

Teres major

T-7

T-12

Sacrum
Iliac crest

SERRATUS ANTERIOR

Origin	Lateral surface of upper 8 or 9 ribs.
Insertion	Anterior surface of medial border of scapula.
Action	Abduct and depress scapula, stabilize scapula against rib cage, forced inhalation.
Nerve	Long thoracic.

LATISSIMUS DORSI

Origin	SP of T7–12, ribs 8–12, thoracolumbar aponeurosis, and posterior iliac crest.
Insertion	Crest of lesser tubercle of humerus.
Action	Extend, adduct, and medially rotate shoulder.
Nerve	Thoracodorsal.

TERES MAJOR

Origin	Lateral, inferior angle and lateral border of scapula.
Insertion	Crest of lesser tubercle of humerus.
Action	Extend, adduct, and medially rotate shoulder.
Nerve	Lower subscapular.

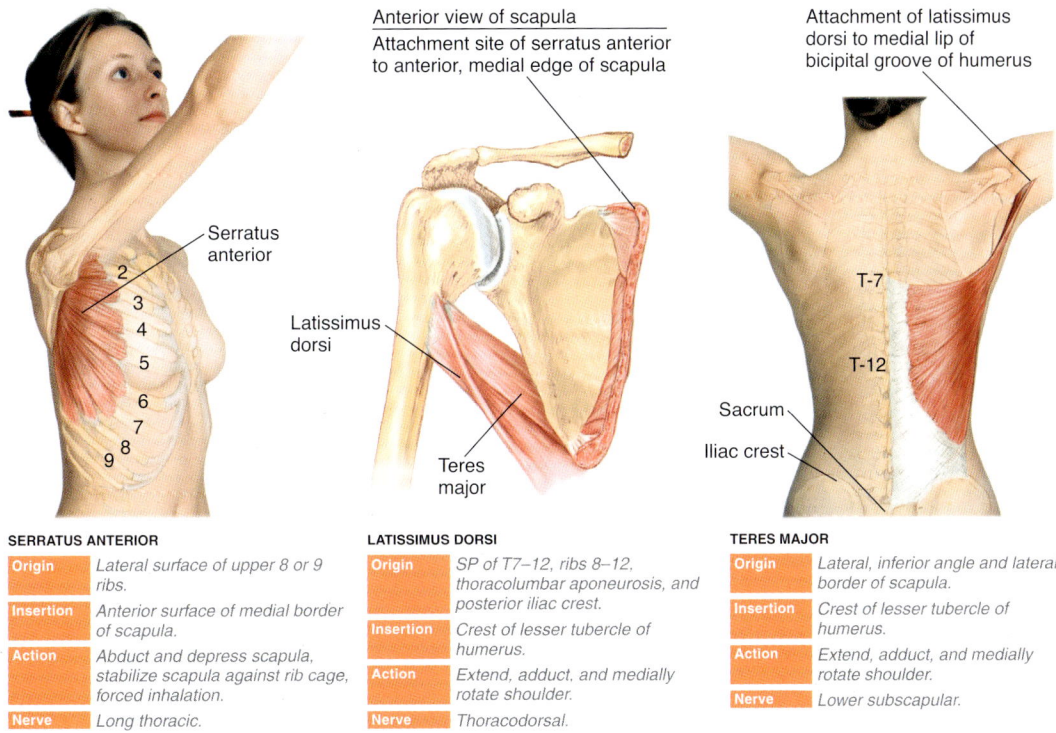

Figure 4-18   Teres major, latissimus dorsi, and serratus anterior. The teres major, latissimus dorsi, and serratus anterior may become hypertonic with hyperkyphosis.

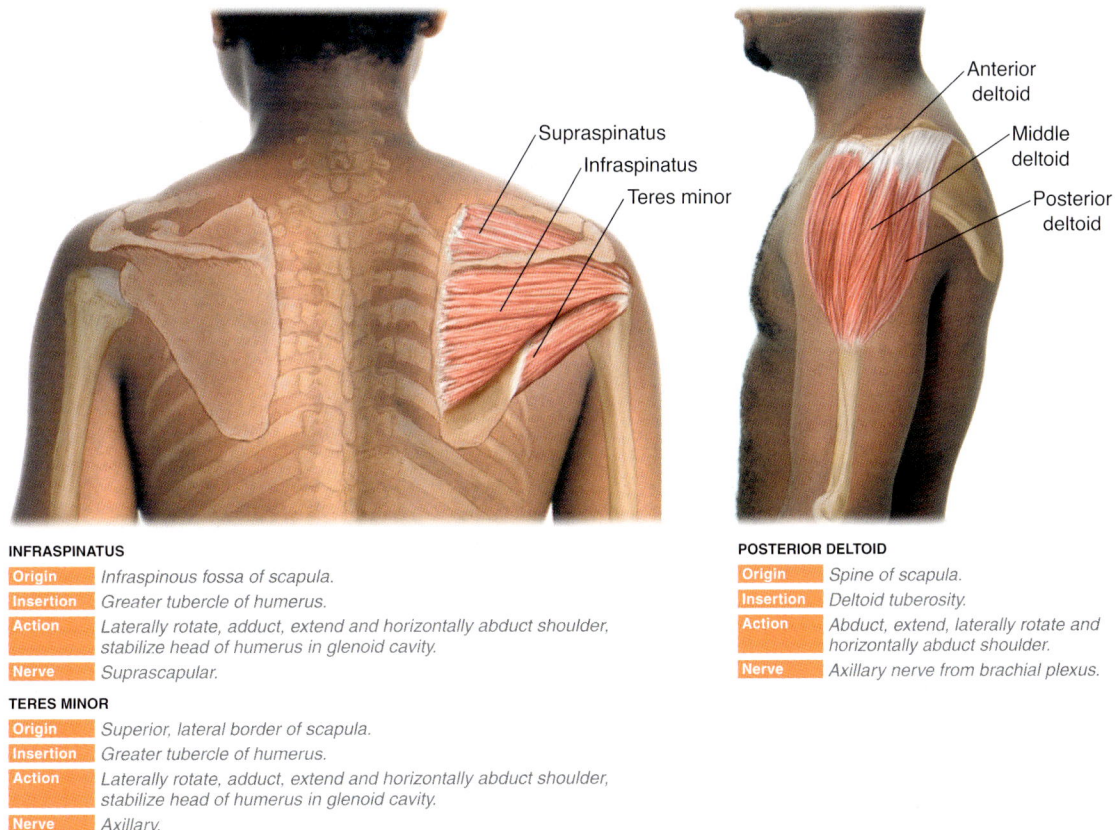

Supraspinatus
Infraspinatus
Teres minor

Anterior deltoid
Middle deltoid
Posterior deltoid

INFRASPINATUS

Origin	Infraspinous fossa of scapula.
Insertion	Greater tubercle of humerus.
Action	Laterally rotate, adduct, extend and horizontally abduct shoulder, stabilize head of humerus in glenoid cavity.
Nerve	Suprascapular.

TERES MINOR

Origin	Superior, lateral border of scapula.
Insertion	Greater tubercle of humerus.
Action	Laterally rotate, adduct, extend and horizontally abduct shoulder, stabilize head of humerus in glenoid cavity.
Nerve	Axillary.

POSTERIOR DELTOID

Origin	Spine of scapula.
Insertion	Deltoid tuberosity.
Action	Abduct, extend, laterally rotate and horizontally abduct shoulder.
Nerve	Axillary nerve from brachial plexus.

Figure 4-19   Infraspinatus, teres minor, and posterior deltoid. The infraspinatus, teres minor, and posterior deltoid may become overstretched with internal rotation of the shoulder.

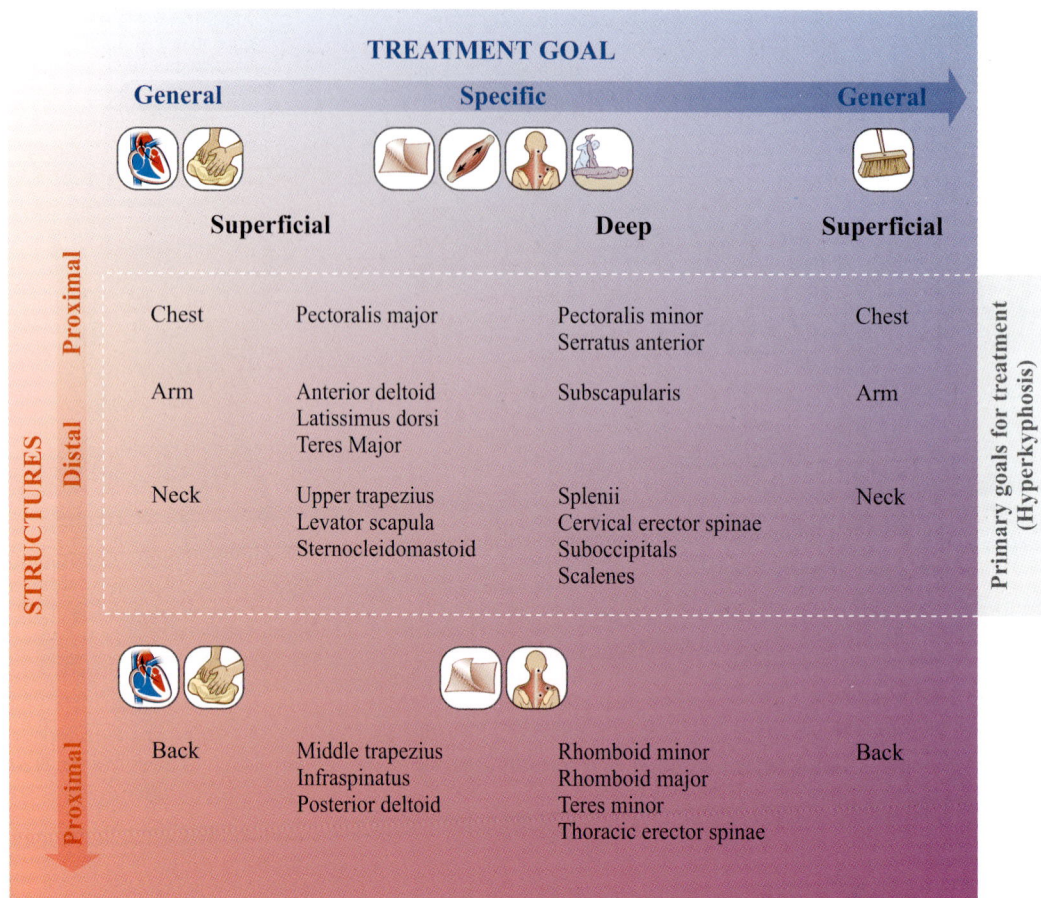

TREATMENT GOAL

General	Specific			General

	Superficial	Deep	Superficial
Proximal Chest	Pectoralis major	Pectoralis minor Serratus anterior	Chest
Proximal Arm	Anterior deltoid Latissimus dorsi Teres Major	Subscapularis	Arm
Distal Neck	Upper trapezius Levator scapula Sternocleidomastoid	Splenii Cervical erector spinae Suboccipitals Scalenes	Neck
Proximal Back	Middle trapezius Infraspinatus Posterior deltoid	Rhomboid minor Rhomboid major Teres minor Thoracic erector spinae	Back

STRUCTURES

Primary goals for treatment (Hyperkyphosis)

Figure 4-20 **Hyperkyphosis treatment overview diagram.** Follow the general principles from left to right or top to bottom when treating hyperkyphosis.

poromandibular joint dysfunction to the jaw, thoracic outlet syndrome to the affected limb, and hyperlordosis to the hip flexors and lumbar erectors. You may not have time to treat all of these fully, but you can give some attention to them in each session as time permits. As the signs and symptoms of hyperkyphosis decrease, you can increase the amount of time you spend on other pain patterns or restrictions in ROM.

■ End with clearing strokes to the full back.

The Treatment Overview diagram summarizes the flow of treatment (Fig. 4-20).

CLIENT SELF-CARE

Avoiding further injury is a primary concern when recommending self-care. Self-care for a client with structural hyperkyphosis should be planned with the client's health care provider. Reducing or eliminating habitual offending activities and other perpetuating factors is crucial for long-term relief of pain related to functional hyperkyphosis. The client with functional hyperkyphosis must learn to recognize when he or she is holding the affected muscle in a shortened position and which of his or her activities of daily living is putting undue stress on the joints and the muscles that cross them. You can help clients learn how to modify such activities to avoid overstressing the affected structures. The following are intended as general recommendations for stretching and strengthening the muscles involved in hyperkyphosis. The objective is to create distance between the attachment sites of muscles that have shortened and to perform repetitions of movements that decrease the distance between the attachments of muscles that have weakened. If you have had no training in remedial exercises and do not feel that you have a functional understanding of stretching and strengthening, refer the client to a professional with training in this area.

Clients often neglect self-care because their daily lives are busy. Encourage them to follow these guidelines:

- Instruct the client to perform self-care activities throughout the day, such as while taking a phone call, reading e-mail, watching television, or during other activities of daily living instead of setting aside extra time.
- Encourage the client to take regular breaks from repetitive actions. Demonstrate gentle self-massage to keep adhesions and hypertonicity at bay between treatments.
- Instruct the client on proper posture in the seated position to keep pressure off the weakened joints.
- Instruct an athlete who is strengthening the pectorals more regularly than he or she is strengthening the rhomboid and middle trapezius to reduce pectoral resistance exercises and increase scapular retraction and thoracic extension to balance strength in the thoracic area.
- Instruct a client who regularly performs heavy lifting to lift with the legs instead of the back.
- Demonstrate all strengthening exercises and stretches to your client and have him or her perform these in your presence before leaving to ensure that he or she is performing them properly and will not harm himself or herself when practicing alone. Stretches should be held for 15–30 seconds and performed frequently throughout the day within the client's limits. The client should not force the stretch. It should be slow and gentle, trying to keep other muscles as relaxed as possible.

Stretching

Instruct the client to stretch the pectoralis major and minor by standing in a doorway with the hands on the frame while stepping forward to bring the arms slightly posterior (Fig. 4-21). It is essential that he or she step rather than lean forward, because leaning will affect the muscles of the neck, back, and hips. The stretch is best performed with the spine straight. The client can raise the hands above the head on the doorway to stretch the lower fibers, at the level of the shoulder to stretch the middle fibers, and below the hips to stretch the upper fibers.

As an alternative stretch that the client can perform during work hours, while reading an e-mail or during a conference call, instruct the client to clasp the fingers behind the head (moderate stretch) or rest the fingers behind the ears (deeper stretch) while drawing the elbows posteriorly within his or her range of comfort (Fig. 4-22). This will also retract the scapulae and reduce the stretch on the rhomboids and middle trapezius.

To stretch the posterior neck muscles, instruct your client to let the head hang so that the chin approaches the chest, without flexing the thoracic spine (Fig. 4-23). The client should not actively force the chin to touch the chest. If he or she wants to increase the stretch, he or she can rest the hands on the back of the head and allow the weight of the arms to gently pull the chin toward the chest. It may help to gently rotate the flexed neck from side to side so that the chin is parallel to the shoulder on either side. Although, for some, it may feel good to include cervical extension into the stretch, this is not advised if the client is at risk for nerve compression or disc herniation. Even in the absence of disc disease or nerve compression, one rotation in extension may be performed after several side-to-side rotations in flexion, but do not instruct the client to do a full, repeated circumduction of the head.

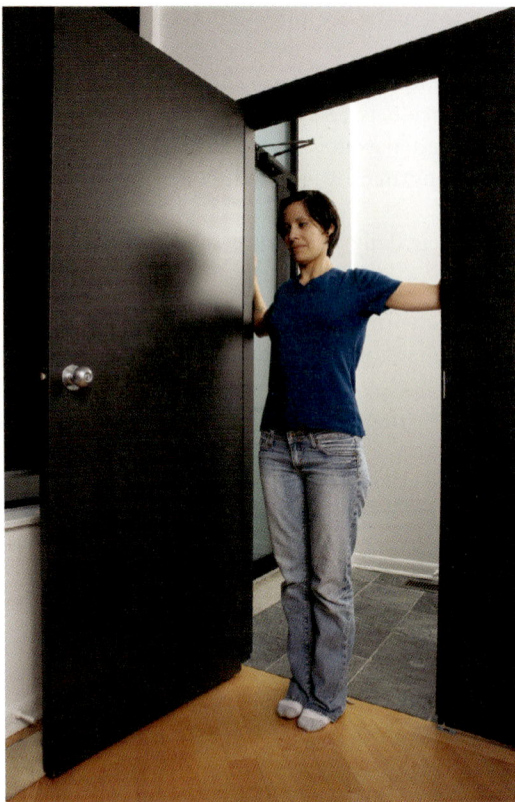

Figure 4-21   **Doorway pectoral stretch.** Instruct the client to step forward rather than lean forward.

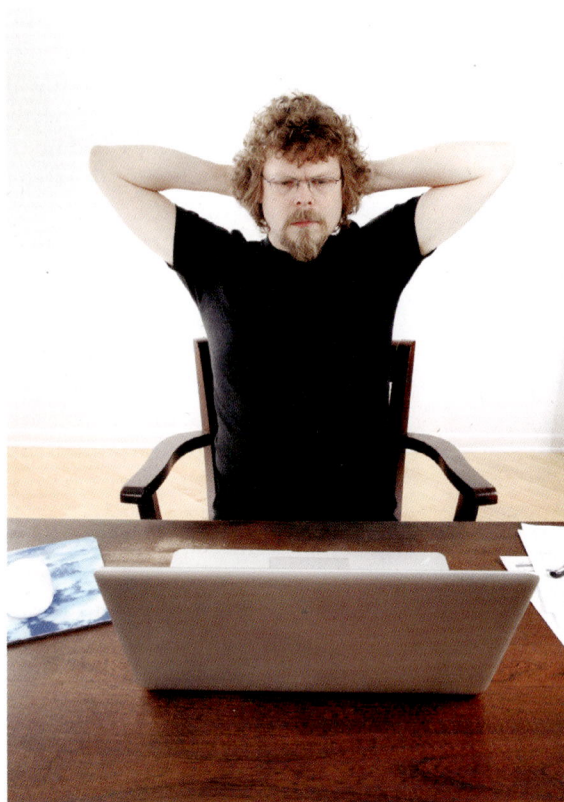

Figure 4-22   **Seated pectoral stretch.** Instruct the client to clasp the fingers together behind the head and gently draw the elbows back.

Strengthening

The client should also strengthen the middle trapezius, rhomboids, and thoracic erector spinae in order to efficiently antagonize protraction of the scapula and flexion of the thorax.

Instruct the client to sit or stand while squeezing the scapulae together (Fig. 4-24). When this is done properly, only the scapulae should retract, and the shoulders should be relaxed. Hold each contraction for 5–10 seconds with 3–5 seconds of rest between contractions. Perform 10 repetitions or as many as are comfortable before feeling fatigue or weakness.

Instruct the client to strengthen the thoracic erector spinae by resting his or her hands behind the head in either a seated or prone position while extending the thoracic spine within his or her limits.

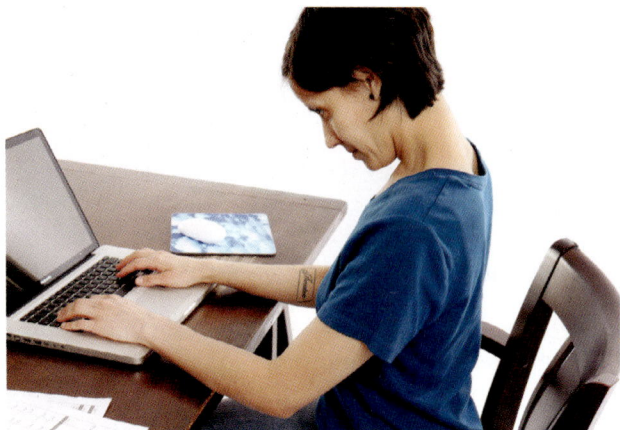

Figure 4-23   **Cervical extensor stretch.** Instruct the client to let the head hang without any force.

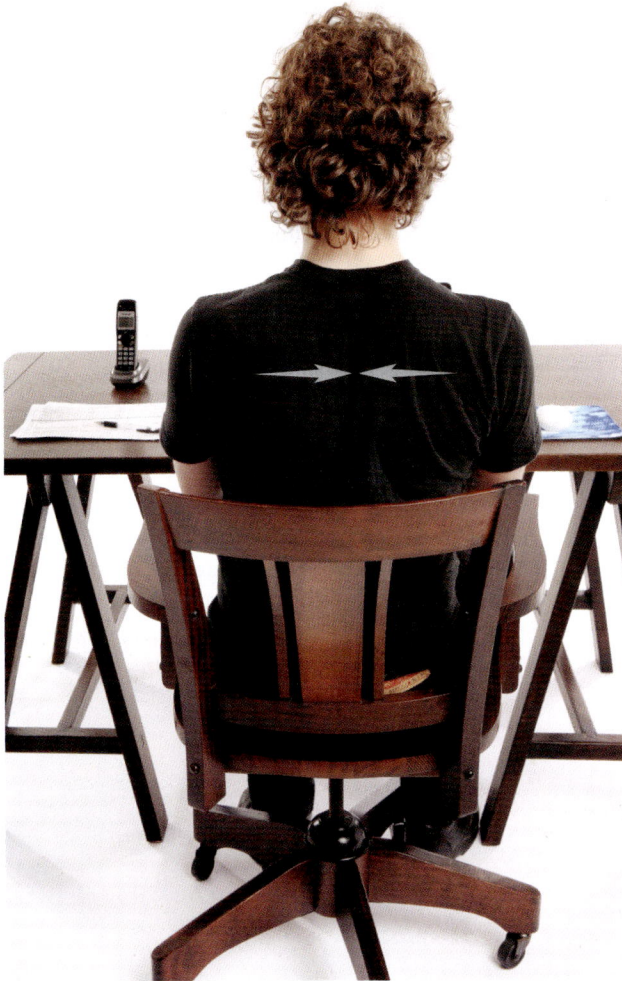

Figure 4-24   Middle trapezius and rhomboid strengthening.
Instruct the client to squeeze the scapulae together without using any
muscles other than middle trapezius and rhomboids.

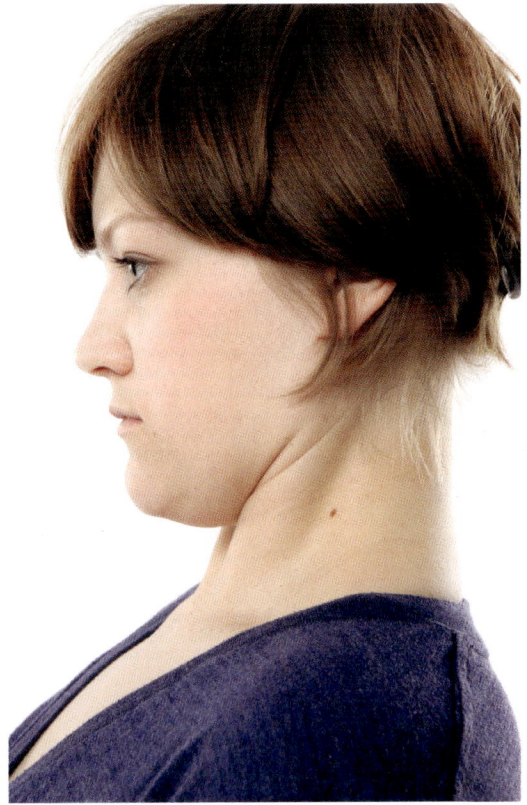

Figure 4-25   Strengthening the deep neck flexors.
Instruct the client to draw the chin inward.

The client can work toward reducing the head-forward posture by tucking the chin inward
(Fig. 4-25). The act of retracting the neck and head may also reduce thoracic flexion. Hold the
posture for about 5–10 seconds with 3–5 seconds of rest between contractions. Perform 10 repetitions or as many as are comfortable before feeling fatigue or weakness in the neck.

SUGGESTIONS FOR FURTHER TREATMENT

Ideally, a client developing hyperkyphosis will have treatments once a week until symptoms are
absent for at least 7 days. A client with more severe signs and symptoms is best treated twice per
week until signs of improvement occur, such as improvement in ROM and reduction in hypertonicity and pain. Reduce frequency to once per week until symptoms are absent for at least
7 days. When the client reports that he or she has been pain-free for up to 7 days, treatment can be
reduced to twice per month. If the client is pain-free for 2 or more weeks at a time, he or she can
then schedule an appointment once per month or as necessary. With functional hyperkyphosis,
there should be some improvement with each session. If this is not happening, consider the following possibilities:

- There is too much time between treatments. It is always best to give the newly treated tissues
  24–48 hours to adapt, but if too much time passes between treatments in the beginning, the
  client's activities of daily living may reverse any progress.

- The client is not adjusting his or her activities of daily living or is not keeping up with self-care. As much as we want to fix the problem, we cannot force a client to make the adjustments we suggest. Explain the importance of the client's participation in the healing process, and encourage the client to follow your recommendations, but be careful not to judge or reprimand a client who does not.
- The condition is advanced or involves other musculoskeletal complications that are beyond your basic training. Refer this client to a massage therapist with advanced training. Continuing to treat a client whose case is beyond your scope could hinder healing and turn the client away from massage therapy altogether.
- The hyperkyphosis is structural or there is an undiagnosed, underlying condition. Discontinue treatment until the client sees a health care provider for a medical assessment. Discuss the medical assessment with the client's health care provider to determine cautions or contraindications for future treatments.

If you are not treating the client in a clinical setting or private practice, you may not be able to take this client through the full program of healing. Still, if you can bring some relief, it may encourage the client to discuss this change with his or her health care provider and seek manual therapy rather than more aggressive treatment options. If the client agrees to return for regular treatments, the symptoms are likely to change each time, so it is important to perform an assessment before each session. Once you have released superficial tissues in general areas, you may be able to focus more of your treatment on a specific area. Likewise, once you have treated the structures specific to hyperkyphosis, you may be able to pay closer attention to compensating structures and coexisting conditions.

PROFESSIONAL GROWTH

CASE STUDY

Seth is a 26-year-old recording engineer. He works an average of 50 hours per week, usually beginning in the late afternoon and finishing well after midnight. Seth rides his bicycle 6 miles to work and 6 miles home for daily exercise. He eats a reasonably healthy diet and drinks water throughout the day, but beer is often the drink of choice during a recording session. He has been feeling pain between his scapulae, especially on the left side.

Subjective

The client complained of pain between his shoulder blades, particularly on the left side, with an area of sharp, intermittent pain along his spine about midway between his upper and lower back. He rides a classic 10-speed bicycle on which he must lean forward to hold the handle bars, causing him to bend his neck back in order to look forward. While at work, he spends the first hour or so arranging microphones and equipment but spends the rest of the session in a chair at the recording console. He rarely gets up, except to go to the bathroom. He reports that the symptoms are most aggravating when he gets tired or feels weaker toward the end of a recording session, and he has noticed that he feels less stiff the day after working with a band that does not drink alcohol. When it hurts most, it hurts to turn his head to the right, and he feels like he cannot turn all the way when he tries to turn it to the left. He has no insurance and has not seen a health care provider but has had no history of illness and feels no pain or weakness in any other part of his body. When asked if he has experienced nausea, vertigo, or blurred vision, Seth responded "No." When asked if he had radiating pain or numbness or tingling in the arm, Seth responded "No." He could not recall if he felt pain near the spine when he coughs or sneezes. The symptoms do not keep him from his normal activities. Seth asked for a session focused on his neck and back pain.

Objective

As Seth was explaining his symptoms, he stood with most of his weight on the left leg, the right hip externally rotated, and the thorax slightly laterally flexed to the left. Postural assessment revealed a slight increase in thoracic kyphosis, slight internal rotation of the shoulders bilaterally, and significant head-forward posture with extension of the upper cervical spine, particularly near the occiput. The left shoulder is slightly elevated. The head is slightly rotated to the right and laterally flexed to the left. The left hip is slightly elevated; the right hip is slightly externally rotated.

Valsalva test was negative for herniation or other factors increasing pressure on the spinal cord.

Active rotation of the cervical spine was reduced to the left and caused pain at the end point to the right. Flexion of the cervical spine was reduced but caused no pain. Extension of the thoracic spine was normal and produced no pain.

Palpation revealed hypertonicity in upper trapezius, SCM, scalenes, and pectoralis major bilaterally, and levator scapula, latissimus dorsi, and lower trapezius on the left. The rhomboids minor, serratus posterior superior, middle trapezius, and thoracic erector spinae are taut and tender bilaterally.

Action

I began in the supine position with a rolled towel along the length of the spine and a pillow under the occiput. I performed myofascial release on the tissue around the humeral attachments of the pectoralis major and latissimus dorsi and along the sternum. I used effleurage to warm the pectorals and anterior deltoid and used muscle stripping to lengthen both bilaterally. No trigger points were found.

I performed myofascial release on the posterior neck, particularly near the occiput. I used effleurage to warm the superficial tissues followed by muscle stripping to the upper trapezius and levator scapulae. No trigger points were found. I used pincer grip kneading on the SCM bilaterally. No trigger points were found. I used muscle stripping on the scalenes, splenius muscles, and occipitals bilaterally. Hypertonicity was greater in the left scalenes. A trigger point was found in the left anterior scalene, halfway between the origin and the insertion, that referred toward the left scapula. Referred pain decreased from level 7 to 3 after two rounds of compression followed by muscle stripping. No trigger points were found on the right side. I performed a full cervical rotation to the left and lateral flexion to the right followed by postisometric relaxation to lengthen the left scalenes.

I removed the bolster from the occiput to apply deep petrissage to the occipital muscles. No trigger points were found. I applied a passive stretch to the cervical extensors by bringing the chin toward the chest.

In a prone position, I began with firm effleurage and superficial cross-fiber friction on the latissimus dorsi, particularly on the left side. A tender spot was found slightly medial to the scapula in upper fibers of the left latissimus dorsi. No referral was produced.

I performed superficial, bilateral cross-fiber friction to reduce adhesions around the superior angle of the scapula and at the junction of the lower trapezius and latissimus dorsi. Muscle stripping on the lower trapezius revealed a trigger point slightly medial to the lateral border of the left scapula, which referred around the left scapula and toward the acromion process. Compression of the trigger point produced a local twitch response. Pain reduced from level 6 to 2. I used pin and stretch along the fibers containing the trigger point.

I used deep effleurage from the medial border of the scapula toward the spine along the rhomboids and middle trapezius. Compression slightly inferior to the superior angle of the scapula produced a local twitch response in the rhomboid major but no referred pain. Local pain reduced from level 5 to 2.

I followed deep cross-fiber friction with muscle stripping from superior to inferior along the thoracic erector spinae. No trigger points were found. The client reported feeling no pain, but rather, comfortable relief here.

Following treatment, active left rotation of the cervical spine increased by approximately 10° compared to pre-treatment, and right rotation caused no pain. Flexion of the cervical spine improved by approximately 25° compared to pre-treatment.

Plan

I demonstrated stretches for the pectoral muscles and posterior neck, and strengthening exercises for the rhomboids and middle trapezius that can be performed during work hours. Seth rescheduled for 1 week from today. If improvement is significant enough to allow time for treatment to other areas, I will assess and treat the muscles of the lower back and hips that may be contributing to the elevation and external rotation of the hip and lateral flexion of the trunk. Based on my assessment of the tissues and posture, which are only minimally affected, general maintenance may be sufficient following a second treatment if the client is pain-free and maintains normal ROM for at least 1 week. I encouraged the client to drink plenty of water following treatments to flush out metabolites and keep the muscles hydrated. I recommended avoiding alcohol during flare-ups if it intensifies symptoms. I recommended that Seth consider switching to a bicycle, like an upright cruiser, which allows him to sit erect without extending his neck.

CRITICAL THINKING EXERCISES

1. Develop a 10-minute stretching and strengthening routine for a client, which covers all of the muscles involved in hyperkyphosis. Use Table 4-1, Box 4-1, and Figure 4-8 as a guide. Remember that a stretch increases the distance between the origin and insertion of a muscle and is important for those muscles that are shortened, while strengthening is performed by actively bringing the origin and insertion closer together and is important for the antagonists of shortened muscles. Describe each step of the routine in enough detail that the client can perform it without your assistance.

2. A client calls to schedule a massage for pain between the shoulder blades and in the neck. She explains that she had open heart surgery 5 years ago that left a scar along the length of her sternum. Although her physician considers her healthy and she has normal activities of daily living, she is regularly monitored for signs of cardiovascular disease. Discuss the impact her surgery may have had in the development of her chronic pain, the essential questions to ask the client and her health care provider before initiating treatment, and the cautions and considerations necessary when planning treatment.

3. Discuss the necessary adjustments to treatment for a client who has a natural or surgical fusion of cervical or thoracic vertebrae.

4. Conduct a short literature review to explain how the following conditions may put a client at greater risk for developing hyperkyphosis:
   - Nerve root compression
   - Obesity
   - Respiratory disorders
   - Rheumatoid arthritis
   - Vitamin D deficiency
   - Hormone imbalance
   - Spondylolisthesis
   - Pott's disease
   - Paget's disease

BIBLIOGRAPHY AND SUGGESTED READINGS

Biel A. *Trail Guide to the Body: How to Locate Muscles, Bones and More*, 3rd ed. Boulder, CO: Books of Discovery, 2005.

Clarkson HM. *Joint Motion and Function Assessment*. Baltimore, MD: Lippincott Williams & Wilkins, 2005.

Greig AM, Bennell KL, Briggs AM, et al. Postural taping decreases thoracic kyphosis but does not influence trunk muscle electromyographic activity or balance in women with osteoporosis. Manual Therapy. 2008;13(3):249–257.

Mayo Foundation for Medical Education and Research. Muscular Dystrophy. Available at http://www.mayoclinic.com/health/muscular-dystrophy. Accessed Summer 2008.

Mayo Foundation for Medical Education and Research. Paget's disease of the bone. Available at http://www.mayoclinic.com/health/pagets-disease-of-bone/DS00485. Accessed Summer 2008.

McKenzie K, Lin G, Tamir S. Thoracic outlet syndrome part I: A clinical review. Journal of the American Chiropractic Association. 2004;41(1):17–24.

Nicholas Institute of Sports Medicine and Athletic Trauma, Plone Foundation. Physical Examination of the Shoulder. Available at http://www.nismat.org/orthocor/exam/shoulder.html. Accessed Summer 2008.

Osar E. *Form & Function: The Anatomy of Motion*, 2nd ed. Evanston, IL: Osar Publications, 2005.

Rattray F, Ludwig L. *Clinical Massage Therapy: Understanding, Assessing and Treating over 70 Conditions*. Toronto, ON: Talus Incorporated, 2000.

Spine Universe. Scheuermann's Kyphosis (Scheuermann's Disease): Abnormal Curvature of the Spine. Available at http://www.spineuniverse.com/displayarticle.php/article593.html. Accessed Summer 2008.

Spondylitis Association of America. Ankylosing Spondylitis. Available at http://www.spondylitis.org/about/as_diag.aspx. Accessed Summer 2008.

Simons DG, Travell JG, Simons LS. *Myofascial Pain and Dysfunction: The Trigger Point Manual*, 2nd ed. Philadelphia, PA: Lippincott Williams & Wilkins, 1999.

Turchaninov R. *Medical Massage*, 2nd ed. Phoenix, AZ: Aesculapius Books, 2006.

U.S. National Library of Medicine and the National Institutes of Health. Ankylosing Spondylitis. Available at http://www.nlm.nih.gov/medlineplus/ankylosingspondylitis.html. Accessed Summer 2008.

U.S. National Library of Medicine and the National Institutes of Health. Kyphosis. Available at http://www.nlm.nih.gov/medlineplus/ency/article/000353.htm. Accessed Summer 2008.

U.S. National Library of Medicine and the National Institutes of Health. Osteoporosis. Available at http://www.nlm.nih.gov/medlineplus/ency/article/000360.htm. Accessed Summer 2008.

U.S. National Library of Medicine and the National Institutes of Health. Spondylolisthesis. Available at http://www.nlm.nih.gov/medlineplus/ency/article/001260.htm. Accessed Summer 2008.

U.S. National Library of Medicine and the National Institutes of Health. Tuberculous Arthritis. Available at http://www.nlm.nih.gov/medlineplus/ency/article/000417.htm. Accessed Summer 2008.

Werner R. *A Massage Therapist's Guide to Pathology*, 4th ed. Philadelphia, PA: Lippincott Williams & Wilkins, 2009.

Tension Headaches

UNDERSTANDING TENSION HEADACHES

Headaches can indicate a wide variety of changes in a person's health. They may result from an injury, occur as a symptom of a systemic condition, or may be a condition in themselves. The International Headache Society classifies headaches as primary headaches, secondary headaches, and cranial neuralgias or other headaches. Tension headaches, migraines, and cluster headaches are commonly categorized as primary headaches; this means that the headache is the pathology itself (Fig. 5-1). Headaches that are caused by underlying pathologies (e.g., sinus headaches) are considered secondary headaches. It is essential to understand the client's health history and to refer the client to a health care provider for diagnosis if you suspect an underlying condition or other contraindications before treating chronic headaches as if the cause is muscle tension. While massage therapy may help relieve symptoms and reduce the occurrence of some secondary headaches, it is not a cure for an underlying condition, and caution should be taken when treating these clients. However, if no other conditions are present, reducing hypertonicity, trigger points, and blood pressure with regularly scheduled massage therapy can decrease the severity and frequency of chronic tension headaches.

Tension headaches are the most common type of headache. Evidence suggests that they may be caused by muscle tension and trigger points, primarily in the shoulders, neck, and head. They respond well to treatments such as over-the-counter pain relievers and manual therapies such as massage. Tension headaches often disrupt the client's activities of daily living, but they are rarely dangerous. Tension headaches are different from migraines, which are believed to have origins that vary but are commonly associated with vascular constriction or a condition of the central nervous system. However, muscle tension often accompanies migraines, and studies have shown that massage can reduce the intensity and frequency of episodes.

Common Signs and Symptoms

Tension headaches are often bilateral but may be unilateral and specific to the referral pattern of one or more trigger points. The pain is dull and aching and is often described as feeling like the pressure of a band or vice around the head or a heavy cape over the head and shoulders. Unlike people with migraines, sufferers of tension headaches do not commonly experience aura, nausea, or vomiting, and physical activity does not usually intensify a tension headache.

In addition to aching in the head, clients sometimes feel pain in the neck or shoulders or between the scapulae. These symptoms may even precede headaches. If the client has hyperkyphosis or hyperlordosis, the common pain patterns that accompany these conditions may also be present. Hypertonicity and trigger points are frequently found in the cervical extensors, particularly the upper trapezius, splenius cervicis, splenius capitis, and the suboccipitals; in cervical

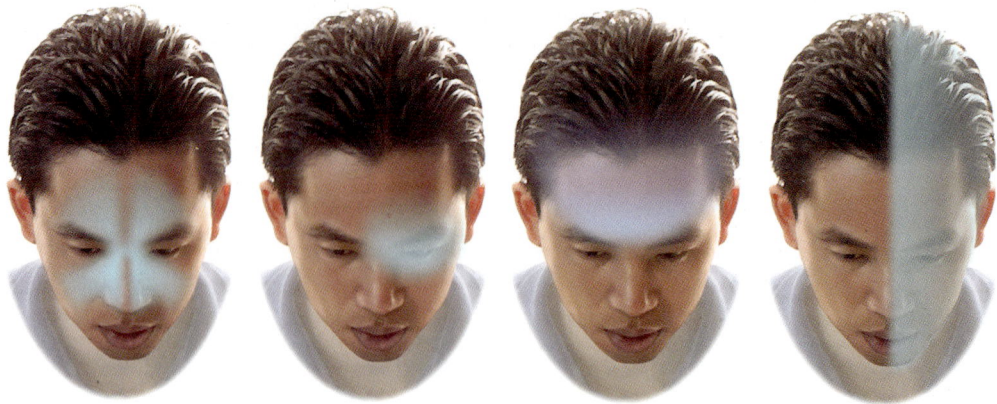

✿A.D.A.M.

Figure 5-1   Primary headaches. The client's pattern of pain may help you understand what type of headache he or she is experiencing. Left to right: sinus headache, cluster headache, tension headache, migraine headache. Used with permission of A.D.A.M.

flexors including the scalenes and SCM; and in the muscles of mastication. Satellite trigger points may be found in the referral patterns of primary trigger points. The muscles of respiration may also be involved, particularly with hyperkyphosis or chronic respiratory conditions. Clients who suffer from tension headaches may also experience tenderness in the scalp, loss of appetite, fatigue, insomnia, mood changes, and problems with concentration.

Chronic tension headaches are likely to arise in adolescence or young adulthood. This may occur because young adults must become more self-sufficient, which can be stressful, and because activities of daily living often become more sedentary, which affects postural changes that may contribute to muscle tension. Tension headaches often last from 30 minutes to several weeks and can come and go or persist without relief. The headache is considered chronic when it occurs two or three times per week over the course of several months. Without treatment, the client may suffer from chronic tension headaches for years. Tension headaches often manifest in the afternoon, when stress and fatigue accumulate and trigger points become active. The client may have difficulty sleeping—a symptom that, if left untreated, may contribute to the cause of tension headaches.

Possible Causes and Contributing Factors

To date, there is no consensus about the precise cause(s) of tension headaches or whether the tension said to contribute is actually due to a contraction of the muscles. Tension in the muscles has been noted in sufferers of both tension and migraine headaches. Fluctuations in levels of chemicals including serotonin have also been found in both. While the cause(s) of these fluctuations remain(s) unclear, researchers now believe that the imbalance activates pain pathways to the brain and impedes natural pain suppression. Nevertheless, headaches are often felt in the referral area of a trigger point, and studies have shown that relaxing tense muscles reduces the frequency of both tension and migraine headaches. However, massage is not likely to improve a migraine that is already in progress, and caution should be used when treating a tension headache in progress to avoid pressure and techniques that could intensify symptoms.

Any postural deviation that affects the cervical or thoracic spine can contribute to muscle tension and resulting headaches. The head-forward posture commonly found in hyperkyphosis is often observed. Temporomandibular joint dysfunction, also often found in clients with hyperkyphosis, is likewise a common contributing factor. Torticollis, disc herniations, whiplash, or other unresolved trauma may be involved. Clients whose activities of daily living include maintaining an inactive posture, such as sitting at a desk or sleeping with the neck in extension, may set the muscles at a high resting tone, contributing to the formation or activation of trigger points. Lack of physical activity—the muscle's enemy—can lead to adhesions, to an accumulation of metabolites, and ultimately to active trigger points. Overuse, fatigue, and stress on the muscles can be culprits of hypertonicity and trigger points. Dehydration, which may cause fatigue and confusion, is one of the most common causes of headaches.

Chemical and hormonal changes, side effects of medications, fluctuations in blood pressure, and hunger or low blood sugar can all contribute to headaches. In these cases, the symptoms are often relieved by addressing the cause. The overuse of pain medication can result in a rebound effect, a phenomenon in which the medication (or suddenly stopping the medication) triggers symptoms it used to relieve. This too can be resolved by decreasing, ceasing, or changing the use of medication under the supervision of a health care provider. Depression and anxiety, which are often related to chemical imbalances and can also cause a client to contract the muscles of the neck and jaw, may play a role in tension headaches.

Insufficient sleep or changes in sleep patterns can affect circadian rhythms and the biological functions they regulate. Sleeping in a cold room or sitting for long periods near a source of cold, such as an air conditioning vent, may activate trigger points that may contribute to headaches. Lifestyle choices including the use of or withdrawal from drugs, alcohol, or caffeine; excessive smoking; and overexertion may contribute to the development of chronic headaches. Cold and flu, eyestrain, nasal congestion, and sinus infections may also be contributing factors.

Chronic tension headaches rarely develop after the age of 50. If so, they may be a red flag for a more serious condition, and the client should be referred to his or her primary health care provider for assessment. In addition, the client should seek medical attention if headaches are severe (thunderclap), get worse, change patterns, or are no longer relieved by pain medication. Similarly, the client should seek emergency medical attention if difficulty speaking, fever, rash, seizures, numbness, or weakness accompanies headache. These signs and symptoms may indicate a stroke, aneurysm, or other serious conditions. Headaches that occur after coughing, straining, or sudden movement may be a symptom of intracranial pressure or pressure on the spinal cord or nerves and should be assessed by a medical professional. If headaches develop following an injury, the client should see a health care provider for medical assessment before receiving a massage.

Table 5-1 lists conditions commonly confused with or contributing to tension headaches.

Contraindications and Special Considerations

- **Headache on the day of treatment.** If the client presents with a headache on the day of treatment, do not work aggressively. Although massage is not contraindicated during a tension headache, you should take care not to aggravate the client's symptoms. Myofascial release, lymphatic drainage, and gentle, superficial strokes are most appropriate. The client may not tolerate the face cradle and may be disturbed by light, scents, or sound. You may also consider a shorter treatment or rescheduling the client. If the client's headache frequently occurs in the late afternoon, consider scheduling on a weekend morning when trigger points may not be activated.
- **Underlying pathologies.** Headaches can be a symptom of a wide variety of underlying conditions. If you suspect any condition (consult Table 5-1 and your pathology book for signs and symptoms), refer the client to his or her health care provider for diagnosis before initiating treatment. If the client is diagnosed with an underlying pathology that is not contraindicated for massage, work with the health care provider to develop a treatment plan. A client who has newly developed chronic headaches after age 50 should be referred to his or her health care provider.
- **Endangerment sites.** Be cautious near the endangerment sites in the neck. Gently palpate for the pulse of the carotid artery before you begin working. Avoid this area, and if you feel a pulse while working, back off slowly.

Table 5-1	Differentiating Conditions Commonly Confused with or Contributing to Tension Headaches		
Condition	**Typical Signs and Symptoms**	**Testing**	**Massage Therapy**
Migraine	Episodic or chronic Moderate or severe Often unilateral Pulsating or throbbing Aggravated by physical activity Aura, nausea, vomiting, sensitivity to light and sound	Diagnosed by signs and symptoms, familial history, and response to treatment MRI or CT to rule out other causes EEG to exclude seizures	Massage may not be appropriate during a migraine, but may reduce frequency when performed regularly between headaches.
Cluster headaches	Usually unilateral Swelling under or around eye, red eye Excessive tears Sudden headache with sharp, steady pain, often during sleep	Diagnosed by signs and symptoms MRI to rule out other pathologies	Massage may not be appropriate during a cluster headache, but may reduce frequency and severity when performed regularly between headaches.
Sinus headache	Pain or pressure at cheeks and brow Tender sinuses Worse when bending forward or lying down Postnasal drip, sore throat, nasal discharge Possible fever, cough, or fatigue Allergic or infectious sinusitis	Diagnosed by signs and symptoms Mucus sample to test for infection CT scan or MRI	Massage is contraindicated if infection or serious underlying pathology is present. Massage is otherwise appropriate within the client's comfort. The face cradle may be uncomfortable.
Brain tumor	Headaches, seizures, decreased sensation or weakness in one part of the body Changes in mental function and personality Clumsiness, tremor Changes in vision, memory, alertness, speech, hearing, or smell Vomiting, fever, or general ill feeling	CT scan MRI EEG Tissue biopsy Cerebrospinal fluid test	Massage is contraindicated until the client is cleared by a health care provider.
Brain aneurysm	Double vision Loss of vision Headaches Eye pain Neck pain When ruptured: Sudden, severe headache Nausea, vomiting Numbness, weakness, or decreased sensation in a body part Vision or speech changes, drooping eyelid(s) Confusion, lethargy, or seizures	CT scan MRI Cerebrospinal fluid test Cerebral angiography EEG	Massage is contraindicated until the client is cleared by a health care provider. Take caution with circulatory techniques.

Table 5-1	**Differentiating Conditions Commonly Confused with or Contributing to Tension Headaches (Continued)**		
Condition	**Typical Signs and Symptoms**	**Testing**	**Massage Therapy**
Stroke or transient ischemic attack	Symptoms are often unilateral, occur suddenly, last a short time, and may occur again	Medical history	Massage is contraindicated when symptoms are present. For a client surviving a stroke or transient ischemic attack, massage is indicated if the client is cleared by the attending medical professional. Avoid rigorous circulatory techniques. Massage around the neck is postponed until the client has returned to pre-stroke activities of daily living.
		CBC	
	Numbness, tingling, weakness, heavy extremities, speech difficulty, vision changes, vertigo, loss of balance or coordination, staggering or falling	CT scan	
		MRI	
		Cerebral arteriogram	
	Facial paralysis		
	Eye pain		
	Confusion		
Trigeminal neuralgia	Usually unilateral, around the eye, cheek, and lower face	MRI	Because of sensitivity to touch, massage is contraindicated without permission and guidance from the client regarding what feels good. The face cradle may be too painful. Massage elsewhere is indicated.
	Pain triggered by touch or sound	Blood tests	
		Rule out other conditions	
	Sharp, electric spasms lasting a few seconds or minutes		
	Pain while brushing teeth, chewing, drinking, eating, or shaving		
Hemicrania continua	Pain on one side of the head, consistent and daily	Idiopathic	Refer to health care provider for assessment. Clients with symptoms of hemicrania continua are unlikely to tolerate massage until the symptoms are under control.
		No definitive test	
	Generally moderate with occasional severe pain	Diagnosed by signs and symptoms and by ruling out other causes of headache	
	Tearing or redness of eye on affected side		
	Nasal congestion		
	Swelling or drooping of eyelid(s)		
Meningitis	Fever and chills	Chest X-ray	Massage is contraindicated until the condition is resolved. Refer client to a health care provider.
	Nausea and vomiting	CT scan	
	Severe headache	Cerebrospinal fluid test	
	Stiff neck		
	Sensitivity to light		
	Confusion or decreased consciousness		
	Rapid breathing		
	Loss of appetite		
	Agitation		

(continued)

Table 5-1	Differentiating Conditions Commonly Confused with or Contributing to Tension Headaches (Continued)		
Condition	**Typical Signs and Symptoms**	**Testing**	**Massage Therapy**
Encephalitis	Fever Headache Stiff neck, muscle weakness, or paralysis Vomiting Light sensitivity Confusion, drowsiness, or clumsiness Irritability Seizure, loss of consciousness, stupor, or coma	Cerebrospinal fluid test EEG MRI CT scan	Massage therapy is contraindicated until the condition is resolved. Refer client to a health care provider.
Temporal arteritis	Usually occurs in patients over age 50 Unilateral throbbing Tenderness in scalp Fever, loss of appetite, sweating, weight loss Muscle aches, weakness, and fatigue Reduced, blurred, or double vision Jaw pain	Palpation of scalp for tenderness Weak or no pulse in affected artery Blood tests Liver function tests Biopsy of temporal artery	Refer a client over age 50 with newly developed chronic headaches to a health care provider.
Paget's disease	Persistent bone pain Joint pain and stiffness Headache, neck pain Bowed legs Locally hot to touch Fractures Hearing loss Loss of height	X-ray Bone scan Blood test for serum alkaline phosphatase and serum calcium	Work with health care provider. Massage may help maintain flexibility. Use caution if bones are fragile.
Nerve root compression (radiculopathy)	Muscle spasm, weakness, or atrophy Pain around the scapula on the affected side Neck pain Pain radiates to the extremities Pain worsens with lateral flexion or rotation or when sneezing, coughing, laughing, or straining	Spurling's test Valsalva's test Neurological exam to test reflexes, sensation, and strength	Massage is indicated if cause and location are understood. Take care not to increase compression or reproduce symptoms.

- **Treatment duration and pressure.** If the client is elderly, has degenerative bone disease, or has a condition that diminishes his or her activities of daily living, you may need to adjust your pressure as well as the treatment duration. Frequent half-hour sessions may suit the client better.
- **Positioning.** Use bolsters to position a client for comfort as well as to correct postures that may contribute to headaches. If the head-forward posture or extension of the neck is evident, using a small bolster under the occiput in the supine position and adjusting the face cradle to reduce the extension of the neck in the prone position may help. If hyperkyphosis is present, bolsters under the shoulders in the prone position will reduce protraction of the scapulae. In the supine position, a bolster along the length of the spine including the occiput reduces protraction of the scapulae and extension of the neck.
- **Hydrotherapy.** Do not use moist heat on the neck or chest if the client has a cardiovascular condition that may be affected by the dilation of blood vessels. Severe hypertension and atherosclerosis are two examples of conditions that are contraindicated for massage. Consult your pathology book for recommendations.
- **Friction.** Do not use deep frictions if the client has a systemic inflammatory condition such as rheumatoid arthritis or osteoarthritis, if the health of the underlying tissues is compromised, or if the client is taking anti-inflammatory medication. Friction creates the inflammatory process, which may interfere with the intended action of anti-inflammatory medication. Recommend that your client refrain from taking such medication for several hours before treatment if his or her health care provider agrees.
- **Tissue length.** It is important when treating myofascial tissues to not stretch already overstretched tissues. Assess for myofascial restrictions first and only treat those that are clearly present. Likewise, overstretched muscles should not be stretched from origin to insertion. If you treat trigger points, use heat or a localized pin and stretch technique to lengthen that area.
- **Hypermobile joints and unstable ligaments.** Be cautious with mobilizations if the client has hypermobile joints or if ligaments are unstable due to injury, pregnancy or a systemic condition.

Massage Therapy Research

In 2002, Quinn et al. published a study titled "Massage Therapy and Frequency of Chronic Tension Headaches." The study involved four nonsmoking adults between the ages of 18 and 55 who had experienced headaches two to three times per week in the prior 6 months; these were diagnosed as chronic or episodic tension headaches according to the International Headache Society guidelines. Baseline headache measures were recorded for 4 weeks, followed by 30-minute massages twice per week for 4 weeks. The treatment plan was very specific and was followed precisely for each participant. Participants were asked to keep a headache diary noting frequency, intensity, and duration of each headache. Compared with baseline headache measures, the frequency of headaches was reduced as early as the first week of treatment, and the frequency reduction was maintained for the duration of the study. Pain was also reduced, although it is not sufficiently clear if the massage techniques, stretching, or relaxation techniques included in the treatment had a more or less direct effect on pain reduction. The duration of headaches became shorter for all four participants, and intensity diminished in three participants. On four occasions, participants arrived for treatment with a headache that was relieved during the 30-minute treatment. In addition, the authors noted that in most sessions, the participants felt headache symptoms when identified trigger points were palpated deeply even when they had not felt the pain prior to palpation; this suggests that the activation of common trigger points may have a strong connection to tension headaches. Although the results are encouraging, a more substantial study with a control group is needed.

In 1990, Puustjärvi et al. published a study titled "The Effects of Massage in Patients with Chronic Tension Headache." The study involved 21 female patients from 21 to 44 years of age who had experienced chronic neck and head pain. Cervical ROM, surface electromyography (EMG) of the upper trapezius and frontalis muscles, pain quality and intensity, and incidence of pain were recorded for 2 weeks before and 2 weeks after treatment, and again at 3 and 6 months during the follow-up period. Each participant received 10 1-hour massage treatments to the upper body over a period of 2.5 weeks and had no other form of therapy during the study. Compared to the initial recordings, the ROM increased in flexion, lateral flexion, and rotation. EMG improvements were noted in the frontalis muscle alone. Pain decreased significantly, and the number of pain-free days doubled. The participants' psychological state was improved immediately following the 2.5 week treatment period, and the improvement continued at the 3- and 6-month follow-ups. Although the evidence is encouraging, this study is not fully reliable because it did not include a control group, and the treatments were not standardized.

In addition, the 1998 study by Hernández-Reif et al. titled "Migraine Headaches Are Reduced by Massage Therapy" and the 2007 case study by Eisensmith titled "Massage Therapy Decreases Frequency and Intensity of Symptoms Related to Temporomandibular Joint Syndrome in One Case Study" suggest that massage therapy may be effective for both migraine headaches and temporomandibular joint syndrome.

WORKING WITH THE CLIENT

Client Assessment

Assessment begins at your first contact with a client. In some cases, this may be on the telephone when an appointment is requested. Ask in advance if the client is seeking treatment for a specific area of pain so that you can prepare yourself. Headaches are a common symptom of a wide variety of conditions. It is essential for your assessment to be thorough. If you suspect an underlying condition that requires medical attention, refer the client to his or her health care provider for assessment. If the client is diagnosed with an underlying condition, research the contraindications or special considerations for the condition. During your assessment, ask questions that will help you differentiate the possible causes of headaches.

Table 5-2 lists questions to ask the client when taking a health history.

POSTURAL ASSESSMENT

Allow the client to enter the room ahead of you while you observe his or her posture and movements. Look for imbalances or patterns of compensation due to pain or weakness. In the absence of a clear cause of tension headaches, such as whiplash or other injury, hyperkyphosis is often a contributing factor. Look for a head-forward posture, neck extension or rotation, elevated shoulders, and slouching. Notice if the client is able to turn the head without involving the shoulders or thoracic spine. This may indicate reduced ROM in the cervical spine. You may also notice hyperlordosis, scoliosis, rotation, or elevation in the hips or pes planus. Figure 5-2 compares the anatomic position to posture affected by hyperkyphosis with the head forward, a common contributing factor to tension headaches.

ROM ASSESSMENT

Test the ROM of the neck, shoulders, and thoracic spine, assessing the length and strength of both agonists and antagonists that cross the joints tested. See Chapter 4 if hyperkyphosis is present. Since it allows the client to control the amount of movement and stay within a pain-free range, only active ROM should be used in the acute stage of injury to prevent undue pain or

Table 5-2	Health History

Questions for the Client	Importance for the Treatment Plan
Do you have a headache now?	Treatment may need to be adjusted to avoid aggravating symptoms. The client may wish to reschedule.
When did you begin experiencing headaches? Have you experienced any other new symptoms coincident with the onset of headaches?	Newly developed chronic headaches, especially when accompanied by other symptoms, may be a sign of an underlying pathology.
How frequently do you get headaches? Do they occur at or near the same time of day or following similar activities?	Differentiate between episodic or chronic tension headaches. Trigger points are often activated in the late afternoon.
Have you seen a health care provider about your headaches? What was the diagnosis? What tests were performed?	A wide variety of conditions cause headache as a symptom. Infection, acute injury, or an underlying pathology may contraindicate massage. Refer the client to his or her primary health care provider if you suspect an underlying condition.
Was there any change in your activities of daily living before you developed headaches?	This helps determine potential contributing factors.
Where do you feel symptoms?	The location of symptoms gives clues to the location of trigger points, injury, or other contributing factors. Tension headaches often follow the referral area of one or more trigger points.
Describe the character of your symptoms.	This helps to differentiate the possible origins of symptoms. Tension headaches often feel like a band or vise around the head or neck. The character of pain is less likely to be throbbing, pulsating, or sharp.
Do any movements make it worse or better?	Locate tension, weakness, or compression in structures involved in such movements. Tension headaches are not commonly made worse with general activity, although the specific movement of a joint crossed by a muscle containing a trigger point may produce or increase symptoms.
What type of work, hobbies, or other regular activities do you do?	Repetitive motions and static postures that increase neck extension, head-forward posture, or pressure on the mandible may contribute to headaches.
Are you taking any prescribed medication or herbal or other supplements?	Side effects of medications of all types may contribute to symptoms, have contraindications, or require special considerations in treatment.
Have you had a cortisone shot in the past 2 weeks? Where?	Local massage is contraindicated.
Have you taken a pain reliever or muscle relaxant within the past 4 hours?	The client may not be able to judge your pressure.
Have you taken anti-inflammatory medication within the past 4 hours?	Deep friction may cause inflammation and should not be performed if the client has recently taken anti-inflammatory medication.

re-injury. Box 5-1 presents the average active ROM results for the joints involved in tension headache.

Active ROM

Compare your assessment of the client's active ROM to the values in Box 5-1. Pain and other symptoms may not be reproduced with active ROM assessment because the client may limit his or her movement to the symptom-free range.

- **Active extension of the thoracic spine** may be reduced when muscle tension, adhesions, and trigger points are the cause of tension headaches. The client may be resistant to full active extension of the thoracic spine if this produces symptoms during activities of daily living.
- **Active flexion of the cervical spine** in the full range may be restricted due to weakened cervical flexors attempting movement against shortened upper cervical extensors.

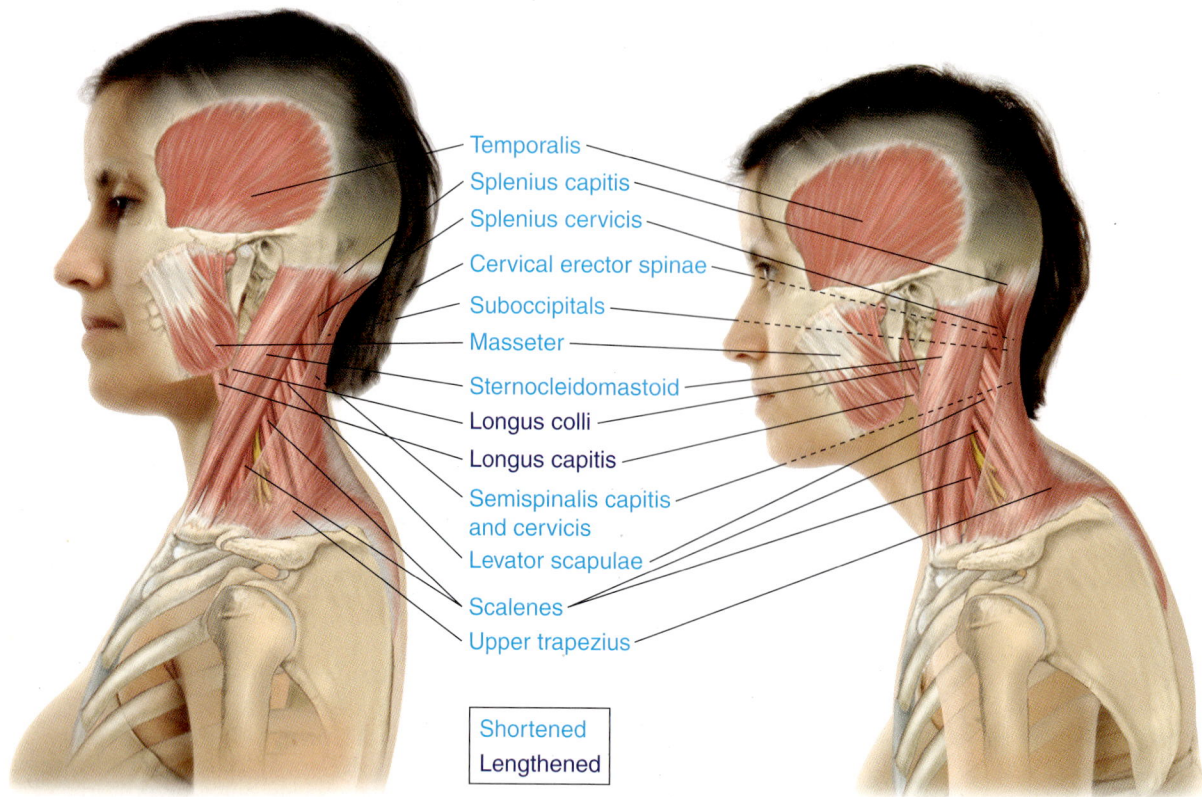

Temporalis
Splenius capitis
Splenius cervicis
Cervical erector spinae
Suboccipitals
Masseter
Sternocleidomastoid
Longus colli
Longus capitis
Semispinalis capitis
and cervicis
Levator scapulae
Scalenes
Upper trapezius

Shortened
Lengthened

Figure 5-2 **Postural assessment comparison. Compare the anatomical posture on the left to the deviated posture on the right.** Notice how the muscles of the upper cross react to the increased kyphotic curve and head-forward posture, which may contribute to chronic tension headaches.

- **Active rotation and lateral flexion** of the cervical spine may be reduced or cause pain due to hypertonicity or spasm in the muscles responsible for rotation or lateral flexion, or weak antagonists.
- **Active mobility of the mandible** may be reduced in any direction when the muscles of mastication are hypertonic or contain trigger points.

PASSIVE ROM

Compare the client's P ROM on one side to the other when applicable. Notice and compare the end feel for each range (refer to Chapter 1 for an explanation of end feel).

- **Passive flexion of the cervical spine** may be restricted due to shortened cervical extensors.
- **Passive lateral flexion or rotation of the cervical spine** may be restricted unilaterally if the client's posture favors lateral flexion or rotation to the opposite side.
- **Passive extension of the cervical spine** will likely occur with ease but may produce pain at the end point.

RESISTED ROM

Use resisted tests to assess the strength of the muscles that cross the joints involved. Compare the strength of the affected side to the unaffected side.

- **Resisted flexion of the neck** may reveal weakness in the anterior neck muscles.
- **Resisted rotation or lateral flexion of the neck** may produce or refer pain if the muscles responsible for that action are tight or contain trigger points, and may reveal weakness in their antagonists.

Box 5-1   AVERAGE ACTIVE ROM FOR JOINTS INVOLVED IN TENSION HEADACHES

Cervical Spine

Flexion 60°
SCM (bilateral)
Anterior scalene (bilateral)
Longus capitis (bilateral)
Longus colli (bilateral)

Extension 55°
Upper trapezius (bilateral)
Levator scapulae (bilateral)
Splenius capitis (bilateral)
Splenius cervicis (bilateral)
Rectus capitis (bilateral)
Obliquus capitis superior (bilateral)
Semispinalis capitis (bilateral)
Longissimus capitis (bilateral)
Longissimus cervicis (bilateral)
Iliocostalis cervicis (bilateral)

Lateral Flexion 20–45°
Upper trapezius (unilateral)
Levator scapulae (unilateral)
Splenius capitis (unilateral)
Splenius cervicis (unilateral)
SCM (unilateral)
Longus capitis (unilateral)
Longus colli (unilateral)
Anterior scalene (unilateral)
Middle scalene (unilateral)
Posterior scalene (unilateral)
Longissimus capitis (unilateral)
Longissimus cervicis (unilateral)
Iliocostalis cervicis (unilateral)

Ipsilateral Rotation 70–90°
Levator scapulae (unilateral)
Splenius capitis (unilateral)
Splenius cervicis (unilateral)
Rectus capitis (unilateral)
Obliquus capitis (unilateral)
Longus colli (unilateral)
Longus capitis (unilateral)
Longissimus capitis (unilateral)
Longissimus cervicis (unilateral)
Iliocostalis cervicis (unilateral)

Contralateral Rotation 70–90°
Upper trapezius (unilateral)
SCM (unilateral)
Anterior scalene (unilateral)
Middle scalene (unilateral)
Posterior scalene (unilateral)

Thoracic Spine
Extension 20–30°
Spinalis
Longissimus
Iliocostalis

Multifidi
Rotatores
Semispinalis capitis
Latissimus dorsi
Quadratus lumborum

Mandible
Elevation (contact of teeth)
Masseter
Temporalis
Medial pterygoid

Depression 35–50 mm
Suprahyoid
Infrahyoid
Digastric
Platysma

Protraction 3–7 mm
Lateral pterygoid
Medial pterygoid

Retraction
Temporalis
Digastric

Contralateral Lateral Deviation 5–12 mm
Lateral pterygoid
Medial pterygoid

SPECIAL TESTS

The following special tests will help you determine when a client should be evaluated by a health care provider using X-ray or other tools, which may reveal conditions that are contraindicated or require special considerations when planning treatment with massage.

The **vertebral artery test** may reveal insufficiency in the vertebral artery and is performed if the client states that he or she experiences vertigo, blurred vision, or light-headedness during activities of daily living (Fig. 5-3).

1. Position the client seated in a chair facing you with the eyes open.
2. Instruct the client to fully rotate and extend the neck to one side for 30 seconds.
3. If, during this time, the client complains of nausea or dizziness or if you notice involuntary motion of the eyes, the test is positive for insufficient circulation through the vertebral artery, and the client should be referred to his or her health care provider.
4. If the test is negative on one side, test the other. Do not test the other side if the first side tests positive.

Spurling's test may reveal compression of a nerve or irritation to the facet joint in the cervical spine and is performed when the client has had an injury, complains of pain that radiates, or experiences numbness and tingling in the arm. Although massage may not be contraindicated for a client with these conditions, refer the client to a health care provider for more detailed information or a massage therapist with advanced training in treating difficult cases. If the client tested positive for vertebral artery insufficiency, do not perform Spurling's test.

1. If the client has recurring symptoms on one side only, begin with that side.
2. Stand behind the seated client and instruct him or her to extend, laterally flex, and rotate the head to the affected side.

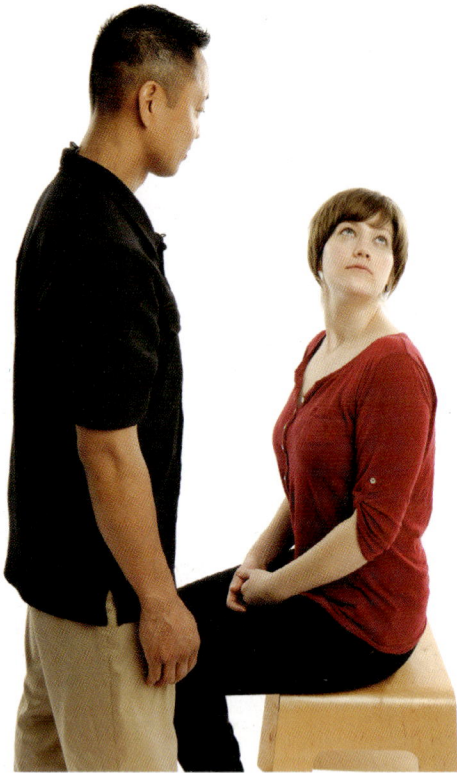

Figure 5-3   **Vertebral artery test.** Watch for involuntary movement of the client's eyes during this test.

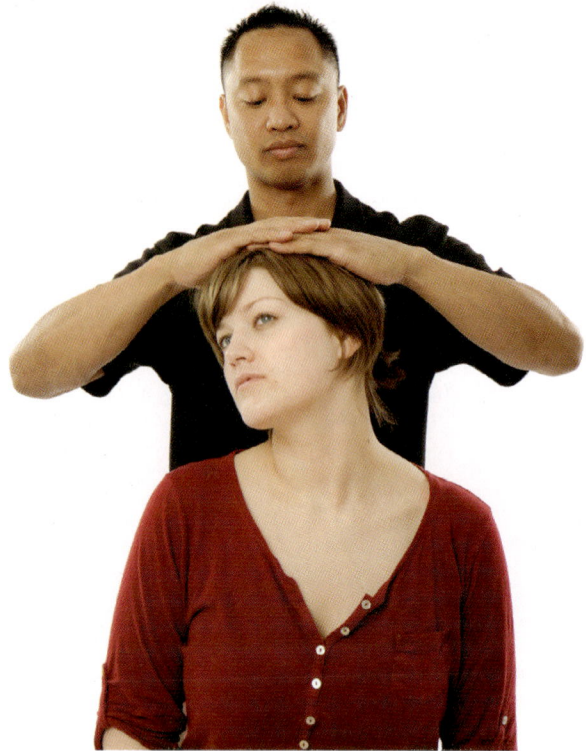

Figure 5-4   **Spurling's test.** With the client's head extended, laterally flexed, and rotated to the affected side, gently and slowly press down on the client's head. Use gentle traction following this test to release pressure.

3. Gently and slowly press down on the client's head (Fig. 5-4). If the client cannot extend, laterally flex, or rotate the neck, perform a simple compression test without these actions.
4. If the client experiences radiating pain, numbness, or tingling in the arm, the test is positive for nerve root compression.
5. Ask the client to describe the location of symptoms because this may suggest which nerve is compressed.
6. If the client feels pain that does not move past the neck, the test is positive for irritation of the facet joint.
7. Applying gentle traction to the neck after the test may relieve symptoms. If traction does relieve symptoms, this is considered reinforcement that Spurling's test was positive for compression of a nerve or facet joint irritation.

PALPATION ASSESSMENT

Muscles that commonly contribute to tension headaches attach at the occiput, mastoid process, ligamentum nuchae, the cervical vertebrae, the upper thoracic vertebrae, and the scapulae. Palpate these areas for tenderness. Carefully palpating the many muscles attached to those bones will give you the most complete picture. The muscles most commonly involved in tension headaches include the trapezius, scalenes, SCM, splenius capitis and cervicis, semispinalis capitis and cervicis, the cervical erector spinae, levator scapulae, and suboccipitals. Palpate these for hyper- or hypotonicity and trigger points.

The muscles of mastication and respiration may also be hypertonic and tender, especially if hyperkyphosis, the head-forward posture, temporomandibular joint dysfunction, or a respiratory disorder is present. Palpate the temporalis, masseter, and pterygoids to assess their involvement. The intercostals and diaphragm may be tender or hypertonic. The occipitofrontalis, which includes the occipitalis, frontalis, and galea aponeurotica between them, may be tender.

Condition-Specific Massage

Because headaches may be a secondary condition or may have a structural cause, it is important to know the health history of the client. If a systemic condition or degenerative bone or disc disease is present, it is advisable to first discuss treatment with the client's health care provider and to adjust accordingly. If hyperkyphosis is present, refer to Chapter 4 for special testing and treatment considerations. Temporomandibular joint dysfunction is another condition that may contribute to tension headaches. Temporomandibular joint dysfunction is not covered in this text, but you may treat the muscles of mastication generally to offer some relief, study this condition in greater detail elsewhere, or refer the client to a massage therapist with training in this area.

It is essential for treatment to be relaxing. You are not likely to eradicate the pain associated with chronic tension headaches, or any of the conditions associated with it, in one treatment. Do not try to do so by treating aggressively. Be sure to ask your client to let you know if the amount of pressure keeps him or her from relaxing. If the client responds by tensing muscles or has a facial expression that looks distressed, reduce your pressure. Remember that you are working on tissue that is compromised.

Ask the client to let you know if any part of your treatment reproduces symptoms. If deep palpation of a trigger point reproduces symptoms, explain this to your client and ask him or her to breathe deeply during the technique. As the trigger point is deactivated, the referral pain will also diminish. Muscles with trigger points that refer pain into the head include the trapezius, SCM, masseter, temporalis, medial and lateral pterygoid, suboccipitals, semispinalis capitis and cervicis, and splenius capitis and cervicis. Common trigger points that refer pain into the head are shown in Figure 5-5.

If any other reproduction of symptoms occurs, adjust the client to a more neutral position, reduce your pressure, or move slightly off the area, and make a note about it, as it may help you understand more clearly exactly which neuromuscular conditions are contributing to the client's symptoms. Instruct your client to use deep but relaxing breathing to encourage calming.

The following suggestions are for the treatment of tension headaches. You may not need a full hour to treat the muscles commonly involved in tension headaches, and overtreating may reproduce symptoms. Treating too many trigger points in one session may increase pain. If time remains, address any other postural deviations or contributing factors you may find in your assessment.

- If light affects the client's condition, cover his or her eyes with an eye pillow or pillowcase. Ask the client if scents or sounds are disturbing, and adjust accordingly. If hyperkyphosis is present, use a rolled towel or other bolster along the length of the spine in the supine position. If the client's neck is in extension, fold a pillowcase or hand towel into a small bolster, and place it under the occiput without obstructing your access to the posterior neck muscles.

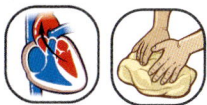

- If it is comfortable for the client, place moist heat on the neck and shoulder muscles.

- If shortened pectorals or hyperkyphosis is a factor, treat this area fully (see Chapter 4). If the pectorals are not involved, treat the area superficially to relax the client, and open the channels of circulation in the thorax.

- Assess the tissues of the lateral neck for myofascial restrictions. These may be found near the mastoid process and along the lateral neck toward the acromion process and lateral clavicle. Reduce adhesions if indicated.

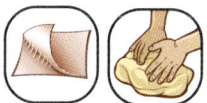

- Assess and treat tissues from the cervical vertebrae to the acromion process to reduce adhesions in the upper trapezius and to begin assessing for taut bands in the cervical muscles. Treat tissues from the cervical vertebrae toward the superior angle of the scapulae to assess and treat the levator scapulae. (Fig. 5-6).

Treatment icons: Increase circulation; Reduce adhesions; Reduce tension; Lengthen tissue; Treat trigger points; Passive stretch; Clear area

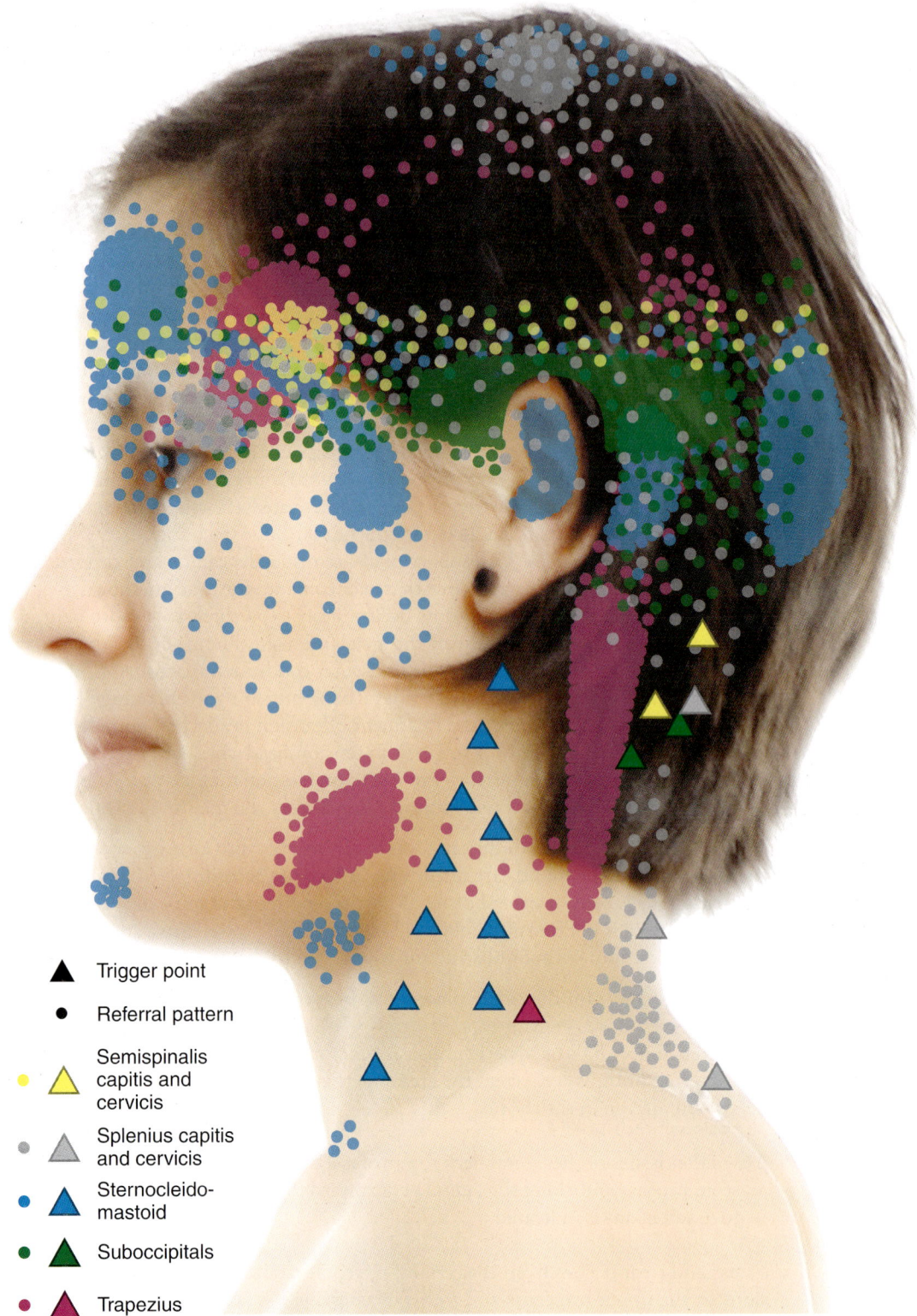

▲ Trigger point

● Referral pattern

○ ▲ Semispinalis capitis and cervicis

○ ▲ Splenius capitis and cervicis

● ▲ Sternocleido-mastoid

● ▲ Suboccipitals

● ▲ Trapezius

Figure 5-5 **Common trigger points and referral.** Common trigger points and referral patterns associated with tension headaches. (*continued*)

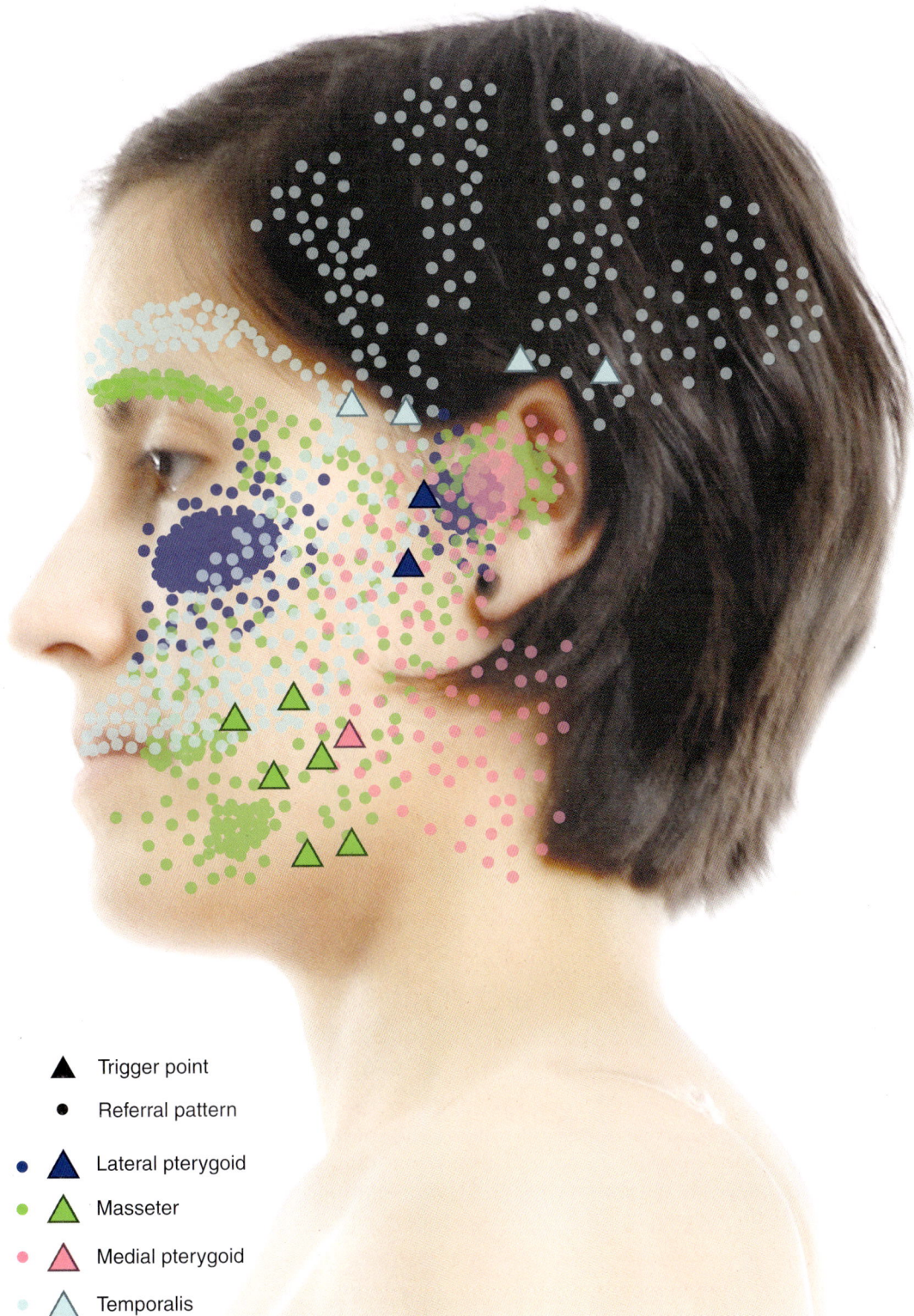

		Trigger point
		Referral pattern
●	▲	Lateral pterygoid
●	▲	Masseter
●	▲	Medial pterygoid
●	▲	Temporalis

Figure 5-5 (*Continued*)

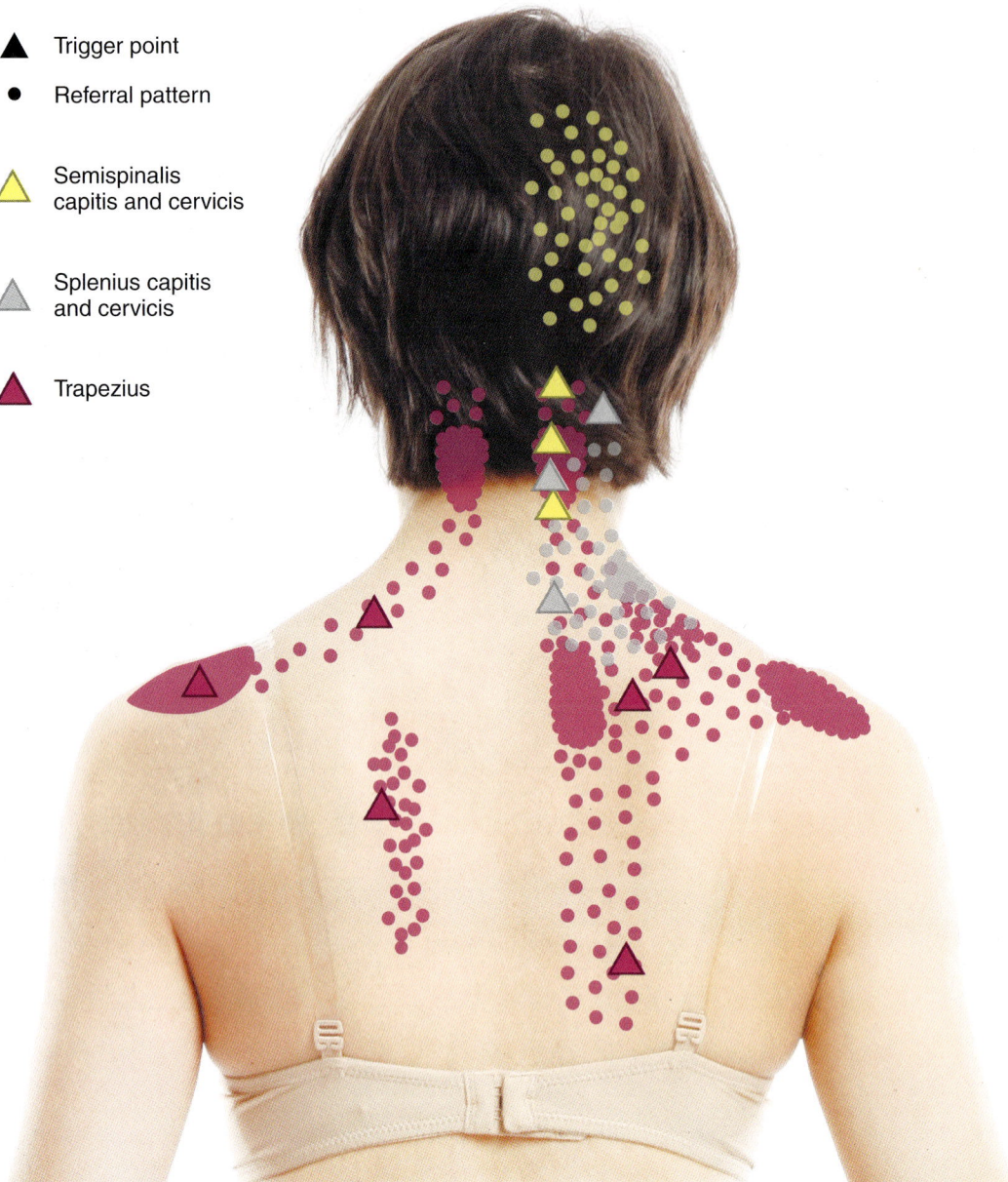

Trigger point

● **Referral pattern**

△ **Semispinalis capitis and cervicis**

△ **Splenius capitis and cervicis**

▲ **Trapezius**

Figure 5-5 (*Continued*)

■ Assess and reduce tension at the attachment sites of all posterior cervical muscles including the acromion process, clavicle, and spine of the scapulae. Follow with the same technique along the transverse and spinous processes of the upper thoracic, all cervical vertebrae, and the occiput.

■ Assess the SCM, suboccipitals, semispinalis capitis and cervicis, and splenius capitis and cervicis for taut bands and trigger points (Fig. 5-7), and treat those you find.

■ Arrange your four fingers of both hands along the occiput and apply pressure to perform Golgi tendon release along the occiput.

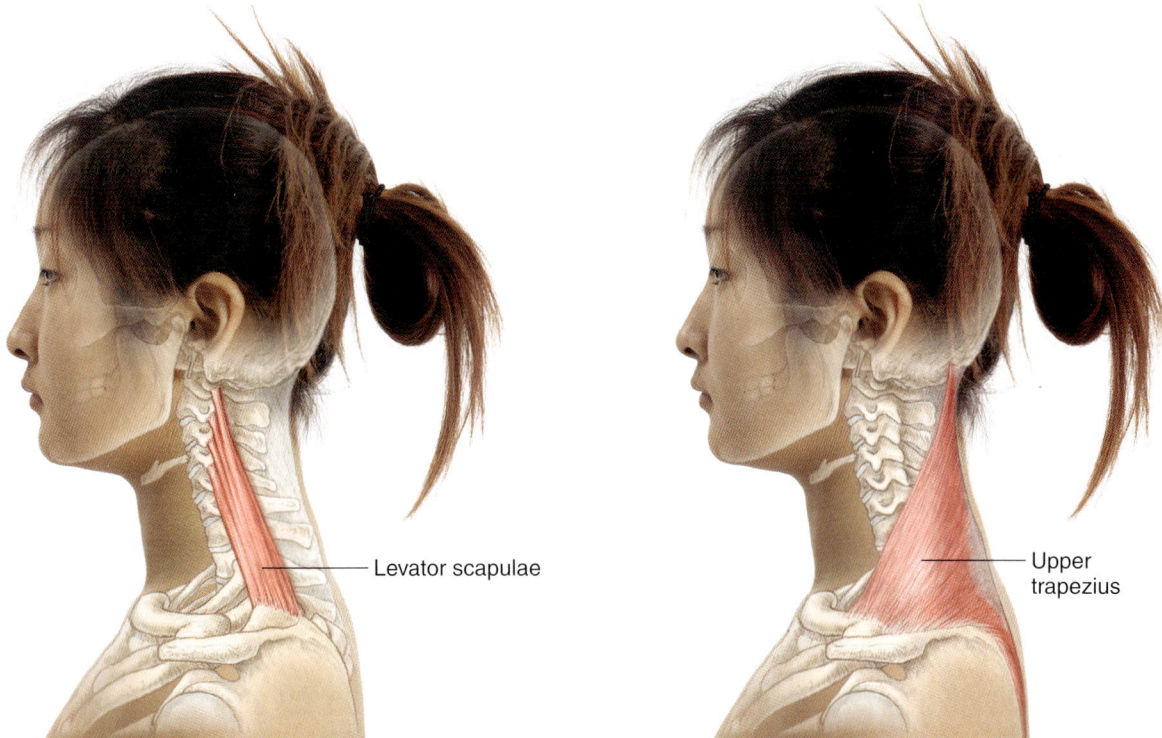

LEVATOR SCAPULA	
Origin	*Transverse process of C1-4.*
Insertion	*Upper medial border and superior angle of scapula.*
Action	***Bilaterally**: extend neck and head; **unilaterally**: elevate scapula, downward rotation of scapula, lateral flexion of neck and head, ipsilateral rotation of neck and head.*
Nerve	*Dorsal scapular and cervical nerves.*

UPPER TRAPEZIUS	
Origin	*External occipital protuberance, medial superior nuchal line of occiput, ligamentum nuchae.*
Insertion	*Lateral third of clavicle, acromion process.*
Action	***Bilaterally**: extend neck and head; **unilaterally**: ipsilateral lateral flexion of neck and head, contralateral rotation of neck and head, elevate scapula, upwardly rotate scapula.*
Nerve	*Spinal accessory and cervical plexus.*

Figure 5-6 **Upper trapezius and levator scapulae.** Reduce adhesions and assess for taut bands in the upper trapezius and levator scapulae. Adapted from Clay JH, Pounds DM. *Basic Clinical Massage Therapy: Integrating Anatomy and Treatment,* 2nd ed. Philadelphia: Lippincott Williams & Wilkins, 2008.

- Thoroughly stretch all muscles that extend and laterally flex the neck.

- Assess and treat the tissues of the anterior neck, in particular the SCM and scalenes (Fig. 5-8). Gently nudge the SCM medially to assess and treat the anterior scalenes. Warm the tissues thoroughly, treat any trigger points found, and follow with a full stretch to the SCM and scalenes.

- Treat the muscles of mastication, including the temporalis, masseter, and pterygoids to reduce tension (Fig. 5-9). Assess for taut bands and treat any trigger points found. Wearing non-powdered or washed gloves, stretch these muscles by gently opening the mouth passively and holding for at least 15 seconds. You can also perform postisometric relaxation techniques by asking the client to close the mouth against your resistance, taking care to instruct the client not to bite down completely, and then releasing the contraction for a full stretch. Intra-oral treatment may be prohibited according to your state regulations.

Figure 5-7   Muscles attached to the occiput. Reduce adhesions and assess for taut bands and trigger points in the SCM, suboccipitals, semispinalis capitis and cervicis, and splenius capitis and cervicis. Adapted from Clay JH, Pounds DM. *Basic Clinical Massage Therapy: Integrating Anatomy and Treatment,* 2nd ed. Philadelphia: Lippincott Williams & Wilkins, 2008.

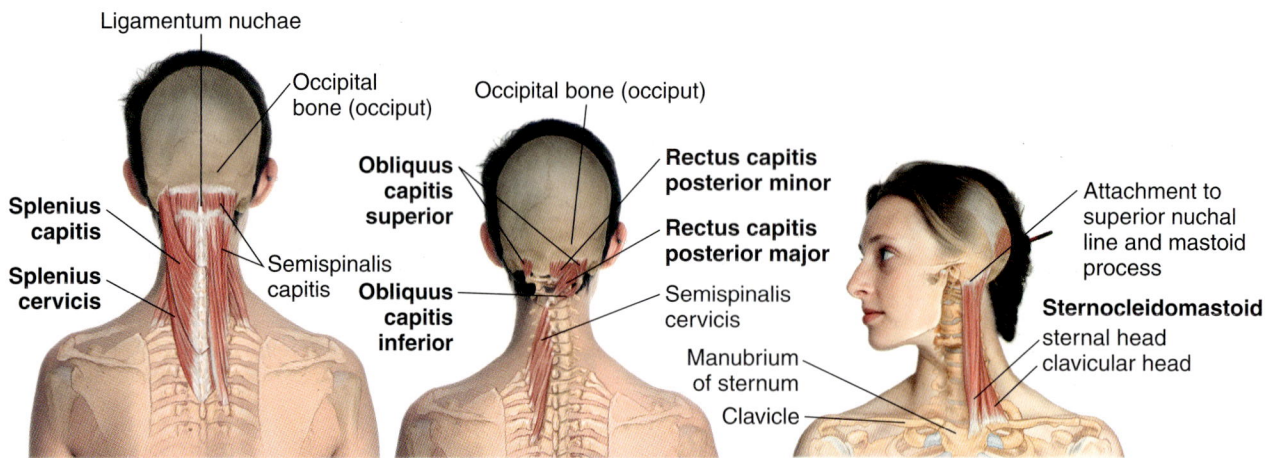

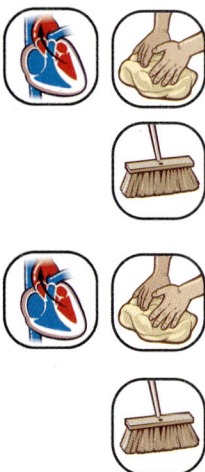

SPLENIUS CAPITIS

Origin	Ligamentum nuchae, SP of C7–T3
Insertion	Mastoid process and lateral superior nuchal line of occiput.
Action	**Bilaterally**: extend neck and head; **unilaterally**: ipsilateral rotation and lateral flexion of head and neck.
Nerve	Branches of dorsal division of cervical nerves.

SPLENIUS CERVICIS

Origin	SP of T3–6.
Insertion	TVP of upper cervical vertebrae.
Action	**Bilaterally**: extend neck and head; **unilaterally**: ipsilateral rotation and lateral flexion of head and neck.
Nerve	Branches of dorsal division of cervical nerves.

SEMISPINALIS CAPITIS

Origin	TVPs of thoracic vertebrae and articular processes of lower cervical vertebrae.
Insertion	SPs of C2–7 and upper thoracic vertebrae, superior nuchal line of occiput.
Action	Extend the vertebral column and head.
Nerve	Dorsal primary divisions of spinal nerves.

SEMISPINALIS CERVICIS

Origin	TVPs of T1–6, articular processes of C4–7
Insertion	SPs of C2–5
Action	**Unilaterally**: lateral flexion of the neck and head; **bilaterally**: extension of the cervical spine.
Nerve	Posterior rami of the cervical nerves.

SUBOCCIPITALS

Origin	SPs and TVPs of C1–2.
Insertion	Nuchal lines of occiput and TVP of C1.
Action	Tilt the head into extension, ipsilateral rotation of head.
Nerve	Suboccipital.

STERNOCLEIDOMASTOID

Origin	Top of manubrium and medial third of clavicle.
Insertion	Mastoid process and superior nuchal line.
Action	**Unilateral**: ipsilateral lateral flexion and rotation of the head and neck; **bilateral**: flexion of the neck, assist in inhalation.
Nerve	Spinal accessory XI.

■ Gently treat the rest of the face, particularly around the sinuses. If you suspect sinus pressure to be a contributing factor, spend a bit more time warming and softening the contents of the sinuses by placing your finger at the sinus and using gentle pressure. You may actually feel movement of fluid during this technique. Follow with gentle tapping at the sinuses, asking the client to hum deeply, explaining that the vibration may help to break up congestion. Follow with superficial gliding strokes moving inferiorly to drain the sinuses.

■ Treat the full scalp to increase circulation and release tension in the occipitofrontalis. If the client tolerates it, pulling the hair very gently may be useful in increasing circulation and reducing tension in the scalp.

■ Apply clearing strokes to the face and head.

■ If time permits and the client can tolerate the face cradle in the prone position, treat the posterior thoracic muscles as needed. If hyperkyphosis is involved, you may find overstretched

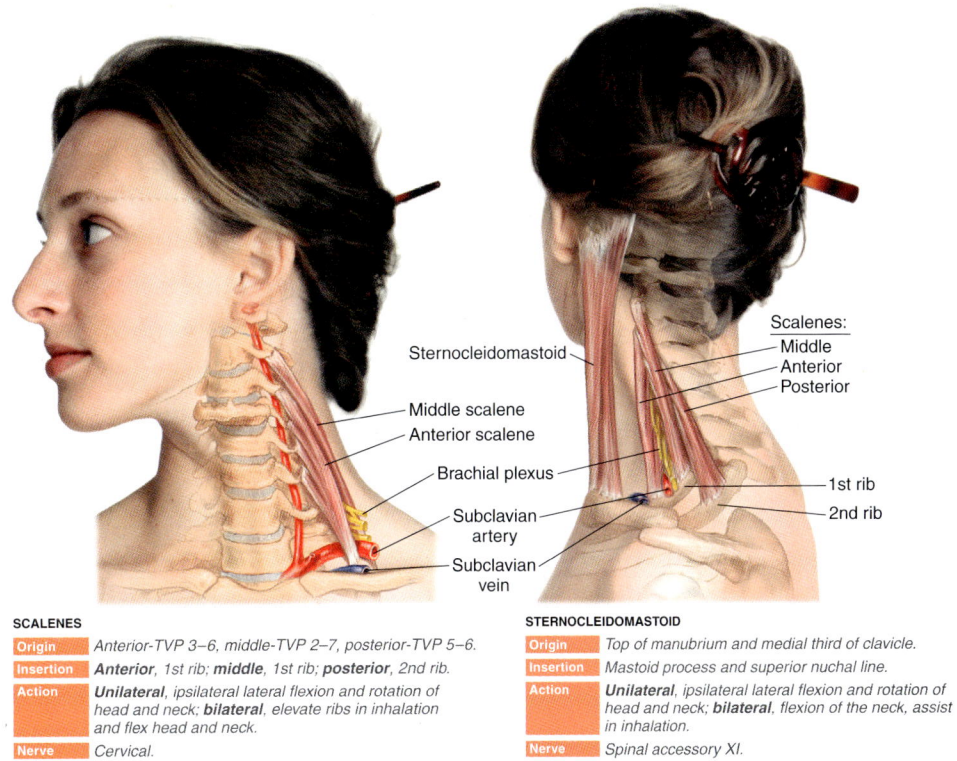

SCALENES

Origin	*Anterior-TVP 3–6, middle-TVP 2–7, posterior-TVP 5–6.*
Insertion	***Anterior**, 1st rib; **middle**, 1st rib; **posterior**, 2nd rib.*
Action	***Unilateral**, ipsilateral lateral flexion and rotation of head and neck; **bilateral**, elevate ribs in inhalation and flex head and neck.*
Nerve	*Cervical.*

STERNOCLEIDOMASTOID

Origin	*Top of manubrium and medial third of clavicle.*
Insertion	*Mastoid process and superior nuchal line.*
Action	***Unilateral**, ipsilateral lateral flexion and rotation of head and neck; **bilateral**, flexion of the neck, assist in inhalation.*
Nerve	*Spinal accessory XI.*

Figure 5-8   Scalenes. The SCM and scalenes may be short and tight with the head-forward posture. Adapted from Clay JH, Pounds DM. *Basic Clinical Massage Therapy: Integrating Anatomy and Treatment,* 2nd ed. Philadelphia: Lippincott Williams & Wilkins, 2008.

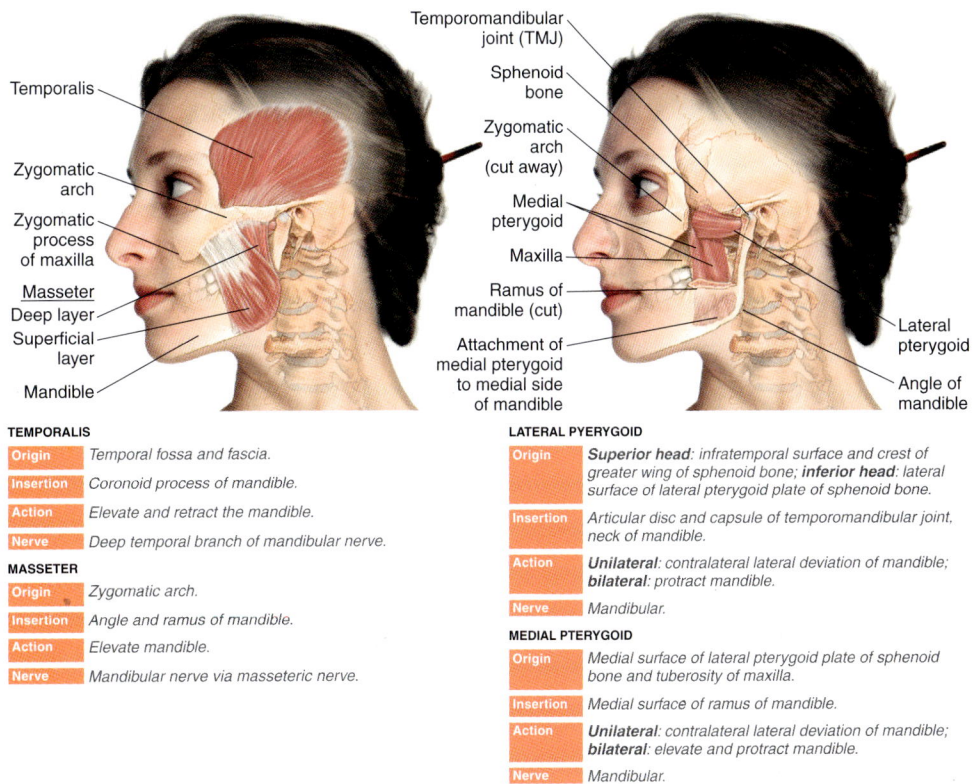

TEMPORALIS

Origin	*Temporal fossa and fascia.*
Insertion	*Coronoid process of mandible.*
Action	*Elevate and retract the mandible.*
Nerve	*Deep temporal branch of mandibular nerve.*

MASSETER

Origin	*Zygomatic arch.*
Insertion	*Angle and ramus of mandible.*
Action	*Elevate mandible.*
Nerve	*Mandibular nerve via masseteric nerve.*

LATERAL PYERYGOID

Origin	***Superior head**: infratemporal surface and crest of greater wing of sphenoid bone; **inferior head**: lateral surface of lateral pterygoid plate of sphenoid bone.*
Insertion	*Articular disc and capsule of temporomandibular joint, neck of mandible.*
Action	***Unilateral**: contralateral lateral deviation of mandible; **bilateral**: protract mandible.*
Nerve	*Mandibular.*

MEDIAL PTERYGOID

Origin	*Medial surface of lateral pterygoid plate of sphenoid bone and tuberosity of maxilla.*
Insertion	*Medial surface of ramus of mandible.*
Action	***Unilateral**: contralateral lateral deviation of mandible; **bilateral**: elevate and protract mandible.*
Nerve	*Mandibular.*

Figure 5-9   Muscles of mastication. Reduce adhesions and assess for taut bands in the temporalis, masseter, and pterygoids. Adapted from Clay JH, Pounds DM. *Basic Clinical Massage Therapy: Integrating Anatomy and Treatment,* 2nd ed. Philadelphia: Lippincott Williams & Wilkins, 2008.

TREATMENT GOAL

STRUCTURES		General	Specific		General
		Superficial		Deep	Superficial
Proximal		Chest			Chest
Distal		Neck	Upper trapezius Levator scapulae Sternocleidomastoid	Semispinalis capitis Semispinalis cervicis Splenius capitis Splenius cervicis Cervical erector spinae Suboccipitals Scalenes	Neck
		Face	Masseter	Medial pterygoid Lateral pterygoid	Face
		Head	Temporalis Occipitofrontalis		Head
Proximal		Back	Middle trapezius Latissimus dorsi	Rhomboids Thoracic erector spinae	Back

Primary goals for treatment (Tension Headaches)

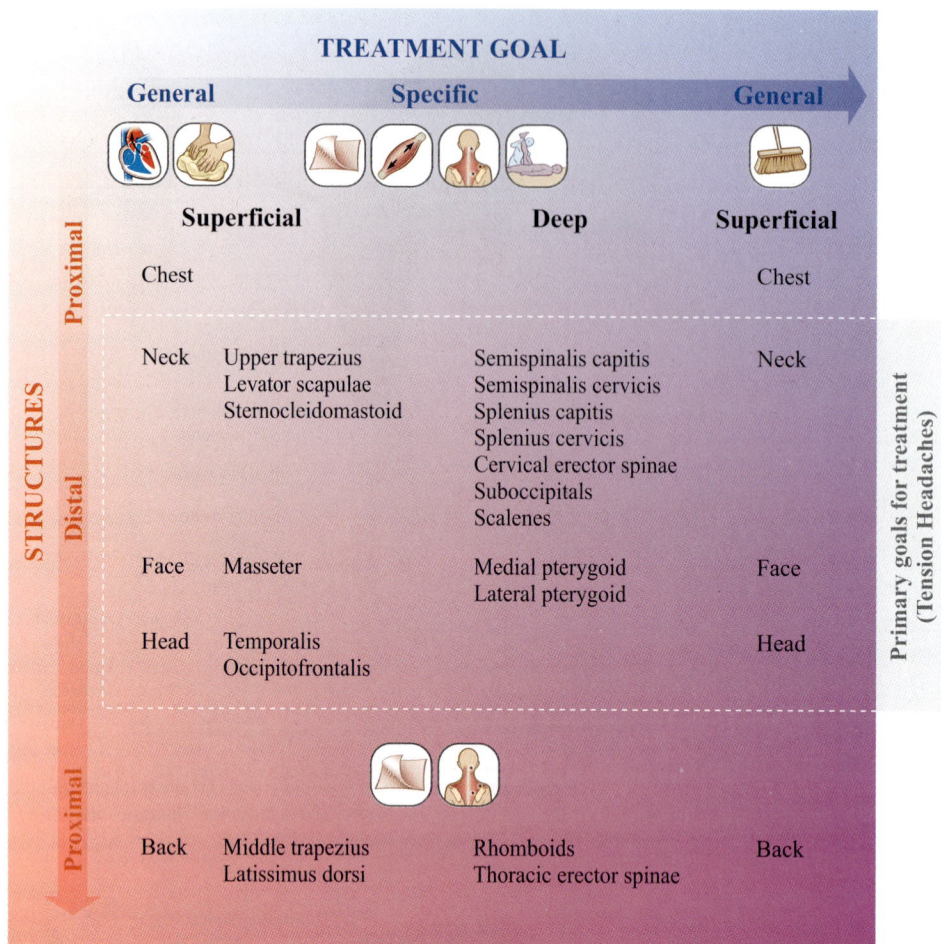

Figure 5-10 **Tension headache treatment overview diagram.** Follow the general principles from left to right or top to bottom when treating tension headaches.

rhomboids, middle trapezius, and thoracic erector spinae and hypertonic cervical erector spinae, lower trapezius, and latissimus dorsi. If a respiratory condition is a factor, be sure to assess and treat the serratus muscles.

The treatment overview diagram summarizes the flow of treatment (Fig. 5-10).

CLIENT SELF-CARE

The following are intended as general recommendations for stretching and strengthening muscles involved in tension headaches. The objective is to create distance between the attachment sites of muscles that have shortened and to perform repetitions of movements that decrease the distance between the attachments of muscles that have weakened. If you have had no training in remedial exercises and do not feel that you have a functional understanding of stretching and strengthening, refer the client to a professional with training in this area.

Clients often neglect self-care because their daily lives are busy. Encourage them to follow these guidelines:

■ Instruct the client to perform self-care activities throughout the day, such as while taking a phone call, reading e-mail, watching television, or performing other activities of daily living instead of setting aside extra time.

- Encourage the client to take regular breaks from repetitive actions.
- Demonstrate gentle self-massage to keep adhesions and hypertonicity at bay between treatments.
- Encourage the client to perform relaxed, deep breathing exercises when pain arises.
- Encourage the client to keep a headache journal, which may help identify patterns and aggravating factors.
- Instruct the client on proper posture to keep pressure off weakened joints. For the client who spends long hours at a desk or on the telephone, it is essential to demonstrate the proper seated posture and to instruct the client not to hold the phone between the ear and shoulder. Recommend a sleeping position that does not stress the client's affected structures.
- Demonstrate all strengthening exercises and stretches to your client and have him or her perform these in your presence before leaving to ensure that he or she is performing them properly and will not harm himself or herself when practicing alone. Stretches should be held for 15–30 seconds and performed frequently throughout the day within the client's limits. The client should not force the stretch. It should be slow and gentle, trying to keep every other muscle as relaxed as possible.

Stretching

To stretch the posterior neck muscles, instruct the client to let the head hang so that the chin approaches the chest (Fig. 5-11). He or she should not force the chin to touch the chest with an active contraction. To increase the stretch, the client can rest the hands on the back of the head and allow the weight of the arms to gently pull the chin toward the chest. It may help to gently rotate the flexed neck to one side to more specifically target muscles that need lengthening.

To stretch the cervical rotators and restore mobility, instruct the client to slowly and gently rotate the neck to one side, hold for 5–10 seconds, then rotate to the other side and hold; repeat this 5–10 times or as often as is comfortable before the client feels fatigue or weakness. For some, it may feel good to rotate the head in extension as well, but this is not advised if the client is at risk for nerve compression or herniation. Even in the absence of disc disease or nerve compression, one rotation in extension may be performed after several side-to-side rotations in flexion, but do not instruct the client to do a full repeated circumduction of the head.

If temporomandibular joint dysfunction is a contributing factor, and the joint does not dislocate during movement, instruct the client to open the mouth as widely as is comfortable and to hold for 15 seconds, relax for 5 seconds, and repeat this stretch 5–10 times. If possible, have the client alternate between opening the mouth straight and then opening the mouth with the lower jaw to the right, then to the left, always coming back to the middle between stretches. You may also instruct the client to perform gentle massage to the muscles of mastication.

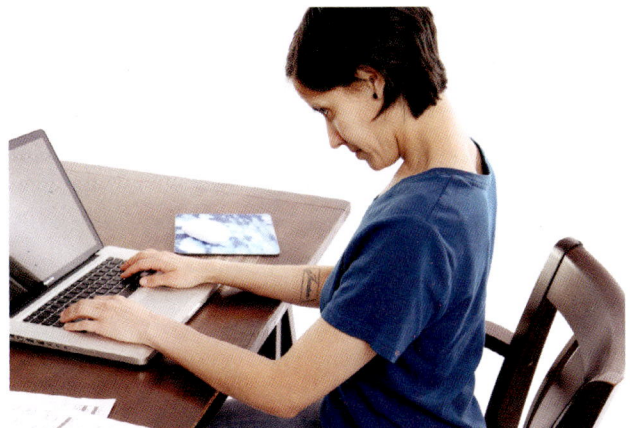

Figure 5-11   Cervical extensor stretch.
Instruct the client to let the head hang without any force.

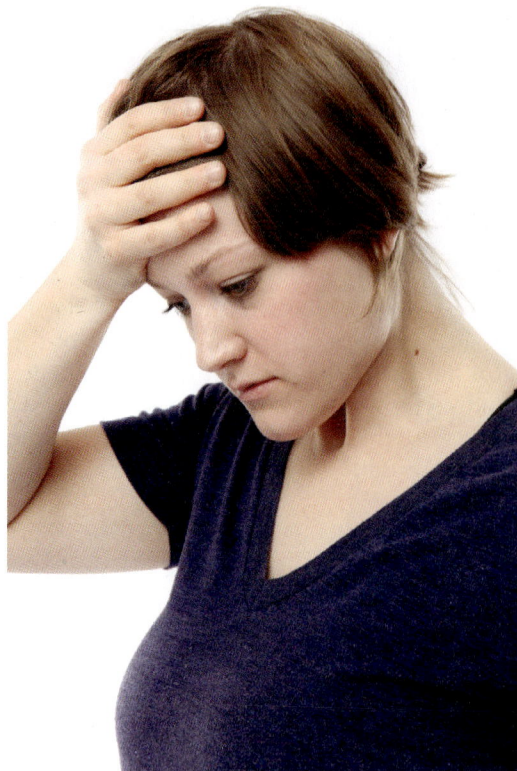

Figure 5-12   **Cervical flexor strengthening.**
Instruct the client to flex the neck against the resistance of his or her hand.

Strengthening

The client can strengthen the deep anterior neck muscles with resisted flexion of the neck. Instruct the client to rest the forehead in the palm of his or her hand, and with the spine erect and thorax in proper alignment, flex the neck against the resistance of the hand (Fig. 5-12). These can be held for approximately 5–10 seconds with 3–5 seconds of rest between each resistance. The client can perform 10 or more repetitions for as long as it is comfortable before feeling fatigue or weakness in the neck.

If hyperkyphosis is a contributing factor, the client must also strengthen the middle trapezius and rhomboids in order to oppose the pull of the shortened pectoral muscles. Instruct the client to stand with the arms comfortably hanging at the sides while squeezing the scapulae together. When this is done properly, only the middle trapezius and rhomboids should contract while the shoulders are relaxed. See Chapter 4 for more detailed instruction and images.

SUGGESTIONS FOR FURTHER TREATMENT

Ideally, the client with chronic tension headaches will have treatments once or twice a week until symptoms are absent for at least 7 days. As treatment continues, the period of symptom-free days should increase until headaches become occasional or are relieved completely. After this, the client can schedule as necessary. If the headaches are caused by muscle tension, there should be some improvement with each session. If this is not happening, consider the following possibilities:

- There is too much time between treatments. It is always best to give the newly treated tissues 24–48 hours to adapt, but if too much time passes between treatments in the beginning, the client's activities of daily living may reverse any progress.
- The client is not adjusting his or her activities of daily living or is not keeping up with self-care. As much as we want to fix the problem, we cannot force a client to make the adjustments we suggest.

- The condition is advanced or involves other musculoskeletal complications that are beyond your basic training. Refer this client to a massage therapist with advanced clinical or medical massage training. Continuing to treat a client whose case is beyond your scope of practice could turn the client away from massage therapy altogether and hinder his or her healing.
- The headaches have an undiagnosed, underlying cause. Discontinue treatment until the client sees a health care provider for medical assessment.

If you are not treating the client in a clinical setting or private practice, you may not be the therapist who takes this client through the full program of healing. Still, if you can bring some relief, it may encourage the client to discuss this change with a health care provider and to consider massage therapy rather than more aggressive treatment options. If the client agrees to return for regular treatments, the symptoms are likely to change each time, so it is important to perform an assessment before each session. Once you have released superficial tissues in general areas, you may be able to focus more of your treatment on a specific area. Likewise, once you have treated the structures specific to tension headaches, you may be able to pay closer attention to compensating structures and coexisting conditions.

PROFESSIONAL GROWTH

CASE STUDY

Grace is a 20-year-old college student. She was an athlete in high school and has tried to continue in sports, but her current responsibilities make it difficult for her to stay active. Grace does her best to choose healthy options when she finds the time to eat a proper meal. She rarely has time for exercise, but walks to and from classes, which are approximately a mile away from her home. She has been getting headaches in the late afternoon a few days a week.

Subjective

Grace stated having headaches that begin in the late afternoon. The headaches get better while she is walking home but sometimes kick up again after dinner when she does her homework and persist until she goes to sleep or takes an aspirin. She does not wake up with the headache. She has had occasional headaches at school for a few months, but recently they have become as frequent as 3 or 4 times per week. She feels the pain on the side of her head as if it wraps around her ear. The pain is often on the left side, but occasionally it feels like it fills her whole head. She also stated that recently she noticed that she feels pain on the left side of her upper back when she gets a headache. She stated that her desk at work is set up with the phone and keyboard to the left of her screen, so she often holds the phone with her left shoulder and has to turn her head to the right to look at the screen when typing. When asked to describe the character and intensity of pain, she stated that it felt as if she were wearing a helmet that is too tight, and that the pain was distracting and slowed her down but did not cause her to stop working. On a scale of 1–10, Grace stated that she felt pain at a level 6 most of the time, occasionally at 7 or 8. When asked, Grace was unsure whether she has the tendency to grind her teeth. When asked, she stated that she has had no numbness, tingling, extremes of temperature, or other unusual sensations in the extremities, has felt no dizziness, vertigo, nausea or changes in vision or speech, and has never experienced an aura or sensitivity to light with her headaches. Grace drinks water regularly throughout the day.

Objective

When I stood to Grace's right, she was able to look toward me by rotating only her head. When I stood to her left, she rotated her whole thorax to look in my direction. Postural assessment revealed a head-forward posture and an elevated left shoulder. Her head is laterally flexed left and rotated to the right. Her thorax is slightly flexed to the left. Her hips are slightly rotated to the right. Palpation assessment revealed that her superficial neck extensors are adhered and dense. It was difficult to distinguish individual muscles or to feel muscle fibers initially.

Action

I began treatment in the supine position with a bolster under the occiput and an eye pillow over the eyes. I performed myofascial release on the superficial adhesions along the occiput toward the mastoid process and down the lateral neck. I spent a significant amount of time warming the lateral and posterior neck with effleurage and cross-fiber friction. I applied muscle stripping to the upper trapezius bilaterally. I found a trigger point approximately 2 inches medial to the left acromion process that referred pain into the head around the ear at a pain level of 8. Compression followed by focused muscle stripping reduced the intensity of the referred pain to level 5. I applied pincer grip petrissage to the SCMs. No trigger points were found. I used cross-fiber friction on the scalenes followed by muscle stripping. I found a trigger point in the left anterior scalene approximately 1 inch superior to the clavicle that referred pain across the left shoulder at level 6. Compression followed by muscle stripping reduced the referred pain to level 2. I applied a deep stretch to the upper trapezius, SCMs, and scalenes bilaterally. I also applied cross-fiber friction to the neck extensors and circular petrissage along the spine of the scapulae, superior angles of the scapulae, and the thoracic and cervical vertebrae. Taut bands were found in the left splenius capitis and levator scapulae. No trigger points were found. I used deep friction on the neck extensors to reduce adhesions and release taut bands. With the remaining time, I paid minor attention to the full length of the erector spinae, latissimus dorsi, internal and external obliques, and quadratus lumborum to assess and begin reducing thoracic flexion and rotation in hips.

Grace stated that she felt less stiff than when she arrived.

Plan

I demonstrated stretches to the neck extensors and rotators. I recommended that she practice these frequently throughout the day, particularly when she is working or studying. I also recommended that she reorganize her desk so that she can look straight ahead instead of rotating her head toward the screen. I recommended that she use, when possible, a speakerphone or headset or to hold the telephone with her hand instead of using her shoulder. I recommended biweekly treatments for 2 weeks followed by reassessment. This will help to keep adhesions at bay so that we can target more specific tissues in subsequent sessions. Grace scheduled a 1-hour session 4 days from today.

CRITICAL THINKING EXERCISES

1. Develop a 10-minute stretching and strengthening routine for a client that covers all of the muscles commonly involved in tension headaches. Use Box 5-1 and Figure 5-5 as a guide. Remember that a stretch increases the distance between the origin and insertion of a muscle and is important for those muscles that are shortened, while strengthening is performed by actively bringing the origin and insertion closer together and is important if the antagonists of shortened muscles have weakened. Describe each step of the routine in enough detail that the client can perform it without your assistance.

2. A potential client explains that about 6 months ago she started feeling stiffness and pain in her neck and shoulders. She associates this pain with being pulled and spun abruptly during a tango class. She saw her doctor when the pain persisted for a week but was released with no injuries found. No X-rays or special tests were performed. The doctor recommended chiropractic treatment, and the client complied. No X-rays were taken, but orthopedic tests were negative for a herniated disc. The chiropractor adjusted the cervical and thoracic vertebrae, which brought relief for only a day or two. Three subsequent visits also resulted in only temporary relief. In the past few weeks, the client has been experiencing chronic headaches. Assuming that the abrupt movement while dancing was the primary contributing factor, what injury may have occurred that would result in chronic pain and headaches? What are some things to consider in your assessment of an injury that was only temporarily

relieved by chiropractic adjustment to the vertebrae? Which structures will you assess and what abnormalities might you expect to find?

3. Discuss special considerations and adjustments to treatment for a client who has chronic tension headaches as well as a condition such as hypertension or atherosclerosis that is currently under control and being monitored by a health care provider.

4. Conduct a short literature review to explain how the following conditions may put a client at risk for chronic headaches:
   - Nerve root compression
   - Diabetes
   - Chronic bronchitis
   - Dental overbite
   - Whiplash
   - Menopause
   - Depression or anxiety
   - Withdrawal from drugs, alcohol, caffeine, or cigarettes

BIBLIOGRAPHY AND SUGGESTED READINGS

Cibulka MT. Sternocleidomastoid muscle imbalance in a patient with recurrent headache. Manual Therapy. 2006;11(1):78–82.

Eisensmith LP. Massage therapy decreases frequency and intensity of symptoms related to temporomandibular joint syndrome in one case study. Journal of Bodywork and Movement Therapies. 2007;11(3):223–230.

Fernández-de-las-Peñas C, Alonso-Blanco C, Cuadrado ML, et al. Myofascial trigger points in the suboccipital muscles in episodic tension-type headache. Manual Therapy. 2006;11(3):225–230.

Fernández-de-las-Peñas C, Ge H-Y, Arendt-Nielsen L, et al. Referred pain from trapezius muscle trigger points share similar characteristics with chronic tension type headache. European Journal of Pain. 2007;11(4): 475–482.

Giacomini PG, Alessandrini M, Evangelista M, et al. Impaired postural control in patients affected by tension-type headache. European Journal of Pain. 2004;8(6):579–583.

Hernandez-Reif M, Dieter J, Field T, et al. Migraine headaches are reduced by massage therapy. International Journal of Neuroscience. 1998;96:1–11.

International Headache Society. IHS Classification ICHD-II. Available at http://ihs-classification.org/en/. Accessed Summer 2008.

International Headache Society. Available at http://www.i-h-s.org/. Accessed Summer 2008.

Mayo Foundation for Medical Education and Research. Sinus Headaches. Available at http://www.mayoclinic.com/health/sinus-headaches/DS00647. Accessed Summer 2008.

Mayo Foundation for Medical Education and Research. Migraine. Available at http://www.mayoclinic.com/health/migraine-headache/DS00120. Accessed Winter 2010.

Mayo Foundation for Medical Education and Research. Tension Headache. Available at http://www.mayoclinic.com/health/tension-headache/DS00304. Accessed Winter 2010.

Moore MK. Upper crossed syndrome and its relationship to cervicogenic headache. Journal of Manipulative and Physiological Therapeutics. 2004;27(6):414–420.

National Institute of Neurological Disorders and Stroke. Hemicrania Continua Information Page. Available at http://www.ninds.nih.gov/disorders/hemicrania_continua/hemicrania_continua.htm. Accessed Summer 2008.

Oksanen A, Erkintalo M, Metsähonkala L, et al. Neck muscles cross-sectional area in adolescents with and without headache—MRI study. European Journal of Pain. 2008;12(7):952–959.

Puustjärvi K, Airaksinen O, Pöntinen PJ. The effects of massage in patients with chronic tension headache. Acupuncture & Electro-Therapeutics Research; The International Journal. 1990;15(2): 159–162.

Quinn C, Chandler C, Moraska A. Massage therapy and frequency of chronic tension headaches. American Journal of Public Health. 2002;92(10):1657–1661.

Rattray F, Ludwig L. *Clinical Massage Therapy: Understanding, Assessing and Treating over 70 Conditions*. Toronto, ON: Talus Incorporated, 2000.

Simons DG, Travell JG, Simons LS. *Myofascial Pain and Dysfunction: The Trigger Point Manual*, 2nd ed. Philadelphia, PA: Lippincott Williams & Wilkins, 1999.

Turchaninov R. *Medical Massage*, 2nd ed. Phoenix, AZ: Aesculapius Books, 2006.

U.S. National Library of Medicine and the National Institutes of Health. Encephalitis. Available at http://www.nlm.nih.gov/medlineplus/ency/article/001415.htm. Accessed Summer 2008.

U.S. National Library of Medicine and the National Institutes of Health. Meningitis. Available at http://www.nlm.nih.gov/medlineplus/ency/article/000680.htm. Accessed Summer 2008.

U.S. National Library of Medicine and the National Institutes of Health. Migraine. Available at http://www.nlm.nih.gov/medlineplus/ency/article/000709.htm. Accessed Summer 2008.

U.S. National Library of Medicine and the National Institutes of Health. Stroke. Available at http://www.nlm.nih.gov/medlineplus/ency/article/000726.htm. Accessed Summer 2008.

U.S. National Library of Medicine and the National Institutes of Health. Temporal Arteritis. Available at http://www.nlm.nih.gov/medlineplus/ency/article/000448.htm. Accessed Summer 2008.

U.S. National Library of Medicine and the National Institutes of Health. Tension Headache. Available at http://www.nlm.nih.gov/medlineplus/ency/article/000797.htm. Accessed Summer 2008.

U.S. National Library of Medicine and the National Institutes of Health. Trigeminal Neuralgia. Available at http://www.nlm.nih.gov/medlineplus/ency/article/000742.htm. Accessed Summer 2008.

Werner R. *A Massage Therapist's Guide to Pathology*, 4th ed. Philadelphia, PA: Lippincott Williams & Wilkins, 2009.

Zito G, Jull G, Story I. Clinical tests of musculoskeletal dysfunction in the diagnosis of cervicogenic headache. Manual Therapy. 2006;11(2):118–129.

Thoracic Outlet Syndrome

UNDERSTANDING THORACIC OUTLET SYNDROME

The thoracic outlet is the space between the base of the anterior lateral neck and the axilla (Fig. 6-1). A neurovascular bundle that includes the brachial plexus, the subclavian artery, and the subclavian vein passes through the thoracic outlet. Thoracic outlet syndrome refers to a collection of symptoms that occur when any of these structures become compressed. The symptoms are often vague, and there is no true consensus about the cause or diagnosis. The condition is called neurogenic thoracic outlet syndrome when the nerves are compressed, and vascular thoracic outlet syndrome when the blood vessels are compressed. Neurogenic thoracic outlet syndrome is most common, although occasionally, both occur simultaneously.

The nerve roots of the brachial plexus exit the spine between C5 and T1. These roots merge to form the superior, middle, and anterior trunks. Each trunk splits into anterior and posterior divisions, which then regroup to form the posterior, lateral, and medial cords; these later split into the branches that innervate the arm. Compression of the nerves slows the transmission of impulses; this can result in pain, burning, numbness, and tingling in the shoulder, axilla, lateral thorax, and down the arm to the hand. The subclavian artery, subclavian vein, and cervical lymph trunk also pass through the thoracic outlet. Compression of these structures can result in decreased blood supply to the arm, insufficient venous return, and lymphatic congestion, causing swelling in the arm, pale or cool skin, and a weakened pulse.

When thoracic outlet syndrome has muscular contributing factors, postures and activities that shorten myofascial tissues and decrease the space through which the nerves and vessels pass may cause symptoms. There are three primary areas where muscular compression of the contents of the thoracic outlet occurs: between the anterior and middle scalenes (anterior scalene syndrome), beneath the clavicle and subclavius (costoclavicular syndrome), and beneath the pectoralis minor (pectoralis minor syndrome). Because common postures like working at a computer for extended periods often result in a head-forward posture, flexion and internal rotation of the shoulder, pronation of the forearm, and extension of the wrist, compression may occur at more than one of these sites, as well as beneath the pronator teres or in the carpal tunnel. Compression occurring at more than one site along the path of a peripheral nerve is called a double crush.

Common Signs and Symptoms

The symptoms of thoracic outlet syndrome usually begin gradually. Symptoms are commonly unilateral but may be bilateral. The signs and symptoms of neurogenic thoracic outlet syndrome include aching, pain, burning, numbness, or tingling in the shoulder, neck, arm, or hand of the

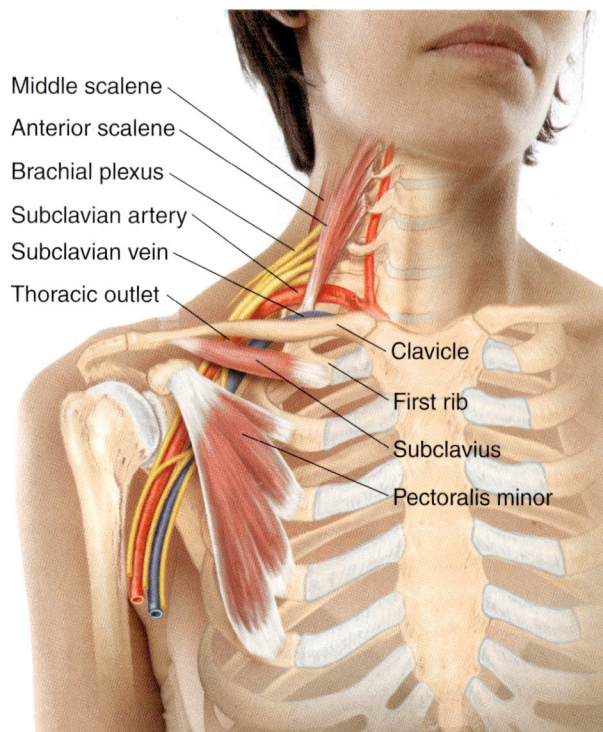

Figure 6-1 **The thoracic outlet.** The brachial plexus, subclavian vein, and subclavian artery pass through the thoracic outlet.

Middle scalene
Anterior scalene
Brachial plexus
Subclavian artery
Subclavian vein
Thoracic outlet
Clavicle
First rib
Subclavius
Pectoralis minor

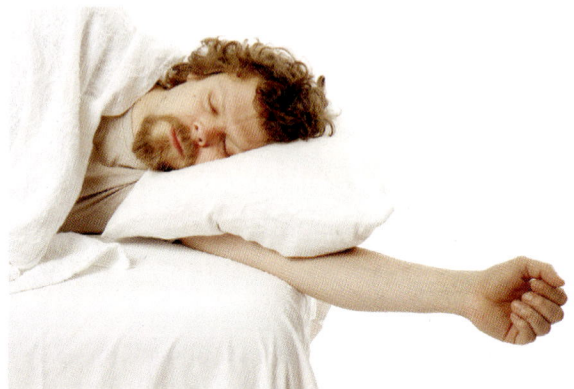

Figure 6-2 **Sleeping on one side.** With the arm raised above the head during sleep, the brachial plexus and blood vessels can become compressed, producing symptoms and waking the client.

affected side. Untreated, reduced innervation may lead to loss of tone, initially in the thenar muscles and eventually in the muscles of the arm and hand, causing reduced strength and fine motor skills. Atrophy may occur in advanced cases.

With vascular thoracic outlet syndrome, the client may experience the symptoms described above in addition to swelling, ischemia, and pain in the arm and hand or sensitivity to temperatures in the hand and fingers. The skin of the hand may be pale or bluish. Symptoms may mimic those of Raynaud's syndrome, namely cold fingers and pallor. The client may have a weak or absent pulse in the affected arm. Black spots on the hand and fingers may be present when decreased circulation affects the health of those tissues. In the worst-case scenario, vascular compression can be caused by blood clots, or can result in blood clots if left untreated. A client with these symptoms should be assessed by a medical professional prior to massage.

Because postural imbalance is often a contributing factor, the client may also have neck pain, chest pain, jaw pain, or frequent tension headaches. Note, however, that chest pain that refers to the jaw, throat, and arm may also be symptoms of a cardiac problem, which requires medical assessment prior to performing massage therapy. See Table 6-1 for conditions commonly confused with or contributing to thoracic outlet syndrome. Raising the arm above the head often intensifies the symptoms, particularly when lifting heavy objects. Lying down or gently moving the head and shoulder into a neutral position may reduce symptoms, particularly in the early stages of the syndrome.

Many people suffering from thoracic outlet syndrome are awakened from sleep by pain or tingling, often because they sleep with the head resting on the raised arm (Fig. 6-2). Disturbed sleep can contribute to a cycle in which fatigue exacerbates symptoms and produces anxiety and depression, which may in turn disturb sleep.

Possible Causes and Contributing Factors

Thoracic outlet syndrome is not a clearly defined condition but a collection of signs and symptoms associated with various contributing factors. Anatomically, a small percentage of people have a cervical rib—a bony prominence that emerges from the C7 transverse process and meets

Table 6-1	Differentiating Conditions Commonly Confused with or Contributing to Thoracic Outlet Syndrome		
Condition	**Typical Signs and Symptoms**	**Testing**	**Massage Therapy**
Herniated disc	Symptoms may increase when coughing, laughing, and straining	Kemp's test	Massage is indicated with caution and proper training. Acute inflammation and acute injury are contraindications. Work with the health care team.
C4-5	Weak deltoid	Spurling's test	
	Shoulder pain	CT scan	
	Usually no radiating pain or paresthesia	Myelography	
		MRI	
C5-6	Weak biceps and wrist extensors		
	Pain and paresthesia in radial distribution		
C6-7	Weak triceps and finger extensors		
	Pain and paresthesia down posterior arm into third digit		
C7-T1	Weak hand grip		
	Pain and paresthesia in ulnar distribution		
Cervical spondylosis (cervical arthritis)	Neck pain that may radiate to the shoulder or arms	X-ray	Massage is indicated with caution. In cases of nerve impingement or spurs that irritate nerves, work with a health care provider. Position client to reduce symptoms, and do not remove protective muscle splinting.
	Loss of or abnormal sensation in the shoulder or arms	CT scan	
	Weak arms	MRI	
	Stiff neck that gradually worsens	Myelogram	
	Loss of balance	EMG	
	Headache		
	Loss of bladder or bowel control		
Nerve root compression (radiculopathy)	Muscle spasm, weakness, or atrophy	Spurling's test	Massage is indicated if cause and location are understood. Take care not to increase compression or reproduce symptoms.
	Pain around the scapula on the affected side	Valsalva's test	
	Neck pain	Neurological exam to test reflexes, sensation, and strength	
	Pain radiates to extremities		
	Pain worsens with lateral flexion or rotation or when sneezing, coughing, laughing, or straining		
Tendinitis (biceps, forearm, or rotator cuff)	Local inflammation and point tenderness	Pain on full passive stretch of the joint that the tendon crosses; pain with resisted activity	See chapter 13
	No muscle wasting		
Pronator teres syndrome	Pain in forearm, worsened by elbow flexion/extension	Resisted pronation of the forearm (excluding resistance to the wrist)	Massage is indicated
	Absence of pain during the night	Tinel's sign at the median nerve as it passes under the pronator teres	

(*continued*)

Table 6-1	Differentiating Conditions Commonly Confused with or Contributing to Thoracic Outlet Syndrome (Continued)		
Condition	**Typical Signs and Symptoms**	**Testing**	**Massage Therapy**
Hypothyroid condition	Weakness, fatigue, intolerance to cold, constipation, unintentional weight gain, brittle hair and nails, dry skin, puffy skin, hoarse voice, sleep disturbance, and mood swings	Physical exam T3, T4, and Serum TSH laboratory tests	Massage is indicated when no other contraindicated condition, such as a circulatory complication, is present.
Rheumatoid arthritis	Fatigue, loss of appetite, low-grade fever, bilateral nonspecific muscle pain, rheumatic nodules, periods of flares and remission	Physical exam Blood tests X-ray	Massage is indicated in nonacute stages. Work with health care team.
Angina pectoris	Chest pain Pain in arms, neck, jaw, shoulder, or back in addition to chest pain Nausea Fatigue Shortness of breath Anxiety Sweating	Physical exam Risk factors Blood test Electrocardiogram Stress test Chest X-ray Echocardiogram CT scan	Trigger points in pectoralis major may mimic some symptoms of angina pectoris. If the client presents with risk factors or the symptoms listed here, refer him or her to a health care provider prior to treatment. When risk factors are present, massage is indicated only if cleared by a primary health care provider, and if client is able to perform normal activities of daily living.
Diabetes	Frequent urination, frequent thirst, increased appetite, fatigue, nausea	Physical exam Fasting blood sugar test	Massage is indicated when tissues and circulation are not compromised.
Cervical stenosis	Pain, weakness, and numbness in the shoulders, arms, and legs Clumsy fine motor skills Balance disturbance	Physical exam X-ray MRI CT scan Myelogram Bone scan	Massage is indicated with caution. Work with a health care provider. Client may receive corticosteroid injections or may be using anti-inflammatory medication.
Tumors (axillary, first rib, pancoast, nerve sheath, and spinal cord)	Signs and symptoms vary depending on type and location of tumor. General characteristics for tumors affecting the thoracic outlet include the following: Pain, often severe and constant, in shoulder and scapula that radiates to the arm and hand Weakening, atrophy, and numbness or tingling in the arm and hand Paraplegia	CT scan MRI Pet scan CBC Biopsy Chest X-ray	Refer client to health care provider if you suspect a tumor. Work with the health care provider if a tumor has been diagnosed. Recommendations for massage depend on the type and location of the tumor.

Table 6-1	Differentiating Conditions Commonly Confused with or Contributing to Thoracic Outlet Syndrome (Continued)		
Condition	**Typical Signs and Symptoms**	**Testing**	**Massage Therapy**
Shoulder injuries (impingement, rotator cuff tears, and adhesive capsulitis)	Often gradual onset with spontaneous resolution	Physical exam	Massage is indicated. Work with the health care team.
	Minor pain at rest; acute pain with activity, which may radiate down the arm	X-ray	
	Pain often worse at night, disrupting sleep	MRI	
	Weakness, reduced ROM in shoulder		
	Tenderness and swelling in shoulder		
	Gradual loss of ROM		
Carpal tunnel syndrome	Pain, numbness, and tingling in thumb, index, and middle fingers, and lateral half of ring finger	Phalen's test	See chapter 7
	Gradual atrophy and reduced fine motor skills	Tinel's sign	
		EMG nerve conduction test	
Temporomandibular joint disorder	Difficulty biting or chewing	Dental exam	Massage is indicated
	Clicking sound when moving jaw	MRI	
	Aching in the jaw and face	X-ray	
	Earache	Palpation of muscles of mastication	
	Headache		
	Reduced ROM in mandible		
Raynaud's disease	Cold hands and feet	Signs and symptoms	Raynaud's that is not linked to an underlying condition is indicated for massage. If Raynaud's disease is associated with another condition, follow the guidelines for that condition.
	White or blue skin	Rule out conditions causing similar symptoms such as nerve damage	
	Dulled sensation	Tests for underlying causes	
	Numbness or pain as extremities warm	Cold simulation test	
		Nail bed or nailfold capillaroscopy	
		Antinuclear antibodies test	
		Erythrocyte sedimentation rate	
Reflex sympathetic dystrophy syndrome (complex regional pain syndrome)	Often preceded by injury	Signs and symptoms	Sufferers of RSDS may not tolerate touch in the affected area. If the client is willing, massage is indicated on or around the affected area.
	Severe, burning pain that is more intense than the severity of injury and gets worse over time	Ruling out other conditions	
	Changes in skin temperature, color, texture, and sensitivity	Bone scans	
	Changes in nail and hair growth		
	Sweating		
	Swelling		
	Joint stiffness		
	Reduced ROM		

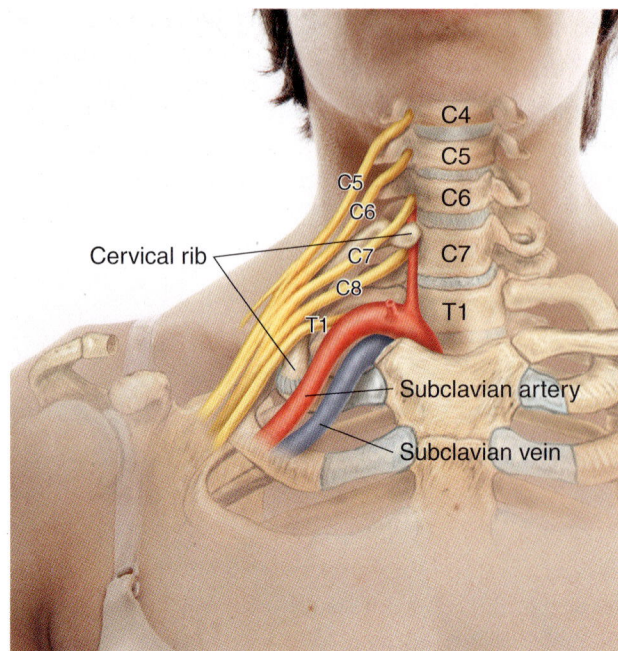

Figure 6-3 **Cervical rib.** An extra rib can develop from the transverse process of C7, connecting to the lateral aspect of the first true rib.

the lateral aspect of the first rib (Fig. 6-3). Cervical ribs are often unilateral but can be bilateral. The presence of a cervical rib, which can be palpated or seen on an X-ray, alters the path of the nerves and vessels as well as the shape of the surrounding soft tissues. In some cases, the C7 transverse process is unusually large, and while it does not form a complete cervical rib, its increased size can displace the tissues around it. Other bony prominences that may develop in the cervical or axillary region as a result of orthopedic disorders can also elicit symptoms. Hyperkyphosis, scoliosis, a subluxed cervical vertebra, or a herniated cervical disc can alter the anatomy of the thoracic outlet and may contribute to symptoms. For example, scoliosis in the thoracic spine will affect the balance of the cervical vertebrae to which the scalenes are attached, potentially shortening the scalenes, which may lead to trigger points and compression of the nerves and vessels passing through the thoracic outlet.

Symptoms of thoracic outlet syndrome may also develop with the use of crutches or any other device or posture that puts pressure on the structures in the axillary region. Weak shoulder muscles may cause a drooping of the shoulder, which causes the clavicle to fall upon the first rib, resulting in compression. Previous traumas including whiplash, rotator cuff injuries, or a fractured clavicle or humerus that were not successfully treated may result in adhesions, scar tissue, compensating patterns, and trigger points that contribute to thoracic outlet symptoms.

The most common postural imbalances that contribute to the symptoms of thoracic outlet syndrome are identical to those of hyperkyphosis. The main difference is that with thoracic outlet syndrome, these postural imbalances have led to the compression of nerves and vessels, causing numbness, tingling, and swelling whereas the symptoms of hyperkyphosis are primarily pain and reduced ROM. Holding postures that include extension and rotation of the neck; head-forward posture; and abduction, flexion, and internal rotation of the shoulder also contribute to the symptoms of this syndrome. People who work at a computer for long periods, teachers who write frequently on a blackboard, cashiers, house painters, and those in any profession in which the neck and shoulders are held in a static position or in which repetitive actions involve flexion and rotation of the shoulder, particularly above the head, are at risk. Athletes whose activities involve forced movement of the shoulder, such as tennis, golf, and volleyball players, are also at risk.

Hypertonicity and trigger points in the anterior and middle scalenes, subclavius, and pectoralis minor are the most common contributing factors and are the focus of the treatment described in this chapter. Any increase in the tone of these muscles can decrease the amount of space through which the brachial plexus and accompanying vessels travel. However, because of the frequent involvement of postural and respiratory abnormalities, nearly all of the muscles attached to the cervical vertebrae, scapulae, or ribs or those that cross the glenohumeral joint may be hypertonic or may develop trigger points. Referral patterns for trigger points in the latissimus dorsi, serratus anterior, and serratus posterior superior can be confused with the symptoms of thoracic outlet syndrome and may be the result of postural deviations that contribute to thoracic outlet syndrome. Other muscles that are not directly involved but may be peripherally involved include the coracobrachialis, anterior deltoid, biceps, upper and middle trapezius, levator scapulae, and SCM because of their attachment sites and their roles in postural imbalances.

Neurogenic thoracic outlet syndrome is a peripheral neuropathy. Systemic disorders including diabetes, hyperthyroid, and rheumatoid arthritis may contribute to the development of peripheral neuropathies. Smoking cigarettes—although not a cause of thoracic outlet syndrome—exacerbates the inflammatory process and can intensify symptoms. In addition, because thoracic outlet syndrome may involve the muscles of respiration, the repeated deep inhalation and exhalation associated with smoking, along with chronic respiratory disorders and coughing, can contribute to hypertonicity in these muscles. Thoracic outlet syndrome may also develop during pregnancy because of increased fluid and postural changes, but this usually resolves itself following delivery. Alcoholism, poor nutrition, vitamin B deficiency, and general stress may also contribute to or exacerbate symptoms.

Because so many factors may potentially contribute to thoracic outlet syndrome, it is important to understand the client's health history before proceeding with treatment. Many of the conditions listed above have contraindications for massage therapy or require adjustments to treatment. Refer the client to his or her health care provider for medical assessment if you suspect any systemic condition. If the client has been diagnosed with a condition that requires special consideration when planning massage, discuss treatment with the client's health care provider and adjust accordingly.

Table 6-1 lists conditions commonly confused with or that contribute to thoracic outlet syndrome.

Contraindications and Special Considerations

- **Underlying pathologies.** The signs and symptoms of thoracic outlet syndrome may result from a wide variety of underlying conditions. If you suspect one of these (consult Table 6-1 and your pathology book for signs and symptoms) or if the client shows signs of vascular compression, refer the client to his or her health care provider for medical assessment before initiating treatment. If the client is diagnosed with an underlying pathology that is not a contraindication for massage, work with the health care provider when necessary to develop an appropriate treatment plan.
- **Edema.** If edema is present, do not work directly on the site. Work proximally, moving the fluid toward the nearest proximal lymph nodes. If vascular compression is a consideration but massage is not contraindicated for the client, do not allow the arm to fall below the heart because gravity may draw fluid into the arm and hand. Bolster the arm if necessary to keep fluid from accumulating.
- **Treatment duration and pressure.** If the client is elderly, has degenerative bone disease, or has been diagnosed with a condition that diminishes activities of daily living, you may need to adjust your pressure as well as the treatment duration. Frequent half-hour sessions may suit the client better.
- **Positioning.** Use bolsters to position a client for comfort as well as to correct postures that may reproduce symptoms. If the head-forward posture or extension of the neck is evident, placing a small bolster under the occiput in the supine position and adjusting the face cradle to reduce the extension of the neck in the prone position may help. A bolster along the length of the spine in the supine position reduces the protraction of the scapulae and the extension of the neck. Bolsters under the shoulders in the prone position reduce the protraction of the scapulae and lengthen the pectoral muscles.

- **Reproducing symptoms.** Symptoms may occur during treatment if you manually compress the neurovascular bundle or if the client's posture causes structures to compress this area. If treatment produces symptoms, first adjust the client to a more neutral posture to relieve compression. If this does not relieve the symptoms, reduce your pressure or move away from the area. You may be able to treat around the site that reproduced the symptoms, but proceed with caution.

- **Hydrotherapy.** Do not use moist heat on the neck or chest if the client has a cardiovascular condition that may be affected by the dilation of blood vessels. Severe hypertension and atherosclerosis are two examples of conditions that are contraindicated for hydrotherapy. Consult your pathology book for recommendations. Do not use heat in areas of edema or inflammation, because heat dilates vessels and may increase the accumulation of fluid.

- **Friction.** Do not use deep frictions if the client has a systemic inflammatory condition, such as rheumatoid arthritis or osteoarthritis, if the health of the underlying tissues is compromised or if the client is taking anti-inflammatory medication. Friction initiates an inflammatory process, which may interfere with the intended action of the anti-inflammatory medication. Recommend that your client refrain from taking such medication for several hours prior to treatment if his or her health care provider is in agreement.

- **Tissue length.** It is important when treating soft tissues that you do not further stretch those that are already overstretched. Assess for myofascial restrictions first and treat only those that are clearly present. Likewise, overstretched muscles should not be stretched from origin to insertion. If you treat trigger points in a muscle that is overstretched, use heat or a localized pin and stretch technique to lengthen that area.

- **Mobilizations.** Be cautious with mobilizations if the client has degenerative disc disease, rheumatoid arthritis, a cervical rib, hypermobile joints, or if ligaments are unstable from pregnancy or a systemic condition.

Massage Therapy Research

Although articles about the benefits of conservative treatment have been published and abundant anecdotal evidence suggests recovery from symptoms is possible following massage, there are currently no extensive experimental investigations into the specific outcomes following massage for the treatment of thoracic outlet syndrome. Much of the research on treatment for thoracic outlet syndrome focuses on pharmaceutical muscle blocks and surgery. Much of the theory behind the use of massage in the treatment of thoracic outlet syndrome has been adapted from other disciplines. Studies conducted by trained therapists into specific outcomes using only massage are needed.

In 1996, Barnes published an article titled "Myofascial Release in Treatment of Thoracic Outlet Syndrome" describing a single treatment program. The client had a 2-year history of chronic pain in her neck, upper extremities, and whole back initiated by an injury to the posterior mid thorax. The client saw many physicians in a variety of specialties and several physical therapists and took dozens of medications in various combinations with no lasting results. Her level of function was reduced; she needed help dressing and grew tired after even minimal writing. Her medical diagnosis at the time she was referred to Barnes' clinic was thoracic outlet syndrome. The client received 30-minute treatments two or three times a day for 2 weeks by a team of physical therapists trained in myofascial release. The client was able to sleep comfortably without using bolsters after the fourth treatment. The client's mobility increased, and she was walking and climbing stairs by the end of the 2-week program. She continued to have difficulty with fine motor skills. Although the positive outcome suggests the benefits of manual therapy for clients with thoracic outlet syndrome, this case study involves a single, severe case complicated by multiple diagnoses that was treated intensively. Further study is needed.

In 1999, Peng published a study titled "16 Cases of Scalenus Syndrome Treated by Massage and Acupoint-Injection." The 16 participants in this study were all female, between 20 and 40 years of age, who had symptoms from 3 months to 4 years prior to treatment. Each had had a previous injury to the shoulder. One of the participants had a cervical rib. All had a positive Adson's test. Of the 16 participants, 12 had vascular symptoms including a cold affected limb, 9 presented with impaired fine motor skills, and 4 showed thenar atrophy. In the seated position with the neck as relaxed as possible, manual manipulations were applied to the shoulder and medial arm followed by kneading and compression of acupoints, which are known in the system of Chinese medicine, while the limb was mobilized. The arm was then shaken and rubbed until the skin warmed. This treatment was performed every day. The study does not state the precise treatment program, only that the relief of symptoms required one or two courses of treatment for 20–40 days. In addition to manual therapy, these clients received an acupoint-injection containing procaine hydrochloride and vitamin B12 once every 5 days followed by infrared radiation. According to the author, all but one client was cured. Only the client with the cervical rib continued to have pain and numbness in the arm, but even this client had a negative Adson's test after treatment. Again, this study did not isolate the effects of massage from another form of treatment, in this case acupoint-injection. In addition, few details are provided regarding relief of neurogenic or vascular symptoms or changes in ROM; it is stated only that the client was cured. Although the results are encouraging, further study is necessary.

In 2006, Michael Hamm published a case study titled "Impact of Massage Therapy in the Treatment of Linked Pathologies: Scoliosis, Costovertebral Dysfunction, and Thoracic Outlet Syndrome." As the title suggests, this case also involved a client with multiple conditions. The client presented with pain and weakness in the right shoulder and arm that had increased progressively over the previous 8 months. She was regularly awakened by symptoms and ultimately had to quit her job as a waitress. Chiropractic diagnoses included scoliosis, costovertebral dysfunction, and thoracic outlet syndrome. The client received eight 60-minute treatments over the course of 4 weeks, which included deep tissue massage, neuromuscular therapy, and muscle energy techniques. Following this treatment plan, the client slept better, ROM increased, postural imbalances in the ilia and spine showed improvement, and pain with shoulder activity reduced by 50%. Other longstanding postural imbalances responded less significantly. As the author suggests, further research is needed. He recommends using more precise measurements of bony alignments that will allow for more accurate results upon follow-up, and using a standard measure for psychological stress to include this dimension of musculoskeletal dysfunction. The author also recommends a larger-scale study of massage to treat linked diseases concurrently. The study offers minimal data regarding increased strength or changes in neurogenic or vascular symptoms common to thoracic outlet syndrome. Although the results are encouraging, further research that considers thoracic outlet syndrome independently is needed.

WORKING WITH THE CLIENT

Client Assessment

Assessment begins with your first contact with a client. In some cases, this may be on the telephone when an appointment is requested. Ask in advance if the client is seeking treatment for a specific pain so that you can prepare yourself. It is essential that your assessment is thorough. If you suspect an underlying condition that requires medical attention, refer the client to a health care provider for assessment. If the client is diagnosed with an underlying condition, research the contraindications or special considerations for the condition. During your assessment, ask questions that will help you to differentiate the possible causes of thoracic outlet syndrome.

Table 6-2 lists questions to ask the client when taking a health history.

POSTURAL ASSESSMENT

Allow the client to enter the room ahead of you while you assess his or her posture and movements. Look for imbalances or patterns of compensation due to pain or restriction. In the case of thoracic outlet syndrome, have the client turn the doorknob to enter the room, pick up a pen, or grasp a cup

Table 6-2	Health History

Questions for the Client	Importance for the Treatment Plan
Where do you feel symptoms?	The location of symptoms gives clues to the location of trigger points, injury, or other contributing factors.
Describe what your symptoms feel like.	Differentiate between possible origins of symptoms, and determine the involvement of nerves or blood vessels.
How long have you had symptoms?	Onset may coincide with an illness or trauma and may help you to assess the extent of the injury.
Do any movements make it worse or better?	Locate tension, weakness, or compression in structures producing such movements.
Have you seen a health care provider for this condition? What was the diagnosis? What tests were performed?	A cervical rib or other bony prominence is most accurately assessed with an X-ray. Vascular insufficiency should be assessed by a health care provider.
Have you been diagnosed with a condition such as diabetes, rheumatoid arthritis, a thyroid condition, or a respiratory condition? Are you pregnant?	Systemic conditions may contribute to signs and symptoms, may require adjustments to treatment, and may impact treatment outcomes. Fluid retention and changes in posture during pregnancy can contribute to signs and symptoms.
Have you had an injury or surgery?	Injury or surgery and resulting scar tissue may cause adhesions, hyper- or hypotonicity, and atypical ROM. The use of crutches may contribute to thoracic outlet syndrome.
What type of work, hobbies, or other regular activities do you do?	Repetitive motions and static postures that increase thoracic flexion, protracted scapulae, cervical extension, or a head-forward posture may contribute to the client's condition.
Are you taking any prescribed medications or herbal or other supplements?	Medication of all types may contribute to symptoms or involve contraindications or cautions.
Have you had a cortisone shot in the past 2 weeks? Where?	Local massage is contraindicated.
Have you taken a pain reliever or muscle relaxant within the past 4 hours?	The client may not be able to judge your pressure.
Have you taken anti-inflammatory medication within the past 4 hours?	Deep friction causes inflammation and should not be performed if the client has recently taken anti-inflammatory medication.

of water without making him or her aware that you have begun your assessment. Do not hand these things to the client but allow him or her to pick them up. If the client performs these tasks clumsily with the affected arm, or performs them with the unaffected arm, particularly if it is the nondominant side, it could indicate a compensation pattern due to weakness in the affected arm.

Because the symptoms of thoracic outlet syndrome can be confused with those of other musculoskeletal conditions, it is important to asses the client's posture thoroughly. If you are performing 30 minutes of treatment in the area of compression, it is best to use the remaining time to target related contributing factors. For example, if your assessment of the client reveals lateral flexion of the thorax, spend some time lengthening the muscles that flex the thorax. Clients with thoracic outlet syndrome may also present with hyperkyphosis. The head-forward posture, a drooped or elevated shoulder, and internally rotated shoulders typically contribute to the compression of the brachial plexus. Figure 6-4 compares the anatomic position to the posture affected by thoracic outlet syndrome.

ROM ASSESSMENT

Test the ROM of the neck and shoulders, assessing the length and strength of both agonists and antagonists that cross the joints being tested. Since it allows the client to control the amount of movement and stay within a pain-free range, only active ROM should be used in the acute stage

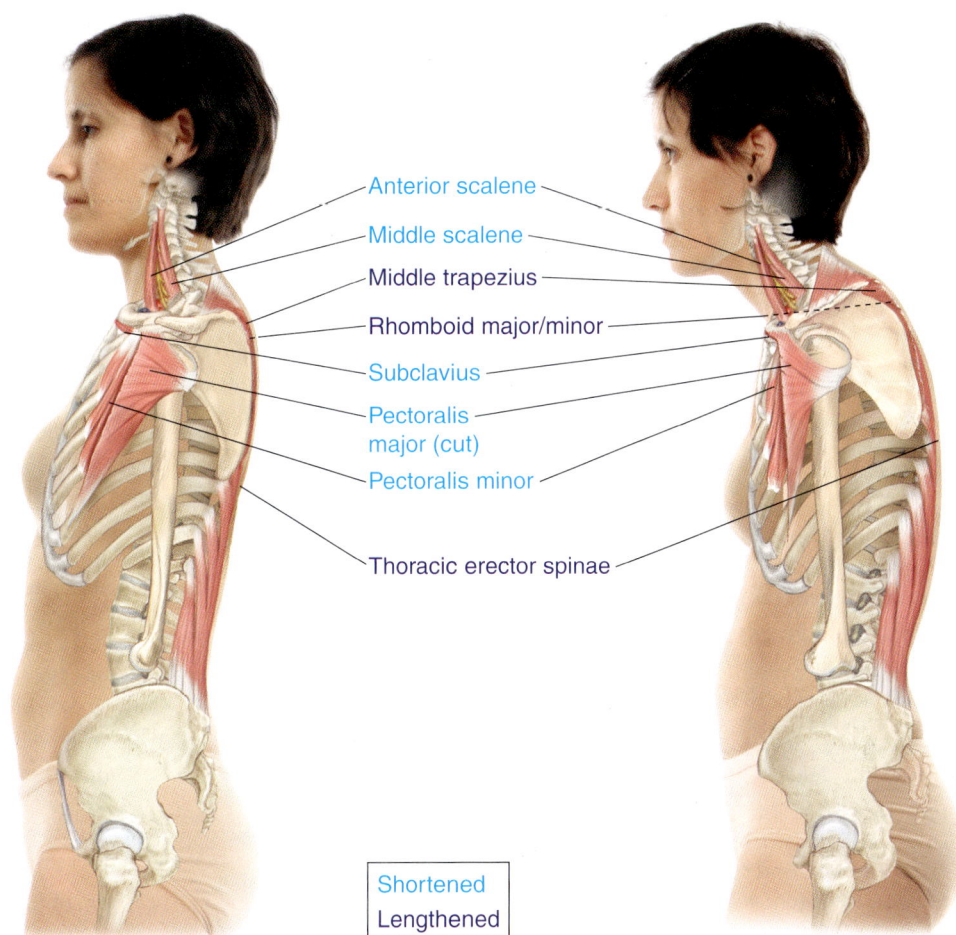

Figure 6-4 **Postural assessment comparison. Compare the anatomical posture on the left to the deviated posture on the right.** Note how the shortened scalenes, subclavius and pectoralis minor may contribute to compression of the contents in the thoracic outlet.

of an injury to prevent undue pain or re-injury. Box 6-1 presents the average active ROM results for the joints involved in thoracic outlet syndrome.

Active ROM

Compare your assessment of the client's active ROM to the values in Box 6-1. Pain and other symptoms may not be reproduced with active ROM assessment, because the client may limit movement to the symptom-free range.

- **Active contralateral rotation and ipsilateral lateral flexion of the cervical spine** on the affected side may cause pain due to trigger points in the scalenes. Ipsilateral rotation and contralateral lateral flexion may also be reduced and produce symptoms when the shortened scalenes are stretched, or cause discomfort on the unaffected side because of weakened antagonists. Active rotation and flexion of the cervical spine may reproduce symptoms.
- **Active extension of the cervical spine** may be reduced or reproduce symptoms and pain when the shortened anterior scalene is stretched.
- **Active external rotation, abduction, and flexion of the shoulder** may be reduced or produce symptoms when trigger points or hypertonicity in the pectorals limits motion in the shoulder.

PASSIVE ROM

Compare the client's P ROM on one side to the other when applicable. Note and compare the end feel for each range (refer to Chapter 1 for an explanation of end feel). The client may resist even

Box 6-1   AVERAGE ACTIVE ROM FOR JOINTS INVOLVED IN THORACIC OUTLET SYNDROME

Cervical Spine

Flexion 60°
SCM (bilateral)
Anterior scalenes (bilateral)
Longus capitis (bilateral)
Longus colli (bilateral)

Extension 55°
Upper trapezius (bilateral)
Levator scapulae (bilateral)
Splenius capitis (bilateral)
Splenius cervicis (bilateral)
Rectus capitis (bilateral)
Oblique capitis superior (bilateral)
Semispinalis capitis (bilateral)
Longissimus capitis (bilateral)
Longissimus cervicis (bilateral)
Iliocostalis cervicis (bilateral)

Lateral Flexion 20–45°
Upper trapezius (unilateral)
Levator scapulae (unilateral)
Splenius capitis (unilateral)
Splenius cervicis (unilateral)
SCM (unilateral)
Longus capitis (unilateral)
Longus colli (unilateral)
Anterior scalene (unilateral)
Middle scalene (unilateral)
Posterior scalene (unilateral)
Longissimus capitis (unilateral)
Longissimus cervicis (unilateral)
Iliocostalis cervicis (unilateral)

Ipsilateral Rotation 70–90°
Levator scapulae (unilateral)
Splenius capitis (unilateral)
Splenius cervicis (unilateral)
Rectus capitis (unilateral)
Oblique capitis (unilateral)
Longus colli (unilateral)
Longus capitis (unilateral)
Longissimus capitis (unilateral)
Longissimus cervicis (unilateral)
Iliocostalis cervicis (unilateral)

Contralateral Rotation 70–90°
Upper trapezius (unilateral)
SCM (unilateral)
Anterior scalene (unilateral)
Middle scalene (unilateral)
Posterior scalene (unilateral)

Shoulder

Flexion 180°
Anterior deltoid
Pectoralis major (upper fibers)
Biceps brachii
Coracobrachialis

Extension 50–60°
Posterior deltoid
Latissimus dorsi
Teres major & minor
Infraspinatus
Pectoralis major (lower fibers)
Triceps brachii

Internal Rotation 60–100°
Anterior deltoid
Latissimus dorsi
Teres major
Subscapularis
Pectoralis major

External Rotation 80–90°
Posterior deltoid
Infraspinatus
Teres minor

Abduction 180°
Deltoids
Supraspinatus

Adduction 50–75°
Latissimus dorsi
Teres major
Infraspinatus
Teres minor
Pectoralis major
Triceps brachii (long head)
Coracobrachialis

Horizontal Abduction 45°
Posterior deltoid
Infraspinatus
Teres minor

Horizontal Adduction 130°
Anterior deltoid
Pectoralis major (upper fibers)

---

passive movement if this movement causes pain in his or her daily life. Symptoms of pain, numbness, and tingling may also occur.

- **Passive ipsilateral rotation and contralateral lateral flexion of the cervical spine** on the affected side may be reduced and may reproduce symptoms as the hypertonic scalenes are stretched.
- **Passive extension of the cervical spine** may be reduced and may reproduce symptoms when the anterior scalene is stretched.
- **Passive external rotation, abduction, or flexion of the shoulder** may be reduced due to myofascial restrictions and hypertonic pectorals.

RESISTED ROM

Use resisted tests to assess the strength of the muscles that cross the joints involved. Compare the strength of the affected side to the unaffected side.

- **Resisted contralateral rotation and ipsilateral lateral flexion of the cervical spine** on the affected side may cause pain and reproduce symptoms. Resisted ipsilateral rotation and contralateral lateral flexion may reveal weakness in the antagonists.
- **Resisted flexion of the cervical spine** may reproduce symptoms.
- **Resisted internal rotation, abduction, or flexion of the shoulder** may reproduce symptoms or result in pain.
- **Resisted extension or external rotation of the shoulder** may reveal weakness in the antagonists with regard to flexion and internal rotation of the shoulder.

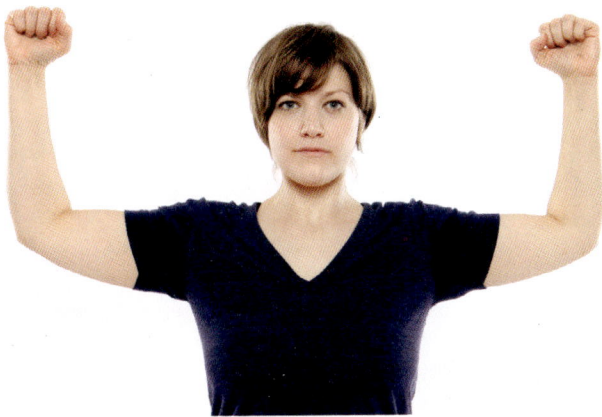

Figure 6-5 **Roos stress test.** Ask the client to abduct and laterally rotate the shoulder, flex the elbows, retract the scapulae, and then flex and extend the fingers repeatedly to test for thoracic outlet syndrome.

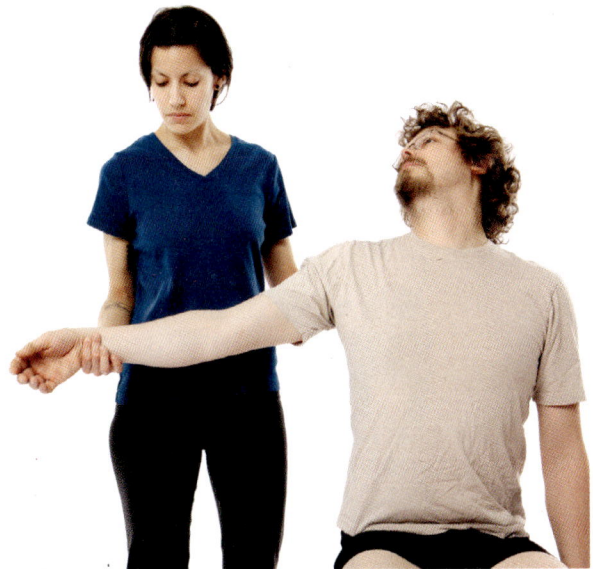

Figure 6-6 **Adson's test.** With the shoulder passively abducted and externally rotated and the cervical spine actively extended and rotated toward the affected side, place your fingers on the radial pulse, and note its strength to assess for compression of the neurovascular bundle by the scalenes.

- **Resisted flexion of the elbow, flexion or extension of the wrist and fingers, and grasping** may reveal weakness if thoracic outlet syndrome has led to atrophy of the muscles involved in those actions.

SPECIAL TESTS

The **Roos elevated arm stress test** is intended to test for thoracic outlet syndrome (Fig. 6-5).

1. Ask the client to abduct the shoulders 90°, laterally rotate the shoulders 180°, flex the elbows 90°, and slightly retract the scapulae.
2. Once in this position, ask the client to flex and extend the fingers (open and close the hands) for as long as the client can tolerate, up to a maximum of 3 minutes.
3. If the client is unable to hold the position for 3 minutes, feels intense heaviness or weakness in the affected arm, or feels numbness and tingling in the fingers of the affected side, the test is considered positive for thoracic outlet syndrome. Minor weakness or fatigue do not suggest thoracic outlet syndrome.

Adson's test assesses the compression of the neurovascular bundle by the scalenes (Fig. 6-6).

1. Stand behind the seated client.
2. Passively abduct and externally rotate the shoulder on the affected side.
3. Place your fingers on the radial pulse and note its strength.
4. Once you have assessed the strength of the pulse, ask the client to extend the neck and rotate it toward the affected side. In this position, the client should take a full, deep breath and hold it for 15–20 seconds or as long as possible, up to 20 seconds. Taking a breath raises the first rib and contracts the anterior scalene.
5. A decreased or absent pulse or the recurrence of pain or tingling in the arm and hand indicates a positive test for compression of the nerves and vessels by the anterior scalene.

The **costoclavicular maneuver** assesses for compression of the neurovascular bundle between the clavicle/subclavius and the first rib (Fig. 6-7).

1. Stand behind the seated client.
2. Place your fingers on the radial pulse, and note its strength.
3. Once you have assessed the strength of the pulse, ask the client to depress and extend the shoulder.

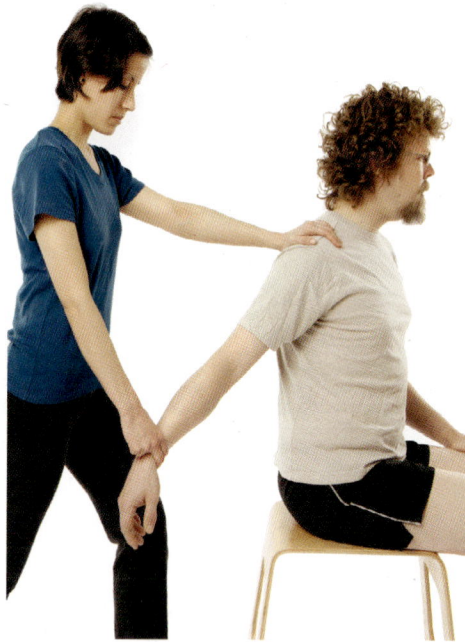

Figure 6-7 **Costoclavicular maneuver.** With the shoulder depressed and extended, place your fingers on the radial pulse, and note its strength to assess for compression of the neurovascular bundle between the clavicle/subclavius and the first rib.

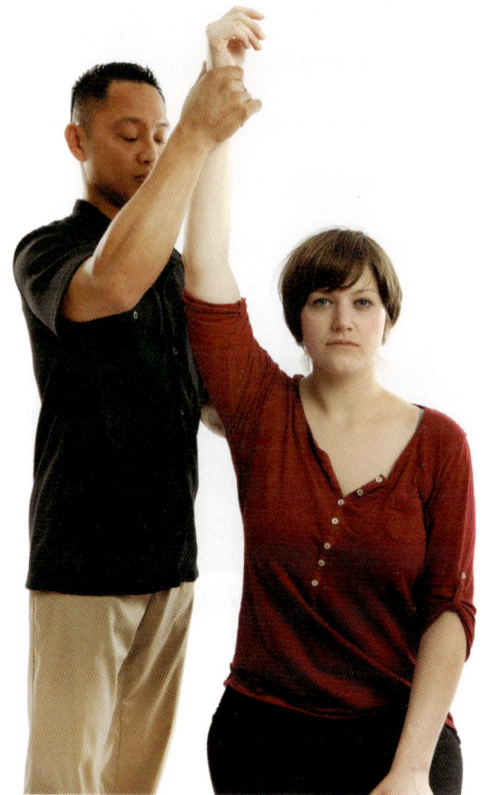

Figure 6-8 **Wright's test.** Assess for compression by the pectoralis minor.

4. In this position, ask the client to take a breath deep enough to expand the chest and hold for 15–20 seconds or as long as possible, up to 20 seconds.
5. A decreased or absent pulse or the recurrence of pain or tingling in the arm and hand indicates a positive test for compression of the nerves and vessels between the clavicle/subclavius and the first rib.

Wright's test assesses compression of the neurovascular bundle by the pectoralis minor muscle (Fig. 6-8).

1. Ask the client to sit in a chair while you stand behind him or her.
2. Place your fingers on the radial pulse, and note its strength.
3. Once you have assessed the strength of the pulse, passively laterally rotate, abduct, and slightly extend the affected arm while keeping your fingers on the radial pulse.
4. A decreased or absent pulse or the recurrence of pain or tingling in the arm and hand indicates a positive test for compression of the nerves and vessels beneath the pectoralis minor.

PALPATION ASSESSMENT

Assess the tissues of the neck, chest, shoulder, arm, forearm, and hand. Compare the affected to the unaffected side. Check the temperature, color, and texture of the superficial tissues. You may find fascial restrictions and tenderness in the lateral neck, beneath the clavicle, or around the anterior glenohumeral joint as well as in the muscles involved in any accompanying postural deviations such as the head-forward posture or hyperkyphosis. Depending on the duration and degree of compression of the brachial plexus, you may find atrophy, pale skin, swelling, reduced hair growth, ulcers, cyanosis, and possibly even necrosis of the tissues of the fingers and hand. If ulcers, cyanosis, or necrosis is present, refer the client to a health care provider for medical assessment.

Condition-Specific Massage

Since the causes of pain, numbness, and tingling in the arm and hand vary, it may be difficult to pinpoint the area of compression. Moreover, it is common for more than one area to be compressed at the same time. A client who works at a desk for long periods everyday is likely to be seated with the head jutting forward (affecting the scalenes), one or both scapulae elevated or depressed, one or both shoulders internally rotated (affecting the pectorals), the forearms pronated (affecting the pronator teres), and the wrists and fingers in flexion, extension, or moving constantly between these (affecting the contents of the carpal tunnel).

It is essential for treatment to be relaxing. You are not likely to eliminate the symptoms of thoracic outlet syndrome, or any of the conditions associated with it, in one treatment. Do not try to do so by treating aggressively. Be sure to ask your client to let you know if the amount of pressure you are applying keeps him or her from relaxing. If the client responds by tensing muscles or has a facial expression that looks distressed, reduce your pressure. Remember that you are working on tissue that is compromised.

It is also important for the client to let you know if any part of your treatment reproduces symptoms. Adjust the client to a more neutral position, reduce your pressure, or move slightly off the area if this occurs, and make a note about it as this may help you understand more clearly exactly which neuromuscular conditions are contributing to symptoms. Instruct your client to use deep but relaxing breathing to help with relaxation.

If deep palpation of a trigger point refers pain elsewhere, explain this to your client, and ask him or her to breathe deeply during the technique. As the trigger point is deactivated, the referred pain will also diminish. Scalene trigger points refer pain across the shoulder and along the medial border of the scapulae, into the chest, and down the lateral arm and forearm into the lateral hand. Subclavius trigger points refer pain across the clavicle, into the areas around the biceps and brachioradialis, and into the lateral hand. Pectoralis minor trigger points refer pain across the chest and into the areas of the anterior deltoid, down the medial arm and forearm, and into the palm and three middle fingers. Other muscles with trigger points that refer pain into the arm, forearm, and hand include the pectoralis major, sternalis, serratus anterior, serratus posterior superior, latissimus dorsi, muscles of the rotator cuff, and the triceps brachii. Most of the muscles of the arm and forearm refer pain into the wrist, hand, and fingers. Common trigger points and their referral patterns are shown in Figure 6-9.

The following suggestions are for treatment that considers several neuromuscular factors involved in producing pain, tingling, or numbness along the arm and into the hand. The section of this treatment that focuses on the anterior and middle scalene, subclavius, and pectoralis minor is specific for thoracic outlet syndrome. If the client has an acute injury, follow the PRICE (protect, rest, ice, compression, elevation) protocol. In this case, you may work conservatively proximal to the site but will have to avoid the injured area until the subacute or chronic stage.

- Begin in the supine position, and initiate treatment on the affected side. If both arms are affected, begin on the dominant side. If edema is present, bolster the arm so that gravity will encourage venous return and the draining of fluid toward the proximal lymph nodes. If hyperkyphosis is a consideration, see Chapter 4 for additional bolstering.

- Moist heat is indicated on the chest, neck, and shoulder unless the client has cardiovascular disease.

- Before applying emollient, assess the tissues of the upper cross for myofascial restrictions, and release them if indicated. Restrictions are often found around the glenohumeral joint, along the anterior deltoid, and along the lateral and posterior neck.

Treatment icons: 🔆 Increase circulation; 🖐 Reduce adhesions; ✋ Reduce tension; 🪶 Lengthen tissue; 🖐 Treat trigger points; 🖐 Passive stretch; 🧹 Clear area

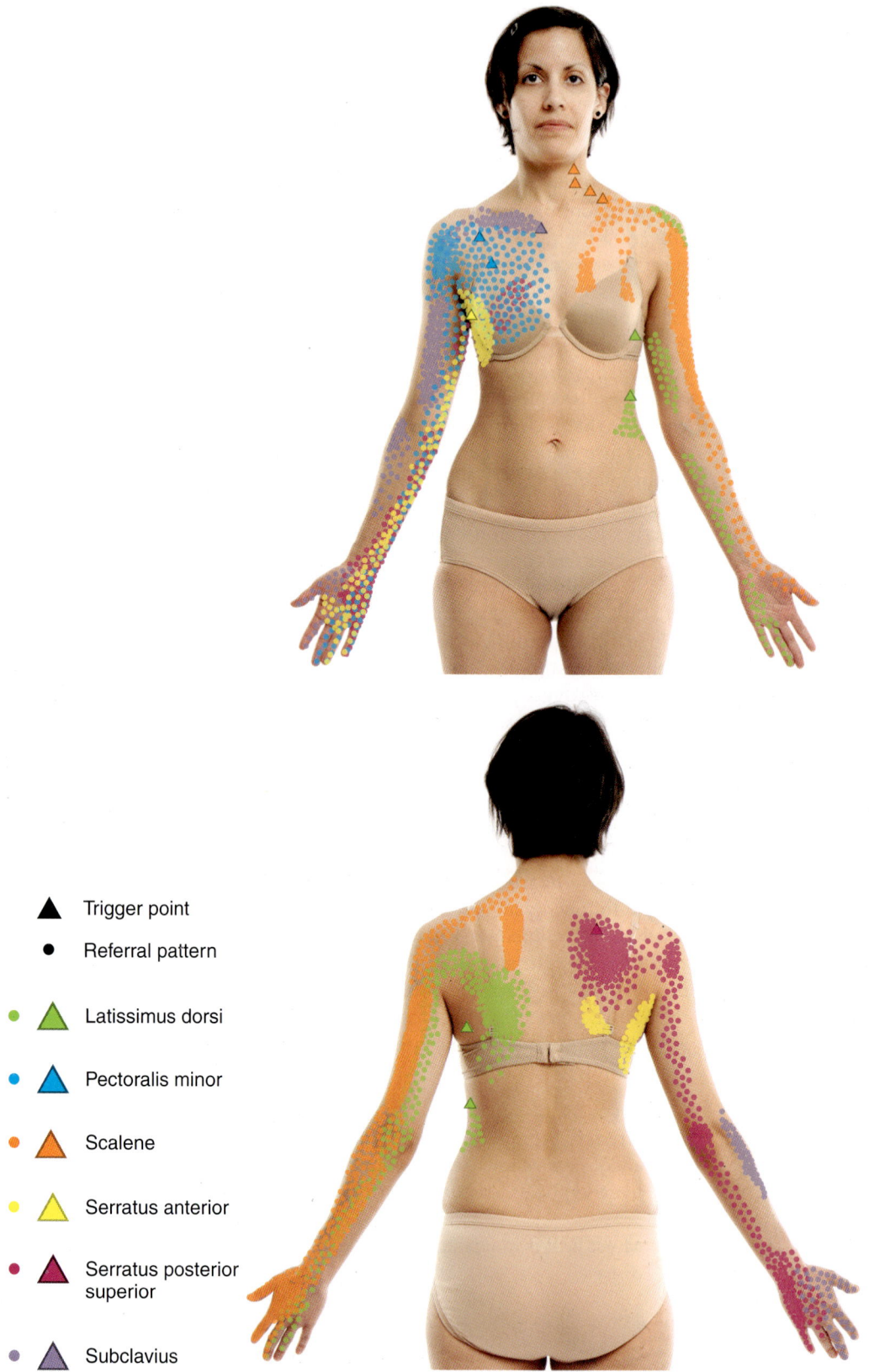

Trigger point

Referral pattern

Latissimus dorsi

Pectoralis minor

Scalene

Serratus anterior

Serratus posterior superior

Subclavius

Figure 6-9 **Common trigger points and referral.** Common trigger points and referral patterns associated with thoracic outlet syndrome.

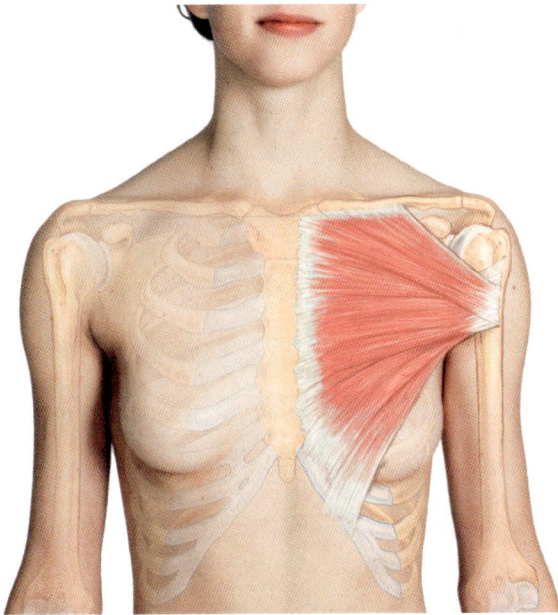

PECTORALIS MAJOR

Origin	Medial half of clavicle, sternum, and cartilage of ribs
Insertion	Crest of greater tubercle of humerus.
Action	**All fibers** adduct shoulder, internally rotate shoulder, assist in elevating thorax in forced inspiration; **upper fibers** flex shoulder, horizontally adduct shoulder; **lower fibers** extend shoulder.
Nerve	Medial and lateral pectoral.

Figure 6-10 **Pectoralis major.** Short, tight pectorals contribute to the internal rotation of the shoulders.

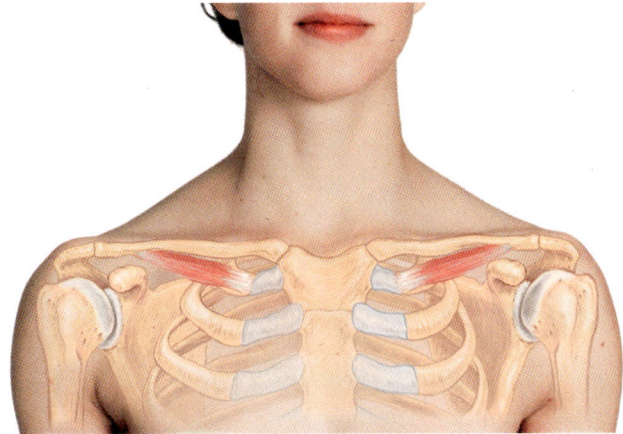

SUBCLAVIUS

Origin	First rib and costal cartilage.
Insertion	Inferior, lateral aspect of clavicle.
Action	Draws rib inferiorly and anteriorly, elevates first rib in inhalation.
Nerve	Subclavian.

Figure 6-11 **Subclavius.** The subclavius may be adhered and hypertonic when the thorax is flexed.

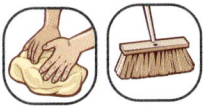

- Use warming strokes to superficially assess the tissues from the neck down to the hand and to begin superficial draining of accumulated fluid toward the nearest lymph nodes. You should be able to minimally assess the degree of tension in each area, which may help you to determine where to focus your time.

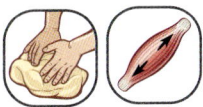

- Use broad strokes along the full length of the pectoralis major (Fig. 6-10) to soften tissues, allowing you to access the deeper structures.

- Assess pectoralis major for trigger points, and treat them if found. Common trigger points in the pectoralis major are found along the mid sternum, at the clavicular attachments, along the inferior fibers, and near the axilla.

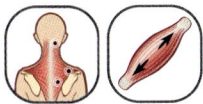

- Assess and treat the subclavius for hypertonicity and trigger points (Fig. 6-11). The subclavius is a slight, thin muscle and may not be easily palpated. Trust your knowledge of anatomy as you palpate along the inferior edge of the middle third of the clavicle toward the costal cartilage of the first rib. If you find and treat trigger points in the subclavius, use a pin and stretch technique to lengthen the muscle fibers.

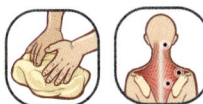

- You can access the pectoralis minor through the pectoralis major or by pushing the lateral fibers of the pectoralis major medially as you palpate ribs 3, 4, and 5 (Fig. 6-12). This may be performed more easily by kneeling next to the client and placing his or her hand on your shoulder nearest the table, which will gently lift the pectoralis major out of the way. This is also preferable to externally rotating the shoulder, which may put tension on the pectorals and reproduce symptoms. Once you believe you have found it, ask the client to depress the shoulder and feel for a contraction. As you assess and treat the pectoralis minor for tension

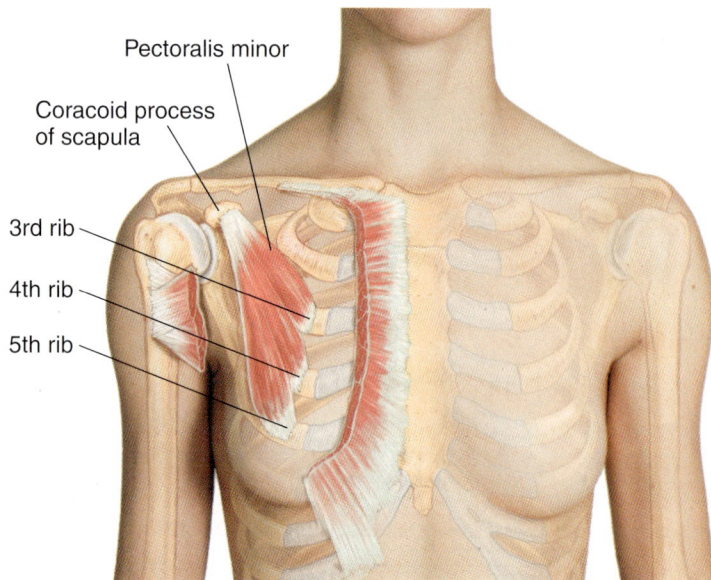

PECTORALIS MINOR

Origin	*Third, fourth, and fifth ribs.*
Insertion	*Coracoid process of the scapula.*
Action	*Depress scapula, protract scapula, tilt scapula anterior, assist in inhalation.*
Nerve	*Medial pectoral.*

Figure 6-12 **Pectoralis minor.** The pectoralis minor may be shortened if the scapulae are protracted. Adapted from Clay JH, Pounds DM. *Basic Clinical Massage Therapy: Integrating Anatomy and Treatment,* 2nd ed. Philadelphia: Lippincott Williams & Wilkins, 2008.

and trigger points, ask the client about the reproduction of symptoms. If they occur, adjust the client to a more neutral position, reduce pressure, or move away from the area. You may be able to revisit the pectoralis minor later in the treatment without reproducing symptoms.

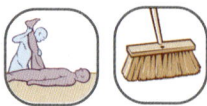

■ If you found myofascial restrictions, hypertonicity, and trigger points in the pectoral area, perform a full stretch to the pectorals and close with clearing strokes. If the tissue is resistant to lengthening, apply postisometric relaxation within the client's tolerance to encourage a normal resting tone. If you found the area to be only minimally affected, close with clearing strokes.

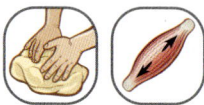

■ Warm and lengthen the superficial neck muscles, namely the upper trapezius. Be careful to avoid endangerment areas, and back away gently if you feel a pulse.

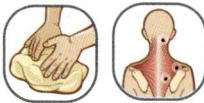

■ Reduce tension in the SCM, and treat any trigger points found. Trigger points in the SCM may cause vertigo, nausea, or ringing in the ears. Ask the client to let you know if he or she feels any unusual sensations, and explain that these are common referrals from SCM trigger points.

■ Once you have softened the SCM and trapezius, you will have greater access to the scalenes (Fig. 6-13). To access the anterior scalene, gently push the SCM medially with one or two fingertips as you feel for the deeper scalenes. As you move the SCM medially, your fingers should gently rest on the transverse processes of the cervical vertebrae. Use this as your guide for palpating the anterior scalene. Once you have found it, ask the client to take a quick, forced breath into the chest and feel for a contraction.

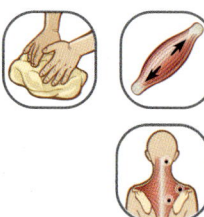

■ Reduce tension and lengthen the anterior scalene. Treat any trigger points found. It is often helpful, once you have found a trigger point in the scalenes, to compress it gently while slowly rotating the head. Trigger points in the anterior scalene are often quite sensitive, and the client may feel cautious about you working deeply in the neck. Begin gently and slowly to avoid frightening the client or causing him or her to jerk the head. Remember that you are working in an area of many nerves and abundant vasculature.

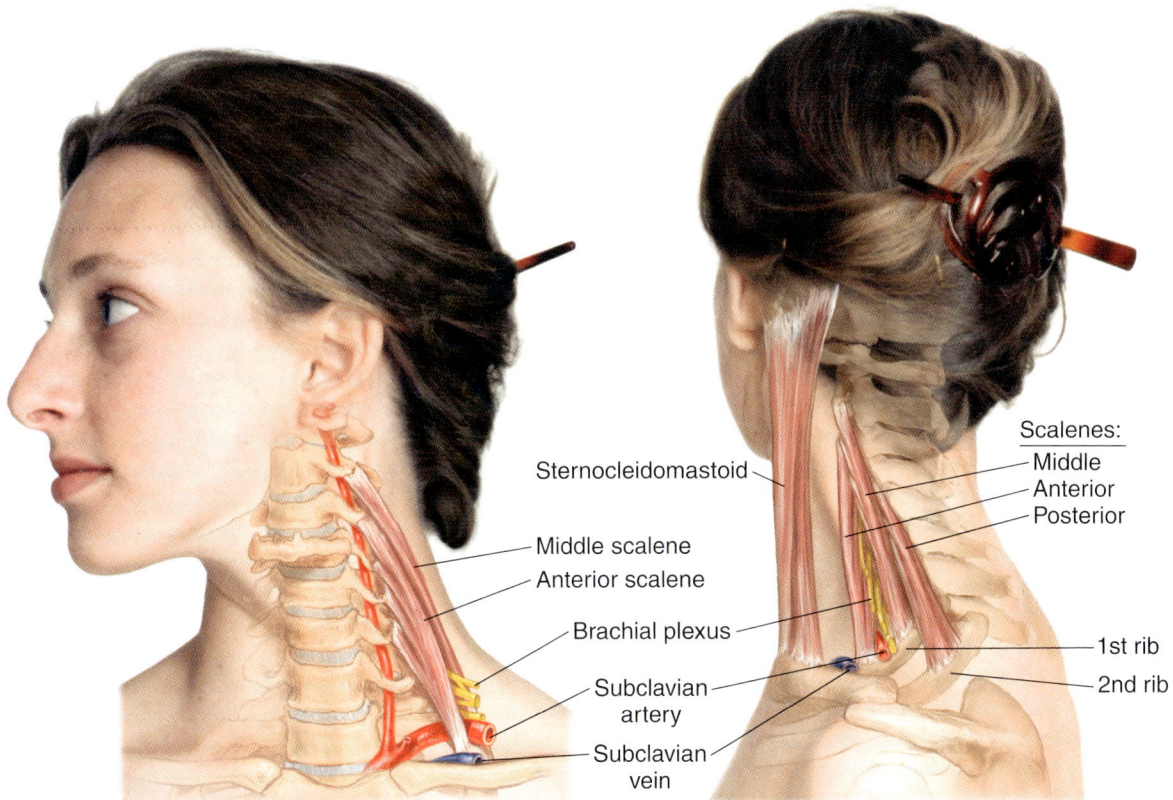

SCALENES

Origin	Anterior-TVP 3–6, middle-TVP 2–7, posterior-TVP 5–6.
Insertion	*Anterior*, 1st rib; *middle*, 1st rib; *posterior*, 2nd rib.
Action	*Unilateral*, ipsilateral lateral flexion and rotation of head and neck; *bilateral*, elevate ribs in inhalation and flex head and neck.
Nerve	Cervical.

STERNOCLEIDOMASTOID

Origin	Top of manubrium and medial third of clavicle.
Insertion	Mastoid process and superior nuchal line.
Action	*Unilateral*, ipsilateral lateral flexion and rotation of head and neck; *bilateral*, flexion of the neck, assist in inhalation.
Nerve	Spinal accessory XI.

Figure 6-13 **SCM and scalenes.** The SCM and scalenes may be short and tight. Adapted from Clay JH, Pounds DM. *Basic Clinical Massage Therapy: Integrating Anatomy and Treatment,* 2nd ed. Philadelphia: Lippincott Williams & Wilkins, 2008.

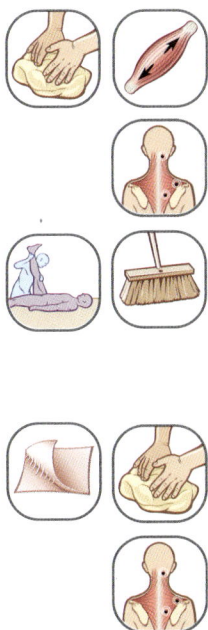

■ Find the middle scalene by gently palpating the transverse processes and then moving slightly posterior. The middle scalene crosses the transverse processes and heads toward the first rib. Once you have found it, ask the client to take a quick, forced breath into the chest and feel for a contraction. Take the same cautions with the middle scalene as with the anterior scalene to avoid frightening the client. Lengthen the muscle and treat any trigger points found.

■ Stretch the scalenes by increasing the distance between their origins and insertions. Options for stretching include contralateral lateral flexion and ipsilateral rotation of the cervical spine (Fig. 6-14). If the tissue resists lengthening, apply postisometric relaxation within the client's tolerance to encourage a normal resting tone. If you found the area to be minimally affected, apply clearing strokes and move on to the arm and hand.

■ Warm the whole arm and assess the muscles for myofascial restrictions, hypertonicity or hypotonicity, and trigger points. If the client has had symptoms for a long time, the muscles of the arm may be compensating. If you suspect pronator teres syndrome or carpal tunnel syndrome to be involved, assess and treat as time permits. You may be able to revisit these areas in a subsequent visit when primary symptoms subside. If you do not find compromised tissue in the arm, be conservative in your treatment of the arm to save time, but do not ignore it. It is important to perform at least the Swedish techniques to the arm to restore neuromuscular memory and function.

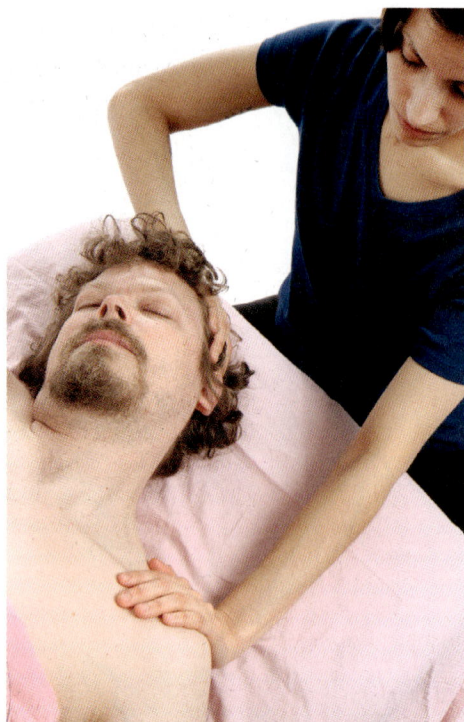

Figure 6-14 **Scalene stretch.** Passively stretch scalenes following trigger point therapy.

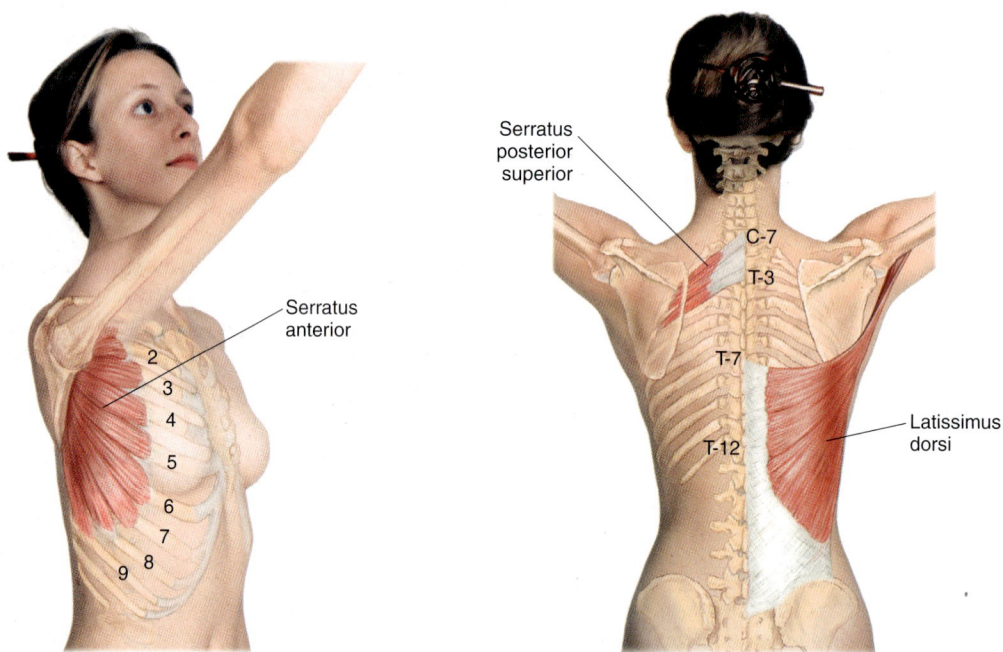

SERRATUS ANTERIOR

Origin	Lateral surface of upper 8 or 9 ribs.
Insertion	Anterior surface of medial border of scapula.
Action	Abduct and depress scapula, stabilize scapula against rib cage, forced inhalation.
Nerve	Long thoracic.

SERRATUS POSTERIOR SUPERIOR

Origin	Spinous processes of C7-T3.
Insertion	Posterior surface of ribs 2-5.
Action	Elevate ribs during inhalation.
Nerve	Spinal nerves 1-4.

LATISSIMUS DORSI

Origin	Spinous process of T7-12, ribs 8-12, thoracolumbar aponeurosis, and posterior iliac crest.
Insertion	Crest of lesser tubercle of humerus.
Action	Extend, adduct and medially rotate shoulder.
Nerve	Thoracodorsal.

Figure 6-15 **Latissimus dorsi, serratus anterior, and serratus posterior superior.** Trigger points in these muscles may mimic the pain involved in thoracic outlet syndrome. Adapted from Clay JH, Pounds DM. *Basic Clinical Massage Therapy: Integrating Anatomy and Treatment,* 2nd ed. Philadelphia: Lippincott Williams & Wilkins, 2008.

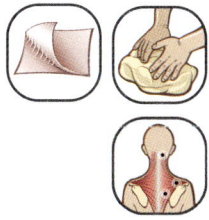

- Treat the unaffected side—superficially if you find no compromised tissue and comprehensively if the client's thoracic outlet syndrome is bilateral.

- Try to leave at least 10 minutes for work in the prone position. Referral patterns for trigger points in the latissimus dorsi, serratus anterior, and serratus posterior superior may be similar to the common pain pattern found in thoracic outlet syndrome (Fig. 6-15). Assess and treat these muscles as time permits.

- Because hyperkyphosis is commonly associated with thoracic outlet syndrome, the muscles of the upper back are likely to be tender or painful, and this may be one of the client's primary complaints along with numbness and tingling in the arm and hand. Treat the back conservatively if time does not allow you to assess and treat trigger points. You can return to this in a subsequent visit once the symptoms of thoracic outlet syndrome begin to subside.

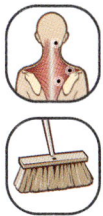

- If the scapulae are protracted, remember to treat the rhomboids and middle trapezius from the scapulae toward the spine to avoid stretching them further. Trigger points can develop in overstretched muscles as well as hypertonic ones.

- Use a local pin and stretch to lengthen fibers that contained trigger points, and clear the area treated.

The treatment overview diagram summarizes the flow of treatment (Fig. 6-16).

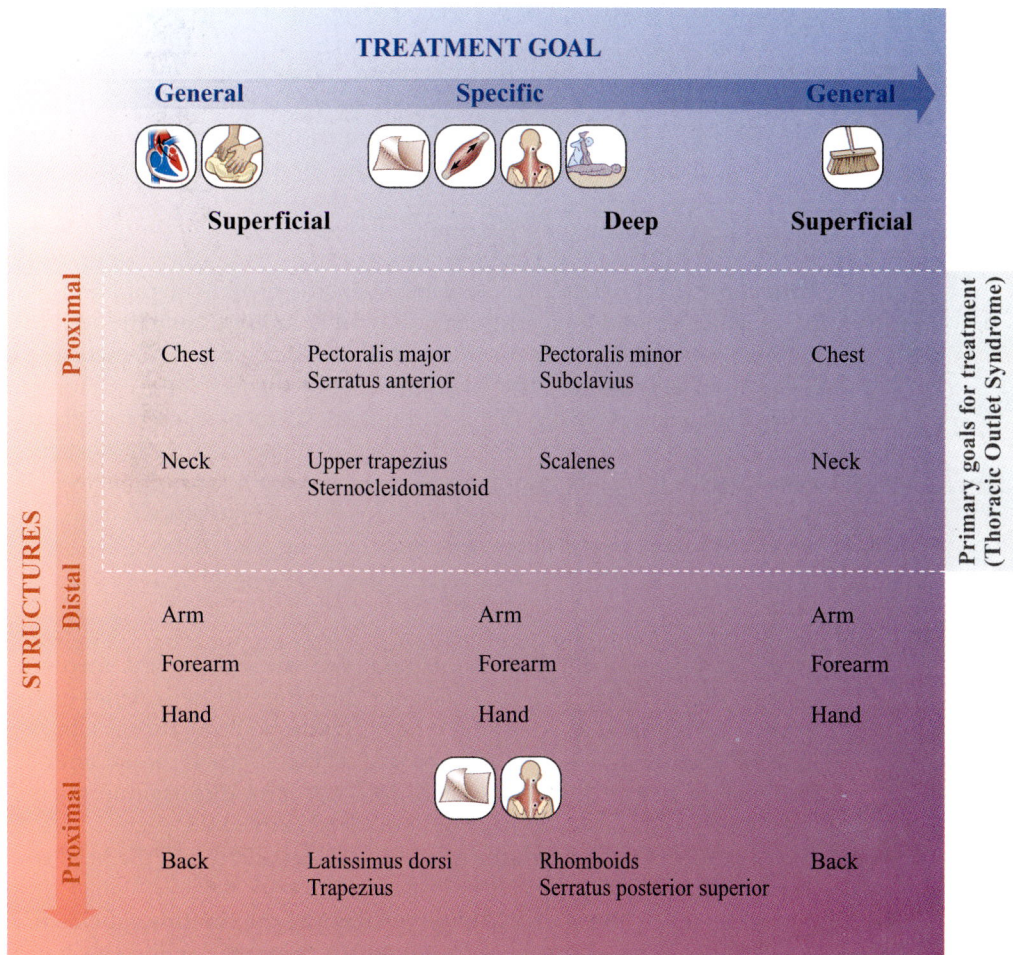

TREATMENT GOAL

STRUCTURES		General / Superficial	Specific / Deep		General / Superficial
Proximal	Chest		Pectoralis major / Serratus anterior	Pectoralis minor / Subclavius	Chest
	Neck		Upper trapezius / Sternocleidomastoid	Scalenes	Neck
Distal	Arm		Arm		Arm
	Forearm		Forearm		Forearm
	Hand		Hand		Hand
Proximal	Back		Latissimus dorsi / Trapezius	Rhomboids / Serratus posterior superior	Back

Primary goals for treatment (Thoracic Outlet Syndrome)

Figure 6-16   Thoracic outlet syndrome treatment overview diagram. Follow the general principles from left to right or top to bottom when treating thoracic outlet syndrome.

CLIENT SELF-CARE

The following are intended as general recommendations for stretching and strengthening muscles involved in thoracic outlet syndrome. The objective is to create distance between the attachment sites of muscles that have shortened and to perform repetitions of movements that decrease the distance between the attachments of muscles that have weakened. If you have had no training in remedial exercises and do not feel that you have a functional understanding of stretching and strengthening, refer the client to a professional with training in this area.

Clients often neglect self-care because their daily lives are busy. Encourage them to follow these guidelines:

- Instruct the client to perform self-care activities throughout the day, such as while taking a phone call, reading e-mail, watching television, or performing other activities of daily living, instead of setting aside extra time.
- Encourage your client to take regular breaks from repetitive actions or static postures.
- Demonstrate gentle self-massage to keep adhesions and hypertonicity at bay between treatments.
- Instruct the client on proper posture in the seated position to keep pressure off the weakened joints. Instruct clients with symptoms of thoracic outlet syndrome to sleep in positions without raising the arm over the head and without lateral flexion or rotation of the cervical spine.
- Instruct an athlete whose sport strengthens the pectorals and internal rotators of the shoulder to reduce pectoral resistance exercises and increase scapular retraction and thoracic extension to strengthen the middle trapezius, rhomboids, and thoracic erector spinae, balancing strength in the thoracic area.
- Instruct a client who regularly performs heavy lifting to lift with the legs instead of the back.
- Demonstrate all strengthening exercises and stretches to your client and have him or her perform these for you before leaving to ensure that he or she is performing them properly and will not harm himself or herself when practicing alone.

Stretching

Instruct the client to stretch the scalenes. Have the client hook the hand of the affected side under the chair while slowly and gently extending and laterally flexing the neck in the opposite direction until he or she feels a deep but comfortable stretch (Fig. 6-17). To increase the stretch, instruct the client to pull gently on the head with the opposite hand.

To stretch the pectoralis major and minor, instruct the client to clasp the hands behind the head, then retract and elevate the scapulae. For a deeper stretch, instruct the client to stand in a doorway with the hands on the frame and then step forward, which will bring the arms slightly posterior. It is essential that the client steps forward rather than leans forward, because leaning would affect the muscles of the neck, back, and hips (Fig. 6-18).

Strengthening

If thoracic outlet syndrome is unilateral and the scalenes are involved, remember that the scalenes of one side antagonize those of the other. If the scalenes of the unaffected side are weak, it is important to strengthen them in order to bring the neck back to a neutral position. Resisted rotation toward the affected side will strengthen the scalenes on the unaffected side. This should be performed only if it does not reproduce symptoms on the affected side or cause pain in the posterior neck or shoulder. Instruct the client to rest the palm of the hand on the side of the head with the affected scalenes and rotate the head toward the affected side (Fig. 6-19).

The client can also strengthen the middle trapezius and rhomboids to reduce protraction of the scapulae. Instruct the client to stand with the arms comfortably hanging at the sides while squeezing the scapulae together (Fig. 6-20). When this is done properly, only the middle trapezius and rhomboids should contract while the shoulders remain relaxed.

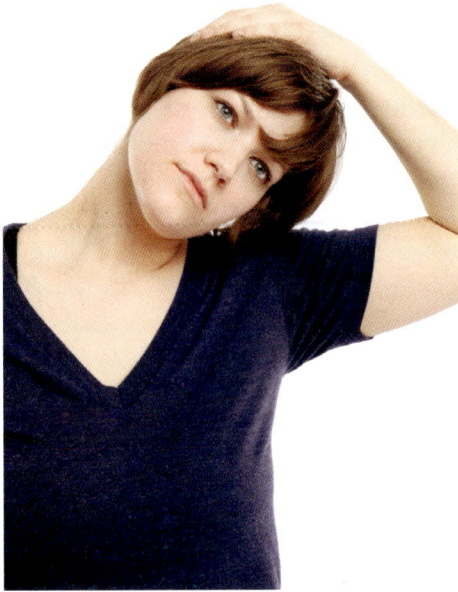

Figure 6-17 **Scalene stretch.** Lateral flexion to the opposite side increases the distance between the origin and insertion of the scalenes.

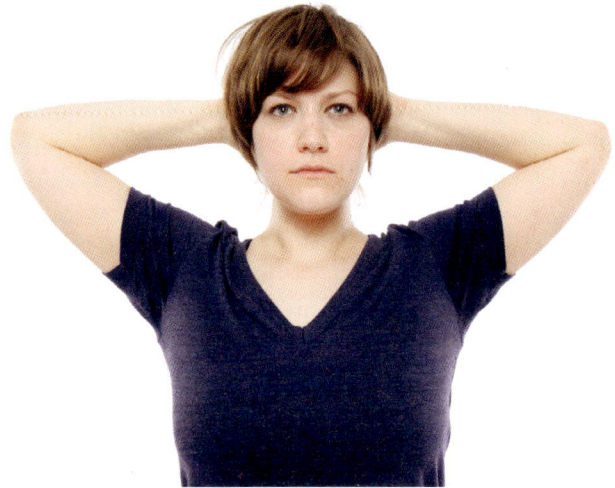

Figure 6-18 **Pectoralis minor stretch.** Increase the distance between the coracoid process of the scapulae and the ribs to stretch the pectoralis minor.

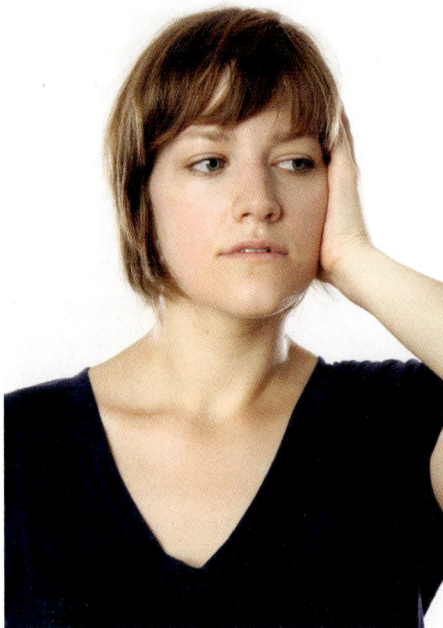

Figure 6-19 **Strengthen contralateral scalenes.** The client rests the flat of the hand on the side of the head with the affected scalenes and rotates the head toward the affected side.

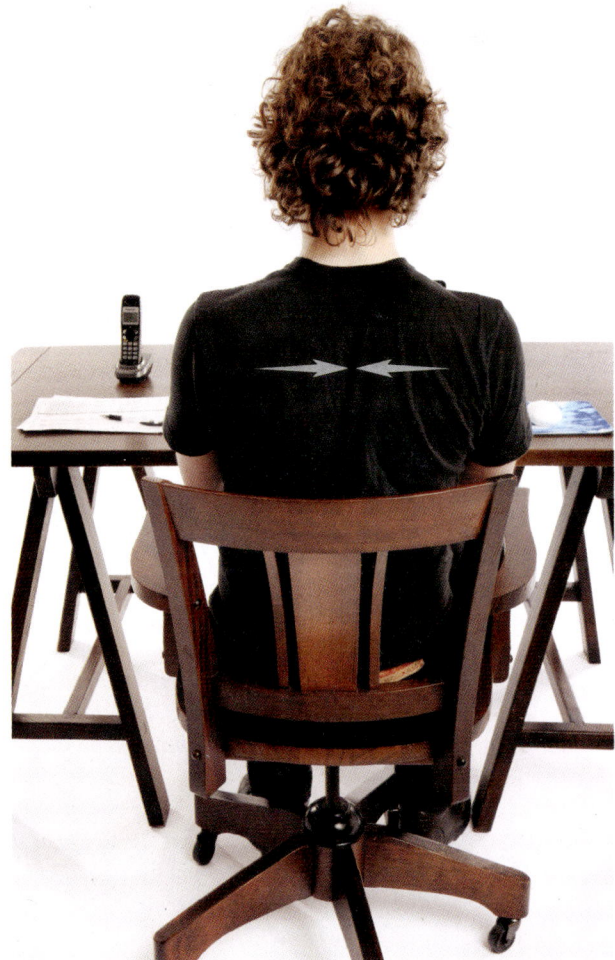

Figure 6-20 **Middle trapezius and rhomboid strengthening.** Instruct the client to squeeze the scapulae together without using any muscles other than the middle trapezius and rhomboids.

SUGGESTIONS FOR FURTHER TREATMENT

Ideally, a client with symptoms of thoracic outlet syndrome will have treatments twice a week for the first week or two or until symptoms are absent for at least 4 days. This should be followed by weekly treatments until the symptoms are absent for at least 7 days and ROM and strength are restored. As treatment continues, the period of symptom-free days should increase until the symptoms become occasional or are relieved completely. After this, the client can schedule appointments as necessary. If the thoracic outlet syndrome is caused by muscle tension, the client should have some improvement with each session. If this is not happening, consider the following possibilities:

- There is too much time between treatments. It is always best to give the newly treated tissues 24–48 hours to adapt, but if too much time passes between treatments in the beginning, the client's activities of daily living may reverse any progress.
- The client is not adjusting his or her activities of daily living or is not keeping up with self-care. As much as we want to fix the problem, we cannot force a client to make the adjustments we suggest.
- The client's thoracic outlet syndrome is advanced or involves other musculoskeletal complications that are beyond your basic training. Refer this client to a massage therapist with advanced clinical or medical massage training. Continuing to treat a client whose case is beyond your training could turn the client away from massage therapy altogether and hinder healing.
- The symptoms have an undiagnosed, underlying cause. Discontinue treatment until the client sees a health care provider for medical assessment.

If you are not treating the client in a clinical setting or private practice, you may not be able to take this client through the full program of healing. Still, if you can bring some relief, it may encourage that client to discuss this change with his or her health care provider and to consider manual therapy rather than more aggressive treatment options. If the client returns for regular treatments, the symptoms are likely to change each time, so it is important to perform an assessment before each session. As the client's symptoms change, you may be able to focus more of your treatment on a specific area or on other postural imbalances.

PROFESSIONAL GROWTH

CASE STUDY

Salim is a 53-year-old father of two adult children. He and his brother own a house painting company. In recent months, business has been slow. To reduce expenses, he and his brother have been doing much of the painting themselves. He began feeling numbness and tingling in his hand a few weeks ago and now feels weak when painting. Salim's primary health care provider, Dr. Johnson, practices in an integrative medicine clinic with massage therapists on staff.

Subjective

Salim stated that a few weeks ago he started feeling pins and needles in his left hand and noticed that from time to time he cannot feel the object he is holding in that hand, as if the tips of his ring finger and little finger had no sensation. During the past week, he has felt fatigue and weakness in his left shoulder and arm, and now his neck is sore on the right side too. In the beginning the symptoms would appear in the middle of the day, but now they happen almost as soon as he starts to paint and sometimes when he sleeps. Recently, he has been awakened from sleep by the sensation. When asked, Salim answered that he has never noticed any swelling in the arm or hand.

Objective

Salim's visit with Dr. Johnson included blood and other tests for systemic conditions, the results of which were negative. Positive Wright and Roos tests suggest thoracic outlet syndrome. Palpation revealed no cervical rib, and no X-ray was ordered. The doctor stated that he believed muscle tension to be the cause and referred Salim to the massage therapy clinic with the caveat that if symptoms were not reduced after two treatments per week for 2 weeks, he would recommend an MRI. Dr. Johnson saw no need to be conservative or cautious with massage.

Salim stood with most of his weight on his left leg while discussing his symptoms, with his pelvis rotated toward the right. The right hip is slightly flexed and externally rotated. The thorax is laterally flexed left, and the left hip is elevated. The right shoulder is elevated compared to the left. The left scapula is tilted anteriorly. The cervical spine is rotated to the right, laterally flexed to the left. The shoulders are internally rotated bilaterally with increased pronation in the right forearm. Slight scoliosis is evident.

The pectoralis major is dense and adhered bilaterally. Nothing is remarkable in either subclavius. The left pectoralis minor is hypertonic and tender to the touch with taut bands but no referral. Superficial fascial restrictions are present along the lateral neck and into the shoulder. The left scalenes are hypertonic. There is a trigger point in both the anterior and middle scalenes with referred pain into the shoulder. The left latissimus dorsi is adhered and tender. No trigger points were found. The left serratus anterior is dense, and the left side of the ribcage is slightly compressed. There is a trigger point in the serratus anterior with referred pain into the forearm. The right levator scapulae and upper trapezius are hypertonic and tender. There is crepitus around the right superior angle of the scapula. The erector spinae are taut bilaterally along the full spine. The left external obliquus and quadratus lumborum are shortened and hypertonic. The right quadriceps femoris and iliotibial band are thick and adhered. I did not investigate the gluteals or lower limbs; these will be revisited in a subsequent visit.

Action

I applied moist heat to the left pectoral area while palpating/assessing tissues around the hips. I moved the heat to the right pectoral area. I performed myofascial release around the glenohumeral joint and across the pectorals bilaterally. With the arm laterally rotated and abducted, I applied effleurage and cross-fiber friction followed by muscle stripping to the pectoralis major, latissimus dorsi, and serratus anterior. I applied trigger point therapy to the serratus. The pain reduced from level 8 to 3 and referral ceased. I applied petrissage to the origin and insertions of the pectoralis minor followed by stripping to the muscle belly. This reproduced symptoms. I returned the client's arm to the neutral position, which eased symptoms, then palpated the pectoralis minor again. No symptoms were reproduced the second time. The pectoralis minor may be too dense to reach trigger points in taut bands. I applied kneading and lengthening strokes to reduce tension, and will attempt to treat trigger points in a subsequent session. I applied a stretch to the pectorals, taking care not to reproduce symptoms. The left scalenes are solid and dense, and the fibers are barely palpable. There are trigger points in the anterior and middle scalene that referred pain across the shoulder but did not reproduce symptoms. I applied cross-fiber friction followed by several rounds of muscle stripping, which reduced referred pain slightly. I used three rounds of brief compression to a trigger point that caused pain at level 7, which then reduced to level 2. I applied general treatment to the upper trapezius, levator scapulae, and neck extensors as well as to the arms bilaterally. In the prone position, I applied general deep tissue massage to the upper back with minor attention to the low back and hips, primarily attempting to lengthen the left latissimus dorsi, abdominals, and quadratus lumborum and to reduce the flexion of the thorax.

The client remained very relaxed throughout the session, seemingly on the verge of sleep if not for my questions regarding symptoms. He stated that he felt looser but a little sore in the pectoral area.

Plan

I recommended taking time throughout that day to mobilize the neck and arm within his comfort level, in positions other than the one(s) he uses while painting. For example, I suggested that he slowly rotate the neck from left to right and bring the ear to the shoulder on both the left and right sides. I demonstrated stretches for pectorals and scalenes and those needed to reduce flexion in the thorax. I demonstrated strengthening for the shoulder retractors and lateral rotators of the shoulder. The client will return for treatment in 3 days and keep an account of symptoms during that time.

As Salim's condition improves and he becomes more able to perform activities of daily living without symptoms, I will focus attention on deviations in his hips and spine that may be contributing to the imbalance in the upper body. I will assess legs, knees, and ankles at that time.

CRITICAL THINKING EXERCISES

1. Develop a 10-minute stretching and strengthening routine for a client covering all of the muscles commonly involved in thoracic outlet syndrome. Use Box 6-1 and Figure 6-4 as a guide. Remember that a stretch increases the distance between the origin and insertion of a muscle and is important for those muscles that are shortened while strengthening is performed by actively bringing the origin and insertion closer together and is important for the antagonists of shortened muscles and otherwise weakened muscles. Describe each step of the routine in sufficient detail that the client can perform it without your assistance.

2. Sometimes an assessment reveals signs and symptoms that differ from the average presentation for a client with thoracic outlet syndrome. The following is a list of possible findings. For each, discuss how or why a client may have developed the imbalance, and how the treatment plan should be adapted:
   - Drooped shoulder on the affected side
   - Elevated shoulder on the affected side
   - Trigger point in the scalenes on the unaffected side, with referred pain, but no other symptoms
   - Lateral flexion of the thorax with internal rotation of the shoulder on the affected side, without scoliosis
   - Symptoms when carrying heavy objects with the arms hanging, no symptoms when raising the arm above the head
   - Previous injury to the shoulder on the unaffected side

3. Your client first had symptoms of numbness, tingling, and weakness in the right arm 6 years ago. Following 2 years of treatment including pharmaceutical injections in the scalenes, oral medications, and 6 months of physical therapy intended to strengthen the muscles of the chest and shoulder, the client had no long-term relief. Ultimately, the client was diagnosed with thoracic outlet syndrome and, after another year of medication and physical therapy with no long-term relief, had decompression surgery that involved dividing the anterior scalene and removing a portion of the first rib. The client had considerable relief, but from time to time, particularly when reaching for something, the tingling would return. Over the past 3 months, the symptoms have worsened. Discuss possible reasons why the injections, physical therapy, and surgery were not successful treatments for the client's symptoms, and explain how manual therapy planned according to a current assessment may reduce the client's symptoms.

4. Discuss special considerations and adjustments to treatment for a client who has been diagnosed with a condition such as hypertension or atherosclerosis that is currently under control and being monitored by a health care provider.

5. Discuss how stress might contribute to the symptoms of thoracic outlet syndrome. Consider possibilities that include nerve conduction, muscle tension, diet and exercise, and life outlook. Knowing that a stressed client will see you for 6 treatments over the course of 4 weeks, plan treatment that takes the client's stress into consideration.

BIBLIOGRAPHY AND SUGGESTED READINGS

American Academy of Family Physicians. Management of Shoulder Impingement Syndrome and Rotator Cuff Tears. Available at http://www.aafp.org/afp/980215ap/fongemie.html. Accessed Fall 2008.

American Academy of Orthopaedic Surgeons. Shoulder Impingement. Available at http://orthoinfo. aaos.org/topic.cfm?topic=a00032. Accessed Fall 2008.

Balakatounis K, Angoules A, Panagiotopoulou K. Conservative treatment of thoracic outlet syndrome (TOS): Creating an evidence-based strategy through critical research appraisal. Current Orthopaedics. 2007;21(6):471–476.

Barnes JF. Myofascial release in treatment of thoracic outlet syndrome. Journal of Bodywork and Movement Therapies. 1996;1(1):53–57.

Hamm M. Impact of massage therapy in the treatment of linked pathologies: Scoliosis, costovertebral dysfunction, and thoracic outlet syndrome. Journal of Bodywork and Movement Therapies. 2006;10(1):12–20.

Lindgren K-A. Conservative treatment of thoracic outlet syndrome: A two-year follow-up. Archives of Physical Medicine & Rehabilitation. 1997;78(4):373–378.

Mayo Foundation for Medical Education and Research. Raynaud's Disease. Available at http://www. mayoclinic.com/health/raynauds-disease/DS00433. Accessed Fall 2008.

Mayo Foundation for Medical Education and Research. Thoracic Outlet Syndrome. Available at http:// www.mayoclinic.com/health/thoracic-outlet-syndrome/DS00800. Accessed Fall 2008.

McKenzie K, Lin G, Tamir S. Thoracic outlet syndrome Part I: A clinical review. Journal of the American Chiropractic Association. 2004;41:17–24.

National Institute of Neurological Disorders and Stroke. Complex Regional Pain Syndrome Fact Sheet. Available at http://www.ninds.nih.gov/disorders/reflex_sympathetic_dystrophy/detail_reflex_sympathetic_dystrophy.htm#105993282. Accessed Fall 2008.

National Institute of Neurological Disorders and Stroke. NINDS Thoracic Outlet Syndrome Information Page. Available at http://www.ninds.nih.gov/disorders/thoracic/thoracic.htm. Accessed Fall 2008.

National Pain Foundation. Thoracic Outlet Syndrome General Information. Available at http://www. nationalpainfoundation.org/cat/871/thoracic-outlet-syndrome. Accessed Fall 2008.

Peng J. 16 cases of scalenus syndrome treated by massage and acupoint-injection. Journal of Traditional Chinese Medicine. 1999;19(3):218–220.

Rattray F, Ludwig L. *Clinical Massage Therapy: Understanding, Assessing and Treating over 70 Conditions.* Toronto, ON: Talus Incorporated, 2000.

Reflex Sympathetic Dystrophy Syndrome Association. About CRPS. Available at http://www.rsds. org/2/what_is_rsd_crps/index.html. Accessed Fall 2008.

Spine Universe. Spinal Stenosis: Lumbar and Cervical. Available at http://www. spineuniverse.com/displayarticle.php/article209.html. Accessed Fall 2008.

Turchaninov R. *Medical Massage*, 2nd ed. Phoenix, AZ: Aesculapius Books, 2006.

U.S. National Library of Medicine and the National Institutes of Health. Cervical Spondylosis. Available at http://www.nlm.nih.gov/MEDLINEPLUS/ency/article/000436.htm. Accessed Fall 2008.

U.S. National Library of Medicine and the National Institutes of Health. Herniated disk. Available at http://www.nlm.nih.gov/medlineplus/ency/article/000442.htm. Accessed Spring 2008.

U.S. National Library of Medicine and the National Institutes of Health. Hypothyroidism. Available at http://www.nlm.nih.gov/medlineplus/ency/article/000353.htm. Accessed Spring 2008.

U.S. National Library of Medicine and the National Institutes of Health. Thoracic Outlet Syndrome. Available at http://www.nlm.nih.gov/medlineplus/thoracicoutletsyndrome.html. Accessed Fall 2008.

U.S. National Library of Medicine and the National Institutes of Health. TMJ Disorders. Available at http://www.nlm.nih.gov/medlineplus/ency/article/001227.htm. Accessed Fall 2008.

U.S. National Library of Medicine and the National Institutes of Health. Tumor. Available at http://www. nlm.nih.gov/MEDLINEPLUS/ency/article/001310.htm. Accessed Fall 2008.

Carpal Tunnel Syndrome

UNDERSTANDING CARPAL TUNNEL SYNDROME

Carpal tunnel syndrome occurs when the median nerve is compressed within the carpal tunnel of the wrist. The carpal tunnel is a small space in the wrist between the carpal bones and the flexor retinaculum (also referred to as the transverse carpal ligament) (Fig. 7-1). The four tendons of flexor digitorum superficialis, the four tendons of flexor digitorum profundus, the tendon of flexor pollicis longus, the ulnar and radial arteries, and the median nerve pass comfortably through this space when the structure and its contents are healthy. When the tissues become inflamed or adhered, or if the structure and its contents are otherwise compromised, the amount of space in the tunnel is reduced and the nerve and the blood vessels may become compressed. Compression of the median nerve slows the impulses transmitted, which results in pain, numbness, and tingling along its distribution. Compression of the blood vessels may reduce circulation, affecting the health and function of the nerve and other tissues nourished by compromised vessels. Movement of the wrist and hand frequently intensifies the symptoms. A client diagnosed with carpal tunnel syndrome often wears a splint to keep the wrist immobilized in an attempt to reduce symptoms.

The carpal tunnel is not the only place where compressed nerves and vessels may result in similar symptoms. The roots of the brachial plexus exit the spine between C5 and T1 (see Chapter 6). These five roots merge, divide, and merge again to form three cords. The median nerve arises from the medial and lateral cords. The nerve wraps around to the front of the neck, travels under the lateral clavicle, passes beneath the coracoid process, and follows down the anterior, medial arm, through the middle of the cubital fossa and forearm, through the carpal tunnel, and into the palm (Fig. 7-2). Because postures and activities that commonly contribute to carpal tunnel syndrome may also involve the elbow, shoulder, and neck, symptoms can be intensified by compression of the nerve at more than one location. This is referred to as "double crush," a condition in which innervation is interrupted at more than one site along the path of a nerve. Trauma, tension, and trigger points in the scalenes, pectoralis minor, or pronator teres can cause similar pain, tingling, and numbness. It is always best to allow time in your treatment to at least superficially treat the whole neck and arm on the affected side.

Muscles innervated by the median nerve include:

- Flexor carpi radialis
- Flexor digitorum superficialis
- Flexor digitorum profundus
- Flexor pollicis brevis
- Flexor pollicis longus
- Palmaris longus

- Pronator teres
- Pronator quadratus
- Opponens pollicis
- Abductor pollicis brevis
- 1st and 2nd lumbricals of the hand

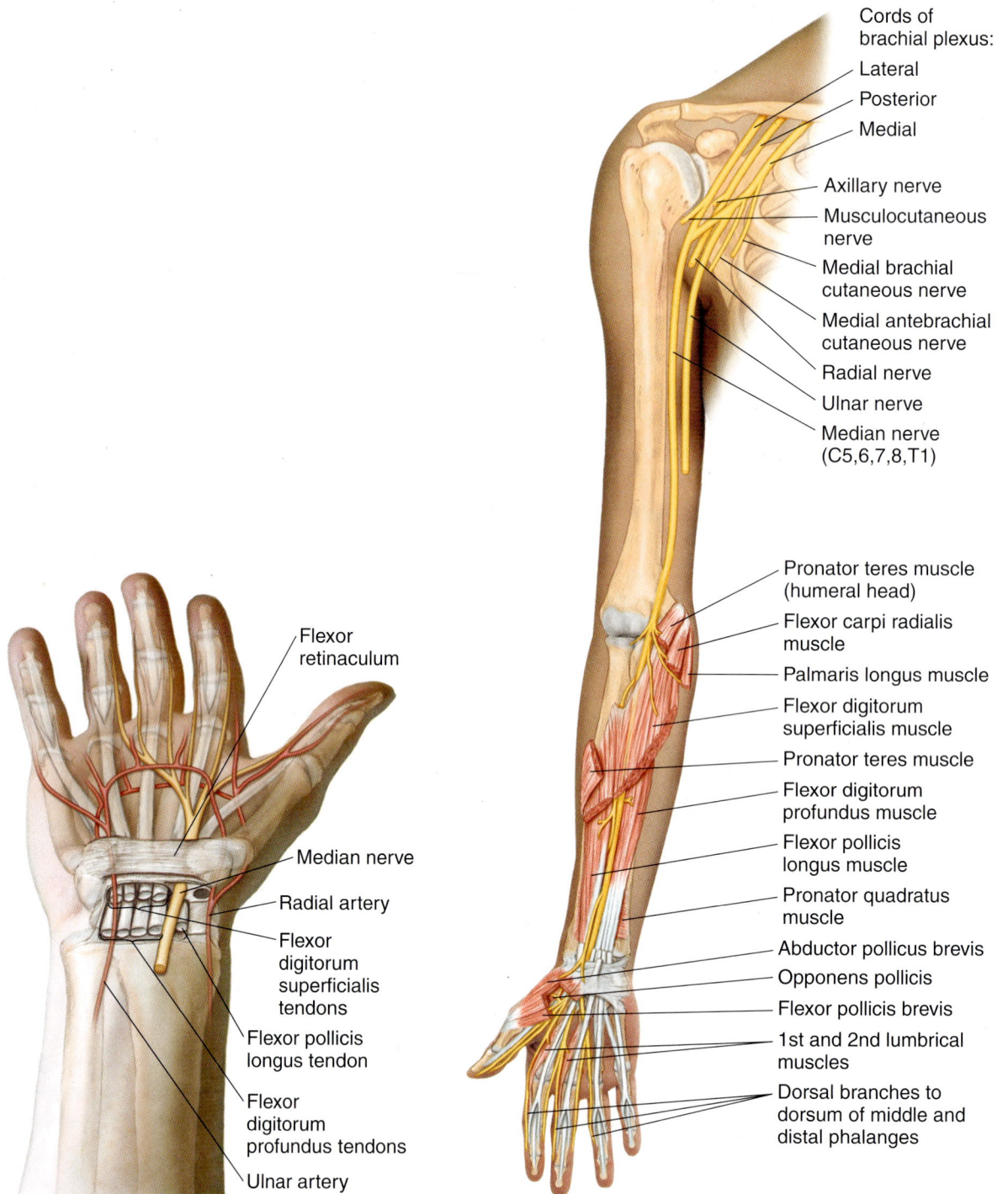

Figure 7-1   **The carpal tunnel.** Several tendons, blood vessels, and the median nerve pass through the carpal tunnel of the wrist. Adapted from Clay JH, Pounds DM. *Basic Clinical Massage Therapy: Integrating Anatomy and Treatment,* 2nd ed. Philadelphia: Lippincott Williams & Wilkins, 2008.

Figure 7-2   **Path of median nerve.** Nerve roots forming the median nerve exit the spine between C5 and T1, merge into trunks, and form divisions and cords. Adapted from Clay JH, Pounds DM. *Basic Clinical Massage Therapy: Integrating Anatomy and Treatment,* 2nd ed. Philadelphia: Lippincott Williams & Wilkins, 2008.

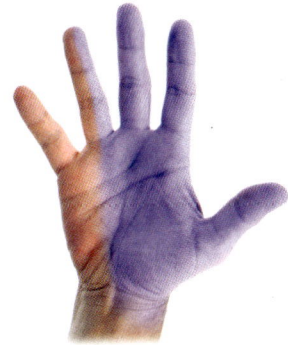

Figure 7-3 **Carpal tunnel symptoms area.** Compression of the median nerve in the carpal tunnel causes pain, numbness, and/or tingling in the thumb, index and middle fingers, the lateral half of the ring finger, and the wrist and palm of the hand. From Clay JH, Pounds DM. Basic Clinical Massage Therapy: Integrating Anatomy and Treatment, 2nd edition. Philadelphia: Lippincott Williams & Wilkins, 2008.

Common Signs and Symptoms

Carpal tunnel syndrome usually begins gradually with pain, numbness, and/or tingling in the thumb, index and middle fingers, lateral half of the ring finger, wrist, and palm of the hand (Fig. 7-3). In the early stages, these symptoms typically occur with movement, especially repetitive movements that cause friction to the structures and increase inflammation, or when the wrist is held in a flexed position for a long time, increasing pressure in the tunnel. Symptoms usually occur in the dominant hand because it is more likely subjected to greater stress but can also occur in the nondominant hand, especially if the nondominant hand has been subjected to trauma or over use, and can occur in both hands. Sleeping with the wrists flexed can intensify symptoms, often waking the person. Disturbed sleep may then become a contributing factor in the progression of the syndrome, possibly contributing to anxiety and depression, which may in turn increase the symptoms. As the syndrome progresses, the client may experience symptoms during the day, with or without movement. With reduced innervation the muscles become weaker, making it difficult to grasp items like a cup or a pen or to perform other fine motor skills. Pain begins to travel up the arm and often reaches the shoulder and neck. Ultimately, the thenar muscles may atrophy and the client may begin to lose sensation in the hand, making it difficult to sense temperature or other normally painful stimuli. Each client may experience this progression differently, with symptoms developing over the course of weeks, months, or years depending on the contributing factors and the client's general health. The further the syndrome progresses, the greater the chance that the nerve itself will become damaged and the muscles innervated by it will lose tone and strength. Therefore, it is important for someone suffering from even mild symptoms of carpal tunnel syndrome to get treatment as soon as possible.

Possible Causes and Contributing Factors

Carpal tunnel syndrome does not have a single primary cause, although certain factors commonly contribute. The minimal space in the tunnel can be reduced by an anatomical variation, bone dislocation, abnormal growth of bone, a cyst, a tumor, or another obstacle. Though massage therapy may reduce the discomfort caused by such obstacles, it cannot eliminate them. Carpal tunnel syndrome may also occur when soft tissues within the tunnel increase in size or change shape because of acute injury, scarring, fibrotic tissue buildup, inflammation, hypertonicity, trigger points, tendinopathy, sprains, and strains. Likewise, the flexor retinaculum may become larger or inflamed because of injury or because adhered tissues increase the amount of friction that occurs with movement. Friction is a common cause of inflammation.

Clients whose activities of daily living include repetitive or forceful actions or vibrations at the wrist are prone to developing carpal tunnel syndrome. Careers in which employees have a high rate of carpal tunnel syndrome include data entry, assembly, meat or fish packing, construction, electrical work, hair styling, driving, and any other job that involves forceful, repetitive actions or that keeps the wrist in flexion for long periods. Unless acute injury is the primary contributing factor, when the cause of carpal tunnel syndrome is neuromuscular, the client may not feel symptoms until long after the contributing postures or activities have become part of his or her activities of daily living. Similarly, once treatment reduces symptoms, the client must diligently address contributing factors to avoid recurrence.

Other factors associated with nerve impairment include obesity, hypothyroid condition, arthritis, diabetes, gout, hormonal changes, lymphedema, rheumatoid arthritis, lupus, and Lyme disease. In these cases, the symptoms may quickly resolve once the associated condition is controlled. During pregnancy, body fluids increase and may contribute to compression, though this is likely to resolve shortly after childbirth. Cigarette smoking, though not a cause of carpal tunnel syndrome, exacerbates the inflammatory process and can intensify symptoms. Alcoholism, poor nutrition, vitamin B deficiency, and general stress may also contribute. Some evidence suggests that genetics may also play a role in carpal tunnel syndrome. Bone structure, abnormal collagen production, and abnormal myelin regulation are genetic factors that may predispose a client to the syndrome. Symptoms are likely to arise in these individuals in adolescence and are more likely to be bilateral.

Because so many factors can contribute to peripheral neuropathies, be sure to understand the client's health history before proceeding with treatment. Many of the conditions listed above have contraindications for massage therapy or require adjustments to treatment. Moreover, when a systemic condition contributes to a peripheral neuropathy, especially if that systemic condition is not being monitored by a health care provider, massage therapy alone may bring only temporary relief of symptoms. Refer the client to his or her health care provider if you suspect a systemic condition or obstruction in the wrist, and discuss treatment with the client's health care provider if such a condition has been diagnosed

Table 7-1 lists conditions commonly confused with or contributing to carpal tunnel syndrome.

Contraindications and Special Considerations

It is essential to understand the factors contributing to carpal tunnel syndrome. If a systemic condition or structural abnormality is present, work with the client's health care provider and consult a pathology text for massage therapists before proceeding. Following are a few general contraindications:

- **Underlying pathologies.** The signs and symptoms of carpal tunnel syndrome may result from a wide variety of underlying conditions. If you suspect one of these (consult Table 7-1 and your pathology book for signs and symptoms), refer the client to his or her health care provider for medical assessment before initiating treatment. If the client is diagnosed with an underlying pathology that is not a contraindication for massage, work with the health care provider when necessary to develop an appropriate treatment plan.
- **Acute injury.** If the client has an acute injury, PRICE (protection, rest, ice, compression, elevation) is the protocol. You may work conservatively proximal to the site but avoid the wrist, hand, fingers, and any other area affected by the injury until it is in the subacute or chronic stage.
- **Edema.** If edema is present, do not work directly on the site. Work proximally, moving the fluid toward the nearest proximal lymph nodes. If vascular compression is a consideration but massage is not contraindicated for the client, do not allow the arm to fall below the heart because gravity may draw fluid into the arm and hand. Bolster the arm if necessary to keep fluid from accumulating.
- **Friction.** Do not use deep frictions if the client has a systemic inflammatory condition such as rheumatoid arthritis or osteoarthritis, if the health of the underlying tissues is compromised, or if the client is taking an anti-inflammatory medication. Friction creates an inflammatory process, which may interfere with the intended action of the anti-inflammatory medication. Recommend that your client refrain from taking such medication for several hours prior to treatment if his or her health care provider is in agreement.
- **Mobilizations.** Be cautious with mobilizations if the client has degenerative disc disease, rheumatoid arthritis, a bony obstruction, hypermobile joints, or if ligaments are unstable due to injury, pregnancy or a systemic condition.

Table 7-1	**Differentiating Conditions Commonly Confused with or Contributing to Carpal Tunnel Syndrome**

Condition	Typical Signs and Symptoms	Testing	Massage Therapy
Herniated disc	Symptoms increase when coughing, laughing, or straining	Kemp's test Spurling's test CT scan Myelography MRI	Massage is indicated with caution and proper training. Acute inflammation and acute injury are contraindications. Work with health care team.
C4-5	Weak deltoid Shoulder pain Usually no radiating pain or paresthesia		
C5-6	Weak biceps and wrist extensors Pain and paresthesia in radial nerve distribution		
C6-7	Weak triceps and finger extensors Pain and paresthesia down the posterior arm into third digit		
C7-T1	Weak hand grip Pain and paresthesia in ulnar nerve distribution		
Thoracic outlet syndrome	Pain in neck, shoulder, chest, arm, and hand Swelling, vascular changes, weakness or clumsiness in arm and hand Paresthesia in ulnar nerve distribution	Adson's test Travell's variation Scalene cramp test Eden's test Wright's hyperabduction Pectoralis minor test Upper limb tension test	See Chapter 6
Pronator teres syndrome	Symptoms can be identical to Carpal tunnel syndrome Pain in forearm—worsened by elbow flexion/extension Absence of pain at night	Resisted pronation of forearm (excluding resistance to wrist) Tinel's sign at the median nerve as it passes under pronator teres	Massage is indicated
Tendinopathy	Local inflammation and point tenderness	Pain on full, passive stretch of joint that tendon crosses; pain with resisted activity	See Chapter 14
Bursitis	Heat and swelling at joint Pain with active and passive movement of joint	Physical examination	Contraindicated locally, peripheral treatment may increase ROM.
Cubital tunnel syndrome	Numbness, pain, paresthesia, or weakness in the ulnar nerve distribution	Symptoms proximal to wrist Tinel's sign at cubital tunnel	Massage is indicated with caution to the area at the elbow where the ulnar nerve is most superficial.
Osteoarthritis	Stiff, painful joints Usually affects more than one joint	Physical examination	Massage is indicated when no acute symptoms are present.

(*continued*)

Table 7-1	Differentiating Conditions Commonly Confused with or Contributing to Carpal Tunnel Syndrome (Continued)		
Condition	**Typical Signs and Symptoms**	**Testing**	**Massage Therapy**
Hypothyroid condition	Weakness, fatigue, intolerance to cold, constipation, unintentional weight gain, brittle hair and nails, dry skin, puffy skin, hoarse voice	Physical examination T3, T4, and serum thyroid-stimulating hormone laboratory tests	Massage is indicated when no other contraindicated condition, such as circulatory complication, is present.
Gout	Red, hot, swollen joints Extreme pain Sudden onset	Physical examination X-ray Synovial fluid test Uric acid blood and urine tests	Massage is contraindicated during acute attacks. Gout may indicate other systemic conditions. Work with health care team.
Lupus	Skin rash Ulcers in mouth, nose, or throat Painful joints Headaches Kidney and nervous system disorders	Physical examination Diagnosis is complex Assessment includes presence of symptoms; blood, kidney, urine tests; chest x-ray; ECG	Massage is contraindicated during flare-ups. Work with health care team.
Lyme disease	Circular, bull's eye rash Red, itchy skin Fever Fatigue Joint pain Irregular heartbeat	Physical examination Assessment of symptoms and antibody tests Laboratory tests may be inconclusive in early stage of disease	Massage is indicated in nonacute stages. Work with health care team.
Rheumatoid arthritis	Fatigue, loss of appetite, low-grade fever, bilateral nonspecific muscle pain, rheumatic nodules, periods of flares and remission	Physical examination Blood tests Radiography	Massage is indicated in nonacute stages. Work with health care team.
Diabetes	Frequent urination, frequent thirst, increased appetite, fatigue, nausea	Physical examination Fasting blood sugar test	Massage is indicated when tissues and circulation are not compromised.

- **Pressure points.** Because pressure points in the hand may induce labor, avoid these in pregnant women.
- **Reproducing symptoms.** Symptoms may occur during treatment if you manually compress the nerve or if the client's posture causes structures to compress the nerve. If treatment reproduces symptoms, first adjust the client's posture to relieve compression. If this does not relieve the symptoms, reduce your pressure or move away from the area. You may be able to treat around the site that reproduced the symptoms, but work with caution.
- **Hydrotherapy.** Do not use heat in areas of edema or inflammation because heat dilates vessels and may increase the accumulation of fluid. Do not use moist heat on the neck or chest if the client has a cardiovascular condition that may be affected by dilation of blood vessels. Severe hypertension and atherosclerosis are two examples. Consult your pathology book for recommendations.
- **Initiating inflammatory process.** If treatment causes inflammation, end with cool hydrotherapy to inhibit the inflammatory process.

Massage Therapy Research

In 2004, Field et al. published a study titled "Carpal Tunnel Syndrome Symptoms Are Lessened Following Massage Therapy." The study involved 16 adults between the ages of 20 and 65 years, of middle socioeconomic status and varied ethnicity. Each participant had been previously diagnosed with carpal tunnel syndrome, worked extensively at a computer, and had unilateral symptoms at the time. The participants were divided randomly into a group that received massage therapy and a group that did not. Those in the massage group received a 15-minute massage to the affected arm once per week for 4 weeks. These participants were also taught self-massage and were instructed to perform it daily before bedtime. The control group received no massage but was taught self-massage after the study was completed. The study's results showed that the group receiving massage had significantly reduced symptoms, increased strength, increased nerve conductivity, and decreased anxiety and depression. The control group showed little change. The study's authors concluded that massage therapy has demonstrable benefits in the treatment of carpal tunnel syndrome. The study further notes that although carpal tunnel release surgery is successful in 75% of cases, complications including injury to the median nerve, scarring, loss of motion, and infection may occur, and symptoms recur in up to 19% of cases.

In 2007, Burke et al. published a study titled "A Pilot Study Comparing Two Manual Therapy Interventions for Carpal Tunnel Syndrome." This study compared the benefits of soft tissue manipulation conducted with the therapist's hands (STM group) to the benefits of manipulation conducted with patented tools used in the Graston Technique (GISTM group). The study involved 22 patients with carpal tunnel syndrome randomly divided into the two groups. On average, each participant received treatment twice per week for 4 weeks, then once per week for 2 weeks. Participants in both groups were treated by the same clinician who was trained in both techniques. Evaluations were made within 1 week of the final treatment, 6 weeks after last treatment, and 3 months after treatment. Although the clinical findings were not significantly different between the STM and GISTM groups, the study showed evidence that manual therapy increased ROM and grip strength in wrists affected by carpal tunnel syndrome. The authors of the study reported that these findings suggest that manual therapy may increase myofascial mobility, increase blood flow, and reduce ischemia, in turn alleviating symptoms of carpal tunnel syndrome.

In 2008, Moraska et al. published a study titled "Comparison of a Targeted and General Massage Protocol on Strength, Function, and Symptoms Associated with Carpal Tunnel Syndrome: A Randomized Pilot Study." In this study, 27 subjects previously diagnosed with carpal tunnel syndrome were randomly assigned to receive 30 minutes of either targeted or general massage therapy twice weekly for 6 weeks. The general protocol was typical of general relaxation massage intended to reduce tension and increase circulation to the back, neck, and both arms. The targeted protocol focused on sites of entrapment of the median nerve by reducing inflammation, adhesions, and hypertonicity along the full course of the brachial plexus and median nerve. Assessments were made at the beginning of the 8th and 12th treatments, and outcome assessments including strength and function were made 2 days after the 7th and 11th sessions. Both groups showed improvement in symptoms, but only the group receiving targeted treatment showed improvement in grip strength. The study's authors concluded that massage therapy may be effective in treating compression neuropathies including carpal tunnel syndrome.

WORKING WITH THE CLIENT

Client Assessment

Assessment begins at your first contact with a client. In some cases, this may be on the telephone when an appointment is requested. Ask whether the client is seeking treatment for specific

Table 7-2	Health History

Questions for the Client	Importance for the Treatment Plan
Where do you feel symptoms?	Location of symptoms gives clues to location of compression, trigger points, injuries, or other contributing factors.
Describe the character of your symptoms.	Differentiate possible origins of symptoms. Nerve compression often results in numbness and tingling along the distribution of that nerve. See Chapter 1 for a more detailed description of symptoms and possible origins.
Do any movements make the symptoms worse or better?	Locate tension, weakness, or compression in structures producing such movements.
Have you seen a health care provider for this condition? What was the diagnosis? What tests were performed?	If no tests were performed by the health care provider making a diagnosis, use the tests described later in this chapter for your assessment. If your assessment is inconsistent with the diagnosis, ask the client to discuss your findings with his or her health care provider, or ask for permission to contact his or her provider directly.
Have you been diagnosed with a condition such as diabetes, hypo- or hyperthyroid condition, rheumatoid arthritis or osteoarthritis, or systemic lupus?	Systemic conditions may contribute to symptoms, may require adjustments to treatment, and may impact treatment outcomes.
Are you pregnant?	Increased body fluid during pregnancy may contribute to symptoms that resolve after childbirth.
Have you had an injury or surgery?	Injury or surgery and resulting scar tissue may cause adhesions, hyper- or hypo-tonicity, trigger points, atypical ROM, and the signs and symptoms of carpal tunnel syndrome.
What type of work, hobbies, or other regular activities do you do?	Repetitive motions and static postures may contribute to the client's condition.
Are you taking any prescribed medication or herbal or other supplements?	Medications of all types may contribute to symptoms or involve contraindications or cautions.
Have you had a cortisone shot in the past 2 weeks? Where?	Local massage is contraindicated.
Have you taken a pain reliever or muscle relaxant within the past 4 hours?	The client may not be able to judge your pressure.
Have you taken an anti-inflammatory medication within the past 4 hours?	Deep friction may initiate an inflammatory process and should not be performed if the client has recently taken an anti-inflammatory medication.

symptoms so that you can review or research treatment options and contraindications to prepare yourself for the session.

Table 7-2 lists questions to ask the client when taking a health history.

POSTURAL ASSESSMENT

Allow the client to walk into the room ahead of you while you assess posture and gait. Look for imbalances or patterns of compensation. If you suspect carpal tunnel syndrome, have the client turn the doorknob to enter the room or pick up a pen or a cup of water without making him or her aware that you have begun your assessment. Do not hand the object to the client, but have the client pick it up himself or herself. If the client performs the task with the unaffected hand, especially if that hand is his or her nondominant hand, this could indicate a compensation pattern due to weakness in the affected hand. A client whose symptoms originate from compression superior to the carpal tunnel is not as likely to lose motor function of the hand unless the condition has existed for a long time without treatment. This client may, however, compensate because of pain.

Because the symptoms of carpal tunnel syndrome are often confused with symptoms from compressions occurring elsewhere in the body, it is important to assess the client in the posture most common in his or her activities of daily living or in the posture or activity that produces symptoms. For example, if your assessment of the standing client reveals exaggerated internal rotation at the shoulder, this could indicate compression of the brachial plexus at the pectoral area. If your assessment of the seated client reveals an exaggerated kyphotic curve with head forward and neck extended, it is possible that the nerve compression begins at the neck, specifically at the scalenes. If you suspect that a client's posture indicates contributing or compensating factors, treat these as much as time and the client's tolerance permit. Figure 7-4 compares the anatomical position to the posture affected by carpal tunnel syndrome.

RANGE OF MOTION ASSESSMENT

Test the range of motion of the elbow, wrist, and fingers, assessing the length and strength of both agonists and antagonists that cross the joints tested. Because the client controls the amount of movement, keeping it within a pain-free range, only active ROM should be used in the acute stage of injury to prevent undue pain or reinjury. Box 7-1 presents the average active ROM results for the joints involved in carpal tunnel syndrome.

Box 7-1 AVERAGE ACTIVE ROM FOR JOINTS INVOLVED IN CARPAL TUNNEL SYNDROME

Elbow
Flexion 140–150°
  Biceps brachii
  Brachialis
  Brachioradialis
  Flexor carpi radialis
  Flexor carpi ulnaris
  Palmaris longus
  Pronator teres
  Extensor carpi radialis longus
  Extensor carpi radialis brevis

Extension 0° (5–10° Hyperextension)
  Triceps brachii
  Anconeus

Radioulnar (Forearm)
Pronation 80–90°
  Pronator teres
  Pronator quadratus
  Brachioradialis

Supination 80–90°
  Biceps brachii
  Supinator
  Brachioradialis

Wrist
Flexion 80–90°
  Flexor carpi radialis
  Flexor carpi ulnaris

  Palmaris longus
  Flexor digitorum superficialis
  Flexor digitorum profundus

Extension 65°
  Extensor carpi radialis longus
  Extensor carpi radialis brevis
  Extensor carpi ulnaris
  Extensor digitorum

Adduction (Ulnar Deviation) 30°
  Extensor carpi ulnaris
  Flexor carpi ulnaris

Abduction (Radial Deviation) 20°
  Extensor carpi radialis longus
  Extensor carpi radialis brevis
  Flexor carpi radialis

Fingers 2–5
Flexion 85–90°
  Flexor digitorum superficialis
  Flexor digitorum profundus
  Flexor digiti minimi brevis
  Lumbricals
  Some interossei

Extension 30–45°
  Extensor digitorum
  Extensor indicis

  Lumbricals
  Some interossei

Abduction 20–30°
  Dorsal interossei
  Abductor digiti minimi

Adduction 0–5°
  Palmar interossei
  Extensor indicis

Thumb
Flexion 55°
  Flexor pollicis longus
  Flexor pollicis brevis
  Adductor pollicis

Extension 20°
  Extensor pollicis longus
  Extensor pollicis brevis
  Abductor pollicis longus

Adduction 30°
  Adductor pollicis

Abduction 60–70°
  Abductor pollicis longus
  Abductor pollicis brevis

Opposition (Flexion and Abduction)
  Opponens pollicis
  Flexor pollicis brevis
  Abductor pollicis brevis

Extensor digitorum

Extensor carpi
radialis longus

Extensor carpi
radialis brevis

Pronator teres

Flexor digitorum
superficialis

Flexor digitorum
profundus

Flexor pollicis
longus

Extensor digitorum

Extensor carpi
radialis longus

Extensor carpi
radialis brevis

Pronator teres

Flexor digitorum
superficialis

Flexor digitorum
profundus

Flexor pollicis
longus

Shortened
Lengthened

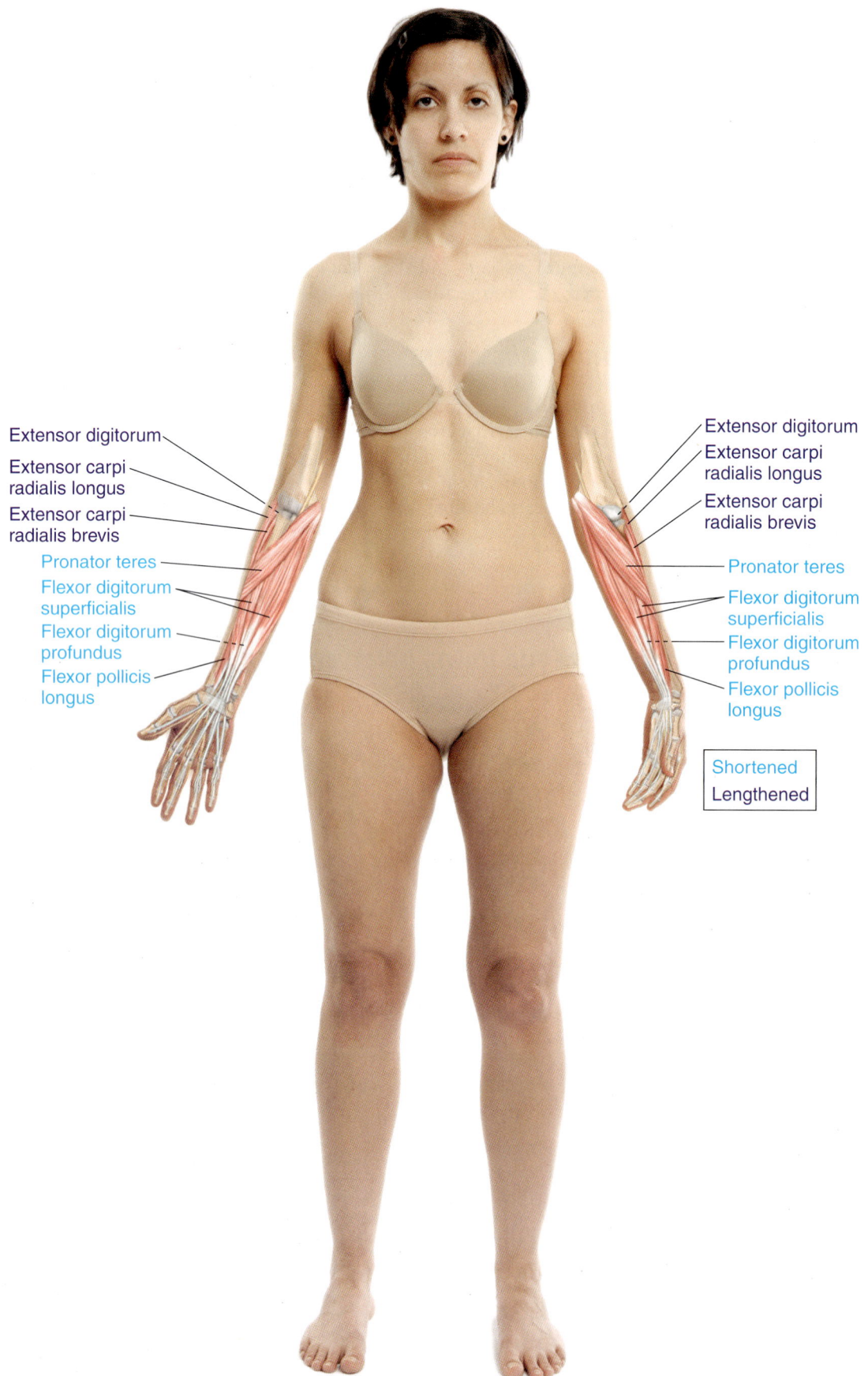

Figure 7-4   Postural assessment comparison. Compare the anatomical posture of the right arm to the deviated posture of the left arm. Note how the shortened flexors may contribute to compression of the contents in the carpal tunnel.

Active ROM

Compare your assessment of the client's active ROM with the ranges in Box 7-1. Carpal tunnel syndrome symptoms may not be reproduced with active ROM assessment because the client may limit his or her movement to the symptom-free range.

- **Active flexion of the wrist.** When muscle tension, adhesions, and trigger points contribute to carpal tunnel syndrome, an active, concentric contraction of the wrist flexors may be reduced. The client will likely be resistant to full, active flexion of the wrist if this produces symptoms during activities of daily living.
- **Active extension of the wrist** may be restricted because tight flexors may not allow the full range of extension in the wrist.
- **Active adduction of the wrist** may be restricted if the abductors of the wrist are shortened and hypertonic.

Passive ROM

Compare the client's passive ROM of the affected wrist with that of the unaffected wrist. Note and compare the end feel for each range in both wrists (refer to Chapter 1 for an explanation of end feel).

- **Passive flexion of wrist.** The client may resist even passive flexion of the wrist if flexion causes pain in daily life. Numbness and tingling may occur with full passive flexion if the space in the carpal tunnel is already reduced by other factors. Pain may be felt at the medial epicondyle of the humerus, on the anterior and medial forearm, and at the wrist itself. A hard end feel may indicate a bony structure as a contributing factor.
- **Passive extension of wrist.** In passive extension, a painful stretch to tight wrist flexors may be felt along the anterior and medial aspect of the forearm and the wrist. Numbness and tingling may occur with full passive extension of the wrist. Pain with full passive extension of the wrist may also suggest tendinopathy of a wrist flexor (see Chapter 14).
- **Passive extension of elbow.** Pain on a full passive extension of the elbow may indicate tendinopathy of the elbow or wrist flexors.
- **Passive adduction of wrist** may cause a painful stretch if the wrist abductors are shortened and hypertonic.

Resisted ROM

Use resisted tests to assess the strength of the muscles that cross the joints involved. Compare the strength of the affected side with that of the unaffected side.

- **Resisted flexion of the wrist** may produce symptoms as tendons passing through the carpal tunnel shorten and widen, further decreasing space in the tunnel.
- **Resisted extension of the wrist** may reveal weakness. This may result from accumulating tension in the flexors, which may lengthen and weaken the extensors reducing their capacity to oppose flexion.
- **Resisted adduction of the wrist** may reveal weakness if the wrist abductors are shortened and hypertonic.
- **Resisted abduction of the thumb** may also reveal weakness, suggesting that the abductor pollicis brevis is affected.

SPECIAL TESTS

Phalen's maneuver may reveal median nerve compression in the carpal tunnel. To ensure that the symptoms originate from the carpal tunnel rather than another area along the median distribution, while performing this test the client must not pronate the forearm, internally rotate the shoulder, or put the neck in flexion, lateral flexion, extension, or rotation.

1. Apply full passive flexion to the affected wrist to test for compression of the median nerve at the carpal tunnel (Fig. 7-5).
2. If symptoms occur within 60 seconds of holding this position, the test is considered positive for median nerve compression with flexion of the wrist.

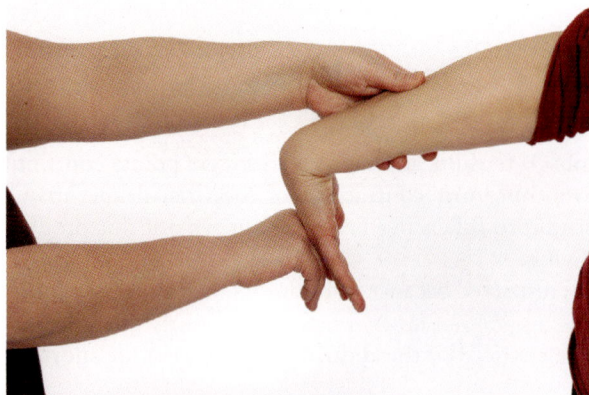

Figure 7-5 **Phalen's test.** Apply full passive flexion to the affected wrist without pronation of the forearm to test for compression of the median nerve at the carpal tunnel.

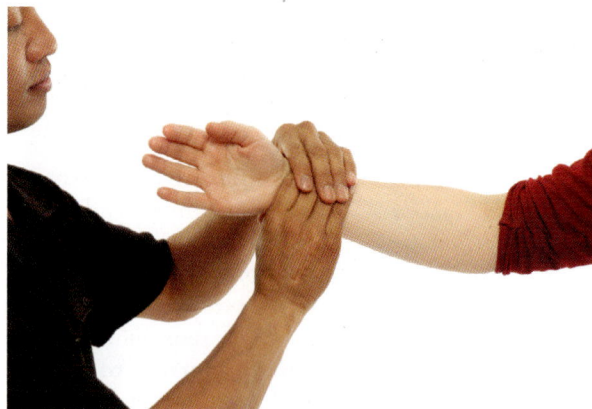

Figure 7-6 **Resisted pronation of the forearm.** Active resisted pronation of the forearm can be used to assess the involvement of pronator teres.

Pronator teres test may reveal compression of the median nerve by pronator teres. Note that unlike carpal tunnel syndrome, pronator teres syndrome does not typically involve symptoms that wake the client from sleep. Symptoms are most noted with repetitive or resisted flexion and extension or pronation and supination of the elbow.

1. Begin with the client's elbow passively flexed. Support the elbow with one hand if the client is unable to keep the flexed elbow relaxed. Instruct the client to pronate the forearm against your resistance, then passively extend the elbow to lengthen the contracting pronator teres. (Fig. 7-6). Apply resistance at the distal forearm instead of the hand to avoid flexion and undue pressure at the wrist and to distinguish between symptoms that originate at pronator teres from those that originate in the carpal tunnel.
2. The test is considered positive for compression of the median nerve under pronator teres if symptoms are reproduced within 60 seconds.

Tinel's sign can be used to test nerve conduction anywhere in the body. When testing for carpal tunnel syndrome, ensure that there is no active contraction producing flexion in the wrist, pronation of the forearm, flexion or internal rotation of the shoulder, or lateral flexion, extension, or rotation of the neck to ensure that any reproduced symptoms are originating from the carpal tunnel.

1. Tap on the median nerve in the carpal tunnel just distal to the crease of the wrist (Fig. 7-7).
2. The test is considered positive for carpal tunnel syndrome if the client feels tingling along the median nerve distribution.

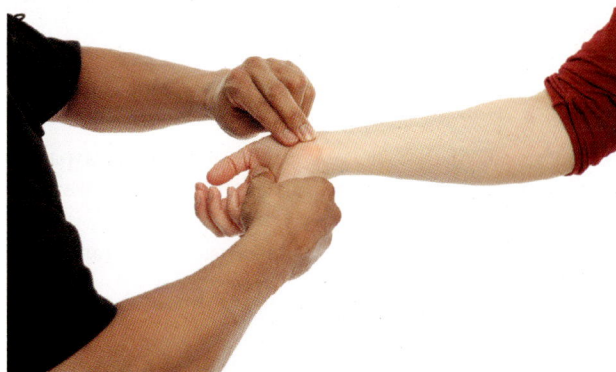

Figure 7-7 **Tinel's sign at the carpal tunnel.** Tap on the carpal tunnel just distal to the crease of the wrist.

PALPATION ASSESSMENT

Assess the fascia along the full forearm, wrist, and hand. Skin rolling is a useful tool for assessing superficial fascial restrictions. Areas of restriction may be found nearest the attachment sites of the forearm flexors, though restrictions are possible anywhere in the forearm.

At the forearm, you may find that the flexors are shortened and hypertonic and the extensors weak and taut. When the extensors are weak, they cannot oppose flexion of the wrist efficiently, allowing exaggerated flexion to continue or worsen.

Check the temperature, color, and texture of the superficial tissues. Compression of the nerve or the vessels may cause cool or warm skin, pale skin, boggy texture, and even reduced hair growth.

Condition-Specific Massage

Because the causes of pain, numbness, and tingling in the wrist and hand vary so widely, it may be difficult to pinpoint a single cause. Moreover, more than one condition may be present at the same time. A client who works at a desk for long periods is likely to sit with the head forward and neck in extension (affecting the scalenes), the shoulder internally rotated (affecting the pectorals), the forearm pronated (affecting the pronator teres), and the wrist and fingers in flexion or extension or moving constantly between these (affecting the contents of the carpal tunnel). Likewise, patterns of compensation for any of these conditions can contribute to symptoms of the others.

It is essential for treatment to be relaxing. You are not likely to eliminate the symptoms of carpal tunnel syndrome, or any of the conditions associated with it, in one treatment. Do not try to do so by treating aggressively. Be sure to ask your client to let you know whether your pressure keeps him or her from relaxing. If the client responds by tensing muscles or has a facial expression that looks stressed, reduce your pressure. Remember that you are working on tissue that is compromised.

It is also important for the client to let you know whether any part of your treatment reproduces symptoms. Adjust the client to a more neutral position, reduce your pressure, or move slightly off the area if this occurs, and make a note about it as it may help you understand more clearly exactly which neuromuscular conditions are contributing to symptoms. Instruct your client to use deep but calming breathing to help him or her relax.

If palpation of a trigger point refers pain elsewhere, explain this to your client and ask him or her to breathe deeply during the technique. As the trigger point is deactivated, the referred pain will also diminish. Common trigger points and their referral patterns are shown in Figure 7-8.

The following suggestions are for treatment of symptoms including pain, tingling, or numbness due to compression of the median nerve at the carpal tunnel in the chronic stage. If the client has an acute injury, follow the PRICE (protect, rest, ice, compression, elevation) protocol. In this case, you may work conservatively proximal to the site but will have to avoid the injured area until the subacute or chronic stage.

- Begin in the supine position and initiate treatment on the affected side. If the affected side is too painful to approach, beginning with the unaffected side may help the affected side to relax. If both arms are affected, begin with the dominant side.
- If inflammation is present, bolster the arm so that gravity encourages venous return and the draining of fluid toward the proximal lymph nodes.

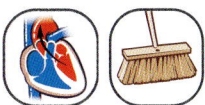

Treatment icons: Increase circulation; Reduce adhesions; Reduce tension; Lengthen tissue; Treat trigger points; Passive stretch; Clear area

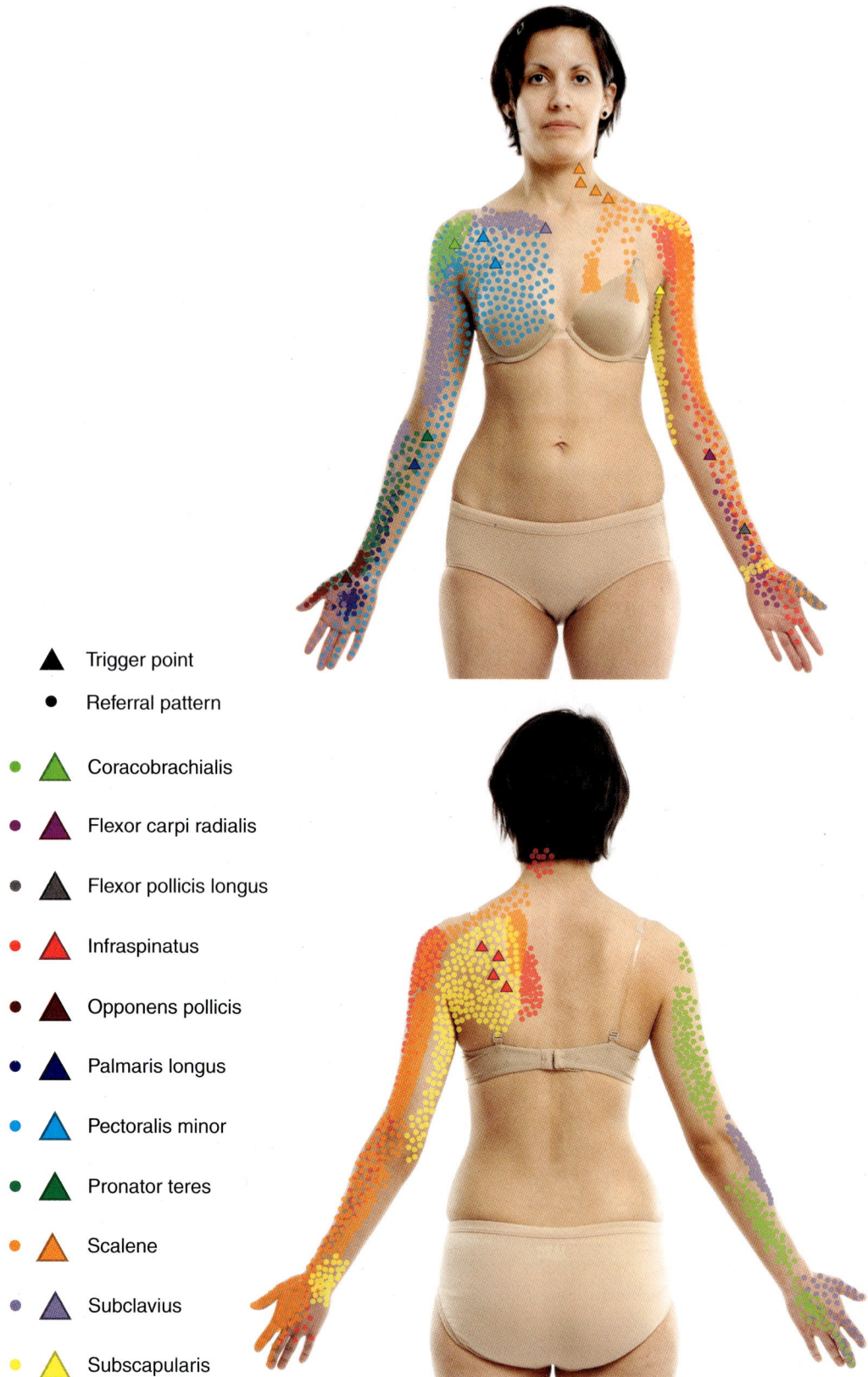

Figure legend:

▲ Trigger point

● Referral pattern

● ▲ Coracobrachialis

● ▲ Flexor carpi radialis

● ▲ Flexor pollicis longus

● ▲ Infraspinatus

● ▲ Opponens pollicis

● ▲ Palmaris longus

● ▲ Pectoralis minor

● ▲ Pronator teres

● ▲ Scalene

● ▲ Subclavius

● ▲ Subscapularis

Figure 7-8 **Common trigger points and referral.** Common trigger points with referrals associated with carpal tunnel syndrome.

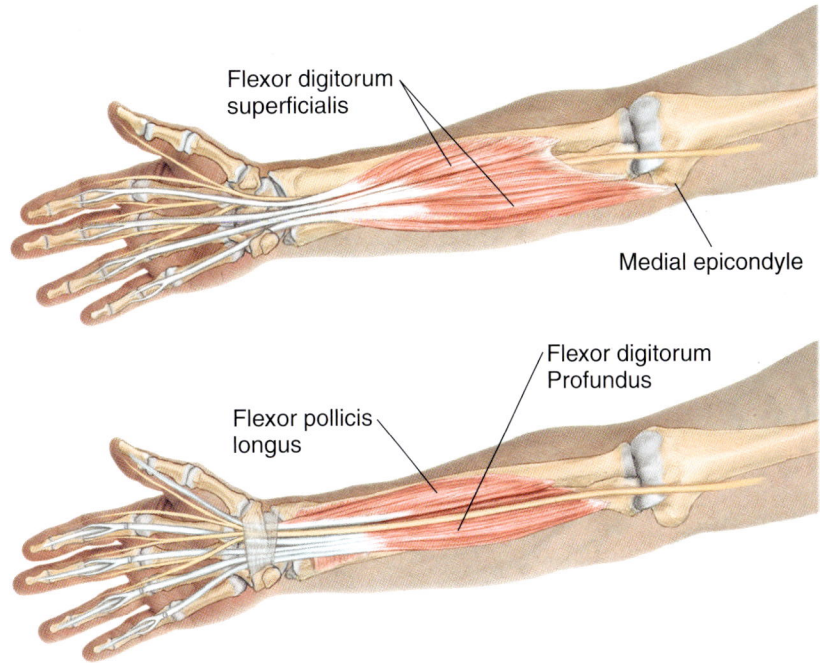

Flexor digitorum
superficialis

Medial epicondyle

Flexor digitorum
Profundus

Flexor pollicis
longus

FLEXOR DIGITORUM SUPERFICIALIS

Origin	*Common flexor tendon at medial epicondyle, coronoid process of ulna and shaft of radius.*
Insertion	*Middle phalanges of digits 2-5.*
Action	*Flex digits 2-5, flex wrist.*
Nerve	*Median.*

FLEXOR DIGITORUM PROFUNDUS

Origin	*Anterior, medial surface of proximal ulna.*
Insertion	*Distal phalanges of digits 2-5.*
Action	*Flex digits 2-5, flex wrist.*
Nerve	*Ulnar and median.*

FLEXOR POLLICIS LONGUS

Origin	*Anterior surface of radius.*
Insertion	*Distal phalange of thumb.*
Action	*Flex thumb.*
Nerve	*Median.*

Figure 7-9   Flexor digitorum superficialis and profundus, flexor pollicis longus. The tendons of flexor digitorum superficialis and profundus, and flexor pollicis longus pass through the carpal tunnel of the wrist. Adapted from Clay JH, Pounds DM. Basic Clinical Massage Therapy: Integrating Anatomy and Treatment, 2nd edition. Philadelphia: Lippincott Williams & Wilkins, 2008.

- If you suspect a double crush that involves compression of the brachial plexus at the neck or the pectoral area, refer to Chapter 6 for suggestions for treating thoracic outlet syndrome.

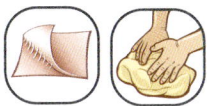

- Assess the arm for adhesions and hypertonicity. The muscles of the arm may be compensating because of pain or weakness in the forearm and hand. If you find nothing remarkable, be conservative in your treatment of the upper arm to spare time. You can come back to this in a subsequent treatment once you have attended to the major contributing factors.

- Assess the wrist flexors for adhesions. Begin with the most superficial muscles and progress to the deepest. Reduce any adhesions found.

- Assess and treat the wrist flexors for hypertonicity. Beginning again with the most superficial tissues and progressing to the deepest, release tension in the wrist flexors.

Coronoid process of ulna

Pronator teres

Radius

Medial epicondyle
of the humerus

Attachment of other flexors

PRONATOR TERES

Origin	*Medial epicondyle of humerus, common flexor tendon, coronoid process of ulna.*
Insertion	*Middle, lateral surface of radius.*
Action	*Pronate forearm, flex elbow.*
Nerve	*Median.*

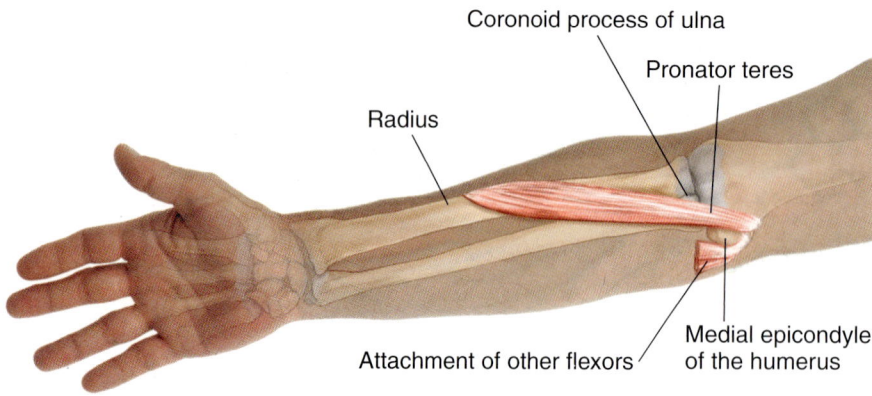

Figure 7-10 **Pronator teres.** The median nerve can become compressed as it passes under pronator teres. Adapted from Clay JH, Pounds DM. Basic Clinical Massage Therapy: Integrating Anatomy and Treatment, 2nd edition. Philadelphia: Lippincott Williams & Wilkins, 2008.

■ Lengthen the individual muscles whose tendons pass through the carpal tunnel. These muscles include the flexor digitorum superficialis, flexor digitorum profundus, and flexor pollicis longus (Fig. 7-9). You may also find the other flexors flexed and shortened. Treat these if indicated. Follow the length of these fibers from origin to insertion to comprehensively assess and lengthen them.

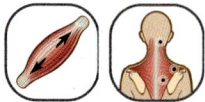

■ Assess the pronator teres for hypertonicity and trigger points because it is a common area for median nerve compression (Fig. 7-10).

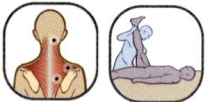

■ Treat trigger points found in the wrist flexors and apply a passive stretch.

■ Assess the flexor retinaculum for adhesions and release them if found (Fig. 7-11). Be sure to work within the client's pain tolerance and to lighten your pressure or discontinue this technique if it reproduces symptoms. It may be necessary to wait until a subsequent treatment to use this technique. As the client's symptoms are reduced with each treatment, the pressure at the carpal tunnel may diminish, allowing for more aggressive treatments such as friction.

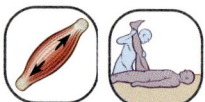

■ Find the attachments of the flexor retinaculum at the pisiform, hamate, scaphoid, and trapezium. Apply lengthening strokes in the direction of the fibers of the retinaculum. Follow this with a gentle stretch to the retinaculum by pinning the tissue at its attachments and gently pulling them away from each other (Fig. 7-12). To avoid repeated injury, be careful not to overstretch a ligament, especially if the client has a history of trauma.

■ If the client has not lost tone or strength in the hand, knead the muscles and tendons in the palm, particularly the thenar muscles. Be careful not to reproduce symptoms when working in the palm. If the tissues of the hand are compromised, you may need to postpone treatment here until innervation and tone are restored. Gentle tapotement may help to build tone in these muscles. If performing tapotement, avoid the carpal tunnel if this action reproduces symptoms.

■ Apply a full passive stretch to the wrist flexors. Extend the elbow and wrist fully and include the fingers and thumb in the stretch to ensure that the whole muscles are lengthened. Perform postisometric relaxation if necessary to encourage greater lengthening of the shortened wrist flexors.

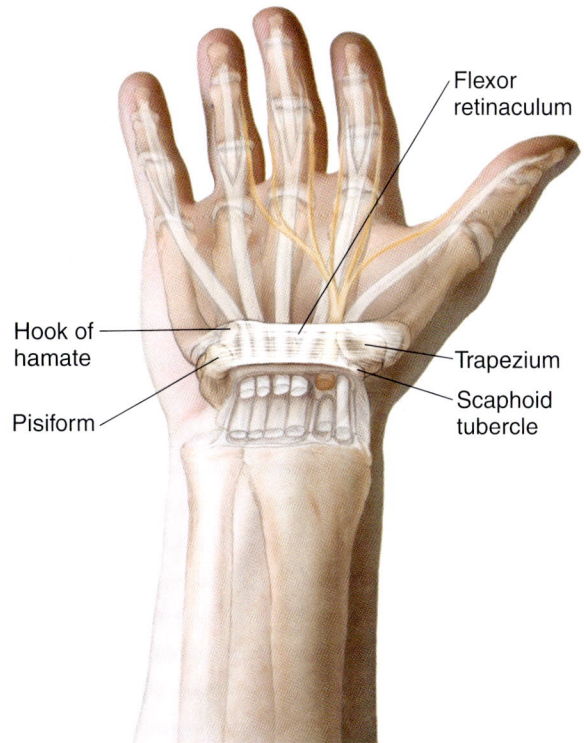

Flexor
retinaculum

Hook of
hamate

Pisiform

Trapezium

Scaphoid
tubercle

Figure 7-11 **Flexor retinaculum.** Adapted
from Clay JH, Pounds DM. Basic Clinical Massage
Therapy: Integrating Anatomy and Treatment, 2nd
edition. Philadelphia: Lippincott Williams & Wilkins,
2008.

FLEXOR RETINACULUM

Attachments	*Pisiform, hook of hamate, scaphoid tubercle, trapezium.*

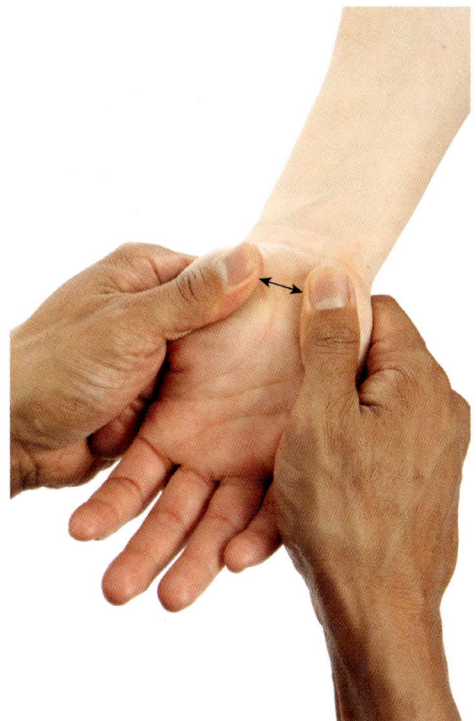

Figure 7-12 **Retinaculum stretch.** Perform a passive
stretch of the flexor retinaculum.

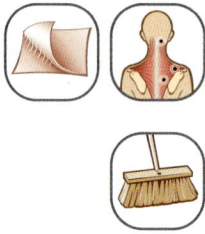

- Assess the wrist extensors for adhesions and trigger points and treat as necessary.

- Clear the whole arm with gentle strokes to move fluid toward proximal lymph nodes and encourage venous return. If inflammation occurred in the area during treatment, bolster the arm and cover the forearm and hand with a cool, wet towel.

- If time remains, consider treating the unaffected arm, neck, chest, or posterior thorax for patterns of compensation that may contribute to pain in these locations. If you do not have time for this in the first session, you may in subsequent sessions when the primary contributing factors require less treatment.

The treatment overview diagram summarizes the flow of the treatment (Fig. 7-13).

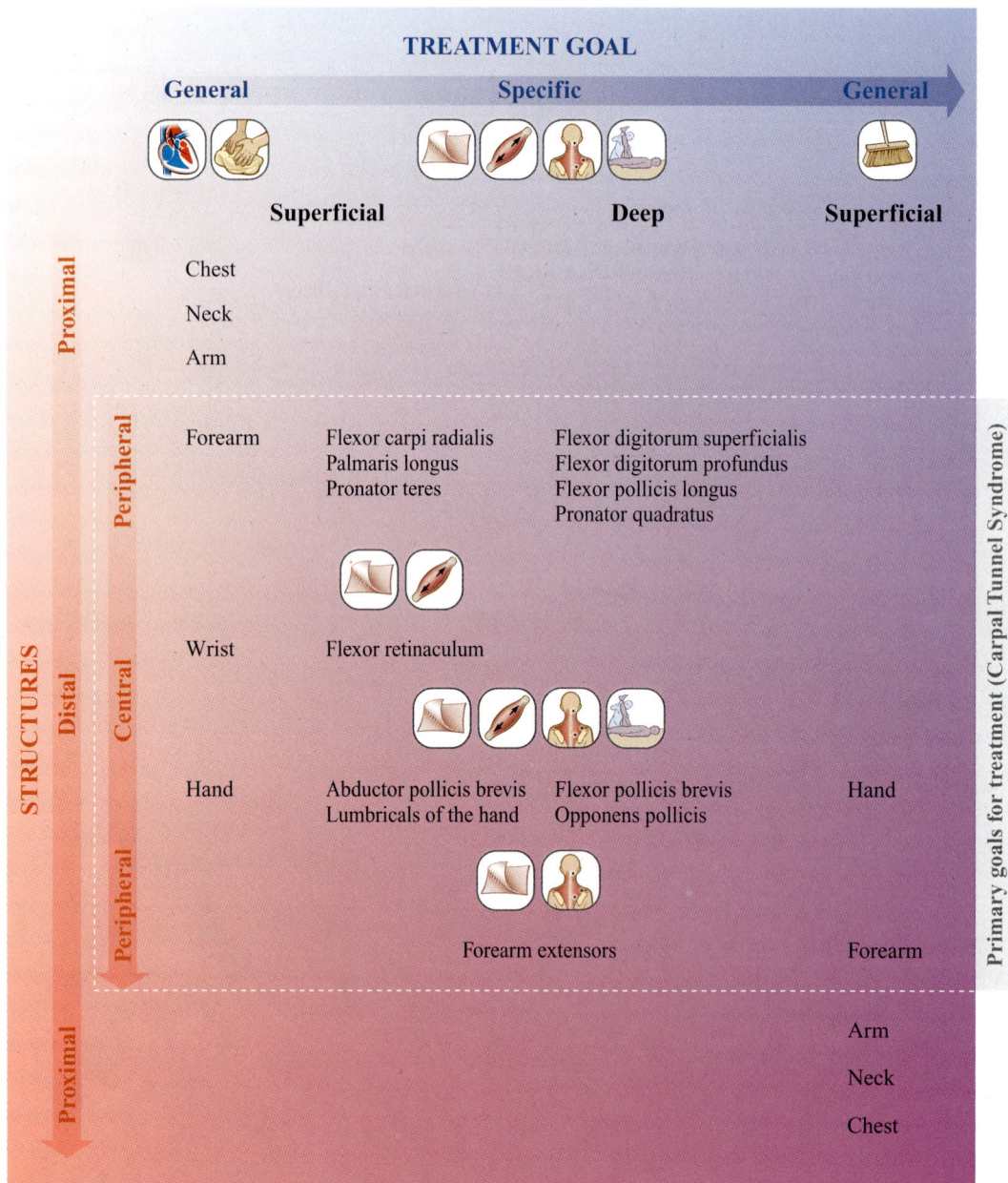

Figure 7-13 Carpal tunnel treatment overview diagram. Follow the general principles from left to right, or top to bottom when addressing carpal tunnel syndrome.

CLIENT SELF-CARE

The following are intended as general recommendations for stretching and strengthening muscles involved in the client's condition. The objective is to create distance between the attachment sites of muscles that have shortened and to perform repetitions of movements that decrease the distance between the attachments of muscles that have weakened. If you have had no training in remedial exercises, or do not feel that you have a functional understanding of stretching and strengthening, refer the client to a professional with training in this area.

Clients often neglect self-care because their daily lives are busy. Encourage them to follow these guidelines.

- When possible, perform self-care activities during the workday, while taking a phone call, or during other activities of daily living instead of setting aside extra time.
- Encourage the client to take regular breaks from repetitive actions.
- Demonstrate gentle self-massage to keep hypertonicity at bay between treatments.
- Instruct the client on proper posture to keep pressure off the weakened joints. Instruct clients with symptoms of carpal tunnel syndrome to sleep in positions without flexing the wrist, and to adjust their workstation to minimize flexion or extension of the wrist while typing.
- Demonstrate all strengthening exercises and stretches to your client and have them perform these for you before leaving to ensure that they are performing them properly and will not harm themselves when practicing on their own.

Stretching

Instruct the client to stretch his or her forearm flexors (Fig. 7-14). Be sure that the elbow is extended, and include the fingers and thumb when performing the stretch. Each stretch should be held at least 15–30 seconds. Extend the wrist only to the point of a comfortable stretch. The stretch should be pain-free with the affected arm fully relaxed. The client should perform stretches frequently throughout the day within his or her tolerance.

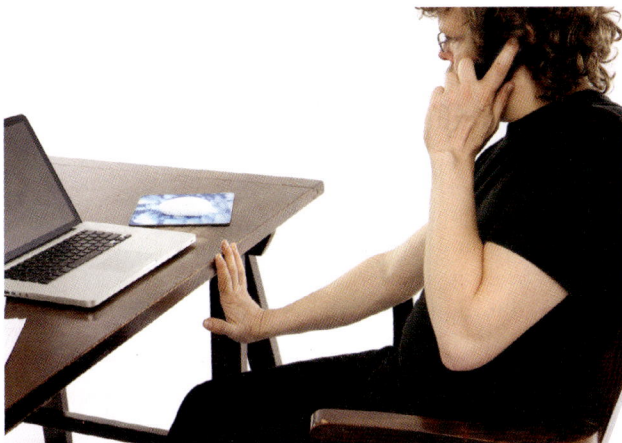

Figure 7-14 **Forearm flexor stretch.** With the elbow extended, extend the wrist and fingers against a surface to stretch the forearm flexors.

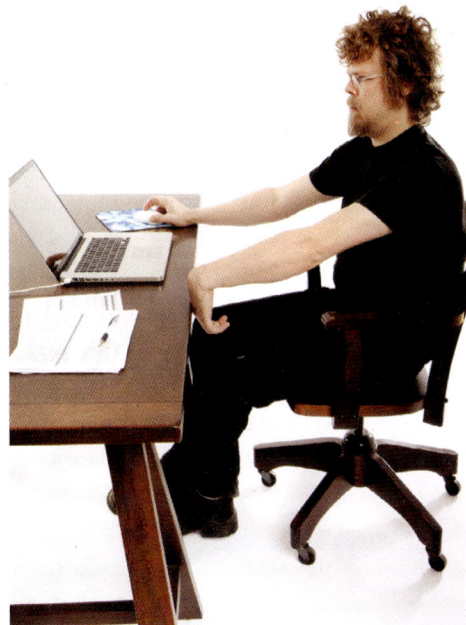

Figure 7-15 **Forearm extensor strengthening.** With the elbow extended and wrist slightly flexed, extend the wrist against resistance to strengthen wrist extensors.

If pronator teres is involved, instruct the client to fully supinate the forearm with the elbow extended to stretch pronator teres. For stretches to other areas along the median nerve, see Chapter 6 on the thoracic outlet syndrome.

Strengthening

Because forearm flexion is opposed by the forearm extensors, it is important to assess the extensors for length and strength. If the forearm extensors are weak and unable to fully oppose flexion of the wrist, the flexors are likely to return to the shortened, hypertonic state following treatment. Encourage the client to strengthen the forearm extensors within his or her tolerance by extending the affected wrist while gently resisting the movement with the opposite hand or a stable surface (Fig. 7-15).

Immobility is often the muscle's enemy. Although splinting is often recommended when a client develops symptoms of carpal tunnel syndrome, if the cause is muscular, immobility may promote the development of adhesions and thickening of the fascia. In addition, splinting the wrist may increase compensatory actions at the elbow and shoulder, putting these areas at greater risk for injury. With consent from his or her health care provider, encourage the client to remove the splint occasionally and gently move the wrist through its full range of motion. The client should not force this movement because forceful movement of the wrist may increase symptoms. Gently drawing the alphabet in the air with the wrist and hand is a helpful exercise, but the client should stop when he or she feels fatigue, pain, or reproduced symptoms.

SUGGESTIONS FOR FURTHER TREATMENT

Ideally, clients with carpal tunnel syndrome will have treatments twice per week for the first week or two, or until symptoms are absent for at least 4 days. This can be followed by weekly treatments until the symptoms are absent for at least 7 days and range of motion and strength have improved. As treatment continues, the period of symptom-free days should increase until the symptoms become occasional or are relieved completely. After this, the client can schedule appointments as necessary. If the cause of symptoms is neuromuscular, some improvement should occur with each session. If the client is not improving, consider the following possibilities:

- There is too much time between treatments. It is always best to give the newly treated tissues 24–48 hours to adapt, but if too much time passes between treatments in the beginning, the client's activities of daily living may reverse any progress.
- The client does not have carpal tunnel syndrome and you may be focusing treatment on the wrong area. Remember that the symptoms may arise from several different points along the neck, shoulder, and arm.
- The client is not adjusting his or her activities of daily living or is not keeping up with self-care. As much as we want to fix the problem, we cannot force a client to make the adjustments we suggest.
- The syndrome is advanced or involves other complications beyond your basic training. Refer this client to a massage therapist with advanced clinical massage training. Continuing to treat a client whose case is beyond your training could turn the client away from massage therapy entirely and hinder his or her healing.
- There is an undiagnosed, underlying condition. Discontinue treatment until the client sees a health care provider for a medical assessment.

If you are not treating the client in a clinical setting or private practice, you may not be the therapist who takes this client through his or her full program of healing. Still, if you can bring some relief, the client may be encouraged to discuss this change with his or her health care provider and to seek manual therapy rather than more aggressive treatment options. If the client returns for regular treatments, the symptoms are likely to change each time, so it is important to perform an assessment before each session.

PROFESSIONAL
GROWTH

CASE STUDY

Caroline is a 34-year-old single mother of one 3-year-old child. She is an assistant to the president of a busy real estate firm, working at a computer an average of 40 hours per week. Caroline is very careful to prepare healthy, home-cooked meals for her family every day. She exercises three or four times per week including 30 minutes of aerobic exercise and 20 minutes of strength training with light weights. She began feeling tingling in her thumb and index finger about 3 weeks ago.

Subjective

Client complained of pain across her shoulder and has had tingling in her thumb and index finger for 3 weeks. She reports that the symptoms are most aggravating at work in the late afternoon and when she cooks. Recently she has been awakened from sleep by the sensation. She also noted that her coffee cup feels heavier in her hand than she had ever noticed before. In her most recent visit to her physician, no systemic conditions were diagnosed, though she was diagnosed with carpal tunnel syndrome and prescribed muscle relaxants and a brace for the wrist. Her physician suggested that if the symptoms do not dissipate, surgery is an option. Caroline requested deep tissue massage to relieve tension in her neck and asked whether massage could help relieve the tingling in her fingers.

Objective

Client wears a brace on her right wrist. She lifted the pen with her left hand and positioned it in her right before filling out her intake form. Shoulders are medially rotated, more notably on the right side. Resisted internal rotation of the shoulder produced no symptoms. There is slight left rotation and right lateral flexion of the neck. Resisted left rotation of neck produced symptoms after 27 seconds. Head is slightly forward. Pronator teres strength test was normal and reproduced no symptoms. Phalen's test is positive for carpal tunnel syndrome. Resisted extension of the right wrist showed weakness. Following the strength test, the client was resistant to other ROM testing of the wrist.

Bilateral pectoralis major and minor are hypertonic and tender to touch. Scalenes are hypertonic, especially right. Trigger point in right anterior scalene referred across shoulder. There is minimal swelling at the hand and wrist. Objective observation suggests "double crush" at scalenes and carpal tunnel.

Action

Right arm bolstered to increase venous return. Warm hydrotherapy applied to neck and shoulders. General warming of tissues from the neck to fingers bilaterally, followed by clearing strokes toward the axillary lymph nodes. Myofascial release across glenohumeral joints bilaterally. Petrissage to bilateral pectorals, followed by muscle stripping. No trigger points found. Full, passive bilateral pectoral stretch followed by clearing strokes toward axillary lymph nodes.

Superficial effleurage to neck bilaterally, especially sternocleidomastoid, followed by deeper effleurage to soften hypertonic neck extensors and scalenes. Slow muscle stripping followed by compression to trigger point 3/4 inch superior to the costal attachment of right anterior scalene. Client reported reduction in pain from level 8 to 6. Full stretch to neck extensors and lateral flexors. Postisometric relaxation to right scalenes. No symptoms reproduced.

Deep effleurage and petrissage followed by clearing strokes to right arm. Nothing remarkable. Myofascial release to right forearm, especially at the medial epicondyle, around the wrist and in the palm. Applied muscle stripping to right forearm flexors. Trigger point found in flexor digitorum profundus. Two rounds of compression for 20 seconds alternating with muscle stripping reduced pain from level 8 to 5.

Cross-fiber strokes to flexor retinaculum. Kneading to retinaculum attachments followed by gentle stripping plus pin and stretch along the length of retinaculum. Deep petrissage to lumbricals and interossei muscles of the hand followed by a full, passive stretch of the wrist, including fingers and thumb. Postisometric relaxation to right wrist flexors. ROM in wrist extension increased slightly. Full, passive stretch with traction to right arm. No symptoms reproduced. Clearing strokes toward axillary lymph nodes.

Remainder of time focused on unaffected arm and posterior torso, ending with relaxing massage to the head and face.

Plan

Demonstrated forearm flexor stretches to client, with care to include the fingers and thumb. Recommended that client discuss with physician the possibility of wearing brace only when performing tasks that aggravate symptoms and at night to avoid prolonged flexion. Also suggested spending a minimum of 1 minute per hour moving the brace-free wrist in its full ROM by gently drawing the alphabet in the air within her tolerance. Scheduled 1-hour appointment 3 days from today, to be followed by reassessment. Depending on improvement, reschedule two times per week until client experiences four consecutive days without symptoms, and once per week following until client experiences longer periods symptom-free. Extensor strengthening exercises may be suggested following next appointment depending on improvement. Recommended drinking water following treatments to flush metabolites and keep the muscles hydrated.

CRITICAL THINKING EXERCISES

1. Activities of daily living, work-related postures, and repetitive motions may increase the risk of carpal tunnel syndrome. Choose a few such postures or activities and consider how they might also contribute to double crush or compression elsewhere that produces similar symptoms. For example, aside from the action at the wrist, what other postures or activities might contribute to numbness and tingling in the hand of a hair stylist?

2. Given evidence that noninvasive manual therapy is indicated for the treatment of carpal tunnel syndrome, discuss its benefits compared with more commonly prescribed treatments including surgery, medication, and immobilization. Are there side effects to medical treatments that can be avoided by treating with massage? What are some limitations of massage therapy in the treatment of carpal tunnel syndrome?

3. Discuss the possible course of treatment of a client who was diagnosed with carpal tunnel syndrome, had surgery to relieve compression of the median nerve, but has had a recurrence of symptoms. What may be some of the reasons that symptoms persist? How will you treat this client?

4. A client calls you the day after treatment and reports that her symptoms have increased. What are some possible reasons for the increase in symptoms? How might you proceed differently in the next treatment?

5. Conduct a short literature review to explain why the following conditions may put a client at greater risk for carpal tunnel syndrome:
   - Poor nutrition
   - Vitamin B deficiency
   - Obesity
   - Hypothyroid
   - Diabetes
   - Gout
   - Hormonal changes
   - Alcoholism

BIBLIOGRAPHY AND SUGGESTED READINGS

Biel A. *Trail Guide to the Body: How to Locate Muscles, Bones and More*, 3rd ed. Boulder, CO: Books of Discovery, 2005.

Bocchese ND, Becker J, Ehlers J, et al. What symptoms are truly caused by median nerve compression in carpal tunnel syndrome? Clinical Neurophysiology. 2005;116:275–283.

Burke J, Buchberger DJ, Carey-Loghmani T, et al. A pilot study comparing two manual therapy interventions for carpal tunnel syndrome. Journal of Manipulative and Physiological Therapeutics. 2007;30:50-61.

Centers for Disease Control and Prevention. Lyme Disease Diagnosis. Available at http://www.cdc.gov/ncidod/dvbid/lyme/ld_humandisease_diagnosis.htm. Accessed Spring 2008.

Clay JH, Pounds DM. *Basic Clinical Massage Therapy: Integrating Anatomy and Treatment*. Baltimore: Lippincott Williams & Wilkins, 2003.

Ettema AM, An K-N, Zhao C, et al. Flexor tendon and synovial gliding during simultaneous and single digit flexion in idiopathic carpal tunnel syndrome. Journal of Biomechanics. 2008;41:292–298.

Field T, Diego M, Cullen C, et al. Carpal tunnel syndrome symptoms are lessened following massage therapy. Journal of Bodywork and Movement Therapies. 2004;8:9–14.

Mayo Foundation for Medical Education and Research. Lupus. Available at http://www.mayoclinic.com/health/lupus/DS00115/DSECTION=6. Accessed Spring 2008.

Meek MF, Dellon AL. Modification of Phalen's wrist-flexion test. Journal of Neuroscience Methods. 2008;170:156–157.

Mell AG, Childress BL, Hughes RE. The effect of wearing a wrist splint on shoulder kinematics during object manipulation. Archives of Physical Medicine and Rehabilitation. 2005;86:1661–1664.

Moraska A, Chandler C, Edmiston-Schaetzel A, et al. Comparison of a targeted and general massage protocol on strength, function, and symptoms associated with carpal tunnel syndrome: A randomized pilot study. Journal of Alternative and Complementary Medicine. 2008;14:259–267.

Muscolino JE. *The Muscular System Manual: The Skeletal Muscles of the Human Body,* 2nd ed. St. Louis, MO: Elsevier Inc., 2005.

National Institute of Neurological Disorders and Stroke (NINDS). Carpal Tunnel Syndrome Fact Sheet. Available at http://www.ninds.nih.gov/disorders/carpal_tunnel/detail_carpal_tunnel.htm. Accessed Fall 2006.

Nidus Information Services, Inc. Carpal Tunnel Syndrome FAQ. Available at http://www.tifaq.com/articles/carpal_tunnel_syndrome-sep98-well-connected.html. Accessed Fall 2006.

Osar E. *Form & Function: The Anatomy of Motion*. Chicago: Evan Osar, 2001.

Rattray F, Ludwig L. *Clinical Massage Therapy: Understanding, Assessing and Treating over 70 Conditions*. Toronto: Talus Incorporated, 2000.

Staehler R, Cervical Herniated Disc Symptoms and Treatment Options. Available at http://www.spine-health.com/ Conditions/Herniated-Disc/Cervical-Herniated-Disc/Cervical-Herniated-Disc-Symptoms-And-Treatment-Options.html. Accessed Spring 2008.

Travell JG, Simons DG, Simons LS. *Myofascial Pain and Dysfunction: The Trigger Point Manual*, 2nd ed. Baltimore: Lippincott Williams & Wilkins, 1999.

Turchaninov R. *Medical Massage*, 2nd ed. Phoenix: Aesculapius Books, 2006.

U.S. National Library of Medicine and the National Institutes of Health. Gout. Available at http://www.nlm.nih.gov/medlineplus/ency/article/000424.htm#Symptoms. Accessed Winter 2009.

U.S. National Library of Medicine and the National Institutes of Health. Herniated Nucleus Pulposus (Slipped Disk). Available at http://www.nlm.nih.gov/medlineplus/ency/article/000442.htm. Accessed Spring 2008.

U.S. National Library of Medicine and the National Institutes of Health. Hypothyroidism. Available at http://www.nlm.nih.gov/medlineplus/ency/article/000353.htm. Accessed Spring 2008.

Werner R. *A Massage Therapist's Guide to Pathology*, 4th ed. Baltimore: Lippincott Williams & Wilkins, 2005.

Hyperlordosis

UNDERSTANDING HYPERLORDOSIS

A healthy spine has four natural curves (Fig. 8-1). The two lordotic curves—cervical and lumbar—arc anteriorly. The two kyphotic curves—thoracic and pelvic—arc posteriorly. These curves are ideal for our species to maintain balance, absorb the impact of movement, and to allow maximum flexibility for our particular types of activity.

Hyperlordosis is an increase in the natural lordotic curve. This chapter focuses on lumbar hyperlordosis: an increased lumbar lordotic curve most often accompanied by shortened hip flexors, anterior pelvic tilt, and shortened lumbar extensors with weakened hamstrings and abdominals (Fig. 8-2). With the hips flexed, such as when sitting, the hip flexors are shortened. If this is a person's common posture, held for hours at a time, day after day, the muscles may develop a high resting tone, making it difficult to lengthen the muscle fully when necessary. As the individual extends the hips, such as when standing from the seated posture, the shortened psoas draws the lumbar vertebrae to which it attaches anteriorly, increasing the lumbar curve, while the iliacus and rectus femoris pull on the pelvis and tilt it anteriorly. The anterior pelvic tilt lengthens and weakens the hamstrings because the distance between the ischium and tibia is increased. The abdominals, which primarily function to maintain posture, weaken and fatigue against the force of the shortened, hypertonic muscles and the associated postural dysfunction. The anterior pelvic tilt and increased lordotic curve decrease the distance between the iliac crests and the ribcage, shortening the lumbar extensors, which may also become hypertonic when they are recruited to maintain an erect posture because the abdominals are not fully able to do so.

In a very short period relative to our evolution, human lifestyle has changed from being highly physical—hunting and gathering, walking, performing manual labor, and so on—to becoming increasingly sedentary. We spend a lot of time driving, sitting, working at a computer, watching television, and so on. These static postures put many of the body's joints in flexion. The hips, knees, thorax, and shoulders are nearly immobile for hours at time. Because of this, hyperkyphosis and hyperlordosis have become two very common postural deviations that lead to chronic pain and limited ROM along the spine and in the shoulders and hips. Both of these postures may lead to other conditions, but you may find that normalizing the curves of the spine and leveling the ilia and scapulae will reduce this client's pain and restriction and may facilitate your treatment of accompanying conditions.

Functional vs. Structural Postural Imbalance

The hyperlordosis described above is functional. Its cause is primarily soft tissue changes and postural deviations that result from an injury to the low back, pelvis, or hip joint or, more commonly, from activities of daily living and poor posture. These deviations can be treated with manual therapy,

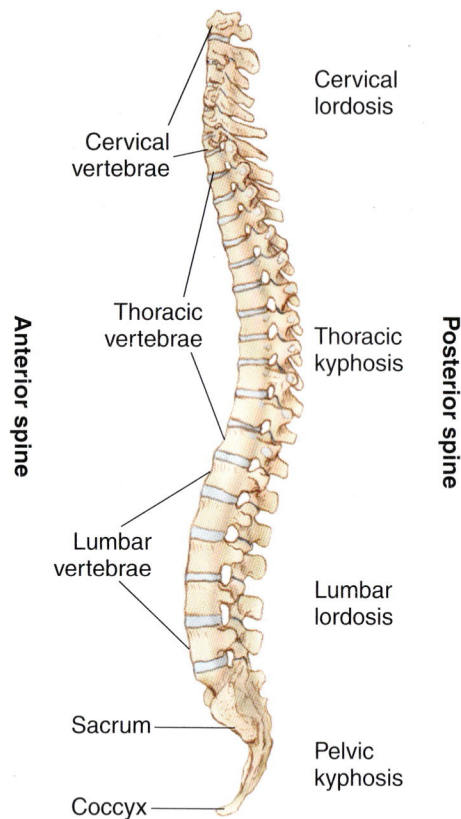

Figure 8-1 **Curves of the spine.** The cervical and lumbar lordotic curves arc anteriorly. The thoracic and pelvic kyphotic curves arc posteriorly.

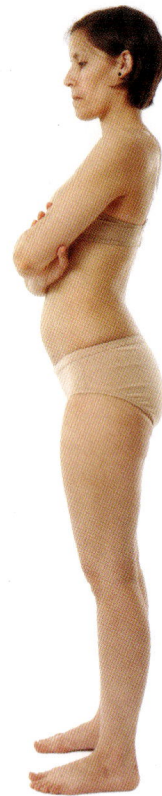

Figure 8-2 **Hyperlordosis.** Hyperlordosis involves an increased lordotic curve most often accompanied by shortened hip flexors, anterior pelvic tilt, and shortened lumbar extensors with weakened hamstrings and abdominals.

self-care, and postural awareness. The therapeutic goal for a client with functional hyperlordosis is to lengthen the muscles that have shortened and become hypertonic and that are pulling the bones out of alignment; to strengthen the muscles that have stretched and become weak; and to reset the neuromuscular system to recognize proper posture and diaphragmatic breathing as normal.

A structural hyperlordotic curve, in contrast, is primarily caused by changes in bones and joints. Bone fusions, bony prominences, bone spurs, fractured bones that were not properly set, osteoporosis, and degenerative disc disease are a few contributing factors. Manual therapy may offer this client pain relief, small increases in ROM, and may slow the progression of postural imbalance but is unlikely to reverse the dysfunction. When hyperlordosis is structural in nature, it is best to discuss the client's condition with his or her health care provider to fully understand the causes. You may need to modify positioning, bolstering, length of treatment, and techniques to accommodate the client's particular needs. In some cases, massage may be contraindicated.

Muscles of the Lower Cross

Lumbar hyperlordosis is also called lower cross syndrome. Coined by Vladimir Janda, MD, DSc, lower cross syndrome refers to an imbalance and dysfunction of the agonists and antagonists that move and support the pelvis (Fig. 8-3). You may find the iliopsoas, rectus femoris, tensor fasciae latae, the lumbar erector spinae, and quadratus lumborum to be short and hypertonic, while the abdominals, gluteus maximus, and hamstrings are stretched and weak. The weakened muscles become less able to oppose the actions of the agonists that function in hip flexion and lumbar extension. As this happens, the imbalance can become more profound and the body less able to reverse the process without intervention (Table 8-1).

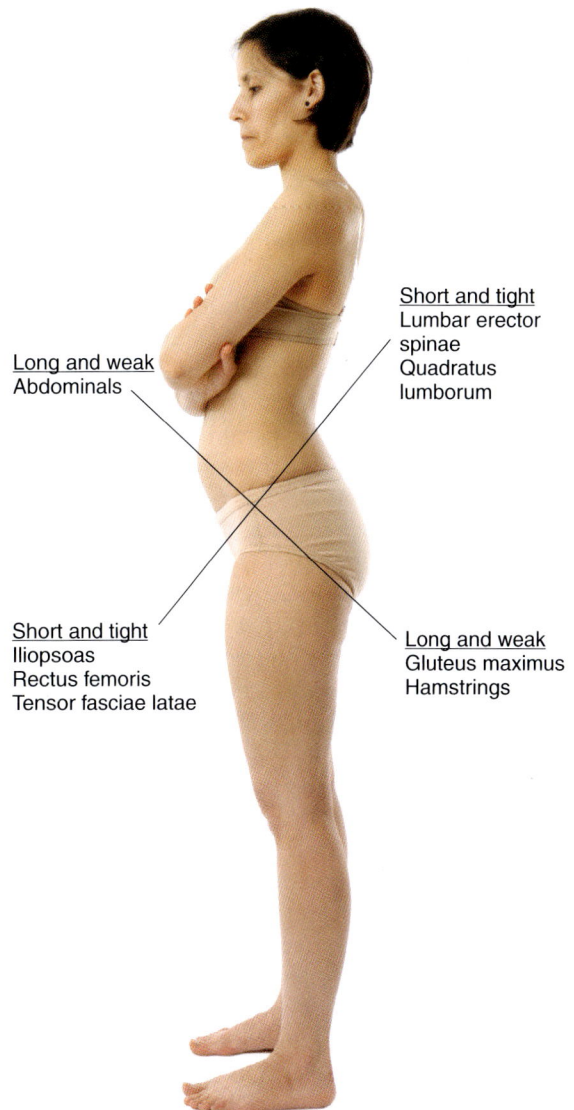

Short and tight
Lumbar erector
spinae
Quadratus
lumborum

Long and weak
Abdominals

Short and tight
Iliopsoas
Rectus femoris
Tensor fasciae latae

Long and weak
Gluteus maximus
Hamstrings

Figure 8-3 **Muscles of the lower cross.** Notice the relationship between the muscles that are short and tight and those that are long and weak.

Table 8-1	Muscles of the Lower Cross with Actions That Contribute to Hyperlordosis
Muscles That are Short and Tight (with Agonist Action)	**Muscles that are Stretched and Weak (with Antagonist Opposition)**
Psoas (hip flexion, increased lumbar curve)	Gluteus maximus (hip flexion)
Iliacus (hip flexion, anterior pelvic tilt)	Hamstrings (hip flexion, anterior pelvic tilt)
Rectus femoris (hip flexion, anterior pelvic tilt)	
Tensor fasciae latae (hip flexion, anterior pelvic tilt)	
Latissimus dorsi (anterior pelvic tilt)	
Quadratus lumborum (lumbar spine extension)	Rectus abdominus (lumbar spine extension)
Lumbar erector spinae (lumbar spine extension)	External abdominal obliques (lumbar spine extension)
	Internal abdominal obliques (lumbar spine extension)

Common Signs and Symptoms

The most common symptom of developing lumbar hyperlordosis is low back pain. The short, hypertonic psoas pulls the lumbar vertebrae anteriorly, increasing the lumbar curve, while the short, tight iliacus tilts the pelvis anteriorly. This stress on the spine and pelvis can reduce the mobility of the vertebrae, sacroiliac joint, and hips. As the muscles of the lower cross shorten or lengthen around these postural deviations, they become less able to perform their actions fluidly. Shortened muscles may not lengthen fully, and weakened muscles may not be able to oppose the actions of the shortened muscles. For example, weak abdominals may not be strong enough to maintain an erect posture when seated or standing, leaving the posterior lumbar muscles to work harder. When standing, lengthened or weakened hamstrings have difficulty opposing the action of the rectus femoris and iliopsoas, which flex the hips and tilt the pelvis anteriorly. The combination of hypertonicity and weakness through the lower cross results in pain when the client needs to recruit these muscles to perform activities or maintain a stable, erect posture.

As the condition progresses, other patterns may develop. The hip adductors may become hypertonic as a result of the increased activity needed to maintain posture or oppose the lateral rotation of the hips. With lateral rotation of the hips, the piriformis shortens and may become hypertonic while the iliotibial band distorts and creates torsional force throughout the thigh. The sacroiliac joint may become hypomobile, and facet joints may become irritated, putting a client who frequently bends and stands at greater risk for a herniated lumbar disc. As the body adjusts to a new center of gravity, the arch of the foot may flatten as the weight of the body is shifted to the ball of the foot. Hip or leg pain may also be present, particularly if another condition such as piriformis syndrome, patellofemoral syndrome, or plantar fasciitis is present (see Chapters 9, 10, and 11). If nerves become compressed by tight muscles or impinged between bones that have deviated from their natural alignment, numbness and tingling may also occur in the lower extremity. Compression of the vasculature or lymph nodes can lead to edema in the lower extremity.

The fascia across the anterior hip and the thoracolumbar fascia may be restricted. During palpation, you may find tenderness in the rectus femoris, particularly near the superior attachment, in the iliacus at the iliac fossa, and in the psoas deep in the abdomen. Tenderness may also be felt along the iliac crests, at the sacroiliac joint, over the sacrum, and around the greater trochanter. When extension of the lumbar spine contributes to hyperlordosis, the area between the lower ribs and iliac crests may be affected. The deep lateral rotators of the hips are likely to be tender if the hips are laterally rotated.

Whether a contributing factor to hyperlordosis or a result of it, compensatory hyperkyphosis may cause any or all of the pain patterns that are common in clients with an increased kyphotic curve, such as internally rotated shoulders and the head-forward posture (see Chapter 4).

Possible Causes and Contributing Factors

Low back pain may be a symptom of a more serious condition such as cancer, kidney stones, infection in the urinary system, endometriosis, spinal stenosis, or infection in the vertebrae. Refer to Table 8-2, and consult your pathology book to identify the client's signs and symptoms, and refer the client to a health care provider for medical assessment if you suspect a more serious condition.

Pathologies that affect the integrity of bones often cause structural hyperlordosis. Porous bones (osteoporosis) become unable to bear weight and may cause the lumbar vertebrae, pelvis, and femur to collapse upon each other, resulting in increased curvature. Herniated discs in the lumbar spine not only cause low back pain but may also cause compensating structures to become stressed and the vertebrae to collapse upon each other, altering the curve of the spine. Scoliosis—a lateral curve in the spine—increases stress on the spine and the structures involved in moving the spine. Spondylolisthesis—a condition in which a vertebra slips forward relative to other vertebrae—may also cause hyperlordosis. This happens most often at L4-5 or L5-S1.

Table 8-2	Differentiating Conditions Commonly Confused with or Contributing to Hyperlordosis

Condition	Typical Signs and Symptoms	Testing	Massage Therapy
Osteoporosis	Bone and joint pain, bone fractures, loss of height, slouching	Bone mineral density test CT X-ray Urinary calcium test	Massage is indicated in the early stages and with the approval of a health care provider in the later stages; may reduce pain. Take care not to use force that may fracture a bone.
Spondylolisthesis	Begins in the lumbar spine and may proceed to the thoracic spine Lumbar hyperlordosis Pain in low back, buttocks, and thighs Stiff back	X-ray Straight leg raise test	Massage is indicated. Stretching and strengthening are encouraged.
Ankylosing spondylitis	Pain often begins in the low back unilaterally and progresses bilaterally to the upper back and throughout the thorax Fatigue and anemia may develop	MRI Blood tests	Massage is indicated to reduce pain, maintain mobility, and slow progress of spinal distortion.
Achondroplasia	Dwarfism Low back pain Abnormal body proportions Bowed legs Decreased muscle tone Prominent forehead Short arms or legs Hyperkyphosis Hyperlordosis	Prenatal ultrasound and amniocentesis Genetic testing X-ray of long bones	Massage is indicated unless an underlying condition such as increased fluid in the brain or spinal stenosis is present.
Urinary and kidney pathologies	Back and flank pain Pain or burning during urination Frequent urge to urinate Fever Pressure in lower abdomen Cloudy, bloody, or foul smelling urine Nausea	Urinalysis or urine culture Ultrasound MRI	Massage is contraindicated until the condition is resolved. Avoid percussive strokes to the back of clients with a history of kidney stones.
Bone cancer	Pain, frequently in the long bones Weak bones easily fractured Swollen, tender joints Fatigue Fever Weight loss Anemia	X-ray CT scan Ultrasound MRI Bone scan Tissue biopsy	Massage may be supportive during treatment and recovery. Work with the health care provider to plan treatment that is best for the individual. A client with bone cancer is susceptible to fractures; take precautions to avoid this risk.

(continued)

| Table 8-2 | Differentiating Conditions Commonly Confused with or Contributing to Hyperlordosis (Continued) | | |

Condition	Typical Signs and Symptoms	Testing	Massage Therapy
Prostate cancer	Urinary problems Blood in urine or semen Swelling in the legs Pelvic pain Bone pain or fractures Compression of the spine	Prostate-specific antigen test Digital rectal exam Ultrasound Biopsy	Massage may be supportive during treatment and recovery. Work with the health care provider to plan treatment that is best for the individual.
Cervical/uterine cancer	Unusual vaginal discharge or bleeding Pelvic/abdominal pain Abdominal mass Pain during intercourse	Pap test HPV exam Ultrasound Cervical/uterine exam Biopsy	Massage may be supportive during treatment and recovery. Work with the health care provider to plan treatment that is best for the individual.
Osteomyelitis	Unrelenting back pain Fever, chills, nausea Swelling and redness Stiffness or pain Weakness, numbness, and tingling in the extremities Drainage at the wound site	X-ray CT scan MRI Blood test Culture to determine bacterial or fungal infection	Massage is contraindicated until infection is resolved and the health care provider approves the massage.
Herniated lumbar disc	Muscle spasm Weakness or atrophy Low back pain Pain in buttocks, legs, and feet, which worsens when coughing, laughing, or straining Numbness and tingling in the legs and feet	Physical exam including muscle reflexes and strength Straight leg raise test X-ray CT MRI EMG Myelogram	Massage is indicated with caution. Work with the health care team.
Nerve root compression	Muscle spasm, weakness, or atrophy Pain radiates to the extremities	Kemp's test Valsalva maneuver Neurological exam to test reflexes, sensation, and strength	Massage is indicated if cause and location are understood. Take care not to increase compression or reproduce symptoms.

Spondylolisthesis can be congenital or may develop from a degenerative disorder such as arthritis, from stress fractures, or from bone disease. Achondroplasia—a genetic disorder that slows the growth of bones—causes a variety of abnormalities affecting the length and shape of bones, particularly in the spine and extremities. Ankylosing spondylitis—an autoimmune disease that causes arthritis or swelling in the spine—may ultimately cause the bones to fuse, limiting the spine's mobility. Nutritional deficiencies of calcium and vitamin D as well as increased consumption of calcium oxalate and carbonated beverages may affect the body's ability to rebuild bone.

In some cases, contributing factors can lead to both structural and functional hyperkyphosis. In these cases, it is important to understand the level of stress to the bones before applying manual therapy to the muscles in order to avoid injury. Age may play a role in developing hyperlordosis because the bones become weaker and activity that keeps the joints mobile decreases with age. A sedentary lifestyle and lack of physical fitness reduce functionality and can lead to pain and dysfunction. Weight gain, particularly when it occurs in the span of a few months or a year, rapidly shifts the center of gravity and increases demands on the musculoskeletal system. The increased size and weight of the abdomen increases the load that the spine must support and may pull the lumbar spine anteriorly, increasing the lordotic curve. Pregnancy may contribute to this pattern, which often resolves itself after delivery. Previous injury or surgery around the low back, pelvis, legs, and abdomen may contribute to hyperlordosis. Injuries that were not properly treated to restore mobility and musculoskeletal function can initiate patterns of compensation that put stress on the muscles and bones. Surgery that produces scar tissue can affect the functionality of fascia and muscle by reducing contractile strength or the ability of those tissues to lengthen sufficiently.

The primary contributing factors in most cases of functional lumbar hyperlordosis, however, are poor posture and repeated activities of daily living. Prolonged standing and prolonged sitting as well as repeated resisted activities that involve bending, twisting, and lifting can cause dysfunction in the muscles of the lower cross and misalignment of the joints that they cross. For example, as mentioned above, when a client sits for long periods, the hip flexors may become shortened as the origins and insertions rest closer to each other while the erector spinae may fatigue from long-term, involuntary contraction in an attempt to keep the posture erect. This is particularly true when the client's abdominal muscles are too weak to contribute to maintaining proper posture. When the client stands, the shortened hip flexors keep the joint from fully extending, and this can leave the hips in varying degrees of flexion. The tight rectus femoris and iliacus pull on the pelvis, causing an anterior pelvic tilt. Without adjusting the posture of the spine, the client's eyes would be facing down. Because hip extension is restricted by the tight hip flexors, the lumbar spine extends without bringing the ilia and sacrum with it, which increases the lordotic curve, shortening the quadratus lumborum and the lumbar erectors.

Try it yourself: Slowly stand up from the seated position without fully extending your hips. Try to stand straight and look ahead. Feel your pelvis stabilized in an anterior tilt while your lumbar spine curves to compensate. You may also notice your knees locking into extension, and the adductors and the gluteal muscles contracting to maintain your center of gravity. When this becomes a common posture, the lumbar spine curves anteriorly. Moreover, when a client regularly holds this posture, the cervical spine must extend to allow the person to look forward, which can lead to hyperkyphosis if it is not already present.

When a person stands for long periods with weight on one leg, the hip on that side is often elevated, causing the sacrum to rotate and tilt. This may cause the sacroiliac joint to become less mobile. Postures that increase lateral rotation or adduction of the hip, as are common with dancers, may increase the risk of hyperlordosis. Wearing high heels displaces the center of gravity and encourages anterior pelvic tilt, increasing lordosis.

Table 8-2 lists conditions commonly confused with or contributing to hyperlordosis.

Contraindications and Special Considerations

- **Underlying pathologies.** Spondylolisthesis, osteoarthritis, osteoporosis, degenerative disc disease, bone spurs, or fusions may be present. If you suspect one of these (consult Table 8-2 and your pathology book for signs and symptoms), refer the client to a health care provider for medical assessment before initiating treatment. If the client is diagnosed with an underlying pathology that is not contraindicated for massage, work with the health care provider to develop a treatment plan that is appropriate for that individual.
- **Endangerment sites.** Be cautious near endangerment sites in the abdomen and femoral area. Gently palpate for the pulse of the abdominal aorta and the femoral artery before you begin working there. If you feel a pulse while working, back off slowly and reposition your stroke to avoid the endangerment site.
- **Menstruation.** Treating iliopsoas when a woman is premenstrual or menstruating may be uncomfortable. Offer to reschedule or to work all other structures, explaining that

lengthening the iliopsoas is an integral part of treatment for hyperlordosis and may require followup after menstruation has ended. If you are unable to massage the iliopsoas, stretching the hip flexors by passively extending the hip is a good alternative.

- **Treatment duration and pressure.** If the client is elderly, has degenerative bone disease, or has a condition that diminishes activities of daily living, you may need to adjust your pressure as well as the treatment duration. Frequent half-hour sessions may suit the client better than prolonged treatment with long intervals.
- **Positioning.** Use bolsters to position a client for comfort as well as to reduce postures that may contribute to hyperlordosis. In the supine position, a bolster under the knees will keep the hip flexors from fully lengthening and may reduce lordosis and pressure on the lumbar spine. In the prone position, a bolster under the anterior superior iliac spines may reduce anterior pelvic tilt, and a bolster under the ankles may reduce stress on the low back.
- **Friction.** Do not use deep frictions if the client has a systemic inflammatory condition such as rheumatoid arthritis or osteoarthritis, if the health of the underlying tissues is compromised, or if the client is taking anti-inflammatory medication. Friction creates an inflammatory process, which may interfere with the intended action of anti-inflammatory medication. Recommend that your client refrain from taking such medication for several hours before treatment if his or her health care provider agrees.
- **Tissue length.** It is important when treating myofascial tissues that you do not lengthen those that are already stretched. Assess for myofascial restrictions first and treat only those that are clearly present. Likewise, overstretched muscles should not be stretched from origin to insertion. For example, because the abdominals and hamstrings tend to be overstretched, it is not advisable to perform myofascial release or a full stretch from origin to insertion on these muscle groups. If you treat trigger points in overstretched tissue, use heat or a localized pin and stretch technique instead of full ROM stretches.
- **Hypermobile joints and unstable ligaments.** Be cautious with mobilizations if the client has hypermobile joints or if ligaments are unstable due to injury, pregnancy or a systemic condition.

Massage Therapy Research

A thorough literature review found no research, case studies, or articles about the specific benefits of massage therapy for the treatment of hyperlordosis, lordosis, or lower cross syndrome. Much of the literature about the use of manual therapies to treat hyperlordosis comes from other disciplines, primarily physical therapy. Closer examination is needed on the benefits of massage therapy to lengthen shortened and hypertonic tissues along with self-care to strengthen lengthened, weak muscles.

Several articles, however, confirm the benefit of massage therapy for low back pain—the most common symptom of hyperlordosis. In 2001, Hernandez-Reif et al. published a study titled "Lower Back Pain Is Reduced and Range of Motion Increased After Massage Therapy." In 2008, Jada Bell described a case study titled "Massage Therapy Helps to Increase Range of Motion, Decrease Pain and Assist in Healing a Client with Low Back Pain and Sciatica Symptoms." These studies are important because of the attention paid to hip flexion and to general areas or specific muscles known to contribute to hyperlordosis. Neither study mentions anterior pelvic tilt, and both also treated muscles that are not directly associated with hyperlordosis.

Hernandez-Reif et al. studied 24 participants who reported low back pain for at least 6 months prior, sought medical attention for the pain, and were cleared by their primary care providers to participate in the study. All participants were free of underlying conditions that can contribute to low back pain. The massage therapy group received 30-minute treatments twice per week for 10 weeks. The relaxation group (control group) was instructed to perform exercises for large muscle groups throughout the body. At the end of the study, the massage group reported less pain, less depression and anxiety, improved sleep, and improved ROM compared to the control group. Serotonin and dopamine levels, which are often depleted in patients with chronic pain, anxiety, and depression, increased in the massage group.

Bell's case study involved a 58-year-old client presenting with a 9-month history of low back pain that radiated into the lower extremity. MRI revealed spondylosis and a herniated disc that caused no nerve root impingement. The client occasionally used nonsteroidal anti-inflammatory medication, muscle relaxants, and narcotic analgesics and was receiving chiropractic care as well as physical therapy. The 45-minute treatments were administered once per week for 6 weeks following a 4-week period during which base line measures were recorded. During the treatment period, activities of daily living and ROM improved and pain was reduced. A significant limitation of this study was the use of physical therapy in addition to massage. Although the client's symptoms improved to a larger extent during the massage treatment period than the physical therapy period, it is impossible to determine whether massage alone or the combination of therapies produced these benefits.

In 2000, Michele Preyde published a study titled "Effectiveness of Massage Therapy for Subacute Low-back Pain: A Randomized Controlled Trial." The study tested 98 subjects between the ages of 18 and 81 with low back pain for 1–8 months prior to the study and no other significant pathology. The subjects were randomly assigned to one of four groups: comprehensive massage therapy (soft-tissue manipulation, remedial exercise, and posture education), soft-tissue manipulation only, remedial exercise with posture education only, or a placebo of sham laser treatment. Participants received six treatments over the course of approximately 1 month. Participants in the comprehensive group received 30–35 minutes of soft tissue manipulation and were taught stretching exercises for the trunk, hips, and thighs. Those in the soft tissue manipulation group received the same soft tissue manipulation as those in the comprehensive group but no remedial exercise, and those in the remedial exercise group performed the same exercises as those in the comprehensive group but received no soft tissue manipulation. Those in the control group received only sham infrared laser treatment. Intensity of pain, quality of pain, and function measures were recorded after each treatment, after 1 month of treatment, and again 1 month after treatment ended. The comprehensive group showed significant improvement in function, pain intensity, and pain quality compared to the other groups. The comprehensive and the soft tissue manipulation groups showed clinically significant improvement in function. At the 1 month follow-up, no pain was reported by 63% of the comprehensive group, 27% of the soft tissue manipulation group, 14% of the remedial exercise group, and 0% of the control group. The authors conclude that massage therapy is beneficial for clients with low back pain. The study does not describe which soft tissues were treated, stating only that "The exact soft tissue that the subject described as the source of pain was located and treated with the specific technique indicated for the specific condition of the soft tissue." Although hip flexion and extension were included in the remedial exercises, and these ROMs are relevant in assessing for hyperlordosis, further research is needed to determine the extent to which massage improves hyperlordosis specifically.

Several literature reviews also explore the benefits of massage for low back pain or compare the benefits of massage to other complementary and alternative therapies. In 2003, Cherkin et al. published a review titled "A Review of the Evidence for the Effectiveness, Safety, and Cost of Acupuncture, Massage Therapy, and Spinal Manipulation for Back Pain." They concluded that massage has been found to be effective for persistent back pain, that spinal manipulation has minimal clinical benefits, and that the effectiveness of acupuncture is unclear. In addition, the review concludes that only massage is cost effective. In 2008, Imamura et al. published a review titled "Evidence-Informed Management of Chronic Low Back Pain with Massage," which concludes that there is strong evidence suggesting massage has long-lasting benefits for nonspecific chronic low back pain and may be cost-effective by way of reducing visits to health care providers. The review also reports that further research into the specific mechanism of improvement with massage therapy is needed.

WORKING WITH THE CLIENT

Client Assessment

Hyperlordosis is a common postural deviation causing chronic pain and restricted ROM in the low back and hips. It involves many joints and all of the muscles that cross them. A wide variety of possible factors can contribute to the development of hyperlordosis. All of these elements add up

Table 8-3	Health History

Questions for the Client	Importance for the Treatment Plan
Where do you feel symptoms?	The location of symptoms gives clues to the location of trigger points, injury, or other contributing factors.
Describe what your symptoms feel like.	Differentiate between the possible origins of symptoms and determine the involvement of muscles, joints, nerves, blood vessels, or viscera. See Chapter 1 for a more detailed description of symptoms and possible origins.
Do any movements make symptoms worse or better?	Locate tension, weakness, or compression in structures producing such movements.
Have you seen a health care provider for this condition? What was the diagnosis? What tests were performed?	Bone density tests, blood tests, and other tests may indicate contributing factors.
Have you been diagnosed with a condition such as osteoporosis, rheumatoid arthritis, or osteoarthritis?	Systemic conditions may contribute to signs and symptoms, may require adjustments to treatment, and may impact treatment outcomes.
Have you had an injury or surgery, or did your symptoms begin during a pregnancy?	Injury or surgery and resulting scar tissue may cause adhesions, hyper- or hypotonicity, and atypical ROM. Changes in the center of gravity during pregnancy or other rapid weight gain may be a contributing factor.
What type of work, hobbies, or other regular activities do you do?	Repetitive motions and static postures that increase flexion of the hips or anterior pelvic tilt may contribute to the client's condition.
Are you taking any prescribed medication or herbal or other supplements?	Medication of all types may contribute to symptoms or involve contraindications or cautions.
Have you had a cortisone shot in the past 2 weeks? Where?	Local massage is contraindicated.
Have you taken a pain reliever or muscle relaxant within the past 4 hours?	The client may not be able to judge your pressure.
Have you taken anti-inflammatory medication within the past 4 hours?	Deep friction initiates an inflammatory process and should not be performed if the client has recently taken anti-inflammatory medication.

to many variations in how a client may present to you. For example, a client with increased lumbar curve and anterior pelvic tilt who often stands with more weight on one leg may present with lateral flexion of the thorax, an elevated iliac crest, sacroiliac joint immobility, and rotation in the hips or spine affecting the abdominal obliques, latissimus dorsi, multifidi and rotatores, and ligaments connecting the sacrum, pelvis, and spine. What follows are common presentations for hyperlordosis. However, it is essential to assess every joint to form an accurate picture for each individual client.

Assessment begins at your first contact with a client. In some cases, this may be on the telephone when an appointment is requested. Ask in advance if the client is seeking treatment for a specific area of pain so that you can prepare yourself.

Table 8-3 lists questions to ask the client when taking a health history.

POSTURAL ASSESSMENT

Allow the client to enter the room ahead of you while you assess his or her posture and movements before he or she is aware that the assessment has begun. Look for imbalances or patterns of compensation for deviations common with hyperlordosis. Watch the client walk and look for reduced mobility in the hips or whether the client appears to be favoring one side. Have the client sit to fill out the assessment form, and watch to see if he or she lowers into the chair cautiously or shifts around to find a comfortable position. Watch also as the client stands up to see if he or she is able to extend the hips fully and if standing from a seated position causes him or her to use the arms to lift themselves or to lean on a stable surface. When assessing the standing posture, be sure that the client is standing comfortably. If the client is asked to stand in the anatomic position, you will not get an accurate assessment of his or her posture in daily life. Look for anterior pelvic tilt, increased curve in the lumbar spine, hip flexion, rotation of the hips, hyperextended knees, and pronation or supination of the ankles.

Figure 8-4 compares healthy posture to a posture affected by hyperlordosis.

ROM ASSESSMENT

Test the ROM of the hips and lumbar spine as both agonists and antagonists. If hyperlordosis is structural in nature, do not perform ROM tests that move the affected joints into ranges that are inhibited by the altered joint structure or that may cause further damage. Since it allows the client to control the amount of movement and stay within a pain-free range, only active ROM should be used in the acute stage of an injury to prevent undue pain or re-injury. Box 8-1 presents the average active ROM results for the joints involved in hyperlordosis.

Active ROM

Compare your assessment of the client's active ROM to the values in Box 8-1. Pain and other symptoms may not be reproduced during active ROM assessment, because the client may limit movement to a symptom-free range.

- **Active posterior pelvic tilt,** particularly when the hip flexors are lengthened as when standing, may be restricted and cause pain.
- **Active extension of the hip** may be reduced when muscle tension, adhesions, and trigger points shorten hip flexors or weaken hip extensors. The client may resist full active extension of the hip if this produces symptoms during activities of daily living.
- **Active medial rotation** of the hip may be reduced or cause pain when shortened or hypertonic muscles hold the hip in lateral rotation.

Passive ROM

Compare the client's P ROM on one side to the other when applicable. Note and compare the end feel for each range (see Chapter 1 for an explanation of end feel).

- **Passive extension of the hips** may be restricted when the hip flexors are shortened or hypertonic.
- **Passive medial rotation of the hips** may be restricted when lateral rotators such as the iliopsoas are short and hypertonic, which could occur if lateral rotation of the hips becomes a compensating pattern.

Resisted ROM

Use resisted tests to assess the strength of the muscles that cross the joints involved. Compare the strength of the affected side to the unaffected side.

- **Resisted extension of the hip** may cause pain in the low back when the hip flexors are short and hypertonic and the hip extensors are weak. The client may rotate the pelvis to compensate.
- **Resisted flexion of the thorax** may be reduced when the abdominals are weak and stretched. This test is best performed with the hips and knees flexed to reduce the contraction of the hip flexors.

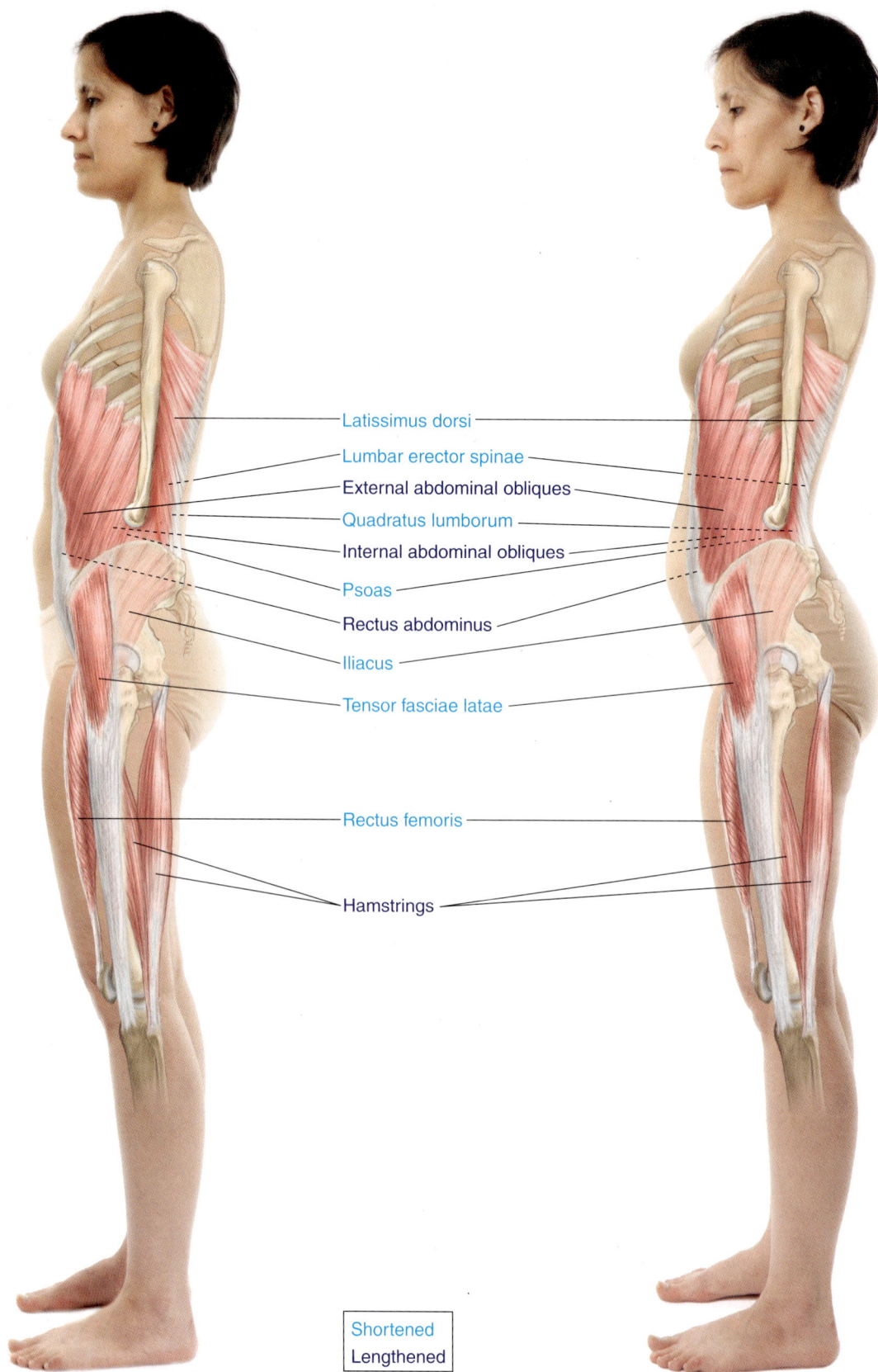

Latissimus dorsi

Lumbar erector spinae

External abdominal obliques

Quadratus lumborum

Internal abdominal obliques

Psoas

Rectus abdominus

Iliacus

Tensor fasciae latae

Rectus femoris

Hamstrings

Shortened
Lengthened

Figure 8-4 **Postural assessment comparison.** Compare the anatomical postures on the left to the hyperlordotic postures on the right. Note how the muscles of the lower cross contribute to the increased lordotic curve and anterior pelvic tilt.

Box 8-1   AVERAGE ACTIVE ROM FOR JOINTS INVOLVED IN HYPERLORDOSIS

Trunk (at Lumbar Spine)

Flexion 50–60°
Rectus abdominis
External oblique (bilateral)
Internal oblique (bilateral)

Extension 25°
Spinalis (bilateral)
Longissimus (bilateral)
Iliocostalis (bilateral)
Multifidi (bilateral)
Rotatores (bilateral)
Quadratus lumborum (bilateral)
Latissimus dorsi (with arm fixed)

Lateral Flexion 25°
Spinalis (unilateral)
Longissimus (unilateral)
Iliocostalis (unilateral)
External oblique (unilateral)
Internal oblique (unilateral)
Quadratus lumborum (unilateral)
Latissimus dorsi (unilateral)

Ipsilateral Rotation 20°
Internal oblique (unilateral)

Contralateral Rotation 20°
External oblique (unilateral)
Multifidi (unilateral)
Rotatores (unilateral)

Pelvis

Anterior Tilt (downward rotation)
(Angle from PSIS to ASIS) 0–10°
Rectus femoris
Iliacus
Sartorius
Tensor fasciae latae

Posterior Tilt (upward rotation)
(Angle from PSIS to ASIS)
0–10°
Biceps femoris
Semitendinosus
Semimembranosus

Lateral tilt (elevation) 0°
Latissimus dorsi (unilateral)
Quadratus lumborum (unilateral)

Hip

Flexion 110–120°
Rectus femoris
Tensor fasciae latae
Sartorius
Psoas major
Iliacus
Gluteus minimus
Gluteus medius (anterior fibers)
Adductor magnus (anterior fibers)
Adductor longus
Adductor brevis
Pectineus
Gracilis

Extension 10–15°
Gluteus maximus
Biceps femoris
Semitendinosus
Semimembranosus
Gluteus medius (posterior fibers)
Gluteus minimus (posterior fibers)
Adductor magnus (posterior fibers)

Lateral Rotation 40–60°
Gluteus maximus
Gluteus medius (posterior fibers)
Gluteus minimus (posterior fibers)
Piriformis
Quadratus femoris
Obturator internus
Obturator externus
Gemellus superior
Gemellus inferior
Sartorius
Biceps femoris (long head)
Psoas major
Iliacus

Medial Rotation 30–40°
Gluteus medius (anterior fibers)
Gluteus minimus (anterior fibers)
Semitendinosus
Semimembranosus
Tensor fasciae latae
Gracilis

Abduction 30–50°
Gluteus medius
Gluteus minimus
Tensor fasciae latae
Sartorius
Gluteus maximus
Piriformis (with flexed hip)

Adduction 30°
Adductor magnus
Adductor longus
Adductor brevis
Pectineus
Gracilis
Gluteus maximus (low fibers)
Psoas major
Iliacus

Knee

Flexion 120–150°
Biceps femoris
Semitendinosus
Semimembranosus
Gracilis
Sartorius
Gastrocnemius
Popliteus
Plantaris

Extension 0–15°
Rectus femoris
Vastus lateralis
Vastus medialis
Vastus intermedius

Medial Rotation (When
Flexed) 20–30°
Semitendinosus
Semimembranosus
Gracilis
Sartorius
Popliteus

Lateral Rotation (When
Flexed) 30–40°
Biceps femoris

SPECIAL TESTS

The following special tests can help you to determine which muscles are contributing to pain and when a client should be evaluated by a medical professional using X-ray or other tools, which may reveal conditions that are contraindications for massage or require special considerations when planning treatment with massage.

The **Valsalva maneuver** may reveal a herniated disc, tumor, or other factor that increases pressure on the spinal cord. This test is used when the client complains of pain in a localized area along the spine, particularly when coughing or sneezing. A herniated disc does not contraindicate massage, but this test is not specific for the cause of increased pressure. For this reason, it is best to refer the client to a health care provider for further testing before performing the massage. To avoid even a temporary reduction in circulation, do not perform this test if the client has tested positive for vertebral artery insufficiency or has a cardiovascular disorder.

1. With the client seated and facing you, ask him or her to take a deep breath and then attempt to forcefully exhale against the closed throat (such as when forcing a bowel movement).
2. The test is positive if the client feels pain in a localized spot along the spine.

Kemp's test may reveal a disc lesion or irritation of the facet joint in the lumbar spine. Neither of these contraindicates massage, but it is best to understand the extent of damage and to be sure that these are not signs of something more serious before performing any deep tissue treatments.

1. With the client standing, ask him or her to slowly extend, laterally flex, and rotate the spine to the affected side as if reaching for the heel (Fig. 8-5). This action increases stress on the nerve root and facet joints.
2. The test is positive for nerve root irritation if the client feels radiating pain or numbness and tingling in the affected leg. Ask the client to describe the area of symptoms to help you determine which nerve root is affected.
3. The test is positive for facet joint irritation if pain is localized along the lumbar vertebrae. Very localized symptoms may help you to determine which vertebrae are affected.

The **Stork test** is intended to assess sacroiliac joint mobility.

1. The client should be standing near a stable surface or wall that he or she can lean on to maintain balance during the test.
2. Begin on the side you suspect is dysfunctional, and then compare the results of both sides.
3. Kneel or sit behind the standing client with one thumb on the posterior superior iliac spine of the affected side and the other thumb on the sacrum at the same level.
4. Instruct the client to flex the hip and knee on the affected side within his or her comfort range. Notice the relative movement of your thumbs while the client flexes the hip (Fig. 8-6).
5. When the sacroiliac joint is normally mobile, the ilium should rotate posteriorly, moving the thumb on the posterior superior iliac spine inferior. The test is positive for decreased sacroiliac joint mobility if the thumb on the posterior superior iliac spine moves superiorly while the client flexes the hip.

The **Thomas test** is intended to assess the client for shortened hip flexors. This test may not be comfortable for clients with severe low back pain.

1. Instruct the client to sit at the edge of the massage table so that the legs can hang freely, then assist the client to lie back.
2. Ask the client to flex one hip by bringing the knee toward the chest (Fig. 8-7). The unflexed hip is the one being tested. If you suspect that one side is primarily responsible for symptoms, instruct the client to flex the unaffected hip first.
3. If the hip flexors are shortened, the straight leg (the affected side) will come off the table, unable to extend fully because the hip flexors are unable to lengthen fully. If the rectus femoris is short and cannot lengthen fully, the knee of the affected leg will be slightly extended. These results indicate a positive test.
4. To assess the degree of the increased lumbar curve and anterior pelvic tilt caused by tight hip flexors, try to slip your hand under the lumbar curve. If your hand moves in easily, this is a sign that the extension of the hips increases the lumbar curve and anterior pelvic tilt because the hip flexors cannot lengthen fully.
5. Repeat the test on the unaffected side for comparison. Although the client may feel symptoms only on one side, these muscles may be short on both.

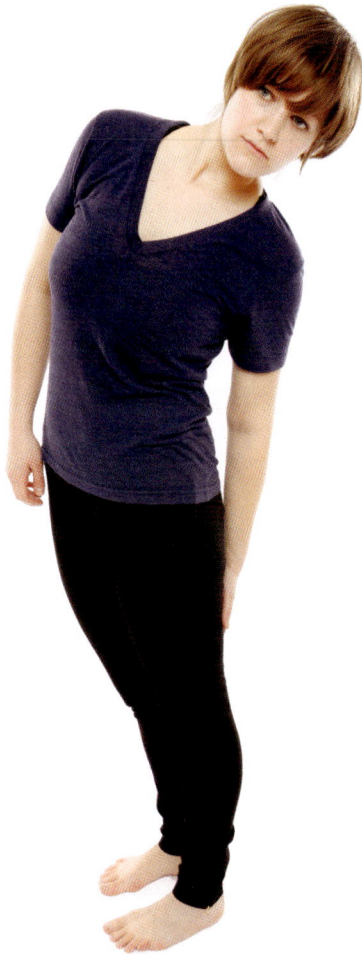

Figure 8-5 **Kemp's test.** With the client standing, ask him or her to slowly extend, laterally flex, and rotate the spine to the affected side as if reaching for the heel.

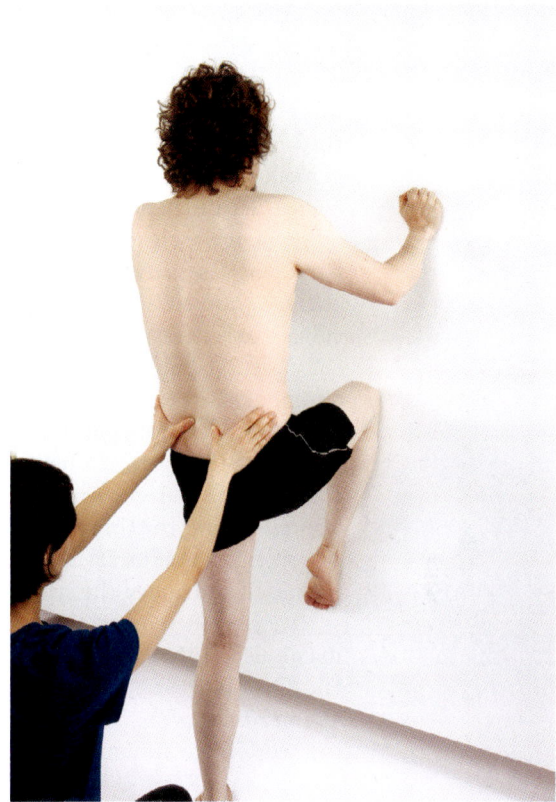

Figure 8-6 **Stork test.** Assess the mobility of the sacroiliac joint with the Stork test.

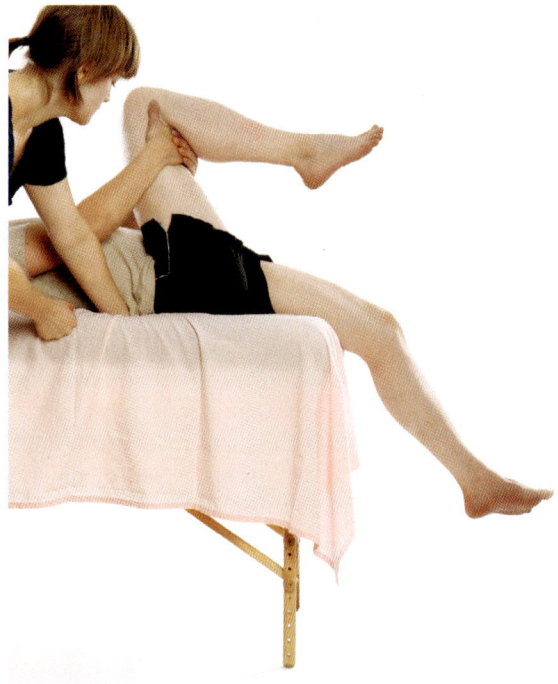

Figure 8-7 **Thomas test.** Assess the involvement of the hip flexors with the Thomas test.

PALPATION ASSESSMENT

Palpate the muscles of the lower cross to assess for hyper- and hypotonicity and myofascial restrictions. You are likely to find myofascial restrictions across the anterior aspect of the hip joint, from the iliac crest down into the quadriceps as well as along the posterior iliac crests and into the thoracolumbar fascia. Shortened, hypertonic muscles that may contain trigger points include the iliacus, psoas major, rectus femoris, sartorius, and tensor fasciae latae anteriorly; posteriorly, these muscles include latissimus dorsi, the lumbar erector spinae and quadratus lumborum. If the client presents with lateral rotation in the hips, assess the lateral rotators of the hips including the piriformis, quadratus femoris, obturator internus and externus, and the gemellus superior and inferior (see chapter 9). While the superficial gluteals may be stretched in clients with hyperlordosis, the deeper gluteal muscles with varied functions may be tight and adhered. If the client presents with an elevated iliac crest or lateral flexion of the thorax or lumbar spine, assess the latissimus dorsi, internal and external obliques, serratus posterior inferior, and the thoracic erector spinae on the affected side. A compromised serratus posterior inferior can also affect respiration. Although the focus here is on the muscles that are directly related to the postural imbalance occurring in hyperlordosis, it is essential to assess the synergists and antagonists in each ROM for these joints. For example, although the rectus femoris is a hip flexor involved in hyperlordosis, it also extends the knee. In this example, you may find adhesions between the rectus femoris, vastus lateralis, and vastus intermedius (see chapter 10). While the internal and external obliques both laterally flex the thorax to the same side, internal obliques rotate the thorax to the same side while external obliques rotate the thorax to the opposite side. When muscles are short or otherwise compromised, any of their actions may be compromised and any of the synergists and antagonists for each of their actions may be affected.

Overstretched muscles that may contain trigger points include the rectus abdominis, gluteus maximus (particularly the lower fibers), and the hamstrings. If lateral rotation of the hip is present, the adductor magnus, longus, and brevis as well as the gracilis, and pectineus may be overstretched and weak. However, if the adductors are regularly recruited to maintain posture or are overworking to antagonize lateral rotation, they may be hypertonic.

Condition-Specific Massage

Because hyperlordosis may have a structural cause, it is essential to understand the client's health history before initiating treatment. If a systemic condition or a degenerative bone or disc disease is present, discuss treatment with the client's health care provider and adjust the treatment accordingly. If hyperkyphosis, piriformis syndrome, patellofemoral syndrome, or plantar fasciitis is present, refer to Chapters 4, 9, 10, and 11, respectively, for special testing and consideration of neuromuscular characteristics.

It is essential for the treatment to be relaxing. You are not likely to eradicate the pain associated with hyperlordosis or any of the associated conditions in one treatment. Do not try to do so by treating aggressively. Be sure to ask your client to let you know if the amount of pressure you are applying keeps him or her from relaxing fully. If the client responds by tensing muscles or has a facial expression that looks distressed, reduce your pressure. Remember that you are working on tissue that is compromised.

Ask the client to let you know if any part of your treatment reproduces symptoms, and always work within his or her tolerance. When deep palpation of a trigger point reproduces symptoms, explain this to your client and ask him or her to breathe deeply during the technique. As the trigger point is deactivated, the referral pain will also diminish. Common trigger points and their referral points are shown in Figure 8-8.

If any other symptoms are reproduced, adjust the client to a more neutral position, reduce your pressure, or move slightly off the area, and make a note about it because this may help you understand more clearly exactly which neuromuscular condition is contributing to the client's symptoms. Instruct your client to use deep but relaxed breathing to assist in relaxation.

▲ Trigger point

● Referral pattern

● ▲ Iliopsoas

● ▲ Quadratus lumborum

● ▲ Rectus femoris

● ▲ Tensor fasciae latae

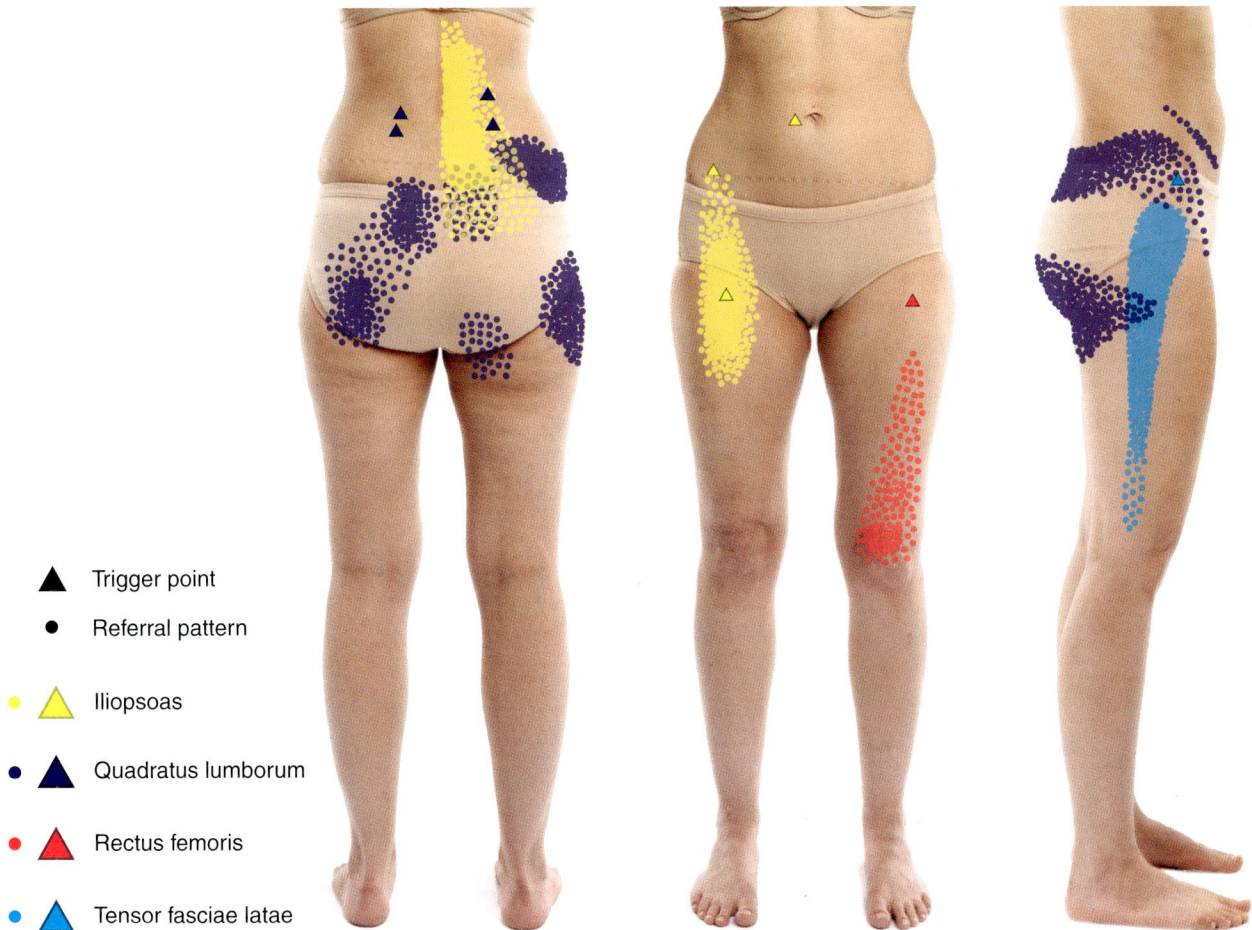

Figure 8-8   Common trigger points and referral. Common trigger points associated with hyperlordosis and their referral patterns.

The following suggestions are for treatment that considers several factors involved in hyperlordosis. Because several joints and many muscles are involved in this condition, your treatment will likely fill the entire session.

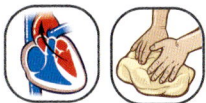

- Begin in the supine position with the knees bolstered.
- If you have access to moist heat, place it on one rectus femoris. After heating one rectus femoris, move the heat to the other side, and begin treating the heated side. After heating the other rectus femoris, you can move the heat to the abdomen.

- Before applying emollient, assess the tissues of the leg and hip for myofascial restrictions, and release them if indicated. A common area of myofascial restriction with hyperlordosis is found where the hip flexor tendons cross the hip joint. You may also find adhesions along the iliac crests. If the rectus femoris is shortened, you may find adhesions anywhere along its length, and it may be adhered to any of the muscles that surround it.

- Treat the thigh generally to soften tissues and reduce hypertonicity.

Treatment icons: 🖐 Increase circulation; 🖐 Reduce adhesions; 🖐 Reduce tension; ✐ Lengthen tissue; 🖐 Treat trigger points; 🖐 Passive stretch; 🖐 Clear area

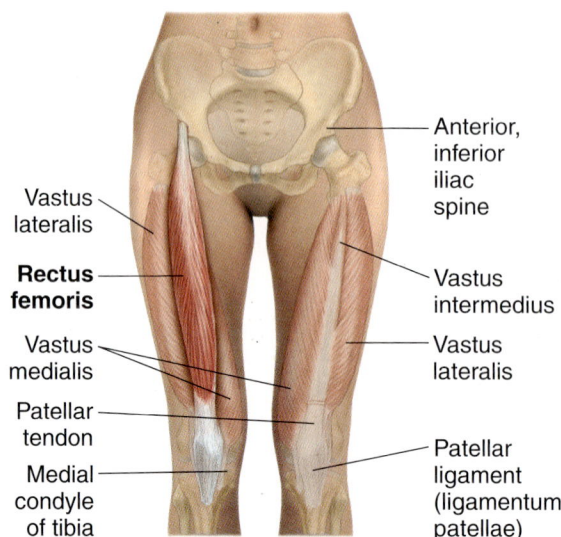

RECTUS FEMORIS

Origin	Anterior inferior iliac spine.
Insertion	Tibial tuberosity.
Action	Flex hip, extend knee, anterior pelvic tilt.
Nerve	Femoral.

Figure 8-9 **Rectus femoris.** A short, tight rectus femoris contributes to hip flexion and anterior pelvic tilt. Adapted from Clay JH, Pounds DM. *Basic Clinical Massage Therapy: Integrating Anatomy and Treatment,* 2nd ed. Philadelphia: Lippincott Williams & Wilkins, 2008.

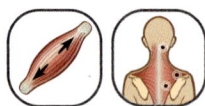

■ Apply lengthening strokes along the rectus femoris and assess for trigger points (Fig. 8-9). Note the varied fiber directions of the rectus femoris. Treat the trigger points if any are found. Common trigger points in the rectus femoris are found near the superior tendon and refer pain along the muscle into the knee.

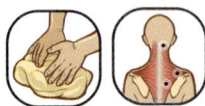

■ Treat the tensor fasciae latae (Fig. 8-10) for hypertonicity and trigger points if found. Because this area may be sensitive or ticklish, begin slowly with firm (not deep) strokes. Trigger points in the tensor fasciae latae refer pain along the iliotibial band.

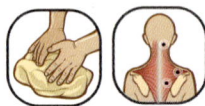

■ If your assessment revealed shortened or hypertonic adductors or iliotibial band, treat these. Assess and treat any trigger points found.

■ Passively Stretch any muscles treated for trigger points.

■ Before treating the iliopsoas, warm the abdominals to be certain that the superficial tissues are prepared to allow you to access the deeper tissues (Fig. 8-11). When warming the abdomen, it is important to work in a clockwise direction to move the contents of the intestines toward the rectum. Your client may feel the need to pass gas during this treatment. Instruct him or her not to hold this back because that would cause muscle tensing.

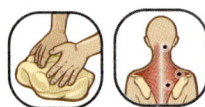

■ With fingers resting on the medial aspect of the iliac crest, instruct the client to take a deep breath into the abdomen, and as he or she exhales, gently move into the iliac fossa to treat the iliacus (Fig. 8-12). The depth of your access into the iliac fossa will depend on the texture of the tissues surrounding it. If you cannot access the fossa, spend a little more time on softening the superficial tissues and try again. Trigger points in the iliacus refer pain into the quadriceps area and into the low back and gluteal muscles.

■ Treating the psoas directly requires proficiency in the anatomy of the abdomen. There are many vessels and viscera that could be damaged when deep pressure is applied to the abdomen, and it is essential to know which structures you may be compressing as you

Anterior, superior
iliac spine

**Tensor
fasciae
latae**

**Tensor
fasciae
latae**

Rectus
femoris

Gluteus
maximus

**Iliotibial
band**

Iliotibial
band

Rectus
femoris

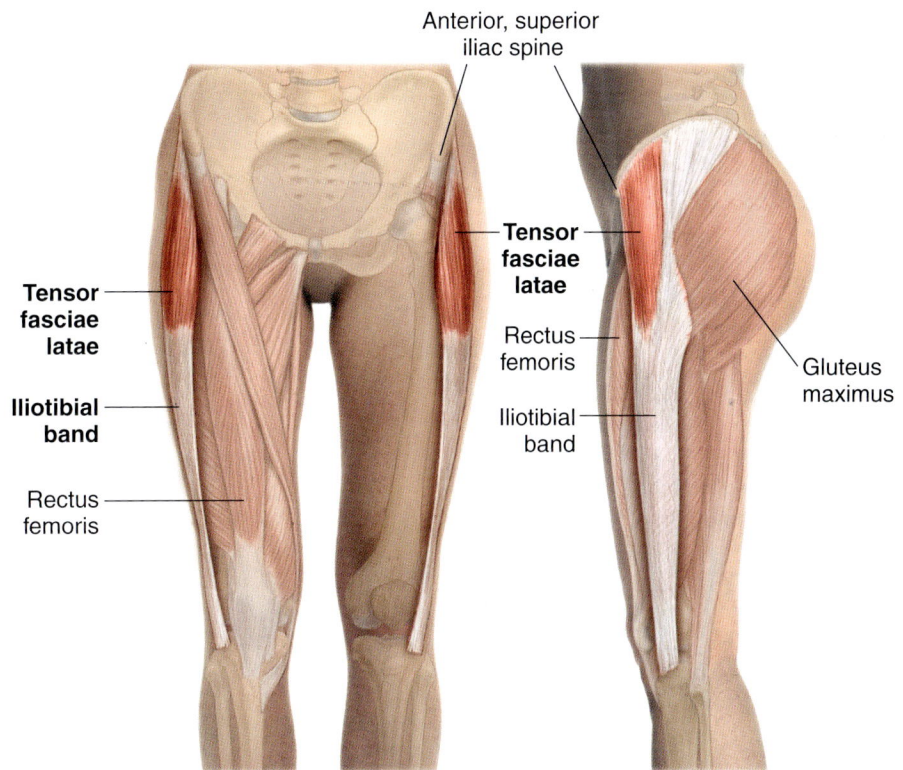

**Figure 8-10   Tensor fasciae
latae.** When the hips are flexed, the
tensor fasciae latae and iliotibial band
may become shortened and hypertonic.
Adapted from Clay JH, Pounds DM.
*Basic Clinical Massage Therapy:
Integrating Anatomy and Treatment,*
2nd ed. Philadelphia: Lippincott
Williams & Wilkins, 2008.

TENSOR FASCIAE LATAE

Origin	*Outer surface of anterior superior iliac spine, outer lip of anterior iliac crest.*
Insertion	*Lateral condyle of tibia via the iliotibial band.*
Action	*Flex hip, medially rotate hip, abduct hip, anterior pelvic tilt.*
Nerve	*Superior gluteal.*

approach the psoas. If you have not had detailed instruction on safely accessing the psoas or do not feel familiar enough with abdominal anatomy to avoid vessels and organs, stretch the psoas by extending the hip when the client is prone.

■ If you have had training in safely accessing the psoas, assess it, and treat it for hypertonicity and trigger points. One safe way to access the psoas is by placing your fingers at the level of the iliac crests and, very slowly, move medially toward the psoas. When you believe you have reached the psoas, ask the client to flex the hip and feel for a contraction.

■ To ensure that the client has control over the amount of movement and pressure applied in the abdomen, ask him or her to slowly flex and extend the hip and feel the psoas move under your fingers. If the client reports nausea, pain, or other sensations that may suggest compression of a vessel or organ, discontinue treatment of the psoas, and give the client a minute to breathe and relax.

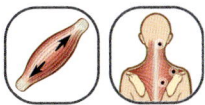

■ Turn the client prone and bolster the ankles. Stretch the rectus femoris and iliopsoas by performing passive hip extension if this does not reproduce symptoms. If you notice the client's hip rotating or elevating during the stretch, stabilize the sacrum and ilium with the palm of your free hand while extending the hip. If hip extension causes pain beyond the client's tolerance, try to stretch the rectus femoris alone by flexing the knee. Apply postisometric relaxation techniques to the hip within the client's tolerance to encourage the lengthening of the hip flexors.

■ Assess and treat any myofascial restrictions found in the thoracolumbar fascia before applying lotions to the back.

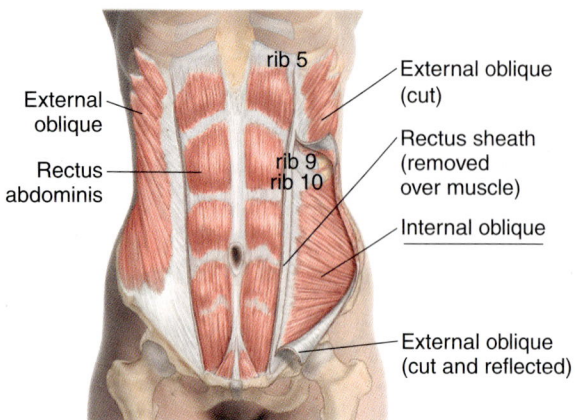

RECTUS ABDOMINIS

Origin	Pubic crest, pubic symphysis.
Insertion	Cartilage of ribs 5, 6, and 7, xiphoid process.
Action	Flex trunk, posterior pelvic tilt.
Nerve	Branches of intercostal nerves.

EXTERNAL OBLIQUES

Origin	Lower 8 ribs.
Insertion	Anterior iliac crest, abdominal aponeurosis to linea alba.
Action	**Unilaterally**: lateral flexion of trunk, contralateral rotation of trunk, ipsilateral rotation of pelvis; **bilaterally**: flex trunk, compress abdominal contents, posterior pelvic tilt.
Nerve	Branches of intercostal nerves.

INTERNAL OBLIQUES

Origin	Lateral inguinal ligament, iliac crest and thoracolumbar fascia.
Insertion	Internal surface of lower three ribs, abdominal aponeurosis to linea alba.
Action	**Unilaterally**: lateral flexion of trunk, ipsilateral rotation of trunk, contralateral rotation of pelvis; **bilaterally**: flex trunk, compress abdominal contents, posterior pelvic tilt.
Nerve	Branches of intercostal nerves.

Figure 8-11   Abdominals. Warm the abdominals and assess for hypotonicity before accessing the psoas. Adapted from Clay JH, Pounds DM. *Basic Clinical Massage Therapy: Integrating Anatomy and Treatment*, 2nd ed. Philadelphia: Lippincott Williams & Wilkins, 2008.

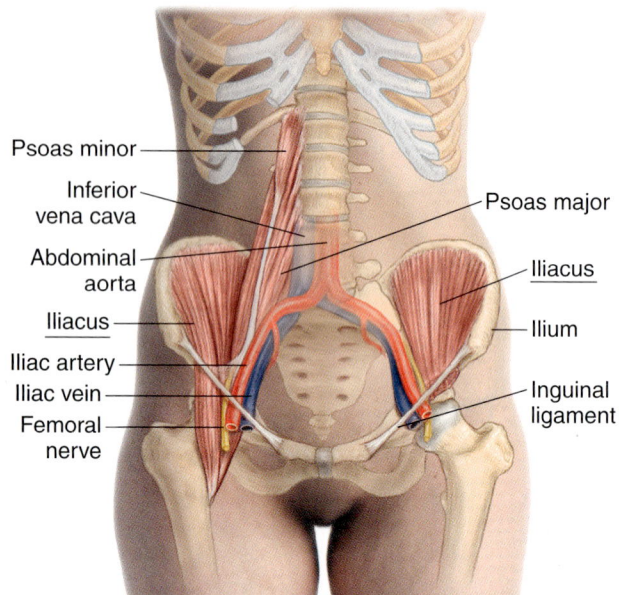

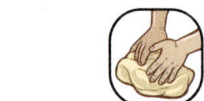

ILIACUS

Origin	Iliac fossa.
Insertion	Lesser trochanter of the femur.
Action	Flex hip, laterally rotate hip, adduct hip, anterior pelvic tilt.
Nerve	Femoral.

PSOAS MAJOR

Origin	Body and transverse processes of lumbar vertebrae.
Insertion	Lesser trochanter of the femur.
Action	Flex hip, laterally rotate hip, adduct hip, flex trunk, anterior pelvic tilt.
Nerve	Lumbar plexus.

Figure 8-12   Iliopsoas. The iliacus and psoas may be short and hypertonic when hip flexion contributes to hyperlordosis. Adapted from Clay JH, Pounds DM. *Basic Clinical Massage Therapy: Integrating Anatomy and Treatment*, 2nd ed. Philadelphia: Lippincott Williams & Wilkins, 2008.

- Once you are ready to apply lotions, warm the full back. If the client has had symptoms in the upper back, treat these as thoroughly as time permits.

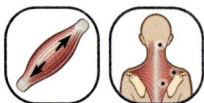

- Treat the latissimus dorsi and serratus posterior inferior for hypertonicity and trigger points (Fig. 8-13).

- Assess and treat the muscles of the lumbar spine. The attachment sites at the iliac crests, transverse and spinous processes, and lower ribs may be tender. Warm and soften the tissues attached to these bones to release tension in these muscles.

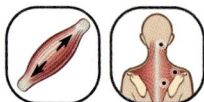

- Treat the bellies of the lumbar erector spinae and the deeper quadratus lumborum for adhesions, hypertonicity and trigger points (Fig. 8-14). Apply cross-fiber strokes to separate the fibers and open the area for deeper work. Treat trigger points if any are found. Follow this with lengthening strokes.

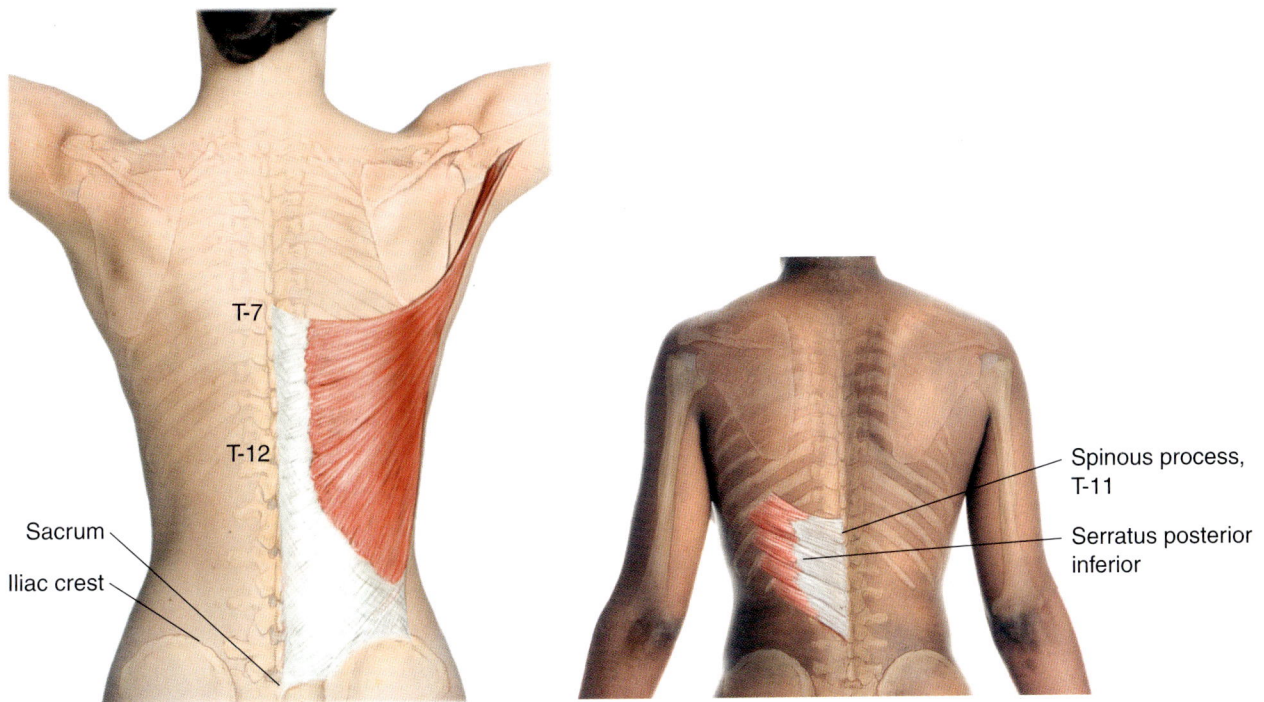

LATISSIMUS DORSI

Origin	*SP of T7-12, ribs 8-12, thoracolumbar aponeurosis and posterior iliac crest.*
Insertion	*Crest of lesser tubercle of humerus.*
Action	*Extend, adduct and medially rotate shoulder.*
Nerve	*Thoracodorsal.*

SERRATUS POSTERIOR INFERIOR

Origin	*Spinous process of T11-L3.*
Insertion	*Ribs 9-12.*
Action	*Depress the ribs during exhalation.*
Nerve	*Spinal nerves 9-12.*

Figure 8-13   **Latissimus dorsi and serratus inferior posterior.** The serratus inferior posterior draws the ribcage down and toward the ribcage, assisting in exhalation. Adapted from Clay JH, Pounds DM. *Basic Clinical Massage Therapy: Integrating Anatomy and Treatment*, 2nd ed. Philadelphia: Lippincott Williams & Wilkins, 2008.

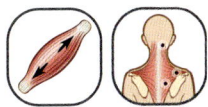

■ Once the erector spinae have softened and allow access to deeper tissues, apply lengthening strokes to the quadratus lumborum. Note the variety of fiber directions in the quadratus lumborum. Common trigger points in the quadratus lumborum are found in the angle formed by the twelfth rib and the spine, as well as in the flank midway between the twelfth rib and the ilium. Take care not to apply excessive force to the floating 11th and 12th ribs.

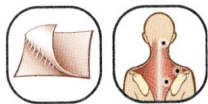

■ Assess the hamstrings for adhesions and trigger points and treat if indicated (Fig. 8-15). It is likely that the hamstrings are overstretched and should not be stretched further by using muscle stripping.

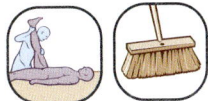

■ From the prone position, ask the client to use the arms to slowly move the body without stressing the low back, bringing the buttocks toward the ankles, to stretch the quadratus lumborum, erector spinae, and the latissimus dorsi (Fig. 8-16). When the client returns to the prone position, end with clearing strokes to the whole back.

■ With the remaining time, consider the other possible conditions that may develop with hyperlordosis and treat these areas. External or internal rotation of the hip suggests treatment to the piriformis and other external rotators or the adductors, respectively. Flat feet suggest treatment to the muscles of the lower leg and feet. If hyperkyphosis is also present, refer to Chapter 4 for additional treatment. You may not have time to treat all of these fully, but you can pay attention to some of them in each session. As the signs and symptoms of hyperlordosis decrease, you can increase the amount of time you spend in other areas.

The treatment overview diagram summarizes the flow of treatment (Fig. 8-17).

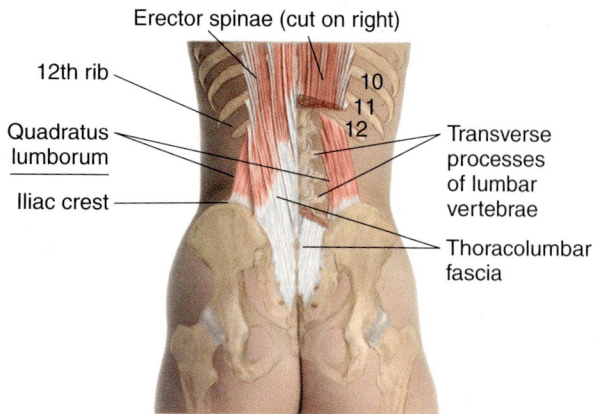

QUADRATUS LUMBORUM

Origin	Posterior iliac crest.
Insertion	Last rib, transverse processes of lumbar vertebrae 1-4.
Action	**Unilaterally**: laterally tilt pelvis, laterally flex spine; **bilaterally**: extend spine, fix last rib during respiration.
Nerve	Branches of first lumbar and 12th thoracic.

ERECTOR SPINAE

Origin	Thoracolumbar fascia, posterior surface of sacrum, iliac crest, SPs of lumbar and a few of the inferior thoracic vertebrae.
Insertion	Posterior ribs, SPs and TVPs of vertebrae.
Action	**Unilaterally**: lateral flexion of spine; **bilaterally**: extend spine.
Nerve	Dorsal primary divisions of spinal nerves.

Figure 8-14 **Quadratus lumborum and the lumbar erector spinae.** Muscles that extend the lumbar spine may become short and hypertonic with hyperlordosis. Adapted from Clay JH, Pounds DM. *Basic Clinical Massage Therapy: Integrating Anatomy and Treatment*, 2nd ed. Philadelphia: Lippincott Williams & Wilkins, 2008.

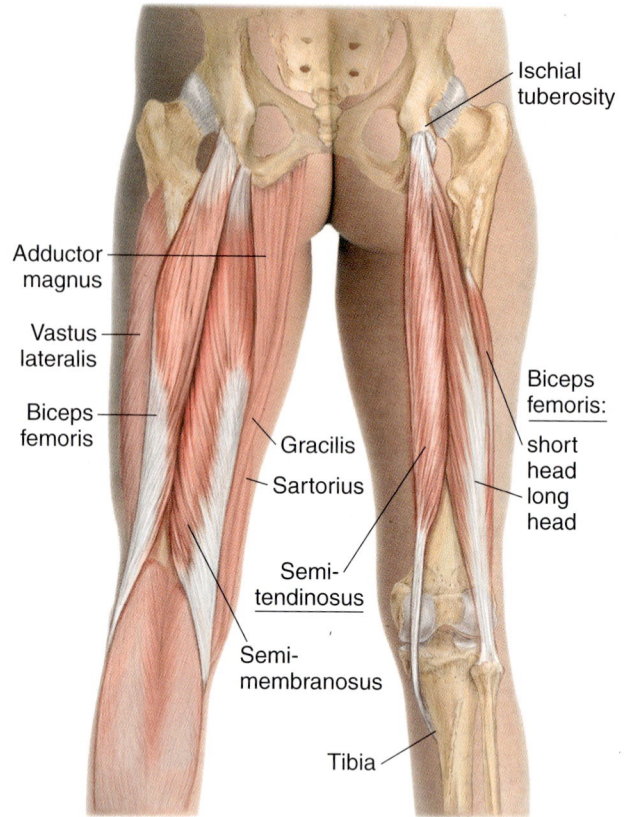

BICEPS FEMORIS

Origin	**Long head**: ischial tuberosity; **short head**: lateral lip of linea aspera.
Insertion	Head of fibula.
Action	Flex knee, laterally rotate flexed knee, extend hip, laterally rotate hip, tilt pelvis posteriorly.
Nerve	Tibial and peroneal.

SEMITENDINOSUS

Origin	Ischial tuberosity.
Insertion	Proximal, medial shaft of tibia at pes anserinus tendon.
Action	Flex knee, medially rotate flexed knee, extend hip, medially rotate hip, tilt pelvis posteriorly.
Nerve	Tibial.

SEMIMEMBRANOSUS

Origin	Ischial tuberosity.
Insertion	Posterior aspect of medial condyle of tibia.
Action	Flex knee, medially rotate flexed knee, extend hip, medially rotate hip, tilt pelvis posteriorly.
Nerve	Tibial.

Figure 8-15 **Hamstrings.** Weak hamstrings cannot adequately oppose flexion of the hip and should be strengthened.

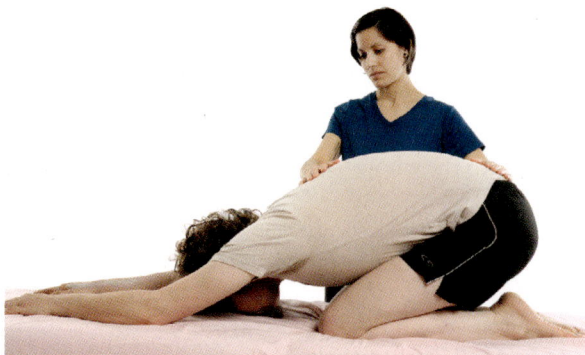

Figure 8-16 **Stretch quadratus lumborum and the lumbar erector spinae.** Instruct the client to bring the buttocks toward the heels to stretch the quadratus lumborum and the erector spinae.

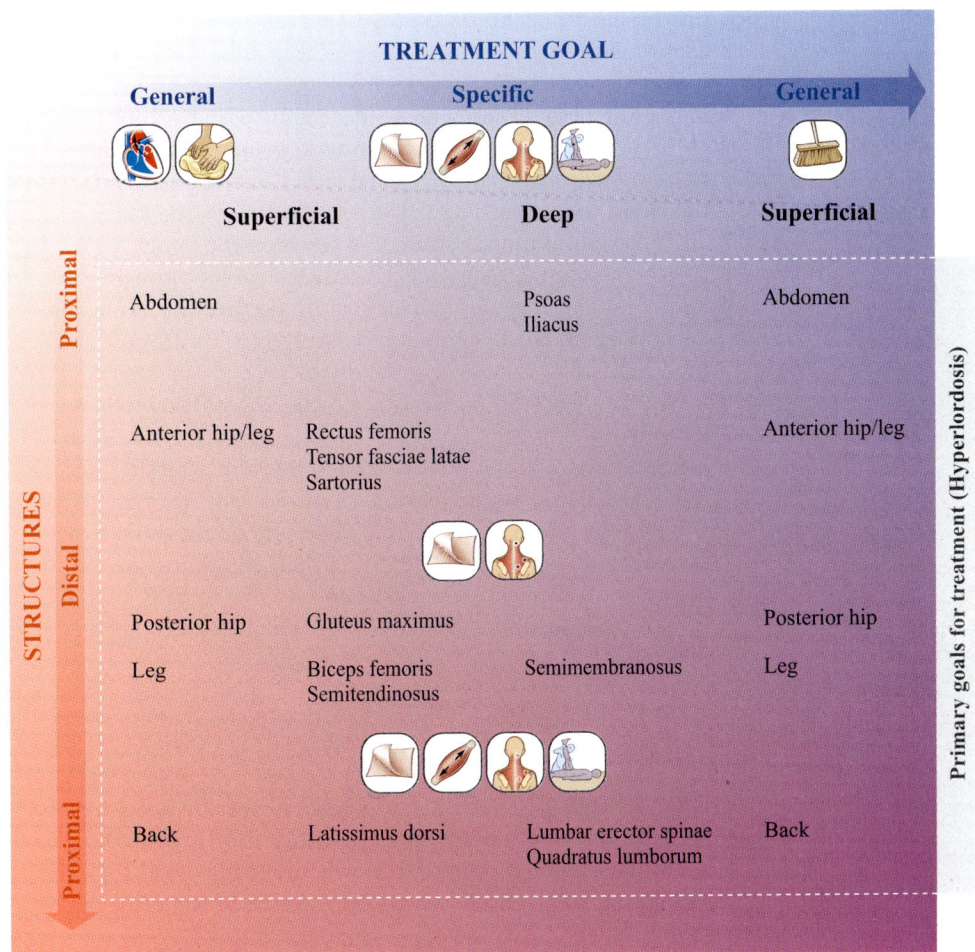

Figure 8-17   Hyperlordosis treatment overview diagram. Follow the general principles from left to right or top to bottom when treating hyperlordosis.

CLIENT SELF-CARE

The following are intended as general recommendations for stretching and strengthening muscles involved in the client's condition. The objective is to create distance between the attachment sites of muscles that have shortened and to perform repetitions of movements that decrease the distance between the attachments of muscles that have weakened. If you have had no training in remedial exercises or do not feel that you have a functional understanding of stretching and strengthening, refer the client to a professional with training in this area.

Clients often neglect self-care because their daily lives are busy. Encourage them to follow these guidelines.

- Instruct the client to perform self-care throughout the day, such as while taking a phone call, reading e-mail, washing the dishes, or watching television, instead of setting aside extra time. When performing activities while standing, contracting the abdominal muscles or "sucking in the stomach" as well as tilting the pelvis posteriorly by squeezing the gluteal muscles may decrease pain and weakness in addition to toning these weakened muscles. This should be done only if it is comfortable and if it does not cause the client to breathe shallowly.

- Encourage the client to take regular breaks from repetitive actions.
- Demonstrate gentle self-massage to keep adhesions and hypertonicity at bay between treatments.
- Recommend that the client avoid sleeping with the hips flexed.
- Instruct the client on how to maintain proper posture in the standing and seated positions to keep pressure off the weakened joints. Sitting in a chair that supports the back and allows the client to rest the feet flat on the floor with the knees and hips flexed at approximately 90° may reduce muscle strain and stress on the joints.
- Instruct those whose exercise is focused on strengthening the quadriceps to stretch these and to strengthen the hamstrings by performing extensions of the hip, resisted or not, depending on their capability. Walking is a low-impact activity that helps keep the joints mobile.
- Instruct a client who regularly performs heavy lifting to bend the knees, and lift with the legs instead of the spine.
- Demonstrate all strengthening exercises and stretches and have the client perform these in your presence before leaving to ensure that he or she is performing them properly and will not harm himself or herself when practicing alone. Stretches should be held for 15–30 seconds and are performed frequently throughout the day, within the client's limits, during an active flare-up. The client should not force the stretch or bounce. Exercises should be slow, gentle, and steady while the client tries to keep every other muscle as relaxed as possible.

Stretching

Instruct the client to stretch his or her hip flexors by kneeling with one knee on a soft surface such as a pillow on the floor and the other foot on the floor with the hip and knee flexed (Fig. 8-18). The client should then slowly move the pelvis forward with the spine erect, lengthening the quadriceps and iliopsoas on the side of the unflexed hip. Switch legs to stretch the other side.

It is also important to reduce anterior pelvic tilt. While this may occur when lengthening the hip flexors, for some, it will be necessary to add a little push. Instruct the client, particularly when standing, to squeeze the gluteal muscles together toward the midline. This action will tilt the pelvis posteriorly while strengthening the gluteals.

To lengthen the lumbar erectors and quadratus lumborum, simple forward bends performed periodically throughout the day are helpful. To add an additional stretch with the pelvis stabilized and hip flexion minimized, instruct the client to stand approximately 12 inches from a wall with the dorsal surface of the hands along the edges of the sacrum as shown in Figure 8-19. With the hands on the sacrum, instruct the client to lean his or her back against a wall with the knees slightly bent. The hands help stabilize the sacrum and pelvis while the client extends the knees and slowly bends forward at the hips, stretching the low back.

Strengthening

While it may be important to strengthen the abdominal muscles for core strength, it is essential that these exercises do not include resisted flexion of the hips. Crunches are best performed with the knees bent to inhibit the hip flexors. While performing crunches this way, the client need not flex the thorax completely, since this might place strain on the low back. Small crunches held for 3–5 seconds will strengthen the abdominal muscles without undue stress on the lumbar spine.

Extension of the hip strengthens the hamstrings and gluteal muscles. The hamstrings are also strengthened by flexing the knee. These exercises can be performed while standing and leaning against a wall or other stable surface for balance or while positioned on the hands and knees (Fig. 8-20). An elastic band around the ankles can be used to add resistance within the client's tolerance.

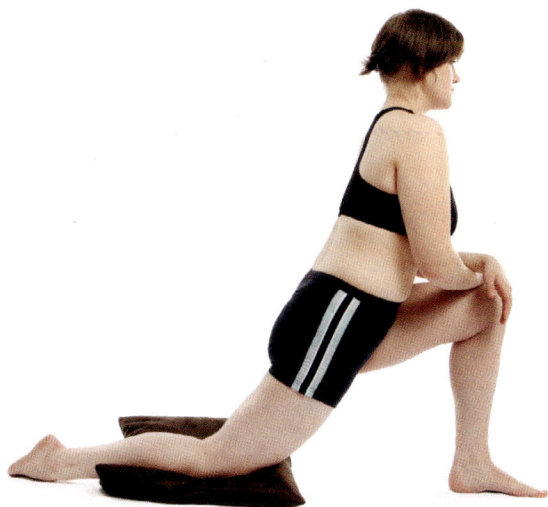

Figure 8-18   **Hip flexor stretch.** Instruct the client to stretch the hip flexors by kneeling with one knee on a soft surface such as a pillow, placing the other foot on the floor with the hip and knee flexed; then slowly move the pelvis forward with the spine erect.

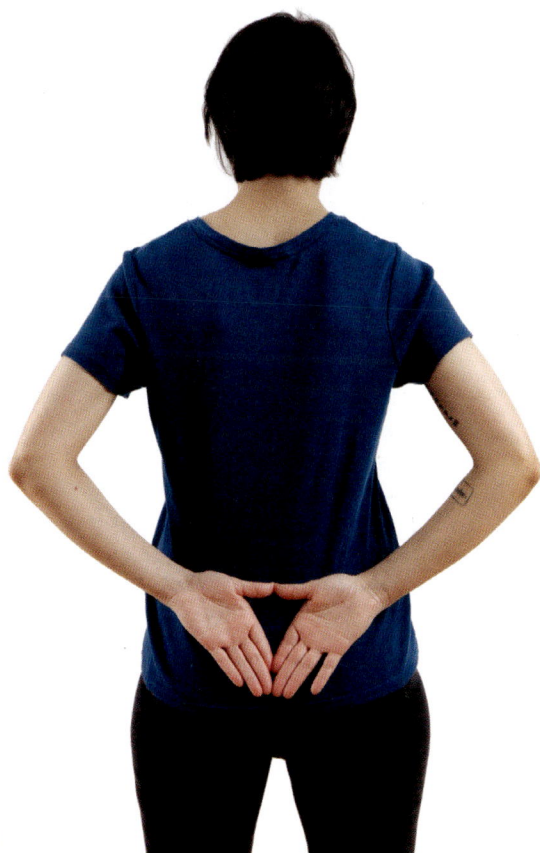

A

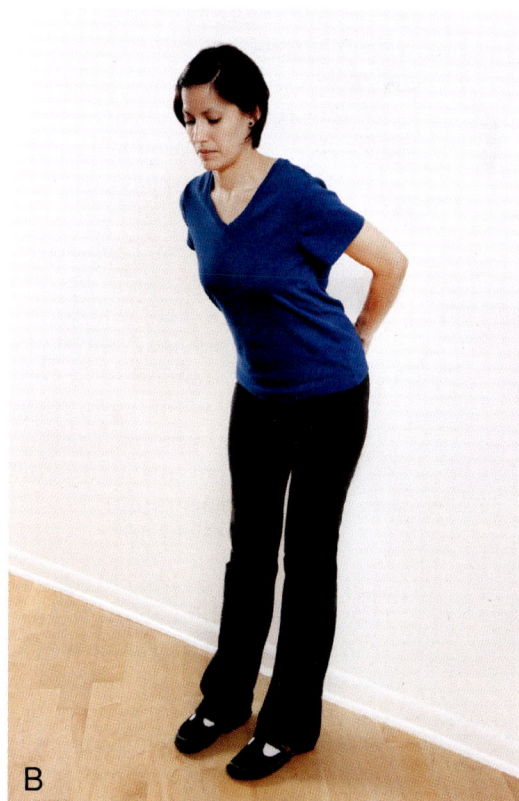

B

Figure 8-19   **Lumbar stretch.** Stabilize the sacrum while bending forward to stretch the low back muscles.

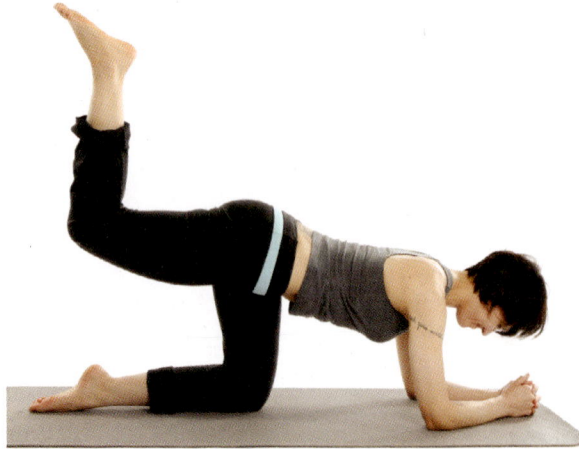

Figure 8-20 **Strengthen hamstrings and gluteal muscles.** Instruct the client to strengthen the hamstrings and gluteal muscles by extending the hip. This exercise will also stretch the hip flexors.

SUGGESTIONS FOR FURTHER TREATMENT

Ideally, a client with hyperlordosis will have treatments twice a week until the client can perform activities of daily living with minimal or no pain for at least 4 days. Reduce frequency to once per week until symptoms are absent for at least 7 days. When the client reports that he or she has been pain-free for more than 7 days, treatment can be reduced to twice per month. If the client is pain-free for 2 or more consecutive weeks, he or she can then schedule once per month or as necessary. With structural hyperkyphosis, treatment goals are limited to pain relief and minor increases in ROM, and these may be temporary. With functional hyperlordosis, there should be some improvement in both pain and posture with each session. If this is not happening, consider the following possibilities:

- There is too much time between treatments. It is always best to give the newly treated tissues 24–48 hours to adapt, but if too much time passes between treatments in the beginning, the client's activities of daily living may reverse any progress.
- The client is not adjusting his or her activities of daily living or is not keeping up with self-care. As much as we want to fix the problem, we cannot force a client to make the adjustments we suggest. Explain the importance of the client's participation in the healing process and encourage him or her to follow your recommendations, but be careful not to judge or reprimand a client who does not.
- The condition is advanced or involves other musculoskeletal complications that are beyond your basic training. Refer this client to a massage therapist with advanced clinical massage training. Continuing to treat a client whose case is beyond your training could turn the client away from massage therapy altogether and hinder healing.
- The hyperlordosis is structural or there is an undiagnosed underlying condition. Discontinue treatment until the client sees a health care provider for a medical assessment, and work with the health care team to plan massage treatments.

If you are not treating the client in a clinical setting or private practice, you may not be able to take this client through the full program of healing. Still, if you can bring some relief in just one treatment, it may encourage the client to discuss this change with his or her health care provider and seek manual therapy rather than more aggressive treatment options. If the client returns for regular treatments, the symptoms are likely to change each time, so it is important to perform an assessment before each session. Once you have released superficial tissues in general areas, you may be able to focus more of your treatment on a specific area. Likewise, once you have treated the structures specific to hyperlordosis, you may be able to pay closer attention to compensating structures and coexisting conditions.

PROFESSIONAL GROWTH

CASE STUDY

Tangelique is a 38-year-old married mother of two children. She cares for her children during the day, which includes home-schooling, and works evenings in a high-end department store, giving perfume samples to customers. In the past year, she has made the consumption of locally grown, whole foods a priority in her home after her husband received a diagnosis of diabetes. Prior to this, processed food and carbonated drinks had been common in their diet. She has had minor low back pain for years, but recently the pain has intensified, and she feels weak when standing for long periods.

Subjective

The client complained of low back pain and weakness when standing for more than 30 minutes. She has had minor back pain since her first pregnancy, and 2 weeks ago, she felt a sharp but diffuse pain across her low back when standing up from sitting. Since then she has had more severe back pain, sometimes causing her to hunch, and she feels weak after standing. She spends 4–6 hours each day home-schooling her children and 4 hours on 3 nights each week in a department store. When home-schooling, Tangelique is often seated for several hours at a time. At the department store, she stands the whole time and is required to wear contemporary fashions with high-heeled shoes.

The client reported no systemic conditions and is taking no medication currently. She reported having no abdominal pain or difficulty urinating or with bowel movements. When asked if she feels any numbness or tingling or has experienced any swelling in her legs, Tangelique stated only that on occasion she feels "electricity" on the front of her right leg. When asked if she wears hip huggers or tight belts low on the waist, she responded "Yes." The client is not currently pregnant, premenstrual, or menstruating.

Objective

Postural assessment revealed a significant increase in the lumbar curve with anterior pelvic tilt. She displayed a minor lateral rotation of hips bilaterally. Valsalva and Kemp's tests were negative for space-occupying lesions and disc involvement. The Stork test was negative for sacroiliac joint dysfunction. The Thomas test was positive for short hip flexors. Tinel's sign was positive for irritation of the femoral nerve. This may be due to compression by tight clothing around the hips.

Palpation revealed fascial restrictions across the hip joint bilaterally and into the quadriceps area on the right thigh. The thoracolumbar fascia is thickened and adhered. The rectus femoris is dense and adhered bilaterally, but particularly on the right. The right tensor fasciae latae and iliotibial band are tender and adhered. The client was ticklish near the iliac fossa initially but was able to relax enough to reveal hypertonicity in the iliacus. Moderate pressure to the psoas caused pain in the low back. The latissimus dorsi contained adhesions at the lateral ribcage bilaterally. The quadratus lumborum and the lumbar erector spinae are tender, hypertonic, and adhered.

Action

I began in the supine position with a bolster under the knees. I applied myofascial release to tissues across the anterior hip joint and leg, taking care not to compress the femoral nerve. I applied general effleurage and petrissage to the anterior leg followed by muscle stripping to the rectus femoris, vastus lateralis, tensor fasciae latae, and the iliotibial band. There was a trigger point in the superior aspect of rectus femoris that referred down into the anterior leg. The client stated that this referral was similar to the area where she occasionally felt "electricity." Muscle stripping did not reduce the referred pain. I followed two rounds of compression with effleurage, which reduced the referred pain from level 6 to 2. I then applied clearing strokes to the legs and the hips.

I applied slow but firm petrissage around the anterior iliac crest to reduce tickling followed by deep petrissage in the iliac fossa. The area was very tender to the client at first, but the tenderness reduced quickly as each layer of tissue was released. No trigger points were found in the iliacus, and there was no reproduction of symptoms. I applied superficial, clockwise effleurage to the abdomen to warm the tissues. The psoas was hypertonic bilaterally, particularly on the right. I applied muscle stripping to the psoas in 1-inch increments. A trigger point was found in the mid belly of the right psoas, which referred into the back. Compression reduced the referred pain from level 8 to 6. I cleared the area, and then instructed the client to turn to the prone position, using the arms as much as possible to reduce the possibility of straining the low back.

I applied a passive stretch to the hip flexors bilaterally. I used myofascial release including skin rolling across the thoracolumbar fascia. I applied petrissage to the muscle attachment sites along the iliac crests, sacrum, and lower ribs. I also applied petrissage and firm effleurage to the latissimus dorsi bilaterally. No trigger points were found here. I used deep effleurage followed by muscle stripping to the lumbar erector spinae and quadratus lumborum. A trigger point was found in the mid muscle belly of the lateral portion of the right quadratus lumborum. Compression followed by muscle stripping reduced the referred pain from level 8 to 4. I cleared the area. I followed deep petrissage to the lateral rotators of the hip with a passive stretch.

Following treatment, the client reported feeling "looser" but stated that getting off the table did cause some discomfort in her low back.

Plan

I explained that the shortened hip flexors pull on the spine and pelvis when she stands because they are unable to lengthen fully. I demonstrated the stretches for the hip flexors and the lumbar spine. I demonstrated strengthening for hamstrings and abdominals but encouraged her to wait for 24–48 hours to see how she responded to treatment before stressing the low back with abdominal strengthening exercises. I advised her to proceed cautiously, with the hips and knees flexed, if she chose to do the strengthening exercises.

I explained that tight clothing around her ilia may be compressing the femoral artery, causing the "electricity" she feels. I suggested that she wear looser clothing or bands and belts that do not rest on the pelvis. I also explained that high heels may be contributing to the postural imbalance, although I understand that this is part of her uniform, and she may not be able to stop wearing them. I recommended wearing lower heels as much as possible and to practice posterior pelvic tilt and calf stretches after wearing high heels.

The client is unable to schedule treatments biweekly, but she scheduled one appointment for next week and stated that frequency will depend on financial restrictions. A sliding scale was offered if she felt she needed more frequent treatments, and I encouraged her to call if she had questions about more intensive self-care if she is unable to return regularly for treatment.

CRITICAL THINKING EXERCISES

1. Develop a 10-minute stretching and strengthening routine for a client that covers all of the muscles involved in hyperlordosis. Use Table 8-1, Box 8-1, and Figure 8-4 as a guide. Remember that a stretch increases the distance between the origin and insertion of a muscle and is important for those muscles that are shortened while strengthening is performed by actively bringing the origin and insertion closer together and is important for the antagonists of shortened muscles. Describe each step of the routine in enough detail that the client can refer to these descriptions in your absence and perform them without harm.

2. A client calls to schedule a massage for low back pain. She explains that she had a caesarian section 7 years ago that left a scar above her pelvis. Discuss the role her surgery may have had in the development of her chronic pain, the essential questions to ask her and her health care provider before initiating treatment, and the cautions and considerations to take when planning treatment.

3. In the assessment of a client with chronic low back pain, he tests negative for short hip flexors and has no anterior pelvic tilt. The client has a right rotation of the pelvis, his left hip is elevated, his thorax is flexed to the left, his right hip is laterally rotated, and his left ankle is everted. His left hamstrings are hypertonic compared to his right. Use Table 8-1 to determine

which muscles are short and which may be lengthened. Put yourself in this posture to figure out how this client's activities or posture may be contributing to his pain. Design a treatment plan describing massage therapy as well as self-care.

4. Conduct a short literature review to learn how the following conditions may put a client at greater risk for developing hyperlordosis:
   - Nerve root compression
   - Obesity
   - Rheumatoid arthritis
   - Vitamin D deficiency
   - Spondylolisthesis

BIBLIOGRAPHY AND SUGGESTED READINGS

Bell J. Massage therapy helps to increase range of motion, decrease pain and assist in healing a client with low back pain and sciatica symptoms. Journal of Bodywork and Movement Therapies. 2008;12(3): 281–289.

Biel A. *Trail Guide to the Body: How to Locate Muscles, Bones and More*, 3rd ed. Boulder, CO: Books of Discovery, 2005.

Cherkin DC, Sherman KJ, Deyo RA, et al. A review of the evidence for the effectiveness, safety, and cost of acupuncture, massage therapy, and spinal manipulation for back pain. Annals of Internal Medicine. 2003;138(11):898–906.

Clarkson HM. *Joint Motion and Function Assessment*. Baltimore, MD: Lippincott Williams & Wilkins, 2005.

Hernandez-Reif M, Field T, Krasnegor J, et al. Lower back pain is reduced and range of motion increased after massage therapy. International Journal of Neuroscience. 2001;106(3–4):131–145.

Imamura M, Furlan AD, Dryden T, et al. Evidence-informed management of chronic low back pain with massage. The Spine Journal. 2008;8(1):121–133.

Mayo Foundation for Medical Education and Research. Herniated Disk. Available at http://www.mayoclinic.com/health/herniated-disk/HD99999. Accessed Winter 2009.

Mayo Foundation for Medical Education and Research. Prostate cancer. Available at http://www.mayoclinic.com/health/prostate-cancer/PT99999. Accessed Winter 2009.

Mayo Foundation for Medical Education and Research. Urinary Tract Infection. Available at http://www.mayoclinic.com/health/urinary-tract-infection/DS00286. Accessed Winter 2009.

Muscolino JE. *The Muscular System Manual: The Skeletal Muscles of the Human Body*, 2nd ed. St. Louis, MO: Elsevier Mosby, 2005.

Osar E. *Form & Function: The Anatomy of Motion*, 2nd ed. Evanston, IL: Osar Publications, 2005.

Pal P, Milosavljevic S, Sole G, et al. Hip and lumbar continuous motion characteristics during flexion and return in young healthy males. European Spine Journal. 2007;16(6):741–747.

Preyde M. Effectiveness of massage therapy for subacute low-back pain: A randomized controlled trial. Canadian Medical Association Journal. 2000;162(13):1815–1820.

Rattray F, Ludwig L. *Clinical Massage Therapy: Understanding, Assessing and Treating over 70 Conditions*. Toronto, ON: Talus Incorporated, 2000.

Spine Universe. Lumbar Radiculopathy: Low Back and Leg Pain. Available at http://www.spineuniverse.com/displayarticle.php/article1469.html. Accessed Winter 2009.

Spondylitis Association of America. Ankylosing Spondylitis. Available at http://www.spondylitis.org/about/as_diag.aspx. Accessed Summer 2008.

Simons DG, Travell JG, Simons LS. *Myofascial Pain and Dysfunction: The Trigger Point Manual*, 2nd ed. Philadelphia, PA: Lippincott Williams & Wilkins, 1999.

Turchaninov R. *Medical Massage*, 2nd ed. Phoenix, AZ: Aesculapius Books, 2006.

U.S. National Library of Medicine and the National Institutes of Health. Achondroplasia. Available at http://www.nlm.nih.gov/medlineplus/ency/article/001577.htm. Accessed Winter 2009.

U.S. National Library of Medicine and the National Institutes of Health. Ankylosing Spondylitis. Available at http://www.nlm.nih.gov/medlineplus/ankylosingspondylitis.html. Accessed Summer 2008.

U.S. National Library of Medicine and the National Institutes of Health. Bone cancer. Available at http://www.nlm.nih.gov/medlineplus/bonecancer.html. Accessed Winter 2009.

U.S. National Library of Medicine and the National Institutes of Health. Cervical Cancer. Available at http://www.nlm.nih.gov/medlineplus/cervicalcancer.html. Accessed Winter 2009.

U.S. National Library of Medicine and the National Institutes of Health. Lordosis. Available at http://www.nlm.nih.gov/medlineplus/ency/article/003278.htm. Accessed Winter 2009.

U.S. National Library of Medicine and the National Institutes of Health. Osteoporosis. Available at http://www.nlm.nih.gov/medlineplus/ency/article/000360.htm. Accessed Summer 2008.

U.S. National Library of Medicine and the National Institutes of Health. Spondylolisthesis. Available at http://www.nlm.nih.gov/medlineplus/ency/article/001260.htm. Accessed Winter 2009.

U.S. National Library of Medicine and the National Institutes of Health. Uterine Cancer. Available at http://www.nlm.nih.gov/medlineplus/uterinecancer.html. Accessed Winter 2009.

Werner R. *A Massage Therapist's Guide to Pathology*, 4th ed. Philadelphia, PA: Lippincott Williams & Wilkins, 2009.

Piriformis Syndrome

UNDERSTANDING PIRIFORMIS SYNDROME

Piriformis syndrome is a complex condition characterized primarily by myofascial pain with trigger points, which may involve nerve and vascular compression or sacroiliac joint dysfunction. Often, piriformis syndrome is reported as "sciatica," a general term referring to pain along the sciatic nerve, which can result from a variety of causes other than piriformis syndrome including a herniated disc, impingement of the nerve between bones, degenerative disc disease, spinal stenosis, tumors compressing the nerve, and trauma.

Because the piriformis muscle fits precisely in the greater sciatic foramen, increased tone and trigger points that shorten and increase the width of the muscle decreases the space available for the nerves that also pass through the foramen to function optimally. Normally, the sciatic nerve emerges from the sacrum and passes deep to the piriformis muscle. In a small percentage of the population, the sciatic nerve travels through the piriformis or the piriformis muscle is split into two bellies with the sciatic nerve running between them. Although the sciatic nerve is most often affected by piriformis syndrome, the gluteal and pudendal nerves may also become irritated. Compression can also affect the vasculature, reducing circulation and affecting the health of the structures supplied by those vessels.

The sciatic nerve exits the spine as five separate roots between L4 and S3. They converge into one large sciatic nerve at the greater sciatic foramen under the piriformis muscle. From here, the nerve curves toward the hip and passes between the greater trochanter and the ischial tuberosity, then down the middle of the thigh along the length of the femur (Fig. 9-1). The sciatic nerve innervates the skin of the leg and foot, as well as the hamstrings. Just above the knee, the nerve divides into the common peroneal and tibial branches. Generally, these branches innervate the muscles of the anterior and lateral leg and the top of the foot and the posterior leg and the bottom of the foot, respectively.

Muscles innervated by the sciatic nerve and its branches include the following:

- Adductor magnus, posterior head (sciatic nerve)
- Semitendinosus (sciatic nerve)
- Semimembranosus (sciatic nerve)
- Biceps femoris (sciatic nerve)
- Plantaris (tibial nerve)
- Gastrocnemius (tibial nerve)
- Soleus (tibial nerve)
- Tibialis posterior (tibial nerve)
- Flexor digitorum longus (tibial nerve)
- Flexor hallucis longus (tibial nerve)
- Peroneus longus (superficial peroneal nerve)
- Peroneus brevis (superficial peroneal nerve)
- Tibialis anterior (deep peroneal nerve)

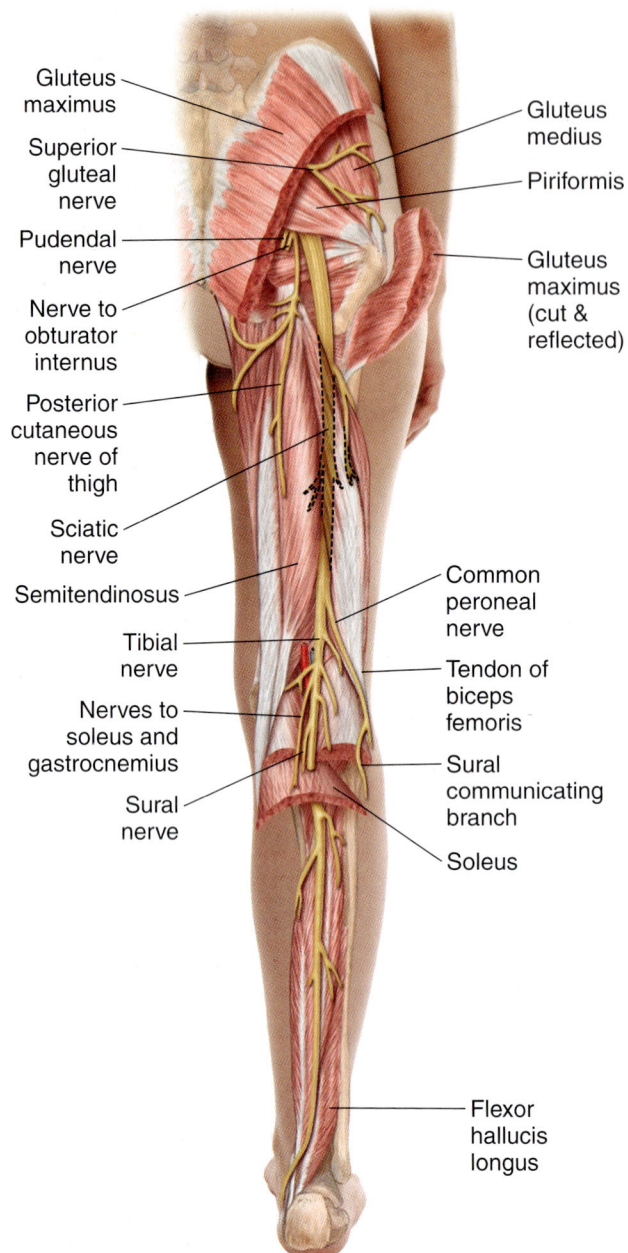

Gluteus maximus

Superior gluteal nerve

Pudendal nerve

Nerve to obturator internus

Posterior cutaneous nerve of thigh

Sciatic nerve

Semitendinosus

Tibial nerve

Nerves to soleus and gastrocnemius

Sural nerve

Gluteus medius

Piriformis

Gluteus maximus (cut & reflected)

Common peroneal nerve

Tendon of biceps femoris

Sural communicating branch

Soleus

Flexor hallucis longus

Figure 9-1 The sciatic nerve and its branches. The sciatic nerve passes under the piriformis muscle.

- Extensor digitorum longus (deep peroneal nerve)
- Extensor hallucis longus (deep peroneal nerve)
- Extensor digitorum brevis (deep peroneal nerve)
- Intrinsic muscles of the foot (medial and lateral plantar nerves)

Common Signs and Symptoms

The symptoms of piriformis syndrome usually begin gradually with pain in the low back, hip, or gluteal area. When the sciatic nerve is involved, radiating pain, numbness, or tingling is felt along the posterior thigh, calf, and foot. Active lateral rotation of the hip, which contracts the piriformis, and active or passive medial rotation of the hip, which stretches the shortened piriformis, may compress the sciatic nerve and intensify symptoms. An absence of numbness and tingling may suggest that the nerves are not involved; this is referred to as non-neurogenic piriformis syndrome. In these cases, referred pain from trigger points as well as weakness due to compensation may present similarly, and the condition can progress to involve the nerves and vessels if the syndrome is not treated.

Trigger points in the piriformis refer pain into the low back, buttocks, hip, and superior posterior thigh. When one piriformis is short, the sacrum may shift laterally toward the affected side and rotate anteriorly, causing sacroiliac joint dysfunction and pain in the low back. In this case, the ilium may be elevated on the opposite side. Sciatic nerve compression may cause pain in the posterior thigh with pain, numbness, and tingling radiating into the leg and foot and impaired proprioception causing an irregular gait and balance. Gluteal nerve irritation may cause pain in the buttocks and atrophy of the gluteal muscles. Pudendal nerve irritation can cause groin and perineal pain, bowel or bladder dysfunction, sexual dysfunction, and impotence. Irritation to the pudendal nerve has also been associated with prostatitis in men.

Sitting, walking, and climbing stairs often worsens the pain. Sitting, particularly with the affected hip flexed and adducted, such as with the legs crossed, often increases pain. Any posture or activity that opposes abduction or lateral rotation, the actions of the piriformis, stretches the muscle and may increase symptoms. If the condition has become chronic or is combined with hyperlordosis, it may be difficult for the person to find a comfortable position when sitting or lying down. Lateral rotation of the hip may relieve symptoms, but maintaining this posture encourages the deviation by keeping the piriformis short and weakening the medial rotators of the hip, decreasing their ability to oppose lateral rotation. Anomalies in posture associated with changes in the piriformis muscle may also decrease mobility in the sacroiliac joint and lead to changes in the muscles that attach to the sacrum and ilium, namely the latissimus dorsi, the lumbar erector spinae, and quadratus lumborum.

The further the syndrome progresses, the greater is the chance that the nerves will become damaged, causing changes in the tone and strength of the muscles innervated by them. In chronic cases, the client may develop an unsteady gait and postural instability due to impaired proprioception and weakening of the muscles from the gluteal region down to the foot. One presentation of this impairment is drop foot or difficulty in dorsiflexing the ankle, which causes the foot to drag or strike hard onto the ground when walking. Chronic compression may also contribute to edema in the lower leg and pallor, cooling, or dryness in the skin of the buttocks and leg. Therefore, it is important for a person suffering from even mild symptoms of piriformis syndrome to be treated as soon as possible.

Possible Causes and Contributing Factors

The piriformis muscle is the biggest of the six lateral rotators of the hip. It originates on the anterior surface of the sacrum and inserts on the superior aspect of the greater trochanter. The piriformis laterally rotates the hip and abducts the flexed hip. The sciatic nerve becomes compressed when the piriformis is shortened; it can also become hypertonic and develop trigger points. The other lateral rotators, namely the quadratus femoris, obturator internus and externus, and the gemellus superior and inferior, are likely involved in the postural deviation and should also be treated.

Standing with one hip laterally rotated with the weight on one leg or squatting with the knees separated also shortens the lateral rotators (Fig. 9-2). Sitting with the knees widely separated—a common posture for pregnant women or clients with a large abdomen—abducts and laterally rotates the hip, and passively shortens the muscles that perform this action. Adding weight or resistance to any of these activities increases the risk of spasm and trigger points in the piriformis.

The piriformis is overactive when the client's posture involves medial rotation of the hips, valgus of the knees, and eversion of the ankle, a posture often referred to as "knock-kneed" (Fig. 9-3). In this posture, the lateral rotators are overstretched and overworked as antagonists to the medial rotation of the hips, particularly when walking, running, or climbing stairs. When hyperlordosis coexists with piriformis syndrome, muscles attached to the ilium, sacrum, and

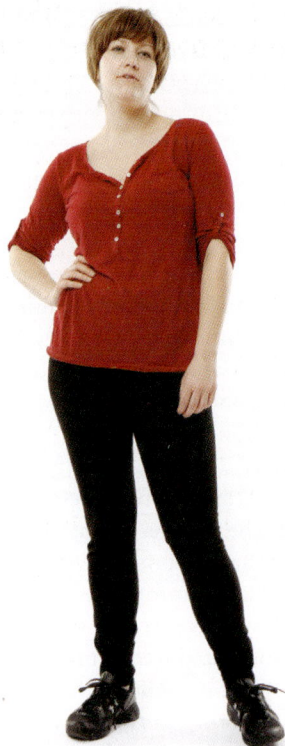

Figure 9-2 **Postural imbalance.** Standing with one or both hips laterally rotated, particularly when the weight is shifted to one side, can contribute to shortening, trigger points, and spasm in the piriformis.

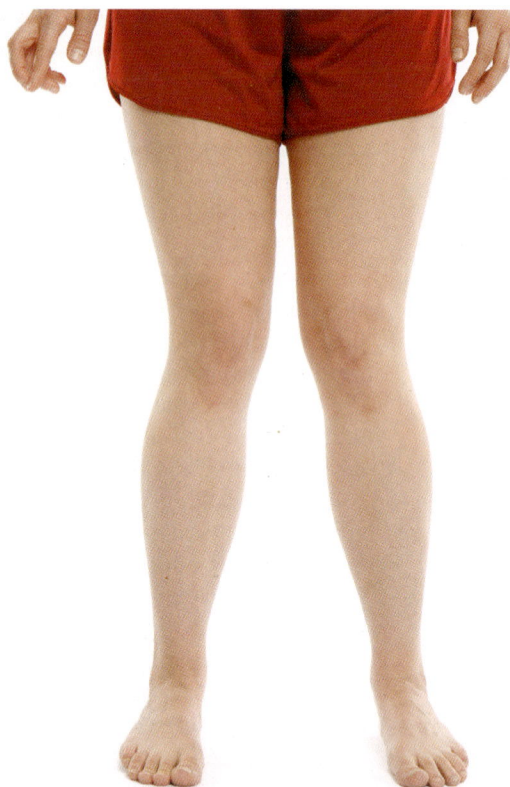

Figure 9-3 **Knee valgus.** With valgus of the knees and medial rotation of the hips, the piriformis may become overactive as an antagonist, resulting in taut bands and trigger points that can irritate the sciatic nerve.

femur work harder to stabilize the joints, which may increase tension. Any increase in the tone of the gluteal muscles may increase the possibility of the sciatic nerve becoming compressed between the piriformis and the pelvis. Postural deviations and the signs and symptoms of plantar fasciitis may also be found in clients with symptoms of piriformis syndrome when these deviations involve rotation of the hips. With each of the postural deviations and activities described above, adhesions and trigger points may develop, reducing the ROM of the hip and sacroiliac joints.

Try these positions yourself. Begin by standing in the anatomic position. Now, laterally rotate one or both hips. Notice changes in the pressure on your pelvis, hips, knees, and ankles. Walk forward, and notice which muscles are compensating. When you stop walking, with the hips still laterally rotated, stand with your weight on one leg and notice how your pelvis, sacrum, and hips feel. With the hips still laterally rotated, sit down. Notice how your spine and pelvis compensate for this posture. If you draw your knees closer together, can you feel a stretch in the piriformis?

Now, stand and medially rotate your hips. Notice the change in distance between your knees, the angle of your femur, and the eversion in your ankle. Did you increase flexion in your knees to keep from straining the joint? While maintaining these deviations, walk forward. Feel the stress on your gluteal muscles and lateral rotators, the relative restriction in the ROM in your hips, and the stress on your knee as you try to move fluidly.

Carrying bulky objects, such as a wallet in a back pocket, can also compress the piriformis and the sciatic nerve, causing irritation, inflammation, spasm, and trigger points. Wearing tight pants low on the hips can put pressure on the sacrum, compressing the sciatic nerve as well as putting pressure on the lateral femoral cutaneous nerve at the anterior superior iliac spine, which may cause numbness and tingling in the anterior and lateral leg. Wearing high heels can contribute to atypical postures that contribute to hyperlordosis and piriformis syndrome. Dancers are often trained to adjust their posture to accentuate lateral rotation in the hips and plantar flexion of the ankle. A dancer who is still performing is unlikely to agree to therapy that restores a more balanced posture. The structures causing pain or other symptoms can be treated, although it may be necessary to omit any techniques intended to adjust posture, such as releasing deep fascial restrictions or fully lengthening the lateral rotators. In this case, the client is at risk for recurring symptoms.

Trauma, such as a fall or car accident, can cause inflammation of the piriformis, irritation to the nerves and vessels, and scar tissue formation. Trauma may also cause myositis ossificans—a calcification in the muscle that can induce symptoms of piriformis syndrome. Consult your pathology book for massage cautions and contraindications for clients with myositis ossificans. Other contributing factors include hip replacement, an aneurysm of the gluteal artery, degenerative disc disease, facet irritation, or bursitis at the greater trochanter. Consult the client's health care provider to determine the best treatment plan in these cases.

Other factors associated with nerve impairment include obesity, hypothyroid condition, arthritis, diabetes, gout, hormonal changes, lymphedema, rheumatoid arthritis, lupus, and Lyme disease. In these cases, the symptoms may quickly resolve once the associated condition is controlled. During pregnancy, body fluids and abdominal size increase while the center of gravity changes, which may contribute to compression that is likely to resolve after childbirth. Smoking cigarettes—although it is not a cause of piriformis syndrome—exacerbates the inflammatory process and thus can intensify the symptoms. Alcoholism, poor nutrition, vitamin B deficiency, and general stress may also contribute to nerve impairment.

Because so many potential factors contribute to peripheral neuropathies, it is essential to understand the client's health history before proceeding with treatment. Many of the conditions listed above involve contraindications for massage therapy or require adjustments to treatment. Moreover, when a systemic condition is a contributing factor for a peripheral neuropathy, particularly if that systemic condition is not being monitored by a health care provider, massage therapy alone may bring only temporary relief of symptoms. Refer the client to his or her health care provider for medical assessment if you suspect a systemic condition, and discuss massage treatment plans with the health care provider if such a condition is diagnosed.

Table 9-1 lists conditions commonly confused with or contributing to piriformis syndrome.

Contraindications and Special Considerations

First, it is essential to understand the cause of sciatic nerve symptoms. If a systemic condition is present, work with the client's physician, and consult a pathology text for massage therapists before proceeding. Following are a few general cautions:

- **Underlying pathologies.** Systemic conditions including diabetes, rheumatoid arthritis, and hypothyroidism may contribute to peripheral neuropathies. Spondylolisthesis or degenerative disc disease may be present. If you suspect an underlying condition (consult Table 9-1 and your pathology book for signs and symptoms), refer the client to his or her health care provider for medical assessment before initiating treatment. If the client is diagnosed with an underlying pathology that is not contraindicated for massage, work with the health care provider to develop a treatment plan that is appropriate for that individual.
- **Endangerment sites.** Be cautious near endangerment sites in the popliteal and femoral areas.
- **Reproducing symptoms.** Symptoms may occur during treatment if you manually compress the sciatic nerve or if the client's posture causes anatomic structures to compress them. If treatment produces symptoms, first adjust the client to a more neutral posture. If this does not relieve the symptoms, reduce your pressure or move away from the area. You may be able to treat around the site that reproduced the symptoms, but proceed with caution.

| Table 9-1 | Differentiating Conditions Commonly Confused with or Contributing to Piriformis Syndrome | | |

Condition	Typical Signs and Symptoms	Testing	Massage Therapy
Sacroiliac joint dysfunction	Pain in the low back, hip, or pelvis Postural deviations Atypical gait	Physical exam Stork (Gillet's) test Gaenslen's test Yeoman's test X-ray	Massage therapy is indicated when the cause is neuromuscular. Consult with the health care provider if an underlying cause is suspected.
Bursitis at greater trochanter	Aching in hip Pain worsens with movement or when lying on the affected side Feeling of swelling or fullness in the hip Skin is warm to the touch	Physical exam X-ray MRI	Massage therapy is systemically contraindicated if bursitis is due to infection. Massage is locally contraindicated in the acute stage to avoid increased swelling. In the subacute stage, massage to structures surrounding the joint is indicated.
Herniated lumbar disc	Muscle spasm Weakness or atrophy Low back pain Pain in buttocks, legs, and feet worsen when coughing, laughing, or straining Numbness and tingling in legs and feet	Physical exam including muscle reflexes and strength Straight leg raise test X-ray, CT, MRI, Electromyography (EMG) Myelogram	Massage therapy is indicated with caution and proper training. Work with the health care team.
Nerve root compression (radiculopathy)	Muscle spasm, weakness, or atrophy Pain radiates to the extremities	Kemp's test Valsalva's test Neurological exam to test reflexes, sensation, and strength	Massage therapy is indicated if the cause and location of the compression are understood. Take care not to increase the compression or reproduce symptoms.
Diabetes	Frequent urination, frequent thirst, increased appetite, fatigue, nausea	Physical exam Fasting blood sugar test	Massage therapy is indicated when tissues and circulation are not compromised.
Myositis ossificans	Local mass that is hard and tender Limited ROM in joint involved	Physical exam X-ray	Massage therapy is locally contraindicated to avoid increased bleeding. Working around the edges of the injury may stimulate reabsorption.
Lumbar spinal stenosis	Pain and cramping in the legs Radiating back or hip pain Numbness, tingling, or weakness in the leg or foot Balance disturbance Loss of bowel or bladder function	Physical exam Spinal X-ray MRI CT scan or myelogram Bone scan	Massage therapy is indicated with caution. Work with the health care provider. Client may receive corticosteroid injections or may be using anti-inflammatory medication.
Spondylolisthesis (begins in the lumbar region and proceeds to the thoracic spine)	Lumbar hyperlordosis Pain in low back, buttocks, and thighs Stiff back	X-ray Straight leg raise test	Massage is indicated. Stretching and strengthening are encouraged.

Table 9-1	Differentiating Conditions Commonly Confused with or Contributing to Piriformis Syndrome (Continued)		
Condition	**Typical Signs and Symptoms**	**Testing**	**Massage Therapy**
Spinal or sciatic tumors	Pain in the back, hips, legs, and feet Loss of sensation or weakness in legs Difficulty walking Decreased sensitivity Loss of bowel or bladder function Varying degrees of paralysis Scoliosis or spinal deformity	MRI CT scan PET scan CBC Myelogram Biopsy	Refer to the health care provider if you suspect a tumor. Work with the health care provider if a tumor is diagnosed. Recommendations for massage depend on the type and location of the tumor.
Pudendal nerve irritation	Pain in the groin, genitals, and rectum Constipation Pain and straining during bowel movements Straining or burning when urinating Painful intercourse Sexual dysfunction	Pudendal nerve motor latency test (PNMLT) Electromyography (EMG) Diagnostic nerve blocks Magnetic resonance neurography (MRN)	Often the muscles of the pelvic floor are involved. Massage is indicated when treatment of these muscles is within the scope of practice for massage therapists. Work with the health care provider.

■ **Treatment duration and pressure.** If the client is elderly, has degenerative disease, or has been diagnosed with a condition that diminishes activities of daily living, you may need to adjust your pressure as well as the treatment duration. Frequent half-hour sessions may suit the client better.

■ **Positioning.** Use bolsters to position a client for comfort as well as to reduce postures that reproduce symptoms. In the supine position, reducing lateral rotation of the hips by placing bolsters at the lateral knee helps to keep the muscle closer to anatomic length and may facilitate access to the piriformis. If hyperlordosis is present, see Chapter 8 for guidelines.

■ **Friction.** Do not use deep frictions if the client has an inflammatory condition such as rheumatoid arthritis or osteoarthritis, if the health of the underlying tissues is compromised, or if the client is taking anti-inflammatory medication. Friction creates an inflammatory process, which may interfere with the intended action of anti-inflammatory medication. Recommend that your client refrain from taking such medication for several hours prior to treatment if the health care provider agrees.

■ **Injections.** If the client has had a steroid, Botox, or analgesic injection within 2 weeks of treatment, avoid that area. These injections reduce sensation and alter the physiology of the muscle, which may prevent the client from assessing your pressure adequately.

■ **Tissue length.** It is important when treating myofascial tissues that you do not further lengthen those that are already stretched. Assess for myofascial restrictions first and treat only those that are clearly present. Likewise, overstretched muscles should not be stretched from origin to insertion. If you treat trigger points in overstretched tissue, use heat or a localized pin and stretch technique instead of full ROM stretches.

■ **Hypermobile joints and unstable ligaments.** Be cautious with mobilizations if the client has hypermobile joints or if ligaments are unstable due to injury, pregnancy or a systemic condition.

Massage Therapy Research

A thorough literature review identified no peer-reviewed studies specifically on the benefits of massage therapy for piriformis syndrome. Much of the literature on the use of manual therapy to treat piriformis syndrome is found in textbooks and originates in other disciplines such as physical medicine, physical therapy, and chiropractic care. A closer examination is needed of the benefits of massage therapy applied to lengthen the tissues that are shortened and hypertonic along with self-care intended to strengthen the muscles that are lengthened and weak.

Several literature reviews explore the use of physical or manual therapy for relieving piriformis syndrome symptoms, although none of these offer specific treatment plans, and most cases involved surgery, Botox or other injections, and other interventions that include manual therapy only in an adjunctive role. The work of Travell and Simons (1999) explaining the role of trigger points in developing piriformis syndrome is sometimes mentioned, but the usual therapeutic intervention described to relieve trigger points is vapocoolant spray. "Massage Therapy and Restless Legs Syndrome" by Meg Russell (2007) mentions a relationship between piriformis syndrome and restless leg syndrome, but that study does not focus on symptoms specific to piriformis syndrome. In 2006, Peggi Honig received the Runner-Up Award from the Massage Therapy Foundation's Student Case Report Contest for her study, "A Case Report of the Treatment of Piriformis Syndrome: Applying Modalities of Therapeutic Bodywork." That study describes the case of a 43-year-old female with a history of chronic pain for a few years prior to this case study, whose symptoms of piriformis syndrome were reduced following massage therapy. Although the case study is unpublished, and a more comprehensive design may result in more conclusive findings, its outcome is encouraging.

WORKING WITH THE CLIENT

Client Assessment

The symptoms of piriformis syndrome can be confused with more serious conditions, and a wide variety of possible factors can contribute to its development. All of these elements add up to many variations in how a client may present. For example, a client with lateral rotation of the hip who tends to stand with more weight on one leg may present with lateral flexion of the thorax, an elevated iliac crest, sacroiliac joint immobility, and rotation in the hips or spine affecting the latissimus dorsi, abdominal obliques, multifidi and rotatores, and the ligaments connecting the sacrum, pelvis, and spine. Hyperlordosis may also be present (see Chapter 8). What follows are common presentations for piriformis syndrome. However, it is essential to assess every involved joint to put together an accurate picture for each individual client.

Assessment begins with your first contact with a client. In some cases, this may be on the telephone when an appointment is requested. Ask in advance if the client is seeking treatment for a specific area of pain so that you can prepare yourself.

Table 9-2 lists questions to ask the client when taking a health history.

POSTURAL ASSESSMENT

Allow the client to walk and enter the room ahead of you while you assess his or her posture and movements. Look for imbalances or patterns of compensation for deviations common with piriformis syndrome. Watch as the client climbs steps, looking for reduced mobility in the hips or whether the client favors one side. Assess for joint instability, limping, drop foot, lateral rotation of the hip, or hyperlordosis. Have the client sit to fill out the assessment form and watch to see if

Table 9-2	Health History

Questions for the Client	Importance to the Treatment Plan
Where do you feel symptoms?	The location of symptoms gives clues to the location of trigger points, injury, or other contributing factors. Radiating pain or numbness and tingling in the extremities indicate nerve involvement.
Describe what your symptoms feel like.	Differentiate between possible origins of symptoms, and determine the involvement of nerves or blood vessels.
Do any movements make it worse or better?	Locate tension, weakness, or compression in structures producing such movements.
Have you seen a health care provider for this condition? What was the diagnosis? What tests were performed?	Medical tests may reveal contributing factors as well as contraindications. If no tests were performed by the health care provider making a diagnosis, use the tests described later in this chapter for your assessment. If your assessment is inconsistent with the diagnosis, ask the client to discuss your findings with the health care provider or for permission to contact the provider directly.
Have you been diagnosed with a condition such as diabetes, osteoporosis, rheumatoid arthritis, or hypothyroid?	Systemic conditions may contribute to signs and symptoms, may require adjustments to treatment, and may impact treatment outcomes.
Have you had an injury or surgery or did your symptoms begin during a pregnancy?	Injury or surgery and resulting scar tissue may cause adhesions, hyper- or hypotonicity, and atypical ROM. Changes in posture during pregnancy may be a contributing factor.
What type of work, hobbies, or other regular activities do you do?	Repetitive motions and static postures that increase lateral rotation or abduction of the hip may contribute to the client's condition.
Are you taking any prescribed medications or herbal or other supplements?	Medication of all types may contribute to symptoms or involve contraindications or cautions.
Have you had a corticosteroid, Botox, or analgesic injection in the past 2 weeks? Where?	Local massage is contraindicated.
Have you taken a pain reliever or muscle relaxant within the past 4 hours?	The client may not be able to judge your pressure.
Have you taken anti-inflammatory medication within the past 4 hours? medication.	Deep friction initiates an inflammatory response and should not be performed if the client has recently taken anti-inflammatory

he or she lowers into the chair cautiously or shifts around to find a comfortable position. Watch also as the client stands up to see if he or she is able to stand without assistance or if he or she lifts out of the chair using the arms or by leaning on a stable surface.

When assessing the standing posture, be sure that the client is standing comfortably and naturally. If he or she deliberately tries to stand in the anatomic position, you will not get an accurate assessment of his or her posture in daily life. In a postural assessment, you may notice a lateral rotation of the hips if the piriformis is short and hypertonic. Lateral rotation of one hip is often accompanied by rotation of the pelvis and slight flexion of that hip. The client may stand with the affected leg anterior to the unaffected leg so that one foot is in front of the other. Compensating patterns may include hyperextension in the knee of the unaffected leg, because the client shifts weight to that leg while favoring the affected hip. The client may also present with hyperlordosis; see Chapter 8 for postural assessment with hyperlordosis. If the client has sacroiliac joint dysfunction, he or she may have an elevated hip, rotation in the pelvis, or lateral flexion of the thoracic and lumbar spine. If the client's symptoms are due to overuse of the piriformis as an antagonist, you may observe medially rotated hips, knee valgus, and eversion of the ankle.

Figure 9-4 compares a healthy posture to a posture affected by piriformis syndrome due to short lateral rotators of the hip.

Shortened
Lengthened

Tensor fasciae latae

Obturator externus

Adductor brevis

Adductor longus

Adductor magnus

Gracilis

Piriformis

Superior gemellus

Obturator internus
and externus

Inferior gemellus

Quadratus femoris

Gluteus maximus

Adductor magnus

Semitendinosus

Semimembranosus

Gracilis

Pectineus

Adductor brevis

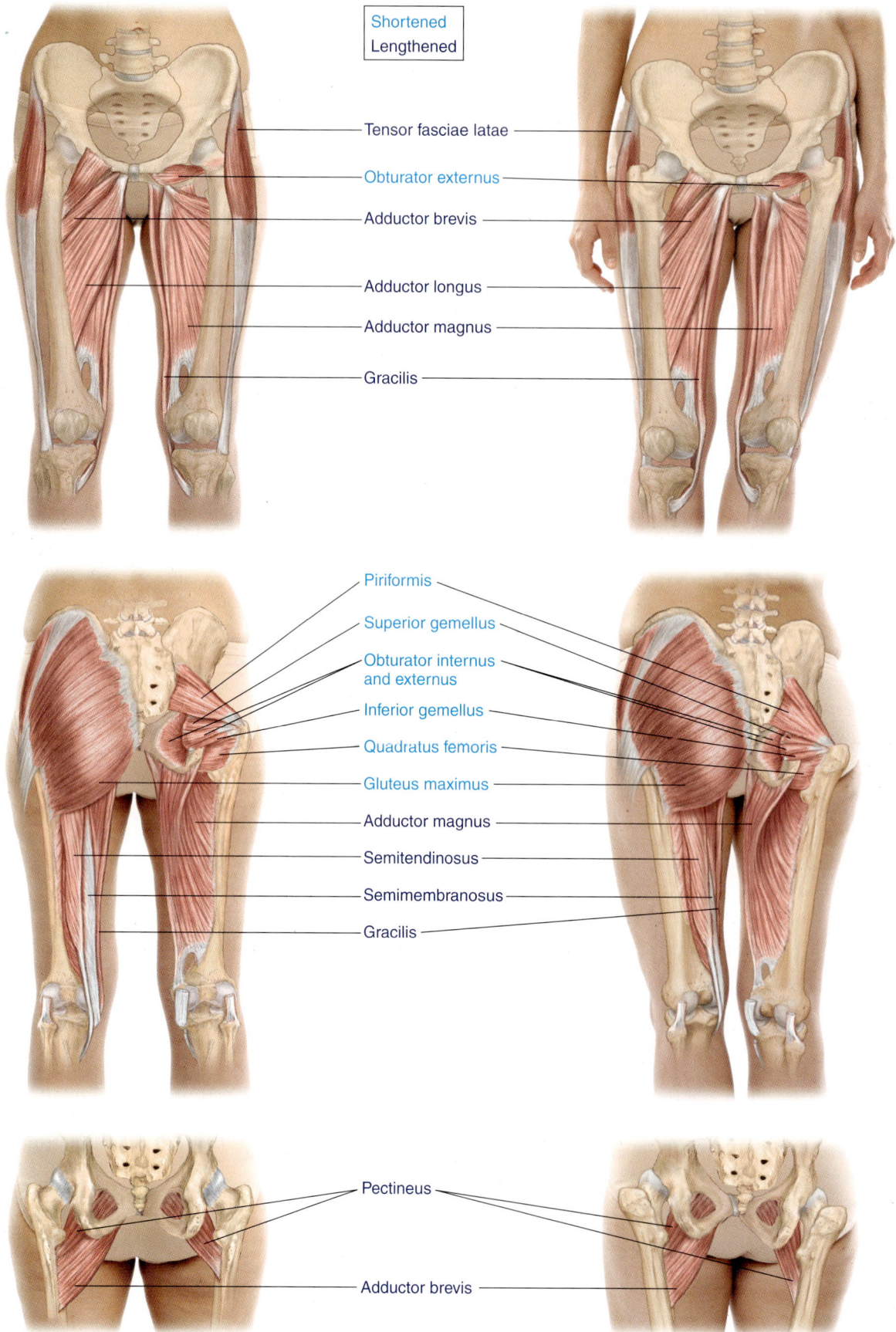

Figure 9-4   Postural assessment comparison. Compare the postures in these images. In the image on the right, note the lateral rotation in the right hip, tilting and rotation of the pelvis, and right lateral flexion of the thorax.

ROM ASSESSMENT

Test the ranges of hip motion that recruit the piriformis as either agonist or antagonist. Since it allows the client to control the amount of movement and stay within a pain-free range, only active ROM should be used in the acute stage of injury to prevent undue pain or re-injury. Box 9-1 presents the average active ROM results for the joints involved in piriformis syndrome.

Box 9-1   **AVERAGE ACTIVE ROM FOR JOINTS INVOLVED IN PIRIFORMIS SYNDROME**

Hip
Flexion 110–120°
- Rectus femoris
- Gluteus medius (anterior fibers)
- Tensor fasciae latae
- Sartorius
- Psoas major
- Iliacus
- Gluteus minimus
- Adductor magnus
- Adductor longus
- Adductor brevis

Extension 10–15°
- Biceps femoris
- Semitendinosus
- Semimembranosus
- Gluteus maximus
- Gluteus medius (posterior fibers)
- Adductor magnus (posterior fibers)

Lateral Rotation 40–60°
- Biceps femoris
- Gluteus maximus
- Gluteus medius (posterior fibers)
- Sartorius
- Piriformis
- Quadratus femoris
- Obturator internus
- Obturator externus
- Gemellus superior
- Gemellus inferior
- Psoas major
- Iliacus

Medial Rotation 30–40°
- Semitendinosus
- Semimembranosus
- Gluteus medius (anterior fibers)
- Gluteus minimus
- Adductor magnus
- Adductor longus
- Adductor brevis
- Gracilis
- Pectineus
- Tensor fasciae latae

Abduction 30–50°
- Gluteus maximus
- Gluteus medius
- Gluteus minimus

- Tensor fasciae latae
- Sartorius
- Piriformis (with flexed hip)

Adduction 30°
- Adductor magnus
- Adductor longus
- Adductor brevis
- Pectineus
- Gracilis
- Psoas Major
- Iliacus
- Gluteus maximus (low fibers)

Trunk (at lumbar spine)
Flexion 50–60°
- Rectus abdominis
- External oblique (bilateral)
- Internal oblique (bilateral)

Extension 25°
- Spinalis (bilateral
- Longissimus (bilateral)
- Iliocostalis (bilateral)
- Multifidi (bilateral)
- Rotatores (bilateral)
- Quadratus lumborum (bilateral)
- Latissimus dorsi (with arm fixed)

Lateral Flexion 25°
- Spinalis (unilateral)
- Longissimus (unilateral)
- Iliocostalis (unilateral)
- External oblique (unilateral)
- Internal oblique (unilateral)
- Quadratus lumborum (unilateral)
- Latissimus dorsi (unilateral)

Ipsilateral Rotation 20°
- Internal oblique (unilateral)

Contralateral Rotation 20°
- Multifidi (unilateral)
- Rotatores (unilateral)
- External oblique(unilateral)

Knee
Flexion 120–150°
- Biceps femoris
- Semitendinosus
- Semimembranosus

- Gracilis
- Sartorius
- Gastrocnemius
- Popliteus
- Plantaris

Extension 0–15°
- Rectus femoris
- Vastus lateralis
- Vastus medialis
- Vastus intermedius

Medial Rotation (when flexed) 20–30°
- Semitendinosus
- Semimembranosus
- Gracilis
- Sartorius
- Popliteus

Lateral Rotation (when flexed) 30–40°
- Biceps femoris

Ankle
Dorsiflexion 20°
- Tibialis anterior
- Extensor digitorum longus
- Extensor hallucis longus

Plantar flexion 50°
- Gastrocnemius
- Soleus
- Tibialis posterior
- Peroneus longus
- Peroneus brevis
- Flexor digitorum longus
- Flexor hallucis longus
- Plantaris

Inversion 45–60°
- Tibialis anterior
- Tibialis posterior
- Flexor digitorum longus
- Flexor hallucis longus
- Extensor hallucis longus

Eversion 15–30°
- Peroneus longus
- Peroneus brevis
- Extensor digitorum longus

Active ROM

Compare your assessment of the client's active ROM to the values in Box 9-1. Pain and other symptoms may not be reproduced during an active ROM assessment because the client may limit movement to a symptom-free range.

- **Active medial rotation of the hip** may be restricted and cause pain, numbness, and tingling when the piriformis is shortened.
- **Active lateral rotation of the hip** may reduce pain caused by medial rotation when the piriformis is short and tight. Although less common, active lateral rotation of the hip may be restricted or cause pain when the piriformis is overactive as an antagonist to the short and tight medial rotators of the hip or when it is recruited to stabilize the hip joint.
- **Active abduction of the hip.** If the piriformis is short and tight, active abduction of the hip may be weak, and the hip may laterally rotate during the movement. This test is best performed in the side-lying position.

Passive ROM

Compare the client's P ROM on one side to the other. Note and compare the end feel for each range (see Chapter 1 for an explanation of end feel).

- **Passive medial rotation of the hips** may be restricted and cause pain for a client whose posture or activities of daily living favor lateral rotation of the hips.
- **Passive lateral rotation of the hip** may reduce pain caused by medial rotation when the piriformis is short.

Resisted ROM

Use resisted tests to assess the strength of the muscles that cross the hip joint. Compare the strength of the affected side to the unaffected side.

- **Resisted lateral rotation and abduction of the hip** may cause pain in the low back, buttocks, and hip and numbness and tingling in the leg and may reveal weakness in the piriformis. The client may rotate the pelvis to compensate.

SPECIAL TESTS

The following special tests help to determine which muscles are contributing to pain and whether the client should be evaluated by a medical professional using X-ray or other tools, which may reveal conditions that are contraindicated or require special considerations when planning treatment with massage.

The **Valsalva maneuver** may reveal a herniated disc, tumor, or other factor that increases pressure on the spinal cord and is used when the client complains of pain in a localized area along the spine, particularly when coughing or sneezing. A herniated disc does not contraindicate massage, but this test is not specific for the cause of increased pressure. For this reason, if Valsalva maneuver is positive it is best to refer the client to a health care provider for further testing before performing the massage.

1. To avoid even a temporary reduction in circulation, do not perform this test if the client has tested positive for vertebral artery insufficiency (see vertebral artery test in Chapter 4) or has cardiovascular disorders.
2. With the client seated facing you, ask them to take a deep breath and then attempt to forcefully exhale against the closed throat (such as when forcing a bowel movement).
3. The test is positive if the client feels pain in a localized spot along the spine. The client should be evaluated by a medical professional prior to receiving the massage.

The **piriformis length test** assesses the length of the piriformis.

1. The client should lie prone with the knees and feet together and the knees flexed to 90°.
2. Instruct the client to keep the knees together while allowing the feet to fall naturally, unforced, to either side, which will medially rotate the hips and lengthen the piriformis (Fig. 9-5).

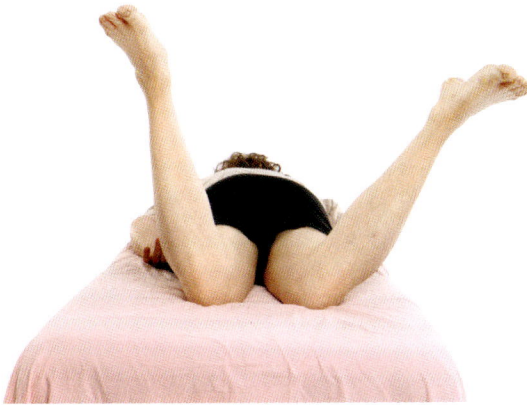

Figure 9-5   **Piriformis length test.** The piriformis is short on the left side, as noted by restricted medial rotation.

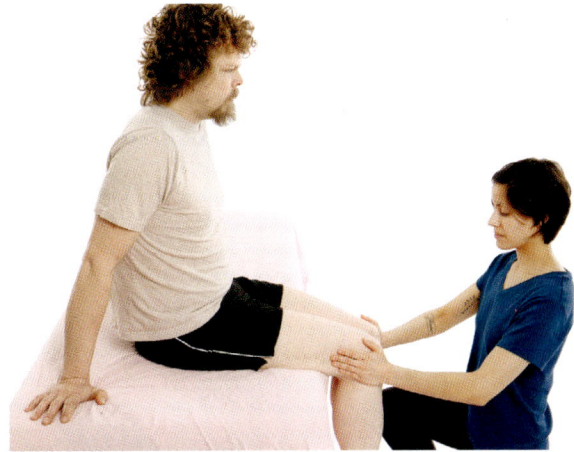

Figure 9-6   **Pace test.** Ask the client to abduct the hips against your resistance to test the strength of the piriformis.

3. Compare the distance that each leg has moved from the midline. Notice whether one has moved further than the other.
4. The test is positive for a shortened piriformis on the side with less movement from the midline.

The **Pace test** is intended to assess the strength of the piriformis.

1. The client should be supine or seated with the knees placed together.
2. Place your hands on the sides of both knees, and ask the client to push the knees apart (abduct) against your resistance (Fig. 9-6).
3. Note weakness on either side. If the syndrome is unilateral, abduction on the affected side will be weaker than on the unaffected side.

The **stork test** is intended to assess sacroiliac joint mobility.

1. The client should stand near a stable surface or wall against which he or she can lean to maintain balance during the test.
2. Begin on the side you suspect is dysfunctional, but it is best to compare the results of both sides.
3. Kneel or sit behind the standing client with one thumb on the posterior superior iliac spine of the affected side and the other thumb on the sacrum at the same level.
4. Instruct the client to flex the hip and knee on the affected side to 90° or within his or her comfort range (Fig. 9-7). Notice the relative movement of your thumbs as the client flexes the hip.
5. When the sacroiliac joint is normally mobile, the ilium should rotate posteriorly, moving the thumb on the posterior superior iliac spine inferiorly. The test is positive for decreased sacroiliac joint mobility if the thumb on the posterior superior iliac spine moves superiorly as the client flexes the hip.

PALPATION ASSESSMENT

Assess the low back, gluteal area, and affected leg for atypical temperature, color, and texture. Compression of the sciatic nerve or the vessels feeding the soft tissues may cause cool skin, swelling, boggy texture, and even reduced hair growth. You may find adhesions around the attachment sites of the gluteal muscles and the lateral rotators of the hips. If bursitis is a contributing factor, the area around the greater trochanter may be hot and tender.

Palpate the gluteal muscles and the lateral rotators of the hip for tenderness, tone, and trigger points. Trigger points in the piriformis refer into the gluteal area and down the posterior thigh. If hyperlordosis is also present, see Chapter 8 for palpation guidelines.

If the client presents with an elevated iliac crest, sacroiliac joint dysfunction, or lateral flexion of the thorax or lumbar spine, assess the latissimus dorsi, quadratus lumborum, internal and external

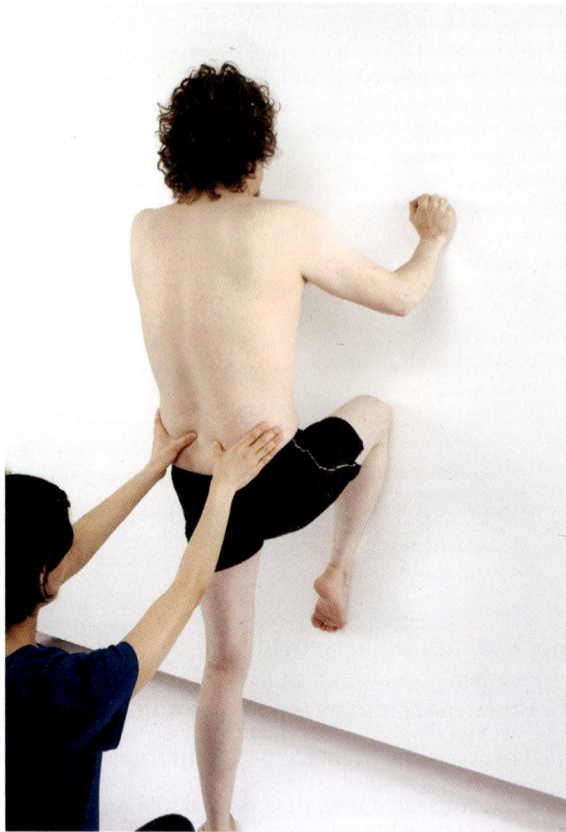

Figure 9-7 **Stork test.** Assess the mobility of the sacroiliac joint with the stork test.

obliques, and thoracic and lumbar erector spinae. Although the focus here is on the muscles that are directly related to the postural imbalance seen in piriformis syndrome, it is essential to assess the synergists and antagonists in each ROM for these joints. For example, although the piriformis is a lateral rotator of the hip, it also abducts the hip. When it is short or otherwise compromised, any of its actions may be compromised, and any of the synergists and antagonists for each of its actions may be affected. In this example, you may find adhesions in the gluteal muscles and the lateral rotators. The biceps femoris, sartorius, and iliopsoas, which laterally rotate the hip, may also be short, adhered, or hypertonic. The medial rotators of the hip may be stretched due to the postural imbalance favoring lateral rotation and taut as a result of overwork as antagonists to lateral rotation. Overstretched muscles that may be adhered and contain trigger points include the semimembranosus, semitendinosus, adductor magnus, adductor longus, adductor brevis, gracilis, and pectineus.

Condition-Specific Massage

Since the causes of pain, numbness, and tingling in the low back and leg vary widely, the exact cause can be difficult to pinpoint and more than one condition may coexist. Systemic conditions such as diabetes may be a contributing factor to neuropathies and involve cautions or contraindications for massage therapy. If you feel uncertain whether the client's symptoms are caused by piriformis dysfunction, refer the client to his or her health care provider for medical assessment.

It is essential for the treatment to be relaxing. You are not likely to eliminate the symptoms associated with piriformis syndrome or any of the coexisting conditions in a single treatment. Do not attempt to do so by treating aggressively. Be sure to ask your client to let you know if the amount of pressure you are applying keeps them from fully relaxing. If the client responds by tensing muscles or has a facial expression that looks distressed, reduce your pressure. Remember that you are working on tissue that is compromised. Ask the client to let you know if any part of your treatment reproduces symptoms, and always work within his or her tolerance. Deep palpation of a trigger point may cause pain at the upper end of the client's tolerance. Explain this to

Legend:
- ▲ Trigger point
- ● Referral pattern
- ● ▲ Gluteus medius
- ● ▲ Gluteus minimus
- ● ▲ Piriformis

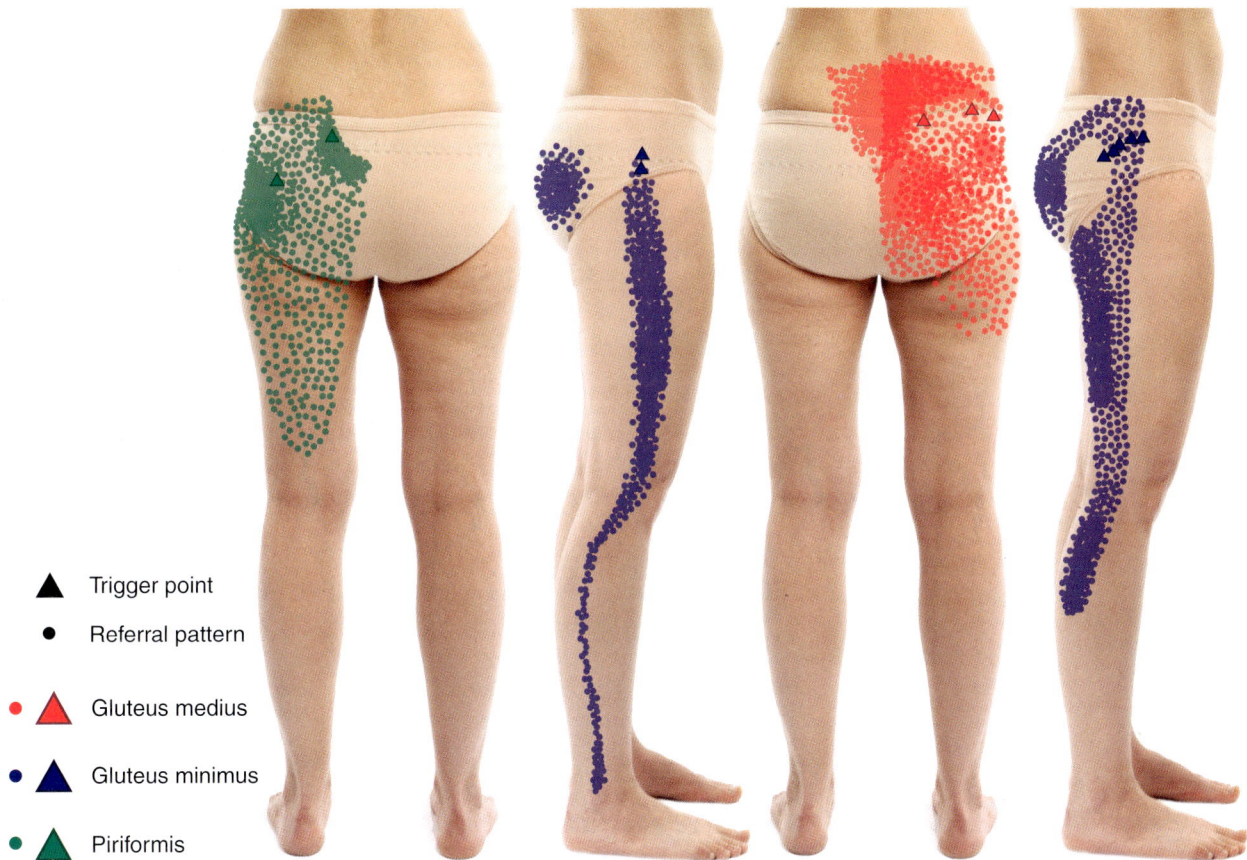

Figure 9-8 Common trigger points associated with piriformis syndrome and their referral patterns.

your client, describe a pain scale, and suggest the level of pain that should not be exceeded; ask them to breathe deeply during the application of the technique. As the trigger point is deactivated, the referred pain will also diminish. Common trigger points and their referral patterns are shown in Figure 9-8.

If symptoms such as numbness and tingling are reproduced, you may be compressing the sciatic nerve. Adjust the client to a more neutral position, reduce your pressure, or move slightly off the area, and make a note about it, because this may help you understand more clearly exactly which neuromuscular condition is contributing to the client's symptoms.

The following are treatment suggestions for the more common presentation of piriformis syndrome caused primarily by the short, tight piriformis irritating the sciatic nerve. If the client has an acute injury, PRICE (protection, rest, ice, compression, and elevation) is the protocol. You may work conservatively proximal or distal to the site, but avoid the area of injury until the subacute or chronic stage.

- Begin with the client in a prone position with the ankles bolstered. If one or both heels of the feet fall closer to the midline than the toes, suggesting that the hip is laterally rotated, try to straighten the leg and minimize rotation by placing bolsters on the outside of the thigh just above the knee.
- Apply moist heat to the gluteal area of the affected side if indicated. If both sides are affected, move the heat to the gluteal area on the other side after heating the first.

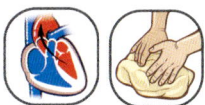

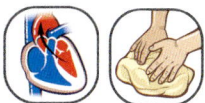

- Use your initial warming strokes to superficially assess the tissues from the trunk down to the feet. You should be able to minimally assess the tissues of the mid and low back, gluteal area, thigh, leg, and feet, which may help you to determine where to focus the time remaining after treating the lateral rotators of the hip.

Treatment icons: 🖐 Increase circulation; 🖐 Reduce adhesions; 🖐 Reduce tension; 🖐 Lengthen tissue; 🖐 Treat trigger points; 🖐 Passive stretch; 🖐 Clear area

■ If you notice swelling around the low back or gluteal area, apply superficial draining strokes toward the nearest lymph nodes.

■ Before applying emollient, assess for and treat myofascial restrictions across the thoracolumbar aponeurosis.

■ Assess and treat hypertonicity and trigger points in the latissimus dorsi, lumbar erector spinae, and quadratus lumborum, particularly if hyperlordosis is also present. Assess and treat these briefly for the moment. You can return to treat the area again if time permits.

■ Remove moist heat, and assess the tissues around the sacrum and greater trochanter for myofascial restrictions and release them. It may be difficult to assess the gluteal area for superficial myofascial restrictions because of the presence of adipose tissue. Superficial restrictions around the attachment sites may be addressed more readily.

■ Treat the gluteal muscles for hypertonicity and trigger points (Fig. 9-9). Knead the tissues along the full length of the iliac crest and sacrum and around the greater trochanter to treat the attachments of the gluteal muscles and lateral rotators. To release adhesions in the deeper gluteal muscles, use cross-fiber friction beginning at the sacrum and move toward the greater trochanter. Lengthen tissues in each of the fiber directions of all three gluteal muscles to assess and treat hypertonicity and trigger points.

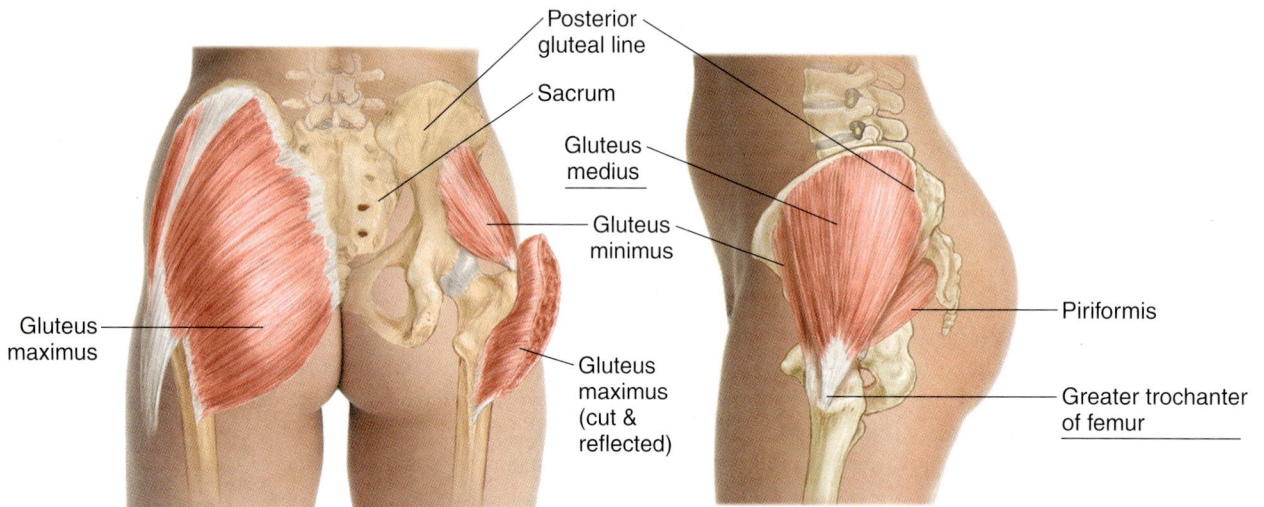

GLUTEUS MAXIMUS

Origin	*Coccyx, lateral sacrum, posterior iliac crest, sacrotuberous and sacroiliac ligaments.*
Insertion	***Upper fibers**: iliotibial band; **lower fibers**: gluteal tuberosity.*
Action	***All fibers**: extend hip, laterally rotate hip, posterior pelvic tilt; **upper fibers**: abduct hip; **lower fibers**: adduct hip.*
Nerve	*Inferior gluteal.*

GLUTEUS MEDIUS

Origin	*Surface of ilium between iliac crest gluteal lines.*
Insertion	*Greater trochanter of the femur.*
Action	***All fibers**: Abduct hip; **anterior fibers**: flex hip, medially rotate hip; **posterior fibers**: extend hip, laterally rotate hip, posterior pelvic tilt.*
Nerve	*Superior gluteal.*

GLUTEUS MINIMUS

Origin	*Ilium between gluteal lines.*
Insertion	*Anterior aspect of greater trochanter.*
Action	*Abduct hip, medially rotate hip, flex hip.*
Nerve	*Superior gluteal.*

Figure 9-9   The gluteal muscles. Warm and treat the gluteal muscles before working on the deeper piriformis. Adapted from Clay JH, Pounds DM. *Basic Clinical Massage Therapy: Integrating Anatomy and Treatment*, 2nd ed. Philadelphia: Lippincott Williams & Wilkins, 2008.

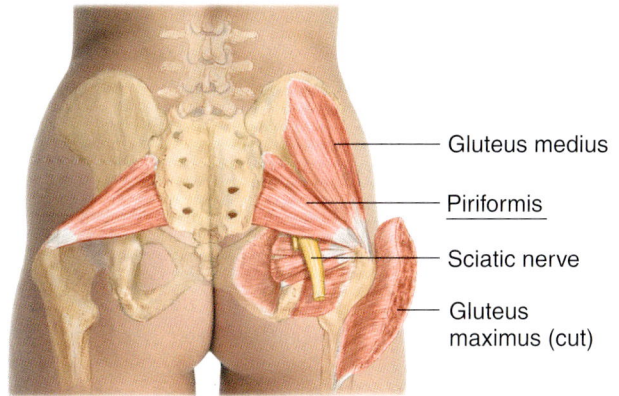

- Gluteus medius
- Piriformis
- Sciatic nerve
- Gluteus maximus (cut)

Figure 9-10   Piriformis. Find and then treat the piriformis for hypertonicity and trigger points. Adapted from Clay JH, Pounds DM. *Basic Clinical Massage Therapy: Integrating Anatomy and Treatment*, 2nd ed. Philadelphia: Lippincott Williams & Wilkins, 2008.

PIRIFORMIS

Origin	*Anterior surface of sacrum.*
Insertion	*Greater trochanter of the femur.*
Action	*Laterally rotate hip, abduct the flexed hip.*
Nerve	*L5-S2 nerve roots of sacral plexus.*

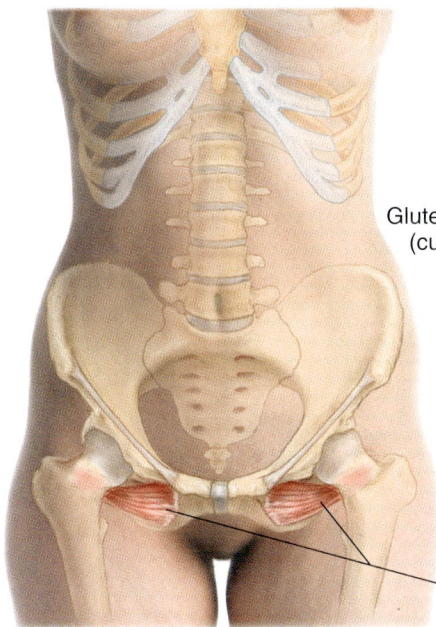

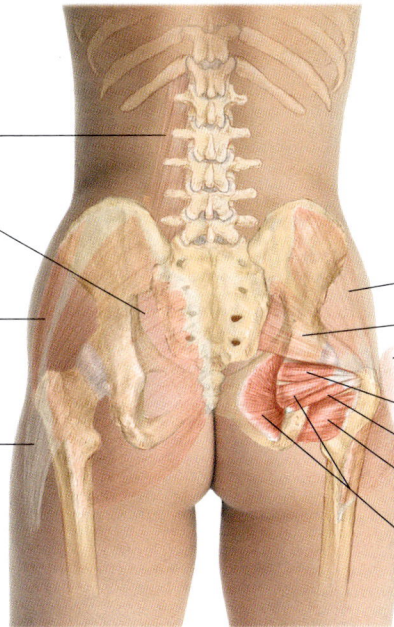

- Psoas major
- Gluteus maximus (cut & reflected on right)
- Tensor fasciae latae
- Iliotibial band
- Obturator externus
- Gluteus medius
- Piriformis
- Gluteus maximus (cut & reflected)
- Superior gemellus
- Inferior gemellus
- Quadratus femoris
- Obturator internus (attachment)

QUADRATUS FEMORIS

Origin	*Lateral ischial tuberosity.*
Insertion	*Crest between greater and lesser trochanter of the femur.*
Action	*Laterally rotate hip.*
Nerve	*L4-S1 nerve roots of sacral plexus.*

OBTURATOR INTERNUS

Origin	*Inferior surface of obturator foramen.*
Insertion	*Medial surface of greater trochanter of the femur.*
Action	*Laterally rotate hip.*
Nerve	*L5-S2 nerve roots of sacral plexus.*

OBTURATOR EXTERNUS

Origin	*Rami of pubis.*
Insertion	*Trochanteric fossa.*
Action	*Laterally rotate hip.*
Nerve	*Obturator.*

SUPERIOR GEMELLUS

Origin	*Ischial spine.*
Insertion	*Upper border of greater trochanter of the femur.*
Action	*Laterally rotate hip.*
Nerve	*L5-S1 nerve roots of sacral plexus.*

INFERIOR GEMELLUS

Origin	*Ischial tuberosity.*
Insertion	*Upper border of greater trochanter of the femur.*
Action	*Laterally rotate hip.*
Nerve	*L5-S1 nerve roots of sacral plexus.*

Figure 9-11   Other lateral rotators of the hip. Assess and treat the deep lateral rotators for hypertonicity and trigger points. Adapted from Clay JH, Pounds DM. *Basic Clinical Massage Therapy: Integrating Anatomy and Treatment*, 2nd ed. Philadelphia: Lippincott Williams & Wilkins, 2008.

■ Once the gluteal muscles are treated sufficiently to access the deeper piriformis, begin your specific work (Fig. 9-10). To find the piriformis, place your fingers midway between the middle of the sacrum and the greater trochanter. Flex the client's knee to 90°, and ask the client to pull the foot away from you against your resistance. This lateral rotation will cause the piriformis to contract under your finger.

■ Once you have found the muscle, slowly lengthen it from origin to insertion. Assess for trigger points as you slowly stroke along the length of the piriformis.

■ Treat trigger points if any are found. Trigger points in the piriformis are frequently found near the greater trochanter and near the sacrum. If your treatment reproduces symptoms, adjust the client's posture, lighten your pressure, or move slightly off the area. As you proceed with the treatment, symptoms may lessen allowing you to treat more directly.

■ Assess the quadratus femoris, obturator internus and externus, and the gemellus superior and inferior for hypertonicity and trigger points (Fig. 9-11). These are small, deep muscles that may be difficult to distinguish. Familiarize yourself with their fiber directions and work generally to increase their length if you are unable to access each one individually. Lengthen these muscles manually, and treat any trigger points found.

■ Stretch the lateral rotators by stabilizing the sacrum with one hand while bending the client's knee to 90° and gently pulling the leg toward you with the other hand (medial rotation) (Fig. 9-12).

■ If the lateral rotators seem resistant to stretch, use postisometric relaxation to encourage lengthening. Bend the knee 90° and minimally rotate the hip medially by bringing the leg closer to you to lengthen the lateral rotators. Instruct the client to laterally rotate the hip by pulling the leg away from you against your resistance and hold for 10 seconds, or less if you feel a tremor or other sign that the muscles are fatiguing. Hold the leg steady while the client releases the contraction; then slowly rotate the hip medially by drawing the leg closer to you as fully as you can within the client's tolerance.

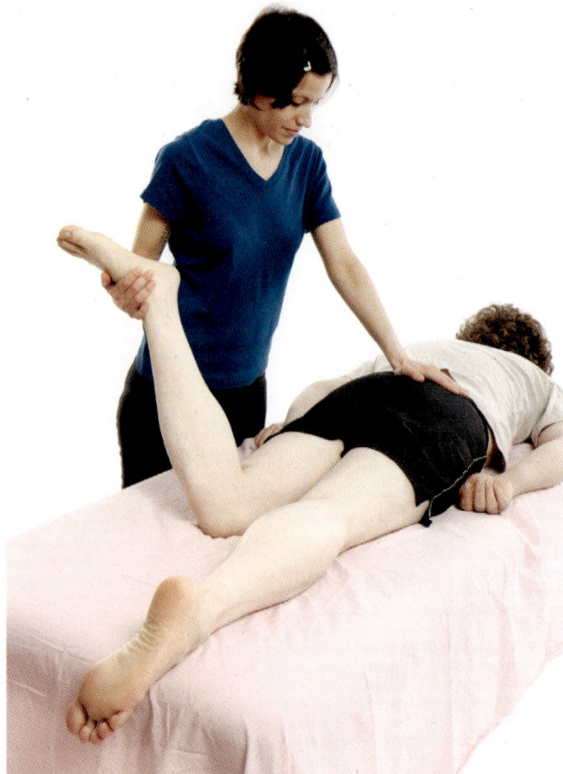

Figure 9-12 **Passively stretch piriformis.**
Stabilize the sacrum, bend the knee to 90°, and draw the client's foot toward you to passively stretch the piriformis.

TREATMENT GOAL

	General	Specific		General
	Superficial		**Deep**	**Superficial**
Mid and low back	Mid and low back	Thoracolumbar Fascia Latissimus dorsi	Erector spinae Quadratus lumborum	
Hip	Hip	Gluteus maximus Gluteus medius	Gluteus minimus Quadratus femoris Obturator internus Obturator externus Gemellus superior Gemellus Inferior Piriformis	
Thigh	Thigh	Sartorius Biceps femoris	Iliopsoas	
		Semitendinosis Gracilis	Adductor magnus Adductor longus Adductor brevis Pectineus Semimembranosis	
Leg	Leg	All muscles of the leg		
Foot	Foot	All muscles of the foot		Foot
				Leg
				Hip and Thigh
				Gluteals
				Mid and low back

STRUCTURES — Proximal / Distal (Central Peripheral) / Peripheral — Proximal

Primary goal for treatment (Piriformis Syndrome)

Figure 9-13 **Piriformis syndrome treatment overview table.** Follow the general principles from left to right or top to bottom when treating piriformis syndrome.

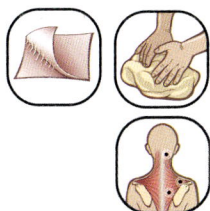

■ Treat the thigh and leg for hypertonicity and trigger points and to restore neuromuscular function. Irritation of the sciatic nerve and its branches can cause changes in the tone and strength of any of the muscles innervated by it. Assess for adhesions, hyper- or hypotonicity, and weakness, and treat accordingly. If the tone is diminished, use stimulating strokes to encourage an increase in tone.

■ Apply superficial gliding to the leg, thigh, and buttocks to clear the areas and encourage venous return.

■ With the remaining time, consider the other possible conditions that may develop with piriformis syndrome and treat these. Hyperlordosis suggests treatment to the hip flexors and lumbar spine extensors. Eversion or inversion of the ankle suggests treatment to the muscles of the lower leg and feet. You may not have time to treat all of these fully, but you can pay attention to some of them in each session, and as the signs and symptoms of piriformis syndrome decrease, you can increase the amount of time you spend in these other areas.

The treatment overview diagram summarizes the flow of treatment (Fig. 9-13).

CLIENT SELF-CARE

The following are intended as general recommendations for stretching and strengthening muscles involved in the client's condition. The objective is to create distance between the attachment sites of muscles that have shortened and to perform repetitions of movements that decrease the distance between the attachments of muscles that have weakened. If you have had no training in remedial exercises and do not feel that you have a functional understanding of stretching and strengthening, refer the client to a professional with training in this area.

Clients often neglect self-care because their daily lives are busy. Encourage them to follow these guidelines:

■ Instruct the client to perform self-care throughout the day, such as while taking a phone call, reading e-mail, washing the dishes, or watching television instead of setting aside extra time. When performing activities while standing, ask the client to notice if he or she is shifting weight to one leg and whether the feet point outward (laterally rotated hips). If so, instruct the client to focus on distributing weight evenly to both legs and on keeping the toes pointed forward within his or her comfort level.

■ Instruct the client on proper seated posture to keep pressure off the weakened joints. Sitting in a chair that supports the back and allows the client to rest the feet flat on the floor with the knees and hips flexed approximately 90° may reduce muscle strain and stress on the joints. To reduce lateral rotation in the hips while sitting for long periods of time, the client can place a band around the knees to keep them from separating.

■ Encourage the client to remove any bulky objects from the back pockets of his or her pants, particularly when sitting.

■ Encourage the client to take regular breaks from repetitive actions.

■ Demonstrate gentle self-massage of the hip to keep adhesions and hypertonicity at bay between treatments.

■ Demonstrate all strengthening exercises and stretches, and have the client perform these in your presence before leaving to ensure that he or she is performing them properly and will not be harmed when practicing alone. Stretches should be held for 15-30 seconds and performed frequently throughout the day, within the client's limits, during an active flare-up. The client should not force the stretch or bounce. It should be slow, gentle, and steady, trying to keep every other muscle as relaxed as possible.

Stretching

To stretch the lateral rotators of the hip, instruct the client to sit at the edge of the chair with the hips medially rotated by bringing the knees together and the feet resting away from the midline, and then have him or her lean forward (Fig. 9-14). Hold the stretch for 15–30 seconds, and then stand and take a few steps to mobilize the hip.

Alternatively, instruct the client to lie supine with the hip and knee of the affected side flexed and the hand of the opposite side rested on the flexed knee. Pull the knee of the affected side medially into a twist until a stretch is felt (Fig. 9-15). Hold the stretch for 15–30 seconds, and then stand and take a few steps to mobilize the hip.

Figure 9-15 **Piriformis stretch.** Draw the flexed knee of the affected side toward the opposite shoulder to stretch the piriformis.

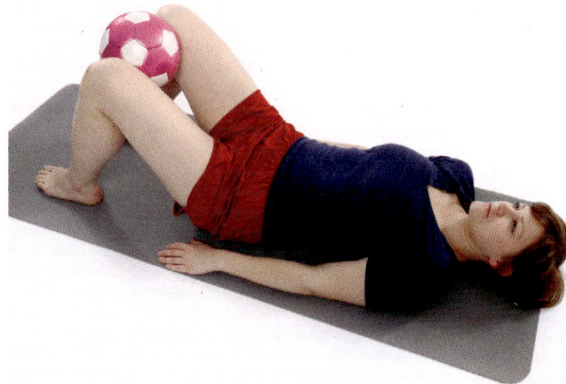

Figure 9-16 **Strengthen adductors.** Instruct the client to squeeze the knees together against the resistance of a ball or other object to strengthen the adductors.

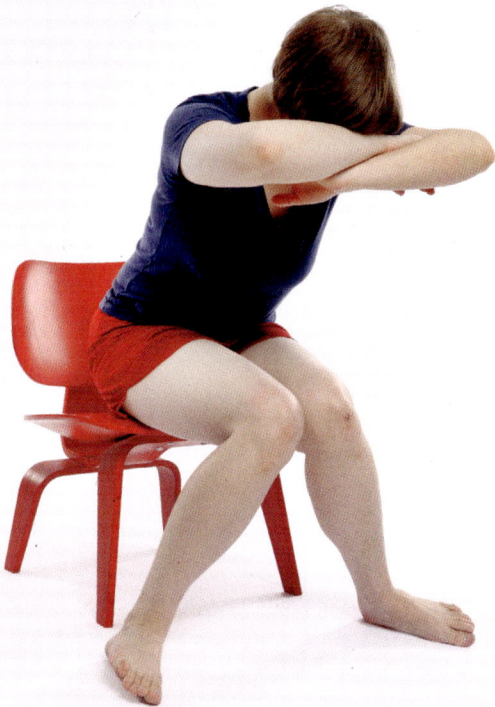

Figure 9-14 **Piriformis seated stretch.** Sit with the knees together and the hips medially rotated while leaning forward to stretch the piriformis.

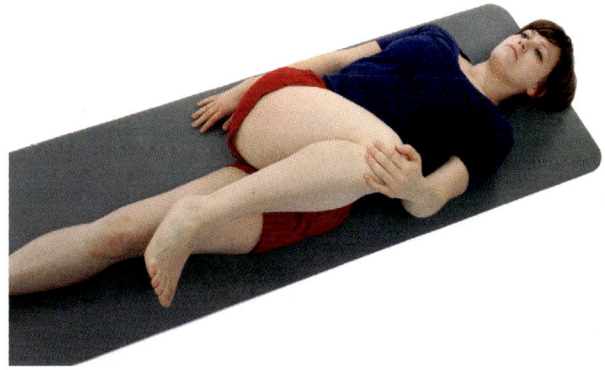

Strengthening

The choice of strengthening exercises depends on which structures are lengthened or have lost tone. Compensating patterns may differ depending on the client's contributing factors and posture. Nearly all of the muscles of the posterior thigh, leg, or foot can lose tone and strength when innervation by the sciatic nerve is reduced. Assess the client thoroughly to determine which structures are affected before assigning strengthening exercises.

Because lateral rotation is the most common postural deviation, you may find the medial hamstrings and adductors lengthened, taut, and weak. To strengthen these, instruct the client to lie supine with his or her feet on the floor, knees bent, and a ball or other object adding resistance between the knees (Fig. 9-16). Instruct the client to adduct and medially rotate the hip by squeezing the knees together against the resistance of the ball and hold for 10 seconds, or less if he or she feels fatigue. The contraction can be repeated 5–10 times.

If the Pace test is positive for weak abduction, recommend strengthening the abductors. Instruct the client to stand with the support of a wall or chair while lifting the affected leg away from the midline (Fig. 9-17). It is important not to laterally rotate the hip when performing this exercise to keep the piriformis from shortening.

SUGGESTIONS FOR FURTHER TREATMENT

Ideally, a client with piriformis syndrome will have treatments twice a week until the client can perform activities of daily living with minimal or no pain for at least 4 days. When this occurs, reduce frequency to once per week until symptoms are absent for at least 7 days. When the client

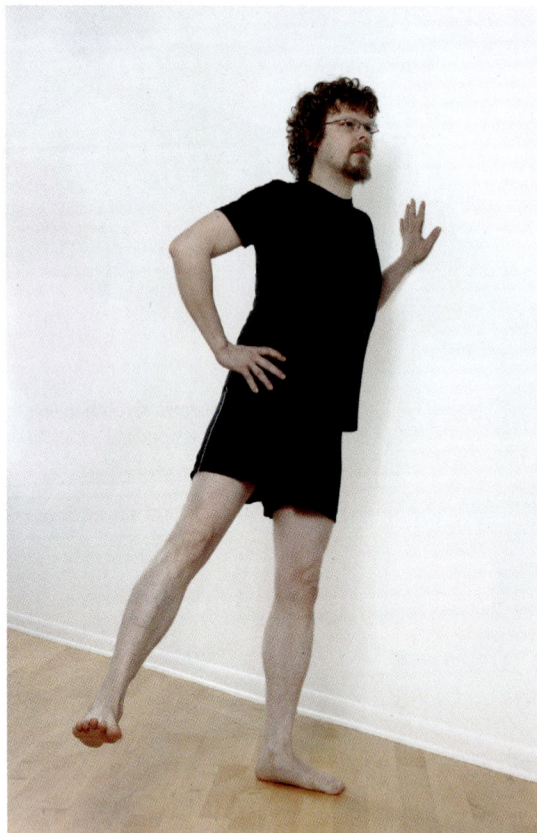

Figure 9-17 Strengthen abductors. Instruct the client to stabilize themselves against a wall or chair, and lift the leg to strengthen the abductors.

reports that he or she has been pain free longer than 7 days, treatment can be reduced to twice per month. If the client is pain-free for 3 or more consecutive weeks, he or she can then schedule once per month or as necessary. In the treatment of piriformis syndrome that is neuromuscular in nature, there should be some improvement with each session. If this is not happening, consider the following possibilities:

- There is too much time between treatments. It is best to give the newly treated tissues 24–48 hours to adapt, but if too much time passes between treatments in the beginning, the client's activities of daily living may reverse any progress.
- The client is not adjusting activities of daily living or is not keeping up with self-care. As much as we want to fix the problem, we cannot force a client to make the adjustments we suggest. Explain the importance of his or her participation in the healing process, and encourage the client to follow your recommendations, but be careful not to judge or reprimand a client who does not.
- The condition is advanced or involves other musculoskeletal complications that are beyond your basic training. Refer this client to a massage therapist with advanced clinical or medical massage training. Continuing to treat a client whose case is beyond your training could turn the client away from massage therapy altogether and hinder healing.
- The client has an undiagnosed, underlying condition. Discontinue treatment until the client sees a health care provider for a medical assessment.

If you are not treating the client in a clinical setting or private practice, you may not be able to take him or her through the full program of healing. Still, if you can bring some relief in just one treatment, it may encourage the client to discuss this change with a physician and seek manual therapy rather than more aggressive treatment options. If the client returns for regular treatments, the symptoms are likely to change each time, so it is important to perform an assessment before each session. Once you have released superficial tissues in general areas, you may be able to focus more of your treatment on a specific area. Likewise, once you have treated the structures specific to piriformis syndrome, you may be able to pay closer attention to compensating structures and coexisting conditions.

PROFESSIONAL GROWTH

CASE STUDY

Vittorio is a 35-year-old, single male. He is currently the marketing director for a nonprofit arts organization. Vittorio trained and performed as a professional ballet dancer until his retirement from dance 4 years ago. Within a year of retiring, he began feeling general aches in his hips, knees, and ankles. The symptoms have gotten worse, and he now feels numbness in his left leg and foot.

Subjective

The client complained of pain in his hips, particularly in the left hip, with occasional general aching in his knees and occasional instability in his ankles. Approximately 6 months ago, he began to feel tingling down the back of his left leg and in the left foot after sitting at his desk for an extended period or driving long distances. Within the past 6 weeks, he has felt numbness in the leg and feels like the step of his left foot is heavier than the right. He has lost his balance more than once while taking the first few steps after having been seated for a while. In his job as a marketing director, he spends many consecutive hours seated. He commutes by car for an average of 1 hour in each direction and frequently drives to meetings. On the weekends, he is much more active, rarely uses his car, and has noticed that he has fewer symptoms. He has purchased a new chair with lumbar support and adjustable height to try to relieve symptoms. The use of this chair reduced the pain he had felt in his low back but had no effect on the pain, numbness, or tingling in his leg.

Vittorio visited his health care provider for a general checkup and to discuss the symptoms in his leg. He was concerned that changes in his diet, which now includes more packaged and take-out food, may be affecting his nervous system. A physical exam and blood tests revealed no underlying pathologies. He is considered to be in "excellent health." His health care provider explained that while his current food choices may contribute to his symptoms and may make healing less efficient, they are not the cause of his pain. The health care provider prescribed physical therapy, which largely focused on strengthening exercises and reduced the pain in his knees and ankles, but Vittorio noticed that the numbness and tingling was often worse after sessions. His former dance instructor referred him to this clinic. When asked about changes in bladder or bowel movements, he replied that nothing had changed. He has no pain in the groin area. He has noticed no swelling, and does not feel unusual heat, cold, or fullness in the extremities.

Objective

The client very clearly protects his left leg. He climbed the stairs using the rail on the left side, lifting his weight with the right leg for each step. When seated, his knees are widely separated. A bulge in the left pocket of his jeans suggests a large wallet or other object. A faded area of fabric around the edges of this bulge suggests that he carries this object in the same pocket regularly. Vittorio had no trouble sitting in the chair. He stood without assistance, but paused for a second, seemingly to check his balance, before walking again. Other than the widely separated knees, his seated posture is well balanced and erect.

Postural assessment revealed a significant lateral rotation of the hips bilaterally. When this was pointed out to Vittorio, he stated that he had trained for years to establish that posture, which is essential for a ballet dancer. I have worked with several dancers who specifically requested that the lateral rotation of the hips not be realigned, but Vittorio responded, "I don't need it anymore," with no apparent regret. He has minor hypolordosis and valgus of the knees. The ankles are everted bilaterally, and the lateral two or three toes are slightly extended (i.e., not fully rested on the floor). The posture of the upper body is normal.

His Valsalva test was negative for space-occupying lesions. The Pace test revealed significant weakness with abduction of the left hip. When asked to try to increase the strength of the contraction in the left hip, Vittorio rotated his trunk to compensate. Although his right hip is stronger, this result is relative. The stork test was negative for sacroiliac joint dysfunction. Active medial rotation of the hips reproduced no symptoms at first, but tingling began at 24 seconds.

Palpation revealed fascial restrictions across the hip joint bilaterally and at the thoracolumbar fascia. No swelling or temperature difference was apparent between the hips. The lateral rotators of both hips have increased tone. Only the lateral rotators of the left hip were tender to the touch. With deep palpation, pain reached a level 8 out of 10. Trigger points near both attachments referred pain within the gluteal area. Pain with compression to a trigger point near the trochanter reduced from level 8 to 5. Pain with compression to a trigger point near the sacrum reduced from level 7 to 3. The iliotibial bands are dense and adhered bilaterally, particularly on the superior aspect of the left. The left vastus lateralis is also dense with superficial adhesions. The adductors and medial hamstrings are tender to the touch (level 4 of 10) with taut bands. There is point tenderness near the adductor tubercle and medial condyle of the femur and the medial tibial plateau (level 6 of 10). The peroneus longus and brevis and extensor digitorum longus are hypertonic bilaterally. Distal tendons of the extensor digitorum longus are thick and short. Biceps femoris and ankle dorsiflexors are slightly hypotonic, and sensation is reduced compared to the right side.

The assessment suggests possible piriformis syndrome—neurogenic in the left hip and non-neurogenic in the right hip. The client was encouraged to discuss this assessment with his health care provider for a specific diagnosis.

Action

Treatment focused on reducing hypertonicity and restoring the proper length of the lateral rotators of the hip bilaterally with the additional goal of reducing irritation to the left sciatic nerve. I performed myofascial release to the thoracolumbar fascia and around the greater trochanters. I used cross-fiber friction on the iliotibial bands and vastus lateralis bilaterally. I softened the superficial tissues moderately, but the fibers were still obscured by adhesions. I applied general warming to the gluteal area followed by muscle stripping and trigger point therapy on the lateral rotators of the hips bilaterally. P ROM in the right hip increased by approximately 15° with no pain upon medial rotation. P ROM in the left hip increased by less than 10° with pain at a level 5 out of 10 upon medial rotation and with tingling in the thigh after 15 seconds in the initial attempt. PIR increased P ROM by only a few degrees, and all successive passive medial rotation of the left hip was confined to 10 seconds. No trigger points were found in the taut bands of the adductors semimembranosus and semitendinosus. Adhesions and warmth at the medial knee suggest strain on the pes anserinus tendon due to excessive lateral rotation and attempts by the medial rotators to oppose the action. The client felt no tenderness in the anterior leg, but the density of the peroneals and extensor digitorum and the minimal change in tissues following the application of superficial techniques limited the depth and pressure attempted in this session. The client felt an intense stretch with a passive inversion of the ankle. I applied stimulating strokes to the left biceps femoris and ankle dorsiflexors.

Following treatment, the client stated that he felt greater mobility in the hips and legs but did not feel confident enough to stop favoring the left leg. I explained that rushing into false confidence in his strength and stability could have negative consequences and that he should trust his instinct and sense of balance when standing or walking but do his best not to favor one side if it is not necessary.

Plan

I demonstrated a stretch for the lateral rotators of the hips while seated. I recommended wrapping a band around the knees while he is seated for long periods to reduce the lateral rotation of the hips. I emphasized the importance of limiting the duration of stretches and removing the band around his knees if numbness, tingling, or pain beyond his tolerance occurs. Results during treatment suggested that stretches should be limited to 10-15 seconds to minimize the reproduction of symptoms. If, at any time, symptoms occur within 5 or fewer seconds, the client was advised to discontinue performing this stretch. We will reevaluate this recommendation in the next session.

I demonstrated stretches to the ankle evertors, emphasizing that these should be performed only if the client feels stable while standing and only with the assistance of a wall or other surface to lean on. If continued treatment reduces symptoms during activities of daily living, and as stability and balance are restored, strengthening exercises for the biceps femoris and the dorsiflexors of the ankle will be introduced.

The client's primary goal is to stop the loss of control he feels in his left leg. His secondary goal is to restore strength. His long-term goals are to realign the hips, knees, and ankles, although this is not a priority. He has agreed to treatments twice a week until symptoms are absent for at least 4 consecutive days, with reassessment at that time. Massage therapy prescribed by a health care provider is covered under his insurance. He will discuss this with his health care provider and request a referral to this clinic.

CRITICAL THINKING EXERCISES

1. Design an assessment and treatment plan that considers the contributing factors for a client with symptoms of piriformis syndrome due to overuse of the piriformis as an antagonist. This client will likely present with medial rotation of the hips, valgus of the knees, and eversion of the ankle. The assessment plan should consider ROMs that may be restricted, testing for muscle weakness, and palpation findings. Treatment goals should include lengthening shortened tissues, strengthening weak muscles, and restoring proper neuromuscular function.

2. A client presents with numbness and tingling in the legs and pain in the hip, low back, and groin. The client also reports having recently developed urinary difficulty. Symptoms suggest both sciatic and pudendal nerve irritation. Conduct a short literature review of manual therapy for restoring the function of the pudendal nerve. Develop a treatment plan for this client with special attention to aspects of treatment both within and outside the massage scope of practice. Include possible referrals to practitioners licensed to treat elements of this condition that are outside the scope of practice for massage therapists.

3. Develop a 10-minute stretching and strengthening routine for a client that covers all of the muscles involved in piriformis syndrome. Use Box 9-1 and Figure 9-4 as a guide. Remember that a stretch increases the distance between the origin and insertion of a muscle and is important for those muscles that are shortened while strengthening is performed by actively bringing the origin and insertion closer together and is important for the antagonists of shortened muscles. Describe each step of the routine in enough detail that the client can refer to these descriptions in your absence and perform them without harm.

4. A client calls to schedule a massage for hip pain with tingling down the back of the leg. She explains that she had a hip replacement following an accident 5 years ago when she was 22 years old. Her physician has cleared her for massage therapy. Discuss the possible relationship between the hip replacement and piriformis syndrome. What questions would you ask this client and her health care provider? What special considerations would you need to make in your treatment plan both for contributing factors and for contraindications? Would a hip replacement affect proprioception at that joint?

5. Conduct a short literature review to explore the relationship between symptoms suggesting compression of one or more nerves in the gluteal area and the following:
   - Facet joint irritation
   - Diabetes
   - Prostatitis
   - Myositis ossificans
   - Rheumatoid arthritis

BIBLIOGRAPHY AND SUGGESTED READINGS

Biel A. *Trail Guide to the Body: How to Locate Muscles, Bones and More*, 3rd ed. Boulder, CO: Books of Discovery, 2005.

Dutton M. *Orthopaedic Examination, Evaluation, and Intervention*. New York, NY: McGraw-Hill, 2004.

Fishman LM, Dombi GW, Michaelsen C, et al. Piriformis syndrome: Diagnosis, treatment, and outcome—A 10 year study. Archives of Physical Medical Rehabilitation. 2002;83(3):295–301.

Honig P. A case report of the treatment of piriformis syndrome: Applying modalities of therapeutic bodywork. Honorable mention, Massage Therapy Foundation 2006 Case Study Competition. Available at http://www.massagetherapyfoundation.org/contest.html. Accessed Fall 2010.

Lowe W. *Orthopedic Massage: Theory and Technique*. St Louis, MO: Mosby-Elsevier, 2003.

Mayo Foundation for Medical Education and Research. Bursitis. Available at http://www.mayoclinic.com/health/bursitis/DS00032. Accessed Winter 2009.

Mayo Foundation for Medical Education and Research. Herniated Disk. Available at http://www.mayoclinic.com/health/herniated-disk/HD99999. Accessed Winter 2009.

Mayo Foundation for Medical Education and Research. Sciatica. Available at http://www.mayoclinic.com/health/sciatica/DS00516. Accessed Winter 2009.

Mayo Foundation for Medical Education and Research. Spinal Stenosis. Available at http://www.mayoclinic.com/health/spinal-stenosis/DS00515. Accessed Winter 2009.

Papadopoulos EC, Khan SN. Piriformis syndrome and low back pain: A new classification and review of the literature. Orthopedic Clinics of North America. 2004;35(1):65–71.

Rattray F, Ludwig L. *Clinical Massage Therapy: Understanding, Assessing and Treating over 70 Conditions*. Toronto, ON: Talus Incorporated, 2000.

Russell M. Massage therapy and restless legs syndrome. Journal of Bodywork and Movement Therapies. 2007;11:146–150.

Simons DG, Travell JG, Simons LS. *Myofascial Pain and Dysfunction: The Trigger Point Manual*, 2nd ed. Philadelphia, PA: Lippincott Williams & Wilkins, 1999.

SpineUniverse.com. Lumbar Radiculopathy: Low Back and Leg Pain. Available at http://www.spineuniverse.com/displayarticle.php/article1469.html. Accessed Winter 2009.

Turchaninov R. *Medical Massage*, 2nd ed. Phoenix, AZ: Aesculapius Books, 2006.

U.S. National Library of Medicine and the National Institutes of Health. Spondylolisthesis. Available at http://www.nlm.nih.gov/medlineplus/ency/article/001260.htm. Accessed Winter 2009.

Werner R. *A Massage Therapist's Guide to Pathology*, 4th ed. Philadelphia, PA: Lippincott Williams & Wilkins, 2009.

Patellofemoral Syndrome

UNDERSTANDING PATELLOFEMORAL SYNDROME

Patellofemoral syndrome refers generally to anterior knee pain primarily due to improper tracking of the patella over the femur. Many factors can affect the tracking of the patella, and the degree of discomfort, pain, or restricted mobility varies widely. To recognize these potential contributing factors, it is important to understand the relationships among the femur, tibia, patella, and the soft tissues responsible for their movement and stability.

The knee joint includes two articulations (Fig. 10-1). The concave plateaus of the tibia and the convex condyles of the femur articulate to form a modified hinge joint (tibiofemoral). The posterior aspect of the patella also has concave surfaces—called the medial and lateral facets—that articulate with the medial and lateral condyles of the femur (patellofemoral). The ridge that separates the medial and lateral facets of the patella glides in the groove between the medial and lateral condyles of the femur. Articular cartilage that covers the condyles of the femur and the tibial plateau, and the menisci that sit between them provide cushioned, friction-free movement of the joint.

Flexion and extension of the knee, which involve both of these articulations, are not simple transverse movements. Some rotation and translation of the bones occurs during flexion and extension of the healthy knee. The angle of the joint and the strength of its surrounding structures influence the amount of rotation and translation. Noncontractile soft tissues including the medial and lateral collateral ligaments and the anterior and posterior cruciate ligaments protect the knee from excessive rotation and translation during movement. Other noncontractile tissues that protect the knee include the joint capsule, menisci, bursae, and fat pads (Fig. 10-2). Contractile soft tissues that both move and stabilize the knee include the quadriceps, hamstrings, gracilis, sartorius, and gastrocnemius. A healthy knee depends on all of these structures working together to create smooth movement.

The lateral condyle of the femur is more prominent anteriorly than the medial condyle, which provides a buffer for excessive lateral movement of the patella. The medial condyle of the femur extends more distally than the lateral condyle, but both lie in the same plane as they articulate with the tibia. This puts the femur at an angle from the inferior medial location of the knee to the superior lateral location of the hip. The angle at the intersection of those differently oriented bones—called the Q angle—partly determines how the quadriceps pull on the tibia in knee extension and how they contract eccentrically in knee flexion. To measure this angle, draw one line diagonally from the middle of the patella to the anterior superior iliac spine (ASIS), and another from the middle of the patella through the middle of the tibial tubercle (Fig. 10-3). The average Q angle is approximately 15°; it is often greater in females than in males, because women generally have a wider pelvis. Because the Q angle affects the line of pull of the quadriceps, significant deviations can have a great impact on how the bones of the knee joint articulate and how the soft

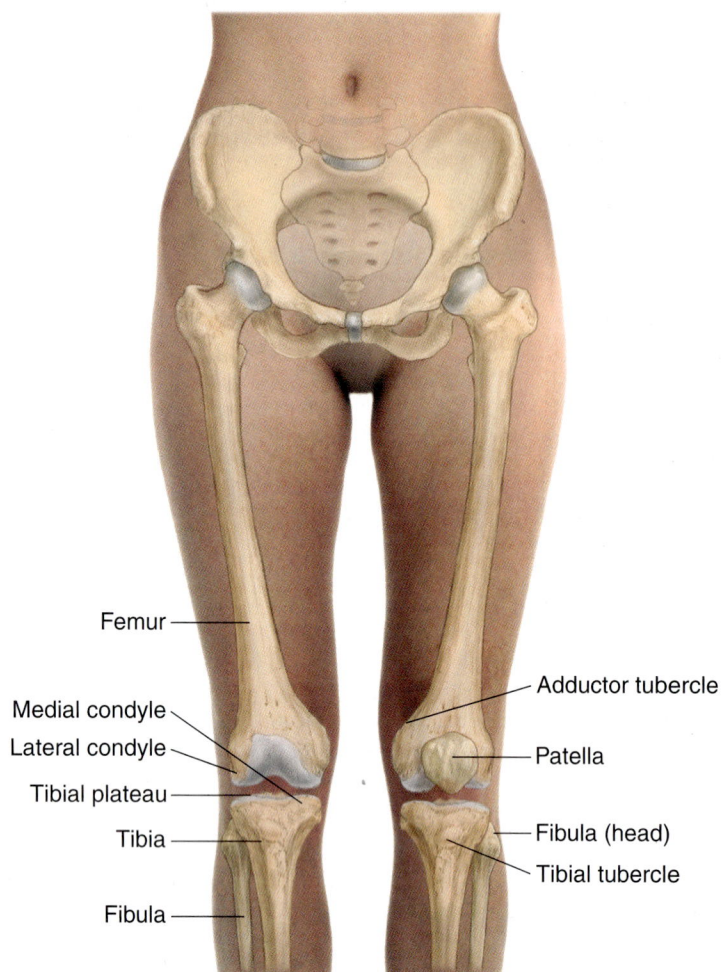

Femur

Medial condyle

Lateral condyle

Tibial plateau

Tibia

Fibula

Adductor tubercle

Patella

Fibula (head)

Tibial tubercle

Figure 10-1 **Articulations of the knee joint.** The tibia articulates with the femur to form the tibiofemoral joint, and the patella articulates with the femur to form the patellofemoral joint. Adapted from Clay JH, Pounds DM. *Basic Clinical Massage Therapy: Integrating Anatomy and Treatment,* 2nd ed. Philadelphia: Lippincott Williams & Wilkins, 2008.

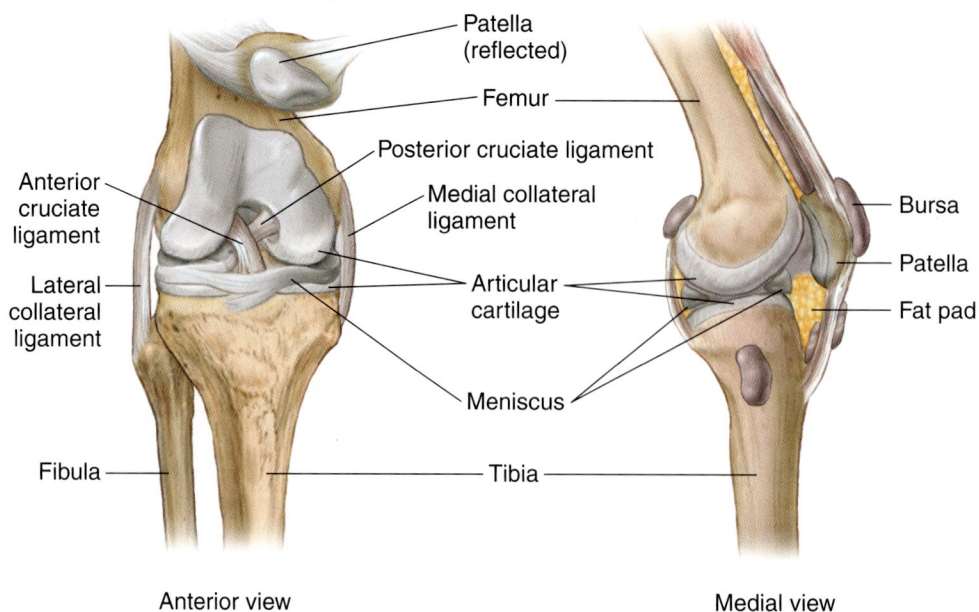

Patella
(reflected)

Femur

Posterior cruciate ligament

Anterior cruciate ligament

Medial collateral ligament

Bursa

Lateral collateral ligament

Articular cartilage

Patella

Fat pad

Meniscus

Fibula

Tibia

Anterior view

Medial view

Figure 10-2 **Supporting structures of the knee.** Ligaments, cartilage, menisci, bursae, and fat pads stabilize and cushion the knee joints.

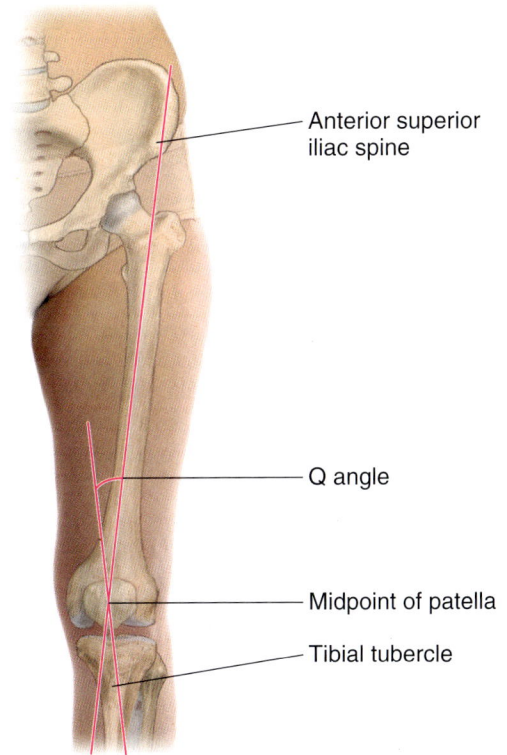

- Anterior superior iliac spine
- Q angle
- Midpoint of patella
- Tibial tubercle

Figure 10-3 **Q angle.** The Q angle is formed by the lines that run from the patella to the anterior superior iliac spine and from the patella to the tibial tubercle.

tissues respond. In the case of patellofemoral syndrome, an increased Q angle—sometimes resulting from an injury, activities of daily living, or postural deviations anywhere from the hips to the feet—may contribute to excessive lateral tracking of the patella.

The quadriceps are also angled, following the line of the femur. The patella is rooted in the quadriceps tendon, is stabilized inferiorly by the patellar tendon, and is further stabilized by the medial and lateral retinacula. In extension and flexion of the knee, the patella moves superiorly and inferiorly over the condyles of the femur. The main function of the patella is to help guide the movement of this joint with differently angled bones by realigning the quadriceps' pull on the tibia. Without the patella, the quadriceps would draw the tibia diagonally, along their line of pull. Instead, the quadriceps move the patella slightly laterally along the line of the femur, while the patellar tendon redirects the line of pull on the tibia, moving it more perpendicularly and minimizing rotation. If the patella is not tracking normally, stress to the joint and the muscles that move it increases.

Because the quadriceps' line of pull is lateral compared to the orientation of the patellar tendon, several other structures are vital for proper tracking of the patella. The distal fibers of the vastus medialis run obliquely, offering ideal resistance to a lateral pull on the patella. The medial patellar retinaculum resists lateral pull while the lateral patellar retinaculum resists medial pull. The medial and lateral collateral ligaments assist in normalizing a valgus or varus position of the knee, which may help to prevent improper tracking of the patella.

Common Signs and Symptoms

The most common symptom of patellofemoral syndrome is pain at the anterior knee, often just above or just below the patella. Pain usually has a gradual onset. Pain may also be felt at the medial or lateral side of the knee depending on which structures are primarily involved. Pain is usually most intense with a weight-bearing extension of the knee. Symptoms are felt when walking, running, squatting and rising from a squat, and when ascending and descending stairs. While sitting for long periods, the knee is flexed, elongating the quadriceps, and pain may be felt upon standing when the lengthened quadriceps need to contract concentrically. The knee may also give way during weight-bearing activities. While instability of the joint may be a complicating factor in patellofemoral syndrome, the knee giving way may also be the result of a neuromuscular reflex inhibition of the quadriceps in response to pain. This inhibition may lead to atrophy of the quadriceps.

Hyper- or hypomobility of the patella in a lateral or medial direction may be present. When structures are pulling the patella laterally, medial mobility may be reduced. When structures are pulling the patella medially, lateral mobility may be reduced. You may notice swelling at the knee when misalignment of the patella and factors contributing to patellofemoral syndrome increase friction and lead to increased inflammation and arthritis. Snapping or grinding may be felt or heard by the client when flexing and extending the knee, particularly during weight-bearing activity.

Patellofemoral syndrome was once called (and is still often confused with) chondromalacia of the patella, which involves degeneration of cartilage. The signs and symptoms listed above are often present without any changes to the cartilage of the patella. However, left untreated, patellofemoral syndrome may lead to degeneration of the patellar cartilage.

Possible Causes and Contributing Factors

There is no single, clearly understood cause of patellofemoral syndrome. Improper tracking of the patella and increased pressure within the patellofemoral joint may involve a variety of coexisting contributing factors. Lateral misalignment of the patella is reported more often than medial misalignment. This is thought to be due to lateral pull by the quadriceps. An increased Q angle may contribute to excessive lateral pull by the quadriceps and rotation of the femur or tibia and may affect proper tracking of the patella. A tight vastus lateralis or iliotibial band, which have distal tissues that blend into the lateral patellar retinaculum, also increase lateral pull on the patella. The distal fibers of the vastus medialis, referred to as vastus medialis obliquus, run at an oblique angle, making them favorable for opposing lateral pull on the patella by the quadriceps and iliotibial band. A weak vastus medialis obliquus may not be optimally effective for this function. In all of these cases, weight-bearing or repetitive activities increase the demand on the knee and the risk of injury to its stabilizing soft tissues.

Try this yourself. Stand on one leg, leaning against a wall or chair for balance. Extend and flex the knee of the opposite leg. If there is no tissue damage, the movement of your knee will be smooth, and you probably will not feel any discomfort. Now, adduct your hip, crossing your free leg over the leg you are standing on, and extend and flex your knee 10 times so that movement of the tibia is straight and directly in front of you. This may not be the exact mechanism of an increased Q angle, but it approximates the rotation of the femur and the increased angle of pull on the quadriceps. Moving the tibia straight and directly in front of you approximates walking. After 10 repetitions of this action, do you feel stress in the medial knee or hip? Now imagine the additional impact on the joint if you added the full weight of your body. Next, without causing discomfort beyond your tolerance, walk around with one ankle everted or inverted. Pay attention to what you feel in that knee and hip compared to the leg with a normally oriented ankle and foot.

Sitting or squatting for long periods lengthens the quadriceps, particularly the distal tendons, which may weaken knee extension causing pain when the individual needs to recruit these muscles to stand. Lengthening may be associated with neuromuscular dysfunction, affecting the tone and strength of the quadriceps, which can cause the knee to give way. It is unclear whether the neuromuscular dysfunction is a cause or result of changes to the quadriceps' muscle tone. Along the same lines, the knee is usually flexed when sitting, which shortens and possibly increases the resting tone of the hamstrings. This may increase the risk of strain during eccentric contractions of the hamstrings such as when extending the knee to stand. Furthermore, if the quadriceps have weakened, they may be less able to oppose the hamstrings that flex the knee.

Although less common, medial misalignment does occur and should be assessed. In fact, any anomaly in the structures of the knee can affect patellar tracking in the femoral groove. Patella alta—a patella that is abnormally high in relation to the femur—is positioned in the more shallow aspect of the femoral groove and may be associated with lateral displacement. Patella baja—a patella that is abnormally low in relation to the femur—increases contact with the tibia and is associated with chondromalacia. Patella alta and patella baja are often associated with an injury to the quadriceps and patellar tendons. A lateral femoral condyle that is smaller than average or that does not protrude sufficiently anteriorly cannot provide an adequate buffer for the patella and may also contribute to excessive lateral tracking.

Pes planus or pes cavus, inversion or eversion of the ankle, and rotation of the femur or tibia may all play a role in improper biomechanics that contribute to patellofemoral syndrome. Injuries, particularly to the ligaments that stabilize the knee, and more so if they are repeated or untreated, may affect the articulation of bones in the joints of the knee and encourage compensating patterns in the soft tissues surrounding the knee. Surgery, including arthroscopic procedures, may damage soft tissues, cartilage, and proprioceptors, resulting in scar tissue and compromised function. Overuse and weight-bearing impact, such as when running and ascending or descending stairs or hills, may contribute to inflammation and degeneration of structures. Weight gain may also be a predisposing factor.

Table 10-1 lists conditions commonly confused with or contributing to patellofemoral syndrome.

Contraindications and Special Considerations

First, it is essential to understand the cause of the client's knee pain. If the client has a history of arthritis, cartilage degeneration, or previously unresolved injuries, or if you suspect the client has a fractured bone or a torn ligament, work with the client's health care provider and consult a pathology text for massage therapists before proceeding. These are a few general cautions:

- **Underlying pathologies.** Arthritis or conditions affecting the cartilage may be contributing factors. If you suspect an underlying condition (consult Table 10-1 and your pathology book for signs and symptoms), refer the client to his or her health care provider for medical assessment before initiating treatment. If the client is diagnosed with an underlying pathology that is not a contraindication for massage, work with the health care team to develop a treatment plan that is appropriate for that individual.
- **Endangerment sites.** Be cautious near endangerment sites in the popliteal area.
- **Producing symptoms.** Symptoms may occur during treatment. If treatment reproduces symptoms, first adjust the client to a more neutral posture. If this does not relieve the symptoms, reduce your pressure or move away from the area. You may be able to treat around the site that reproduced the symptoms, but proceed with caution.
- **Treatment duration and pressure.** If the client is elderly, has degenerative disease, or has been diagnosed with a condition that diminishes activities of daily living, you may need to adjust your pressure as well as the treatment duration. Frequent half-hour sessions may suit the client better.
- **Positioning.** Use bolsters to position the client for comfort as well as to reduce postures that contribute to patellofemoral syndrome or coexisting conditions. Adjusting the alignment of the hips, knees, and ankles helps to keep muscles closer to their anatomic length and may facilitate access.
- **Friction.** Do not use deep frictions if the client has a systemic inflammatory condition such as rheumatoid arthritis or osteoarthritis, if the health of the underlying tissues is compromised, or if the client is taking anti-inflammatory medication. Friction creates an inflammatory process, which may interfere with the intended action of anti-inflammatory medication. Recommend that your client refrain from taking such medication for several hours prior to treatment if the health care provider agrees.
- **Injections.** If the client has had a steroid or analgesic injection within 2 weeks of treatment, avoid the area. These injections reduce sensation, which may prevent the client from assessing your pressure adequately. These injections may also alter the physiology of the soft tissues, increasing the risk of injury from manual pressure.
- **Tissue length.** It is important when treating myofascial tissues that you do not lengthen those that are already stretched. Assess for myofascial restrictions first and treat only those

Table 10-1	Differentiating Conditions Commonly Confused with or Contributing to Patellofemoral Syndrome		
Condition	**Typical Signs and Symptoms**	**Testing**	**Massage Therapy**
Baker's cyst	May be asymptomatic Pain and swelling behind the knee If cyst ruptures, pain, swelling, and bruising at posterior knee and calf	Physical exam Transillumination X-ray MRI	Baker's cyst can be confused with deep vein thrombosis and should be assessed by a medical professional prior to treatment. Massage is locally contraindicated in the popliteal area. Massage elsewhere is indicated.
Bone spur	Pain in knee, particularly on flexion and extension and when kneeling Reduced ROM	X-ray MRI CT scan	Massage will not reduce symptoms of a bone spur. ROM testing or exercises are locally contraindicated. Be cautious with compressions.
Bursitis (pes anserine, infrapatellar, prepatellar)	Heat, redness, and swelling Pain at rest Aching or stiffness with use Significant pain when kneeling and ascending or descending stairs Fever, pain, and swelling if infection occurs	Physical exam ROM tests X-ray MRI	Massage is systemically contraindicated if bursitis is due to infection. Massage is locally contraindicated in the acute stage to avoid increased swelling. In the subacute stage, massage to structures surrounding the joint is indicated.
Chondromalacia	Dull pain and tenderness at the anterior knee Worsens with kneeling, squatting, prolonged sitting, standing from sitting, and ascending or descending stairs Crepitus	Physical exam X-ray MRI	Massage is indicated to reduce stress on the joint by altering soft tissues but will not affect cartilage. Avoid compression to the patella and repeated ROM exercises of the knee.
Gout	Redness, heat, and swelling Sudden, intense pain, often at night, that diminishes gradually over a couple of weeks	Physical exam Blood and urine uric acid concentration tests Synovial fluid test	Massage is contraindicated during acute attacks. Gout may indicate other systemic conditions. Work with health care team.
Iliotibial band syndrome	Sharp or burning pain in lateral knee, particularly following activity Pain resolves with rest in early stages As syndrome progresses, pain with simple activities like walking and ascending or descending stairs	Physical exam ROM tests	Massage is indicated

Table 10-1	**Differentiating Conditions Commonly Confused with or Contributing to Patellofemoral Syndrome (Continued)**		
Condition	**Typical Signs and Symptoms**	**Testing**	**Massage Therapy**
Ligament injury/ sprain	Snapping sound or sensation at time of injury Acute pain that worsens with movement Rapid swelling, heat, and redness Unable to bear weight on the injured leg Knee gives way In the subacute stage, joint may regain function	Physical exam MRI	Massage is indicated and best used following acute stage. See Chapter 13.
Meniscus injury	Pain and stiffness Popping sensation Slowly progressive swelling Reduced ROM Pain with activity Knee may lock in place	Physical exam McMurray's test X-ray MRI Arthroscopy	Massage is indicated to reduce stress on the joint by altering soft tissues but will not affect meniscus. Avoid compression to the injured meniscus and the patella and minimize repeated ROM exercises of the knee.
Osgood-Schlatter disease (primarily affects teenagers)	Pain that worsens with activity Swelling Tenderness at tibial tuberosity Symptoms often resolve when bones stop growing	Physical exam ROM tests X-ray	Techniques that increase circulation are locally contraindicated in the acute stage to avoid increased inflammation. Massage is indicated in chronic stage.
Osteoarthritis	Pain on standing and walking Swelling Tenderness with pressure on joint Stiffness, particularly after rest or inactivity Inflexibility in the knee Grating sensation or sound	Physical exam X-rays Blood tests Synovial fluid tests Arthroscopy	Massage is contraindicated during an acute flare-up. Massage is indicated in the subacute stage.
Plica syndrome	Intermittent anteromedial knee pain Inflammation Edema Thickening of plica Decreased elasticity of plica Snapping sound when dense plica rolls over femoral condyle Knee may lock or give way	TARP sign (Taut Articular band Reproduces Pain) Arthroscopy	Massage is indicated to reduce inflammation or adhesions, restore mobility, and effect a change in the tone of muscles that cross the knee. There is no research to indicate the benefit of massage to the plica itself.

(continued)

Table 10-1	Differentiating Conditions Commonly Confused with or Contributing to Patellofemoral Syndrome (Continued)		
Condition	**Typical Signs and Symptoms**	**Testing**	**Massage Therapy**
Rheumatoid arthritis	Chondromalacia Periods of flare-ups and remission Pain, swelling Aching and stiffness, particularly after rest or inactivity Reduced ROM Distortion of knee joint Rheumatic nodules Occasional low-grade fever and malaise	Physical exam Blood tests Synovial fluid tests X-ray	Massage is indicated in nonacute stages. Work with the health care team.
Septic arthritis	Pain, swelling, redness, and heat around the knee Fever, chills Symptoms may occur without prior injury	Synovial fluid test Blood test X-ray MRI	Massage is systemically contraindicated. Refer to a medical professional.
Tendon injuries	Pain in the knee Swelling Pain worsens with intense weight-bearing activity such as jumping, squatting, or climbing stairs Reduced ROM	Physical exam ROM tests	Massage is indicated. See Chapter 14.

that are clearly present. Likewise, overstretched muscles should not be stretched from origin to insertion. If you treat trigger points in overstretched tissue, use heat or a localized pin and stretch technique instead of full ROM stretches.

■ **Hypermobile joints and unstable ligaments.** Be cautious with mobilizations if the client has hypermobile joints or if ligaments are unstable due to injury, pregnancy, or a systemic condition.

Massage Therapy Research

In 2006, Paul van den Dolder and David Roberts published a study titled "Six Sessions of Manual Therapy Increase Knee Flexion and Improve Activity in People with Anterior Knee Pain: A Randomised Controlled Trial." The participants were 38 individuals between the ages of 18 and 80 with anterior knee pain, who were assigned to either an experimental group that received manual therapy or to a control group whose subjects were placed on a waiting list. Participants were excluded if knee pain was caused by recent trauma, infection, tumor, or acute inflammation or if the participant had knee surgery within 6 weeks of the study. Participants were also excluded if pain was reproduced with extension, flexion, or lateral flexion of the lumbar spine or overpressure to the hip or if there was no tenderness on palpation of the lateral knee. Manual therapy consisted of six 15- to 20-minute treatments over the course of approximately 2 weeks. Therapy focused on transverse frictions to the lateral retinaculum of the knee in the fully extended and fully flexed positions, tilt patellofemoral stretches, and sustained medial glide during extension and flexion. Participants were given no self-care instructions or other healing advice. Pain was measured using Laprade and Culham's patellofemoral pain severity questionnaire. ROM and activity were also assessed. The experimental group reported less average daily pain, less pain, increased speed while ascending or descending stairs, and increased knee flexion compared to the control group. There was no change in knee extension for either group.

In 2009, Pedrelli et al. published a study titled "Treating Patellar Tendinopathy with Fascial Manipulation." All 18 subjects, who were between the ages of 17 and 42 with unilateral, subacute, or chronic patellar tendon pain, received a single treatment using the fascial manipulation technique. Subjects with acute inflammation, meniscus damage, or advanced osteoarthritis were excluded. Prior to treatment, subjects completed the VAS pain questionnaire, describing pain experienced while descending steps and while jumping on flat feet. Subjects were asked to refrain from sports for 4 days following treatment. The same evaluation was repeated after one treatment and again one month after treatment. All treatments were performed by the same therapist and included fascial techniques over the muscular fascia between the vastus lateralis and the rectus femoris with pressure applied toward the vastus intermedius. Client feedback was used to accurately locate the point that produced local pain and referral. All patients reported decreased pain or weakness or increased mobility. All subjects reported a significant decrease in pain immediately following treatment, and progress was maintained or even improved at follow-up by all but three participants. These three subjects had a recurrence of pain, albeit less severe than at pre-treatment levels. It is also noted that these three subjects had more complicated clinical cases compared to other participants.

In 2008, Jennifer Zalta published "Massage Therapy Protocol for Post-Anterior Cruciate Ligament Reconstruction Patellofemoral Pain Syndrome: A Case Report." The study involved a 29-year-old female athlete with a history of injury to her anterior cruciate ligament, medial collateral ligament, and medial meniscus and had surgical repair of all but the medial ligament. After several months following surgery, the subject began experiencing grinding and clicking in the knee. She was later diagnosed as having patellofemoral pain syndrome. She scheduled arthroscopic surgery to remove the damaged cartilage and to reduce crepitus and agreed to participate in the case study beginning 4 days after her arthroscopy. Treatments were performed once a week over the course of 10 weeks, lasting between 60 and 90 minutes to accommodate a wide variety of contributing factors. Subjective pain and function levels were recorded before and after each treatment and daily during the treatment period. Goals included reducing postsurgical inflammation (lymphatic drainage); reducing hypertonicity and lengthening the tensor fasciae latae, iliotibial band, and hamstrings (muscle energy technique); deactivating trigger points in the tensor fasciae latae, vastus lateralis, and biceps femoris (neuromuscular therapy); increasing ROM (PIR and contract relax techniques); and reducing fibrotic tissue around the patella (myofascial release and cross-fiber friction). Strengthening of the vastus medialis oblique and the hip adductors were assigned as self-care. Following the treatment program, the client reported full, pain-free ROM in the affected knee. Pain was reported as 0 on a 0-10 scale by the sixth session. Lateral pull on the patella was reduced, and results of orthopedic tests showed improvement in the Q angle, tensor fasciae latae and iliotibial band contracture, patellar grind, and contracture in the knee flexors. Two weeks before the 1-year follow-up, the subject injured her medial meniscus, but reported that, prior to this most recent injury, she had experienced no pain and had returned to presurgery activity.

WORKING WITH THE CLIENT

Client Assessment

The signs and symptoms of patellofemoral syndrome can present in many different ways. Dysfunction that causes the patella to track laterally is most often reported, but any abnormal tracking that results in pain or dysfunction of the patellofemoral joint may be present. In addition, various repetitive actions, postures, or injuries may be contributing factors; each client will present differently. For example, an increased Q angle may affect the length and strength of the hip adductors and abductors as well as inversion or eversion of the ankles. A tight semitendinosus may contribute to injury of the pes anserine tendon, which in turn may affect the health of the sartorius or gracilis. Tight hamstrings or quadriceps may also affect pelvic tilt and lumbar lordosis. In general, lateral tracking of the patella suggests shortening of the soft tissues of the lateral thigh and weakening of the medial structures that stabilize the knee while medial tracking of the patella suggests shortening of the soft tissues of the medial thigh and weakening of the lateral structures that stabilize the knee. What follows are common presentations for patellofemoral syndrome. However, it is essential to assess every joint involved to put together an accurate picture for each individual client.

Assessment begins during your first contact with a client. In some cases, this may be on the telephone when an appointment is requested. Ask in advance if the client is seeking treatment for a specific area of pain so that you can prepare yourself.

Table 10-2 lists questions to ask the client when taking a health history.

Table 10-2	Health History
Questions for the Client	**Importance to the Treatment Plan**
Was there a precipitating event, or can you remember a specific moment when the pain began?	The details of the activity or posture that initiated the pain may help you to determine contributing factors. A new regimen of running, new activity that requires weight-bearing movement or squatting, or newly developed sedentary postures may contribute to symptoms of patellofemoral syndrome.
Where do you feel symptoms?	The location of symptoms gives clues to the location of trigger points, injury, or other contributing factors. Patellofemoral syndrome generally causes pain in the anterior knee. Although pain elsewhere does not exclude the possibility of patellofemoral syndrome, it may suggest a coexisting condition.
Describe what your symptoms feel like.	Differentiate between possible origins of symptoms, and determine the involvement of bones and soft tissues. See Chapter 1 for descriptions of pain sensations and possible contributing factors.
Do any movements make it worse or better?	Locate tension, weakness, or compression in structures producing such movements. Extension of the knee, ascending and descending stairs, and weight-bearing activity often exacerbate symptoms.
Have you seen a health care provider for this condition? What was the diagnosis? What tests were performed?	Medical tests may reveal contributing factors as well as contraindications. If no tests were performed in making a diagnosis, use the tests described in this chapter for your assessment. If your assessment is inconsistent with the diagnosis, ask the client to discuss your findings with his or her health care provider or for permission to contact the provider directly.
Have you been diagnosed with a condition such as arthritis?	Arthritis may contribute to signs and symptoms, may require adjustments to treatment and may impact treatment outcomes.
Have you had a previous injury or surgery?	Injury or surgery and resulting scar tissue may cause adhesions, hyper- or hypotonicity, and atypical ROM.
What type of work, hobbies, or other regular activities do you do?	Repetitive motions that stress the knee and static postures that increase flexion of the knee may contribute to the client's condition.
Are you taking any prescribed medications or herbal or other supplements?	Medication of all types may contribute to symptoms or have contraindications or cautions.
Have you had a corticosteroid or analgesic injection in the past 2 weeks? Where?	Local massage is contraindicated.
Have you taken a pain reliever or muscle relaxant within the past 4 hours?	The client may not be able to judge your pressure.
Have you taken anti-inflammatory medication within the past 4 hours?	Deep friction may initiate an inflammatory process and should not be performed if the client has recently taken anti-inflammatory medication.

POSTURAL ASSESSMENT

Allow the client to walk and enter the room ahead of you while you assess his or her posture and movements. Look for imbalances or patterns of compensation for deviations common with patellofemoral syndrome. Watch as the client climbs steps, and look for reduced mobility in the knee or whether the client is favoring one side. Assess for joint instability, limping, rotation of the femur or tibia, or hyper- or hypolordosis. Have the client sit to fill out the assessment form and watch to see if he or she lowers into the chair cautiously or shifts around to find a comfortable position for the knee. Watch also as the client stands up to see if he or she can stand without assistance or whether he or she lifts out of the chair using the arms or by leaning on a stable surface.

When assessing the standing posture, be sure that the client stands comfortably. If he or she tries to stand in the anatomic position, you will not get an accurate assessment of his or her posture in daily life. If the patella is tracking laterally, you may notice adduction of the hips, valgus of the knee, increased Q angle, or eversion of the ankle. If the patella is tracking medially, you may notice rotation of the femur and tibia, which appears as lateral rotation of the feet. Other anomalies may include patella alta or patella baja, hyper- or hypoextension of the knees, swelling around the patella, and pes planus or pes cavus.

Figure 10-4 compares a healthy posture to a posture affected by patellofemoral syndrome due to lateral tracking of the patella.

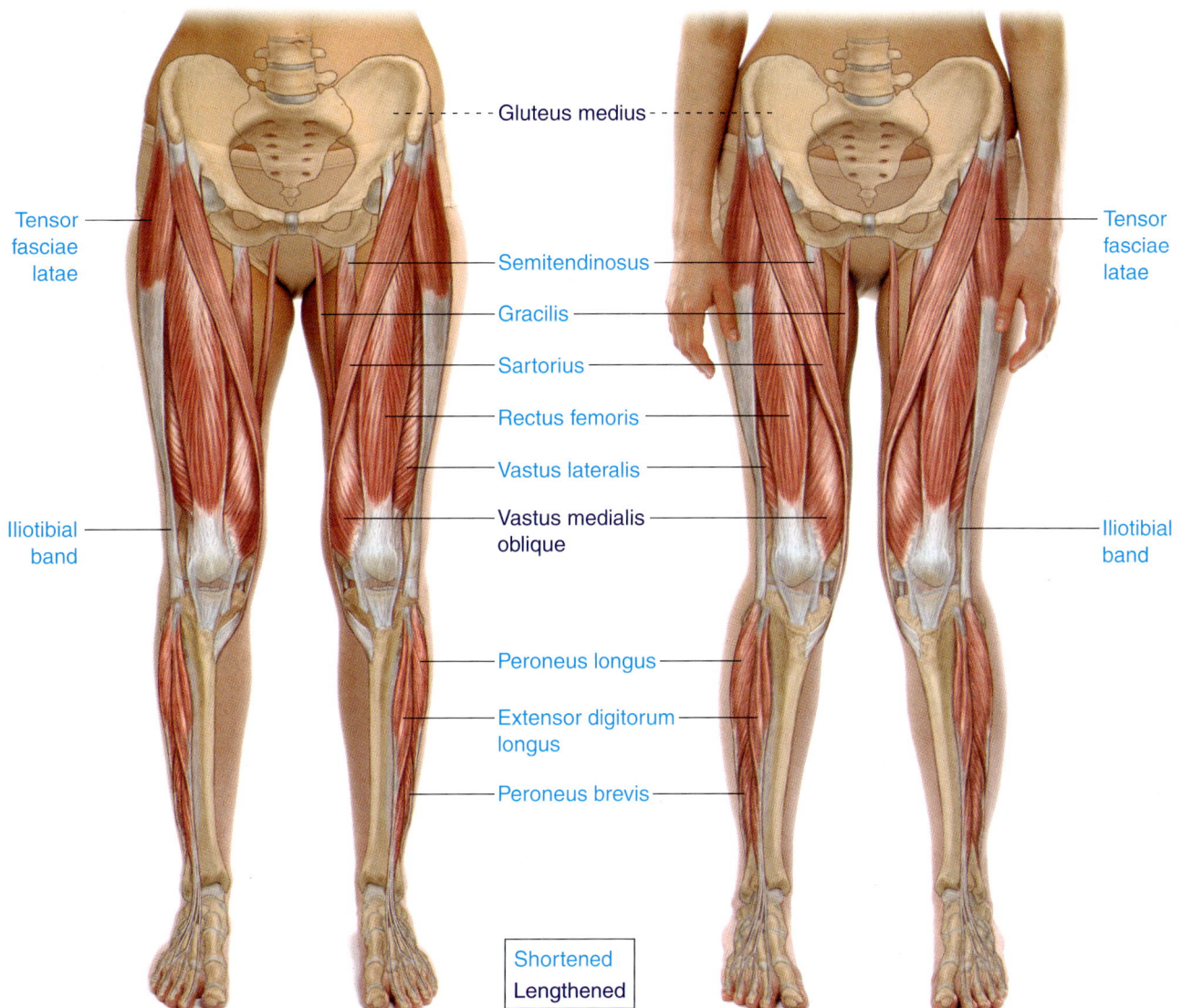

Figure 10-4 **Postural assessment comparison.** Compare the postures in these images. In the figure on the right, note the angle and rotation of the femur and tibia and the orientation of the ankle and the foot.

ROM ASSESSMENT

Test the ROMs of the knee involving muscles as both agonists and antagonists. Since it allows the client to control the amount of movement and stay within a pain-free range, only active ROM should be used in the acute stage of injury to prevent undue pain or re-injury. Box 10-1 presents the average active ROM results for the joints involved in patellofemoral syndrome.

Active ROM

Compare your assessment of the client's active ROM to the values in Box 10-1. Pain and other symptoms may not be reproduced during active ROM assessment because the client may limit movement to a symptom-free range.

  ■ **Active extension of the knee** may be restricted and cause pain when weak quadriceps and shortened hamstrings limit movement and when improper patellar tracking increases bone

---

Box 10-1   **AVERAGE ACTIVE ROM FOR JOINTS INVOLVED IN PATELLOFEMORAL SYNDROME**

Hip
Flexion 110–120°
  Rectus femoris
  Gluteus medius (anterior fibers)
  Tensor fasciae latae
  Sartorius
  Psoas major
  Iliacus
  Gluteus minimus
  Adductor magnus
  Adductor longus
  Adductor brevis

Extension 10–15°
  Biceps femoris
  Semitendinosus
  Semimembranosus
  Gluteus maximus
  Gluteus medius (posterior fibers)
  Adductor magnus (posterior fibers)

Lateral Rotation 40–60°
  Biceps femoris
  Gluteus maximus
  Gluteus medius (posterior fibers)
  Sartorius
  Piriformis
  Quadratus femoris
  Obturator internus
  Obturator externus
  Gemellus superior
  Gemellus inferior
  Psoas major
  Iliacus

Medial Rotation 30–40°
  Semitendinosus
  Semimembranosus
  Gluteus medius (anterior fibers)
  Adductor magnus

  Adductor longus
  Adductor brevis
  Gracilis
  Pectineus
  Tensor fasciae latae

Abduction 30–50°
  Gluteus maximus
  Gluteus medius
  Gluteus minimus
  Tensor fasciae latae
  Sartorius
  Piriformis (with flexed hip)

Adduction 30°
  Adductor magnus
  Adductor longus
  Adductor brevis
  Pectineus
  Gracilis
  Psoas major
  Iliacus
  Gluteus maximus (low fibers)

Knee
Flexion 120–150°
  Biceps femoris
  Semitendinosus
  Semimembranosus
  Gracilis
  Sartorius
  Gastrocnemius
  Popliteus
  Plantaris

Extension 0–15°
  Rectus femoris
  Vastus lateralis
  Vastus medialis
  Vastus intermedius

Medial Rotation (when flexed)
20–30°
  Semitendinosus
  Semimembranosus
  Gracilis
  Sartorius
  Popliteus

Lateral Rotation (when flexed)
30–40°
  Biceps femoris

Ankle
Dorsiflexion 20°
  Tibialis anterior
  Extensor digitorum longus
  Extensor hallucis longus

Plantar Flexion 50°
  Gastrocnemius
  Soleus
  Tibialis posterior
  Peroneus longus
  Peroneus brevis
  Flexor digitorum longus
  Flexor hallucis longus
  Plantaris

Inversion 45–60°
  Tibialis anterior
  Tibialis posterior
  Flexor digitorum longus
  Flexor hallucis longus
  Extensor hallucis longus

Eversion 15–30°
  Peroneus longus
  Peroneus brevis
  Extensor digitorum longus

to bone contact. Grinding or clicking may be heard or felt by the client. Active extension of the knee may also reveal lateral tracking of the patella when the rectus femoris and vastus lateralis contract with greater force than the vastus medialis.

- **Active abduction of the hip** may be restricted if medial rotation of the femur and knee valgus are present.
- **Active dorsiflexion of the ankle** may be restricted if the plantar flexors of the ankle are short and tight.

Passive ROM

Compare the client's P ROM on one side to the other when applicable. Note and compare the end feel for each range (see Chapter 1 for an explanation of end feel).

- **Passive flexion and extension of the knee** may reveal crepitus.
- **Passive extension of the knee** may reveal lateral tracking of the patella when the lateral retinaculum is tight or medial tracking if the medial retinaculum is tight.

Resisted ROM

Use resisted tests to assess the strength of the muscles that cross the knee. Compare the strength of the affected side to the unaffected side.

- **Resisted extension of the knee** may reveal weakness in the quadriceps and cause pain in the anterior knee.
- **Resisted flexion of the knee** may cause pain in the anterior knee.
- **Resisted abduction of the hip** may reveal weakness in the gluteal muscles.

SPECIAL TESTS

The following special tests can help you to determine which structures are contributing to pain and when a client should be evaluated by a medical professional using X-ray or other tools, which may reveal conditions that are contraindications or require special considerations when planning treatment with massage.

The patellar glide test is used to assess the medial and lateral mobility of the patella (Fig. 10-5). This test may also reveal crepitus.

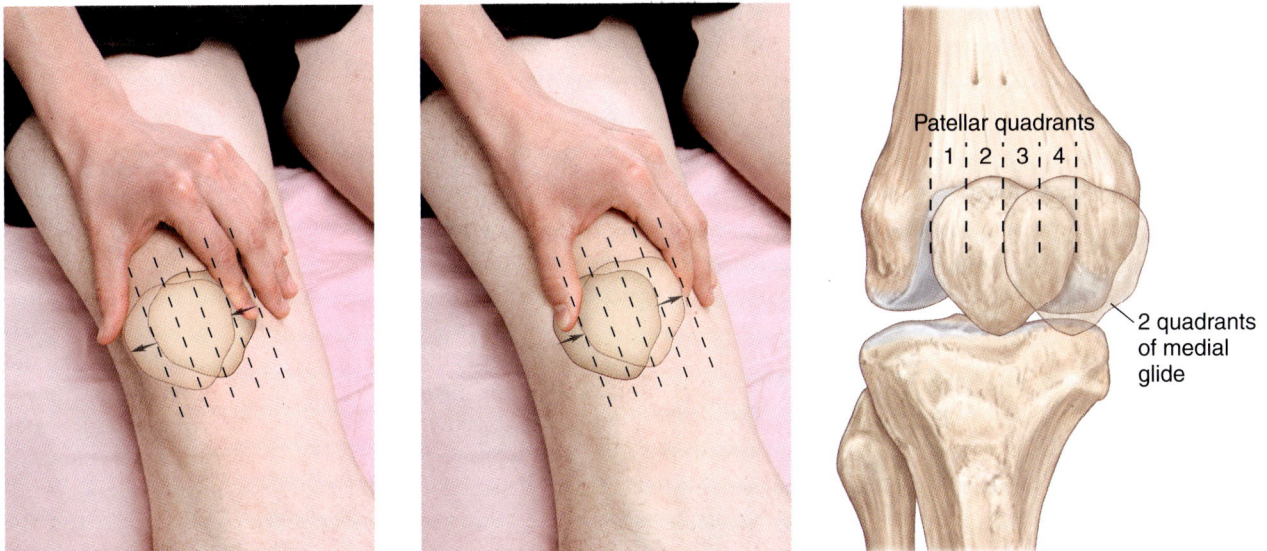

Figure 10-5   Patellar glide test. Slowly and gently, glide the patella laterally and medially to assess its mobility.

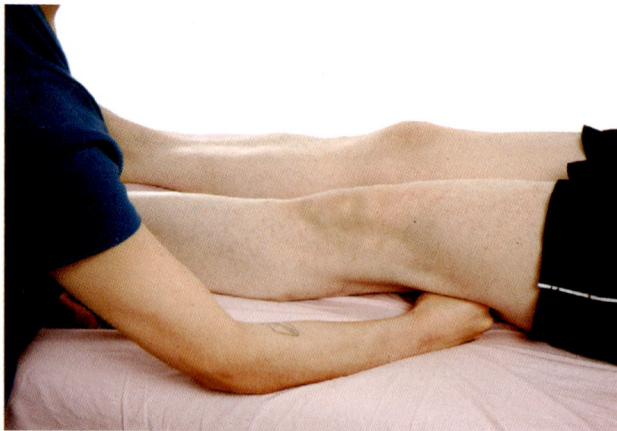

Figure 10-6 **Vastus medialis coordination test.** Test the functioning of the vastus medialis with resisted extension.

1. The client should be supine with a bolster under the knees and the quadriceps relaxed.
2. Place your thumb on one side of the patella and one or two fingers on the other side.
3. Slowly and gently glide the patella laterally and medially to assess its mobility. Ideally, the patella should move a distance equal to approximately half of its width in either direction.
4. Limited medial glide suggests that lateral structures are restricting movement. Limited lateral glide suggests that medial structures are restricting movement.

The vastus medialis coordination test is intended to isolate and assess the function of vastus medialis during extension of the knee (Fig. 10-6).

1. The client is supine with the knees extended and the quadriceps relaxed.
2. Place your fist under the distal thigh, superior to the affected knee.
3. Ask the client to slowly extend the knee without moving other joints while you assess the coordination of that action.
4. If you feel the client pushing the thigh into your fist or pulling away from your fist or if he or she flexes the hip to raise the leg, ask him or her to perform the action again by extending only the knee. You may also be able to see the orientation of the teardrop-shaped vastus medialis.
5. The test is considered positive for vastus medialis oblique dysfunction if the client has difficulty extending the knee or if he or she recruits muscles other than the quadriceps to perform this action.

PALPATION ASSESSMENT

Dysfunction in any joint from the sacroiliac to the metatarsals may cause or result from patellofemoral dysfunction. Because contributing factors may vary widely, it is essential to assess the tissues of each individual client from the ilium to the toes. It should not be surprising to find minor or even major differences in the way the tissues respond to this dysfunction.

Assess the knee for atypical temperature, color, and texture. You may find inflammation, adhesions, and tenderness around the patella. If the patella is tracking laterally, you may find the lateral retinaculum, iliotibial band, vastus lateralis, rectus femoris, and tensor fasciae latae tight and adhered; they may contain trigger points. The vastus medialis oblique may be hypotonic, and the semitendinosus, gracilis, and sartorius—muscles that blend into the pes anserinus tendon—may be dense and adhered with trigger points. Crepitus, fibrotic tissue, or a plica cord may be palpated at the medial knee. The hamstrings may feel tight and dense due to flexion contracture. Depending on the biomechanical factors involved, the adductors may be dense and adhered and the abductors taut or weak.

The gastrocnemius may also be tight due to flexion contracture at the knee. If eversion of the ankles is a factor, the peroneus longus and brevis and the extensor digitorum longus may be short and tight. These two factors may also play a role in developing plantar fasciitis, in which case the plantar flexors may be short and tight, and the tissues of the plantar surface of the foot may be thick, dense, and tender. Chapter 11 covers plantar fasciitis in more detail. If the client has a long history of knee pain or injury or has had surgery, you may find scar tissue and adhesions in the affected areas.

Trigger points that refer pain into the anterior knee may be found in the sartorius, rectus femoris, vastus medialis, vastus lateralis, adductor brevis, and adductor longus. See Figure 10-7 for common trigger points with referrals into the anterior knee.

Condition-Specific Massage

Because the causes of knee pain vary widely, the exact cause can be difficult to pinpoint, and more than one of these conditions may coexist. Systemic conditions that involve cautions or contraindications for massage may be the underlying cause of knee pain. If you feel uncertain that symptoms are caused by improper tracking of the patella or any of the soft tissue dysfunctions listed above, refer the client for medical assessment by a health care provider prior to treatment with massage.

It is essential for the treatment to be relaxing. You are not likely to eliminate the symptoms associated with patellofemoral syndrome or any of the coexisting conditions in a single treatment. Do not attempt to do so by treating aggressively. Be sure to ask your client to let you know if the amount of pressure you are applying keeps him or her from fully relaxing. If the client responds by tensing muscles or has a facial expression that looks distressed, reduce your pressure. Remember that you are working on tissue that is compromised. Ask the client to let you know if any part of your treatment reproduces symptoms, and always work within his or her tolerance. Deep palpation of a trigger point may cause pain at the upper end of the client's tolerance. Explain this to your client, describe a pain scale with a level of pain that should not be exceeded, and ask him or her to breathe deeply during the application of the technique. As the trigger point is deactivated, the referral pain will also diminish. Common trigger points and their referral patterns are shown in Figure 10-7.

The following suggestions are for treating the more common presentation of patellofemoral syndrome, caused primarily by improper lateral tracking of the patella. If the client has an acute injury, the protocol is PRICE (protection, rest, ice, compression, and elevation). You may work conservatively proximal or distal to the site, but avoid the area of injury until the subacute or chronic stage.

- Begin in the supine position with the knees bolstered.

- If you notice swelling, apply superficial draining strokes toward the nearest lymph nodes.

- If swelling is minor or absent, apply moist heat to the anterolateral thigh above the knee on the affected side. Do not use heat if swelling is significant.

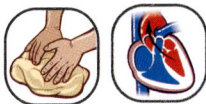

- Use your initial warming strokes to increase superficial circulation, soften tissues, and to assess the tissues from the ASIS down to the feet. You should be able to minimally assess tissues of the thigh, leg, and foot, which may help you to determine where to focus the time remaining after treating the knee.

Treatment icons: Increase circulation; Reduce adhesions; Reduce tension; Lengthen tissue; Treat trigger points; Passive stretch; Clear area

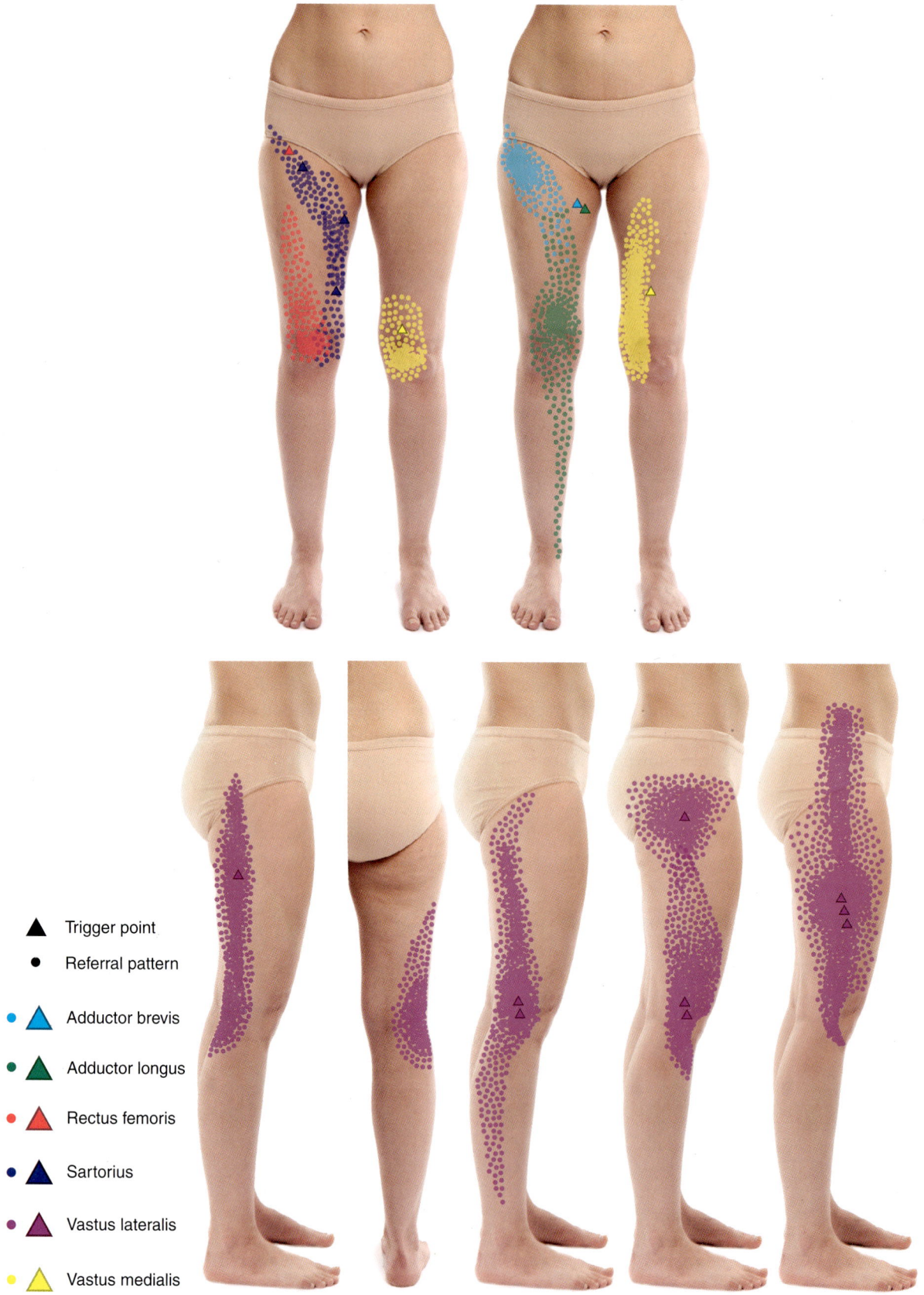

Trigger point

Referral pattern

Adductor brevis

Adductor longus

Rectus femoris

Sartorius

Vastus lateralis

Vastus medialis

Figure 10-7 **Common trigger points and referral.** Common trigger points associated with patellofemoral syndrome and their referral patterns.

■ Before applying emollient, assess for and treat myofascial restrictions in the thigh. You may find restrictions along the length of the iliotibial band, in the lateral quadriceps, and at the medial thigh and knee.

■ Treat the tissues of the thigh generally to reduce tension and to continue reducing adhesions.

■ Once the superficial tissues are pliable enough to allow for deeper work, lengthen tissues that are short and tight, and reduce tension in tissues that are taut. These may include the rectus femoris, vastus lateralis, tensor fasciae latae, iliotibial band, gracilis, sartorius, semi-tendinosus, and the adductors (Fig. 10-8).

■ Treat any trigger points that are found.

■ Assess the tissue surrounding the patella and knee joint for crepitus, adhesions, and fibrous tissues. Tissues affected may include the medial and lateral retinacula of the knee, the pes anserine tendon, the quadriceps tendon, the patellar tendon, and the iliotibial band (Fig. 10-9). Use small, focused strokes to release these tissues. If the structures are short and tight, follow this by long strokes in the direction of each muscle's fibers to restore length and tone. Take your time with this step, and treat the area thoroughly within the client's tolerance.

■ If you found the adductors and medial hamstrings to be short and tight, stretch them by passively abducting the hip. Perform PIR, if necessary, to relax and lengthen these muscles if a passive stretch is insufficient.

■ If eversion is a contributing factor, assess and treat the peroneal muscles and extensor digitorum longus for adhesions, increased tone, and trigger points (Fig. 10-10, p. 252).

■ Use clearing strokes to the entire lower extremity to increase venous return.

■ Turn the client prone with a bolster under the ankles. Stretch the lateral quadriceps by bringing the heel toward the buttocks and gently pulling the leg toward you. Use PIR to encourage lengthening if you note resistance.

■ If time permits, assess and treat the gluteal muscles, hamstrings, and plantar flexors for adhesions, hypertonicity, and trigger points if found.

■ Use clearing strokes to the entire lower extremity to increase venous return.

The treatment overview diagram summarizes the flow of treatment (Fig. 10-11, p. 253).

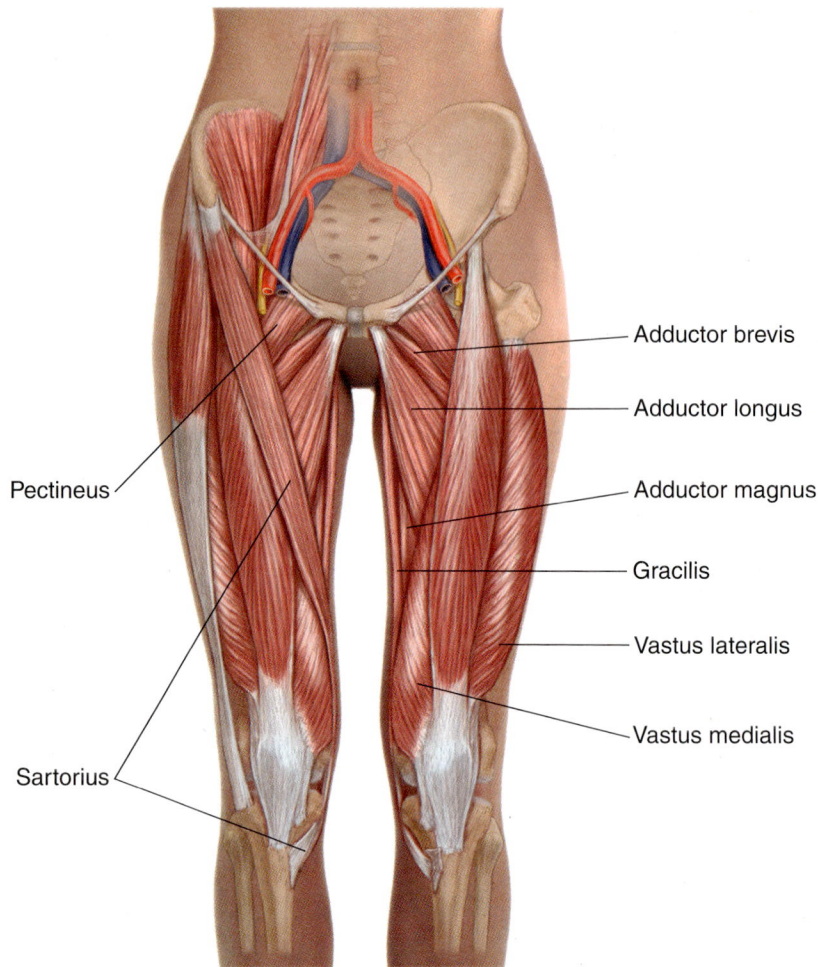

VASTUS LATERALIS

Origin	Lateral linea aspera, gluteal tuberosity.
Insertion	Tibial tuberosity.
Action	Extend knee.
Nerve	Femoral.

GRACILIS

Origin	Inferior ramus of pubis, ramus of ischium.
Insertion	Proximal, medial tibia at pes anserine.
Action	Adduct hip, medially rotate hip, flex knee, medially rotate flexed knee.
Nerve	Obturator.

ADDUCTOR MAGNUS

Origin	Inferior ramus of pubis, ramus of ischium, ischial tuberosity.
Insertion	Medial linea aspera, adductor tubercle.
Action	Adduct hip, medially rotate hip, assist to flex hip, posterior fibers extend hip.
Nerve	Obturator and tibial.

ADDUCTOR BREVIS

Origin	Inferior ramus of pubis.
Insertion	Pectineal line and medial linea aspera.
Action	Adduct hip, medially rotate hip, assist to flex hip.
Nerve	Obturator.

VASTUS MEDIALIS

Origin	Medial linea aspera.
Insertion	Tibial tuberosity.
Action	Extend knee.
Nerve	Femoral.

SARTORIUS

Origin	Anterior superior iliac crest.
Insertion	Proximal, medial tibia at pes anserine.
Action	Flex hip, laterally rotate hip, abduct hip, flex knee, medially rotate flexed knee.
Nerve	Femoral.

ADDUCTOR LONGUS

Origin	Pubic tubercle.
Insertion	Medial linea aspera.
Action	Adduct hip, medially rotate hip, assist to flex hip.
Nerve	Obturator.

PECTINEUS

Origin	Superior ramus of pubis.
Insertion	Pectineal line of femur.
Action	Adduct hip, medially rotate hip, assist to flex hip.
Nerve	Femoral and obturator.

Figure 10-8   Muscles of the anterior thigh. Assess and treat the thigh for myofascial restrictions, hypertonicity, and trigger points. Adapted from Clay JH, Pounds DM. *Basic Clinical Massage Therapy: Integrating Anatomy and Treatment,* 2nd ed. Philadelphia: Lippincott Williams & Wilkins, 2008.

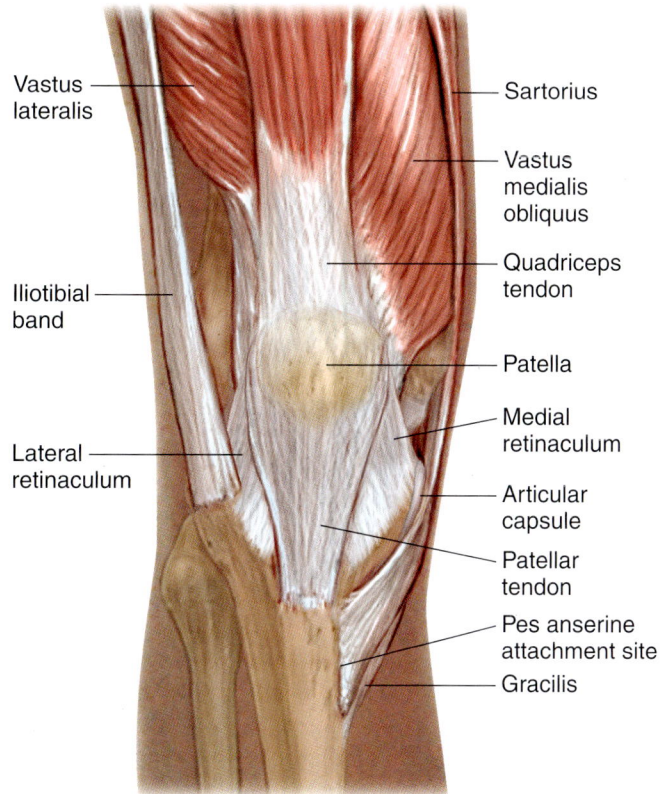

Figure 10-9   Soft tissues surrounding the knee. Adapted from Clay JH, Pounds DM. *Basic Clinical Massage Therapy: Integrating Anatomy and Treatment,* 2nd ed. Philadelphia: Lippincott Williams & Wilkins, 2008.

CLIENT SELF-CARE

A client with patellofemoral pain may benefit from wearing a knee brace during activity, in particular if his or her activities include sports, repetitive actions, or weight-bearing motions of the knee such as squatting and lifting heavy objects. If the client wears a brace, recommend that he or she remove the brace during periods of inactivity to avoid reduced circulation to the area if the health care provider agrees. Clients with pes planus or eversion of the ankle may benefit from corrective arch support. Refer the client to a podiatrist for an assessment and fitting for corrective arch support.

The following are intended as general recommendations for stretching and strengthening muscles involved in the client's condition. The objective is to create distance between the attachment sites of muscles that have shortened and to perform repetitions of movements that decrease the distance between the attachments of muscles that have weakened. If you have had no training in remedial exercises and do not feel that you have a functional understanding of stretching and strengthening, refer the client to a professional with training in this area.

Clients often neglect self-care because their daily lives are busy. Encourage them to follow these guidelines:

- Instruct the client to perform self-care throughout the day, such as while taking a phone call, reading e-mail, washing the dishes, or watching television instead of setting aside extra time. When performing self-care while standing, ask the client to notice if he or she is shifting weight to one leg, if the knees are close together, and if the femur is medially rotated. If so, instruct the client to focus on distributing weight evenly to both legs and to keep the toes pointed forward within his or her comfort level.
- Encourage your client to take regular breaks from stationary postures or repetitive actions. If the client's daily activities include hours of sitting, suggest moving for at least a few minutes every hour. If the client's daily activities require repetitive actions affecting the knee, suggest resting for at least a few minutes every hour.

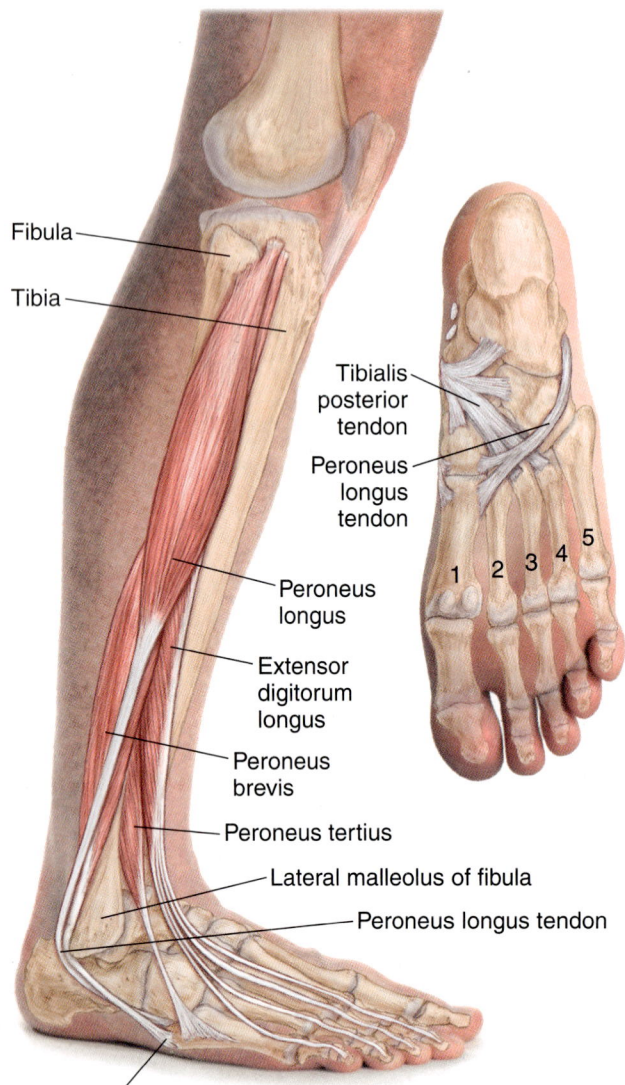

Fibula

Tibia

Tibialis posterior tendon

Peroneus longus tendon

1 2 3 4 5

Peroneus longus

Extensor digitorum longus

Peroneus brevis

Peroneus tertius

Lateral malleolus of fibula

Peroneus longus tendon

Peroneus brevis attachment to 5th metatarsal

PERONEUS LONGUS

Origin	Proximal, lateral fibula.
Insertion	Base of 1st metatarsal and medial cuneiform.
Action	Evert foot, assist in plantar flexion of ankle.
Nerve	Superior peroneal.

PERONEUS BREVIS

Origin	Distal lateral fibula.
Insertion	Tuberosity of 5th metatarsal.
Action	Evert foot, assist in plantar flexion of ankle.
Nerve	Superior peroneal.

EXTENSOR DIGITORUM LONGUS

Origin	Proximal anterior fibula, interosseus membrane.
Insertion	Middle and distal phalanges of toes 2–5.
Action	Extend toes 2–5, dorsiflex ankle, evert foot.
Nerve	Deep peroneal.

Figure 10-10 Muscles that evert the ankle. Adapted from Clay JH, Pounds DM. *Basic Clinical Massage Therapy: Integrating Anatomy and Treatment,* 2nd ed. Philadelphia: Lippincott Williams & Wilkins, 2008.

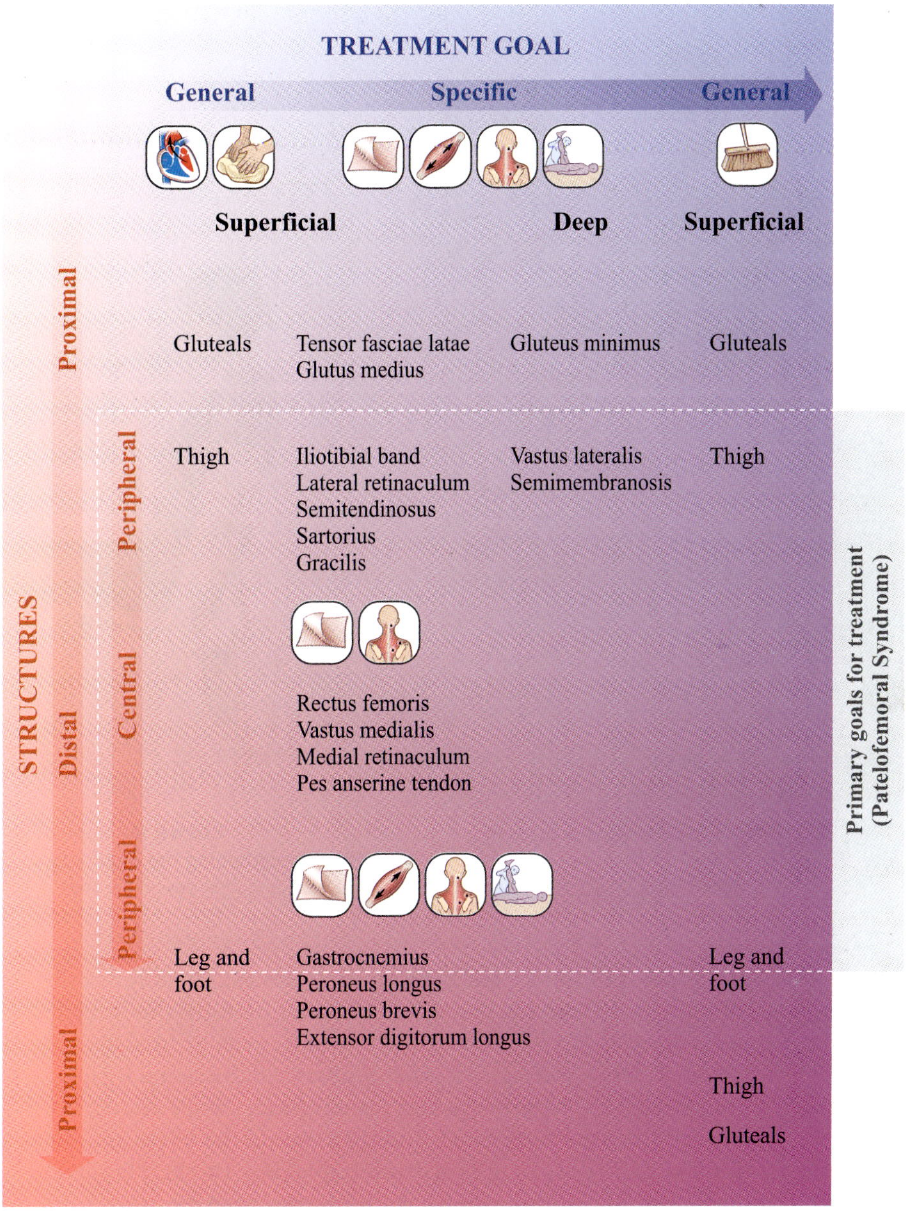

Figure 10-11 **Patellofemoral syndrome treatment overview diagram.** Follow the general principles from left to right or top to bottom when treating patellofemoral syndrome.

- Demonstrate gentle self-massage of the tissues surrounding the knee to keep adhesions and hypertonicity at bay between treatments.
- Demonstrate all strengthening exercises and stretches to your client and have him or her perform these in your presence before leaving to ensure that he or she is performing them properly and will not cause harm when practicing alone. Stretches should be held for 15–30 seconds and performed frequently throughout the day within the client's limits. The client should not force the stretch or bounce. Stretching should be slow, gentle, and steady, trying to keep every other joint as relaxed as possible.
- Stretching and strengthening exercises should be recommended according to your findings in ROM testing and palpation. Because patellofemoral syndrome may present differently with each client, self-care should be tailored to specific needs.

Stretching

To stretch the lateral structures that may contribute to drawing the patella laterally, instruct the client to stand at an arm's length from a wall with the affected side toward the wall. Rest one hand

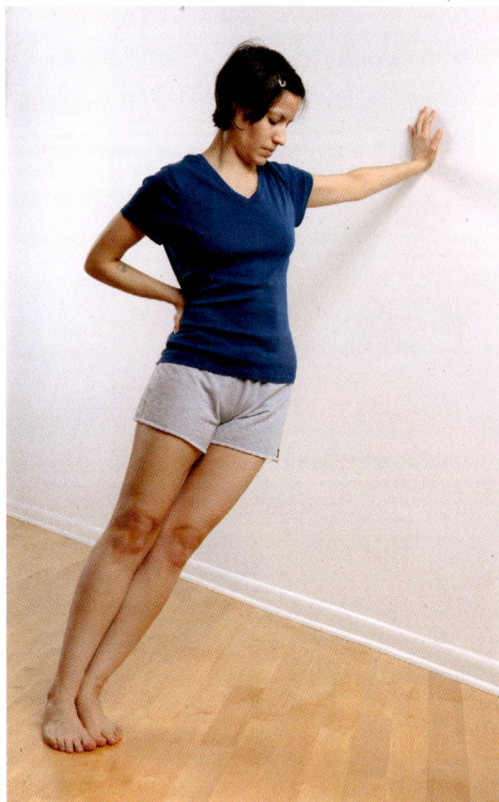

Figure 10-12 **Stretch the lateral structures of the leg.**

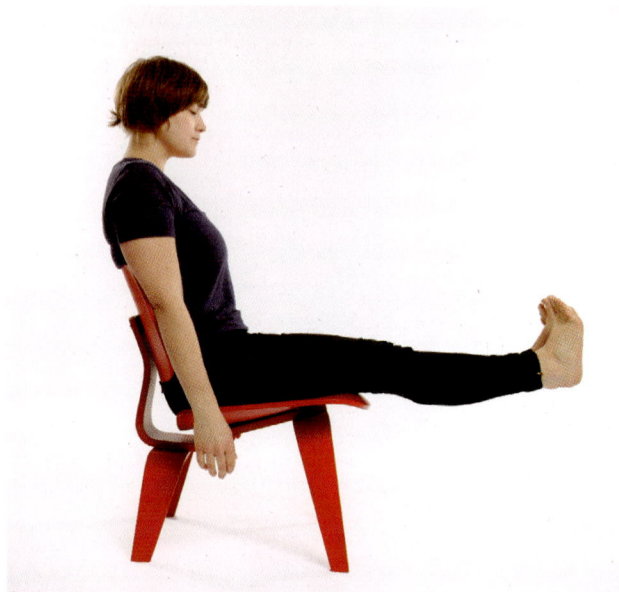

Figure 10-13 **Stretch the hamstrings and plantar flexors while strengthening the quadriceps.** Sit comfortably with the back supported, and then extend the knee and dorsiflex the ankle.

on the wall for support, and with the feet together, laterally flex the trunk away from the wall and hold for 15–30 seconds (Fig. 10-12). Do not perform this stretch if it increases pressure on the medial knee. If you found the gluteus medius weak or stretched, instruct the client to adjust their posture in this stretch until it is felt primarily in the lateral leg instead of in the gluteal muscles.

To stretch the hamstrings and plantar flexors while seated, instruct the client to sit comfortably with the back supported, and then extend the knees and dorsiflex the ankles and hold for 15–30 seconds or as long as is comfortable (Fig. 10-13). This action also helps to strengthen the quadriceps. Repeat this action a few times, and then get up and walk around to mobilize the knee.

If eversion contributes, instruct the client to simultaneously stretch the evertors and strengthen the invertors by actively inverting the ankle fully and holding for as long as is comfortable. Repeat this action a few times, and then get up and walk around to mobilize the ankle.

Strengthening

While it is difficult to isolate the vastus medialis oblique from the other quadriceps, it is important to restore its strength and tone so that it can antagonize lateral tracking of the patella. The seated hamstring stretch described above also strengthens the quadriceps. Repeating the steps of the vastus medialis coordination test (Fig 10-6) with a rolled towel or other bolster under the thigh just above the knee will also strengthen the vastus medialis.

SUGGESTIONS FOR FURTHER TREATMENT

Ideally, a client with patellofemoral syndrome will have treatments twice a week until the client can perform activities of daily living with minimal or no pain for at least 4 days. Once this is achieved, reduce frequency to once per week until symptoms are absent for at least 7 days. When the client reports that he or she has been pain-free for more than 7 days, treatment can be reduced to twice per month. If the client is pain-free for 3 or more consecutive weeks, he or she can then schedule once per month or as necessary. If the client's symptoms are localized and other postural deviations are minimal, half-hour treatments may be sufficient to effect a change in patellofemoral function. In the treatment of patellofemoral syndrome that is muscular in nature, there should be some improvement with each session. If this is not happening, consider the following possibilities:

- There is too much time between treatments. It is always best to give the newly treated tissues 24–48 hours to adapt, but if too much time passes between treatments in the beginning, the client's activities of daily living may reverse any progress.
- The client is not adjusting activities of daily living or is not keeping up with self-care. As much as we want to fix the problem, we cannot force a client to make the adjustments we suggest. Explain the importance of the client's participation in the healing process, and encourage the client to follow your recommendations, but be careful not to judge or reprimand a client who does not.
- The condition is advanced or involves other musculoskeletal complications that are beyond your basic training. Refer this client to a massage therapist with advanced clinical massage training. Continuing to treat a client whose case is beyond your training could turn the client away from massage therapy altogether and hinder healing.
- The client has an undiagnosed, underlying condition. Discontinue treatment until the client sees a health care provider for a medical assessment.

If you are not treating the client in a clinical setting or private practice, you may not be able to take this client through the full program of healing. Still, if you can bring some relief in just one treatment, it may encourage the client to discuss this change with his or her health care provider and seek manual therapy rather than more aggressive treatment options. If the client agrees to return for regular treatments, his or her symptoms are likely to change each time, so it is important to perform an assessment before each session. Once you have released superficial tissues in general areas, you may be able to focus more of your treatment on deeper tissues in a specific area. Likewise, once you have treated the structures specific to patellofemoral syndrome, you may be able to pay closer attention to compensating structures and coexisting conditions.

PROFESSIONAL GROWTH

CASE STUDY

Ronja is a 64-year-old, married female. She is a retired accountant. Ronja and her husband moved from suburban Chicago to San Francisco following their retirement last year. Over the past 2 months she has had knee pain, which is becoming worse. Currently, the pain makes it difficult for her to walk the hills of San Francisco to run her errands.

Subjective

Ronja complained of knee pain that began approximately 2 months ago and has been increasing gradually. She feels aches, sometimes throughout the day, in both knees and feels pain around her right kneecap and on the inside of her knee when she walks. The pain keeps her from performing some activities on some days. She moved from a suburban setting where she worked sitting at a desk all day and had to drive everywhere, because everything was far from her home. She and her husband made a complete lifestyle change that included moving to a more natural environment where locally grown foods are readily available, and they could walk or ride a bike instead of driving. It was difficult at first for her to adjust to the increased activity, but she did not have any pain until recently. Her physician diagnosed chondromalacia and said that she would eventually need knee replacement surgery. He said that while nothing showed up on an MRI, it is probably in the early stages and will show up later. He gave her a prescription for physical therapy. She was referred by a friend who was treated at this clinic and experienced a full recovery from similar symptoms.

Objective

Ronja appears very healthy and vibrant and looks many years younger than her age. She climbed the stairs very slowly, mainly relying on the left leg to lift her weight. She also stood up from a seated position very cautiously but without leaning on the table or chair for support.

Postural assessment revealed increased lordotic curve with anterior pelvic tilt, slight lateral rotation of the hips bilaterally, flexion of the knees bilaterally, and ankle eversion bilaterally. The four lateral toes of the right foot are hyperextended. The Q angle appears within normal range. Medial patellar glide is reduced. ROM testing resulted in reduced active extension of the knees bilaterally, which is possibly a protective measure. The client felt pain in the medial knee with resisted extension of the knee and resisted adduction of the hip. During passive extension of the right knee, Ronja tensed up at the end range. Crepitus was noted during extension and flexion of the right knee. There was weak abduction of the right hip and minimal active inversion of the ankles. There was only slightly greater range with passive inversion.

Palpation revealed tension in rectus femoris which is adhered to a hypertonic vastus lateralis and a dense, fibrous iliotibial band on the right. Fascial restrictions along the lateral right thigh from ASIS to tibiofibular joint. The medial aspect of the patellofemoral joint was tender to the touch with considerable crepitus and possible plica cord. The vastus medialis feels fibrous and hypotonic. The semitendinosus, sartorius, and gracilis, along with the pes anserine tendons, are taut and tender with adhesions at the distal fibers. The hamstrings feel dense and adhered only at the distal, medial fibers. The peroneals and extensor digitorum longus are short, tight, and adhered. The ankle invertors are taut and weak.

Signs and symptoms suggest patellofemoral syndrome with mild hyperlordosis.

Action

Treatment today focused on reducing knee pain. If the client agrees, future treatment will include restoring proper knee function, pelvic tilt, orientation of the femur and the tibia, and ankle function.

On the right thigh, I performed myofascial release from the ASIS to the tibiofibular joint. I used cross-fiber friction on the iliotibial band. I then used petrissage followed by muscle stripping to the rectus femoris, vastus intermedius and vastus lateralis, and IT band. A trigger point was found at the superior fibers of the rectus femoris that referred into the anterior knee. Two rounds of compressions reduced referral pain from level 7 to 2. I applied cross-fiber strokes to the medial knee to release metabolites and reduce crepitus followed by clearing strokes toward the inguinal lymph nodes. I applied general kneading to the medial thigh. I used cross-fiber strokes from the pes anserine along the path of the sartorius and again along the path of the gracilis and the medial hamstrings to separate the fibers of the muscles of the medial thigh, followed by long gliding strokes. I used muscle stripping to lengthen the sartorius and medial hamstrings and performed a stretch to the medial hamstrings. I applied myofascial release, superficial cross-fiber strokes, and muscle stripping to reduce adhesions and lengthen ankle evertors.

I used similar, although less aggressive, treatment to the left thigh and leg. I also applied general deep tissue techniques to the low back, gluteals, calves, and feet.

Following treatment, the client stated feeling looser and less protective with steps. Ronja descended the stairs with less caution, although she did use the handrail.

Plan

I demonstrated a hamstring stretch with knee extension and hip flexor stretches with lunges. I recommended speaking with a podiatrist about shoes with good arch support or being fitted for orthotics to reduce eversion. I demonstrated strengthening for ankle invertors and vastus medialis and emphasized the importance of limiting exercises to a pain-free range. I suggested slowly reintroducing activities that had previously resulted in pain.

I explained that reducing symptoms at the knee alone is manageable with half-hour sessions but that biomechanical factors at the hip and ankle likely contribute to her pain and a more complete recovery would best be managed with 1-hour sessions. Ronja has agreed to 1-hour treatments twice a week until symptoms are absent for at least 4 consecutive days with reassessment at that time.

CRITICAL THINKING EXERCISES

1. In general, the most common presentation of patellofemoral syndrome emerges when the lateral structures that move and stabilize the knee in extension are stronger than the medial structures. Create a SOAP chart with a history, assessment, and treatment plan that describes a case of patellofemoral syndrome due to excessive medial tracking of the patella. This client likely presents with pain and tenderness at the lateral knee, weakening of structures that affect lateral tracking, and tension in structures that affect medial tracking. Treatment goals should include lengthening shortened tissues, strengthening weak muscles, and restoring proper neuromuscular function.

2. Develop a 10-minute stretching and strengthening routine for a client, covering all of the muscles involved in patellofemoral syndrome. Use Box 10-1 and Figure 10-4 as a guide. Remember that a stretch increases the distance between the origin and insertion of a muscle and is important for those muscles that are shortened while strengthening is performed by actively bringing the origin and insertion closer together and is important for the antagonists of shortened muscles. Describe each step of the routine in enough detail that the client can refer to these descriptions in your absence and perform them without harm.

3. A client calls to schedule a massage for knee pain. He states that he hears crunching and clicking in his knee when he stands up and sometimes when he walks. He explains that he has sprained the ankle of the affected leg twice and the ankle of the opposite leg once. He has also had an episode of myositis ossificans to the tibialis anterior after being kicked during a soccer game. Discuss the possible relationship between the injuries and patellofemoral syndrome. What questions would you ask this client? Are there questions that you need to ask his health care provider? What special considerations would you need to include in your treatment plan both for contributing factors and for contraindications?

4. Conduct a short literature review to explain the relationship between symptoms suggesting patellofemoral syndrome and the following:
   - Pes cavus
   - Arthritis
   - Insufficient anterior prominence of the lateral femoral condyle
   - Depth of the patellar groove
   - Patellar taping

BIBLIOGRAPHY AND SUGGESTED READINGS

Bhave A, Baker E. Prescribing quality patellofemoral rehabilitation before advocating operative care. Orthopedic Clinics of North America. 2008;39(3):275–285.

Biel A. *Trail Guide to the Body: How to Locate Muscles, Bones and More*, 3rd ed. Boulder, CO: Books of Discovery, 2005.

Hertling D, Kessler RM. *Management of Common Musculoskeletal Disorders: Physical Therapy Principles and Methods*, 4th ed. Philadelphia, PA: Lippincott Williams & Wilkins, 2006.

Holt G, Nunn T, Gregori A. The vastus medialis obliquus insertion: A classification system relevant to minimally invasive TKA. Orthopedics. 2008;31(11):1090.

Hudson Z, Darthuy E. Iliotibial band tightness and patellofemoral pain syndrome: A case-control study. Manual Therapy. 2009;14(2):147–151.

Juhn M. Patellofemoral pain syndrome: A review and guidelines for treatment. American Family Physician. 1999;60:2012–2022.

Lowe W. *Orthopedic Massage: Theory and Technique*. St Louis, MO: Mosby-Elsevier, 2003.

Mayo Foundation for Medical Education and Research. Bursitis. Available at http://www.mayoclinic.com/health/bursitis/DS00032. Accessed Winter 2009.

Mayo Foundation for Medical Education and Research. Chondromalacia Patella. Available at http://mayoclinic.com/health/chondromalacia-patella/DS00777. Accessed Winter 2009.

Mayo Foundation for Medical Education and Research. Knee Pain. Available at http://www.mayoclinic.com/health/knee-pain/DS00555. Accessed Winter 2009.

Mayo Foundation for Medical Education and Research. Osgood-Schlatter Disease. Available at http://mayoclinic.com/health/osgood-schlatter-disease/DS00392. Accessed Winter 2009.

Mayo Foundation for Medical Education and Research. Osteoarthritis. Available at http://www.mayoclinic.com/ health/osteoarthritis/DS00019. Accessed Winter 2009.

Mayo Foundation for Medical Education and Research. Rheumatoid Arthritis. Available at http://www.mayoclinic.com/health/rheumatoid-arthritis/DS00020. Accessed Winter 2009.

Mayo Foundation for Medical Education and Research. Septic Arthritis. Available at http://www.mayoclinic.com/health/bone-and-joint-infections/DS00545. Accessed Winter 2009.

Mayo Foundation for Medical Education and Research. Torn Meniscus. Available at http://mayoclinic.com/health/torn-meniscus/DS00932. Accessed Winter 2009.

Medscape. Plica Syndrome. Available at http://emedicine.medscape.com/article/1252011-overview. Accessed Winter 2009.

Nijs J, Van Geel C, Van der auwera C, et al. Diagnostic value of five clinical tests in patellofemoral pain syndrome. Manual Therapy. 2006;11(1):69–77.

Oatis C. *Kinesiology: The Mechanics & Pathomechanics of Human Movement*, 2nd ed. Baltimore, MD: Lippincott Williams & Wilkins, 2009.

Pedrelli A, Stecco C, Day JA. Treating patellar tendinopathy with fascial manipulation. Journal of Bodywork and Movement Therapies. 2009;13(1):73–80.

Rattray F, Ludwig L. *Clinical Massage Therapy: Understanding, Assessing and Treating over 70 Conditions*. Toronto, ON: Talus Incorporated, 2000.

Simons DG, Travell JG, Simons LS. *Myofascial Pain and Dysfunction: The Trigger Point Manual*, 2nd ed. Philadelphia, PA: Lippincott Williams & Wilkins, 1999.

U.S. National Library of Medicine and the National Institutes of Health. Baker's Cyst. Available at http://www.nlm.nih.gov/medlineplus/ency/article/001222.htm. Accessed Winter 2009.

U.S. National Library of Medicine and the National Institutes of Health. Gout. Available at http://www.nlm.nih.gov/medlineplus/ency/article/000424.htm#Symptoms. Accessed Winter 2009.

van den Dolder PA, Roberts DL. Six sessions of manual therapy increase knee flexion and improve activity in people with anterior knee pain: A randomised controlled trial. Australian Journal of Physiotherapy. 2006;52(4):261–264.

Ward SR, Terk MR, Powers CM. Patella alta: Association with patellofemoral alignment and changes in contact area during weight-bearing. The Journal of Bone and Joint Surgery. 2007;89:1749–1755.

Werner R. *A Massage Therapist's Guide to Pathology*, 4th ed. Philadelphia, PA: Lippincott Williams and Wilkins, 2009.

White LC, Dolphin P, Dixon J. Hamstring length in patellofemoral pain syndrome. Physiotherapy. 2009;95(1):24–28.

Zalta J. Massage therapy protocol for post-anterior cruciate ligament reconstruction patellofemoral pain syndrome: A case report. International Journal of Therapeutic Massage & Bodywork: Research, Education, & Practice. 2008;1(2):11–21.

Plantar Fasciitis

UNDERSTANDING PLANTAR FASCIITIS

Plantar fasciitis is irritation and inflammation of the plantar fascia. The plantar fascia is a strap of connective tissue that connects the calcaneus to the toes (Fig. 11-1). It is thick and strong in the center with thinner, weaker wings along the medial and lateral foot. The central band is often referred to as the plantar aponeurosis. It is attached to the medial calcaneal tubercle proximally and divides into five bands that merge with the flexor tendons at the proximal phalanx of each toe. The collagen fibers of the plantar fascia are oriented mostly longitudinally and are arranged in bundles but are reinforced by transverse fibers just inferior to the metatarsal heads. The plantar fascia and calcaneal tendon both have attachments on the calcaneus, linking their roles in plantar flexion and dorsiflexion.

Structurally, the plantar fascia connects the bones of the foot, supports the arch of the foot, and minimizes impact to the arch during weight-bearing activities. Functionally, the plantar fascia operates similarly to what is called the windlass mechanism: extending the toes puts tension on the fascia, which shortens the arch and creates a spring. In normal gait, plantar flexion initiates the heel-off phase, and the windlass mechanism of the plantar fascia increases the strength of propulsion at the push-off phase as the tension is released. The calcaneal attachment of the plantar fascia is much smaller than the distal attachments at the proximal phalanges. This concentrates a great amount of force on a small area at the calcaneal tubercle when either the support mechanism or the windlass mechanism is activated during weight-bearing activity.

The two heads of the gastrocnemius and the soleus blend into the calcaneal tendon. This grouping of muscles is called the triceps surae. The triceps surae attaches to the tuberosity of the posterior calcaneus via the calcaneal tendon. When the calcaneal tendon shortens during plantar flexion, it pulls the calcaneus posteriorly and superiorly while tensile stress in the plantar fascia draws the calcaneus anteriorly, leaving the small attachment site situated between tensile forces in virtually opposite directions (Fig. 11-2). When these structures are strong, flexible, and unhindered by dysfunction, forces are distributed efficiently to produce smooth movement. Plantar fasciitis is one possible result when biomechanical factors and soft tissue dysfunction keep those forces from being distributed efficiently.

Common Signs and Symptoms

Plantar fasciitis usually develops gradually, but it can appear suddenly and can be acute. It typically occurs unilaterally but can be bilateral. The most common symptom of plantar fasciitis is sharp, burning, or aching pain in the arch of the foot. The worst of the pain is often felt in the push-off phase of gait, when passive extension of the toes increases tensile stress in the plantar fascia. Pain is often most intense near the calcaneal attachment of the plantar fascia where tearing is most likely to occur, but pain sometimes spreads along the medial border of the arch of the

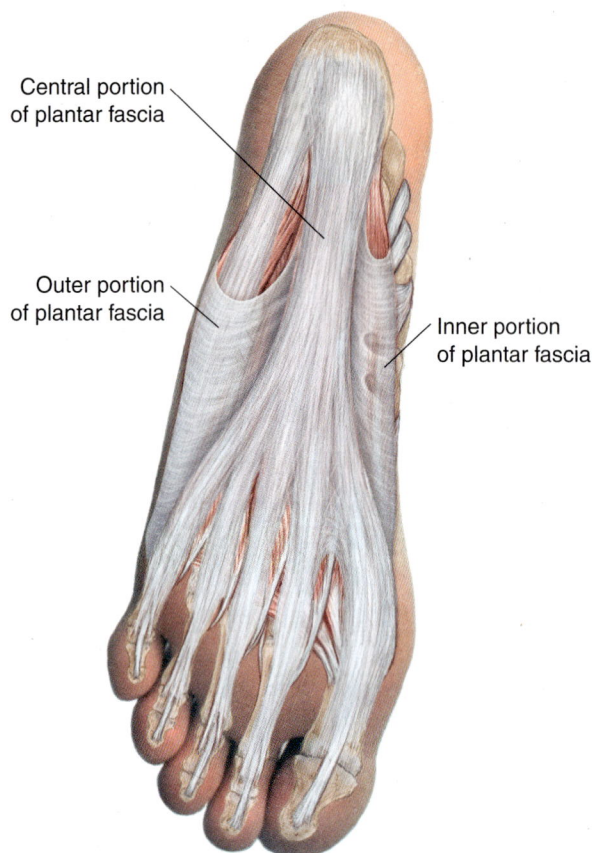

Figure 11-1 **Plantar fascia.** The plantar fascia is thick connective tissue that supports the arch of the foot. Adapted from Clay JH, Pounds DM. *Basic Clinical Massage Therapy: Integrating Anatomy and Treatment,* 2nd ed. Philadelphia: Lippincott Williams & Wilkins, 2008.

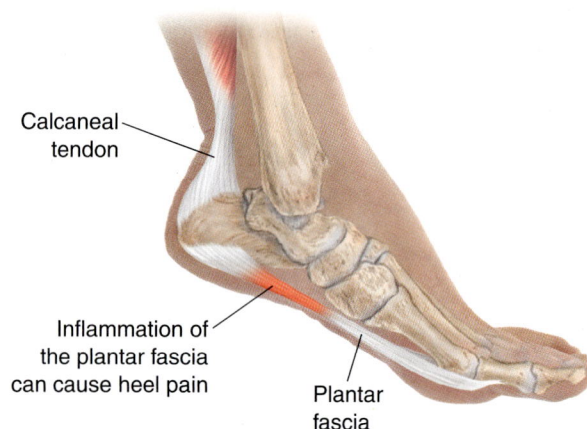

Figure 11-2 **Localized pain characteristic of plantar fasciitis.** The medial calcaneal tubercle is situated between tensile forces in virtually opposite directions, increasing the risk of injury.

foot toward the toes. Symptoms are felt most frequently with the first steps in the morning or after rest. During periods of inactivity, when the injured tissues undergo the process of repair, the plantar fascia contracts and loses flexibility, making those first steps the most painful. As the tissues warm up and become more flexible, symptoms may improve or subside temporarily, but if left untreated, they are likely to return following subsequent periods of rest.

Pain may also be felt while standing, when bearing weight increases tensile stress in the plantar fascia. This is particularly true when the toes are extended either actively or passively. Climbing stairs increases the demand on these structures and may also be painful. Standing on the toes involves plantar flexion of the ankle, which shortens the calcaneal tendon, and passive extension of the toes, which adds tensile stress to the plantar fascia. When the integrity of the plantar fascia is compromised, this action may cause pain, swelling, or tearing of fibers. In all of the cases described above, tension in the plantar fascia increases stress on the periosteum of its small bony attachment on the calcaneus, pulling the tissue away from the bone, which may result in the development of bone spurs. Likewise, stress and tearing of the tissue often result in inflammation of the plantar fascia, which in turn increases sensitivity and pain. When pes cavus is a contributing factor, or if the individual attempts to avoid pain in the arch by walking on the outside of the foot, pain may be felt on the lateral foot due to increased impact during activity.

Possible Causes and Contributing Factors

Many possible factors may contribute to plantar fasciitis, but the factor cited most frequently is overuse. Overuse occurs with any activity in which exaggeration of the normal mechanical function of the tissue may lead to inflammation and tearing. A new or intense exercise regimen that involves running, jumping, or other actions that increase tensile stress on the plantar fascia puts the unconditioned tissues at risk for injury. Standing for long periods on hard, inflexible surfaces increases demand on the spring mechanism of the plantar fascia and also increases the risk of injury. The injured tissue, which repairs itself by forming scars, is continually at risk for further tearing, fibrosis, and inflammation, increasing the risk of bone spurs, and continuing the cycle until the contributing factors are resolved. In addition, because the plantar fascia has a limited blood supply, it heals slowly.

But while plantar fasciitis is often referred to as an overuse injury, underuse may also be a predisposing factor. Inactivity not only decreases circulation to the area, reducing hydration and nutrition to the tissues, but it may also contribute to adhesions, contractures, and joint dysfunction. Sedentary routines may affect the length and strength of the muscles that move the foot as well as the soft tissues that support the structures of the foot. If the foot is not rested flat on the floor while sitting, the ankle may rest in plantar flexion, passively shortening the plantar flexors and the calcaneal tendon, and the toes may be held in passive extension, increasing tension on the plantar fascia. Knee flexion also shortens the gastrocnemius and may affect its resting tone. During sleep or another recumbent position, the ankles generally rest in passive plantar flexion, which may contribute to adhesions and shortening of the plantar flexors, particularly if neuromuscular health is compromised.

Eversion contributes to pes planus, which stretches the plantar fascia taut, reducing its ability to provide the protective spring mechanism during weight-bearing activity. Pes cavus, conversely, brings the origin and insertions together, shortening and thickening the plantar fascia, reducing its ability to absorb shock during weight-bearing activity. Femoral and tibial rotations, common with patellofemoral syndrome, may also affect the orientation of the ankle and contribute to plantar fasciitis. Left untreated, chronic plantar fasciitis continues to affect gait and may contribute to the development of knee, hip, and back pain.

Improper footwear is a common contributing factor to plantar fasciitis. Shoes that do not fit well, that have worn around the edges increasing eversion or inversion, or that do not provide sufficient arch support may alter biomechanics and stress the plantar fascia. When such a deviation exists, an orthotic may be necessary. Orthotics are prescribed, and should be tailored to individual needs and reassessed frequently as gait patterns change and structures adapt. High-heeled shoes also contribute to plantar fasciitis because they increase plantar flexion and passive extension of the toes.

Weight gain, particularly when it occurs rapidly, increases the demand on the plantar fascia primarily by flattening the arch and stretching the fascia. During pregnancy there is rapid weight gain in addition to hormonal changes that loosen connective tissues, which may contribute to increased demand and reduced functionality of the plantar fascia. Some types of arthritis that affect tendons and ligaments may also contribute to plantar fasciitis. Ankylosing spondylitis—a form of arthritis that often begins in the spine and results in fusion of the vertebrae—may progress to affect the hips, knees, and ankles. Reiter's syndrome is an inflammatory disorder of the joints that often occurs following infection in the intestines or urinary tract, causing degeneration at the attachment sites of ligaments and tendons. Although it is unclear why, thickening of the deep tissues of the foot, which contributes to plantar fasciitis, is common among diabetics. Diabetics are also more prone to peripheral neuropathies, which may coexist or be confused with plantar fasciitis. Corticosteroids, which are often injected to relieve the pain and inflammation, may also contribute to the weakening of ligaments, tendons, and bone as well as atrophy of the fat pads in the foot, in turn contributing to chronic cases or the risk of more serious injury. For this reason, the number of repeated injections to a specific area is often limited, and local massage is contraindicated for several days following injections.

Table 11-1 lists conditions commonly confused with or contributing to plantar fasciitis.

Contraindications and Special Considerations

First, it is essential to understand the cause of foot pain. If the client has a history of arthritis, cartilage degeneration, or previously unresolved injuries or if you suspect the client has a fractured bone or significant tearing to the tissues, work with the client's health care provider and

Table 11-1	Differentiating Conditions Commonly Confused with or Contributing to Plantar Fasciitis		
Condition	**Typical Signs and Symptoms**	**Testing**	**Massage Therapy**
Tarsal tunnel syndrome (compression of the posterior tibial nerve)	Tingling, burning, and numbness or sharp, shooting pain in the medial ankle, heel, arch, and toes

Symptoms may extend into the calf

Symptoms may occur at rest, and worsen with activity | Dorsiflexion-eversion test

Tinel's sign

MRI

EMG

Nerve conduction velocity test | Massage is indicated to reduce adhesions and hypertonicity that may contribute to compression. Take caution not to reproduce symptoms or further compress the nerve. |
| Stress fracture (calcaneus, tarsals, or metatarsals) | Symptoms may be mistaken for soft tissue trauma

Swelling, bruising

Pain increases with activity and often persists during rest

Limited ROM | X-ray (stress fracture may not be apparent until symptoms have persisted for weeks)

MRI

Bone scan | Massage is locally contraindicated until bone is healed. Massage peripheral to injury or to reduce compensating patterns is indicated with caution. Circulatory massage distal to a cast is contraindicated to avoid congestion under the cast. |
| Calcaneal tendon injuries | Pain in joint crossed by tendon

Swelling

Pain worsens with weight-bearing activity such as jumping, squatting, or climbing stairs

Reduced ROM | Physical exam

ROM tests | Massage is indicated. See Chapter 14 for suggestions for treating calcaneal tendinitis. |
| Heel fat pad atrophy | Localized heel pain that does not radiate

Deep, dull ache in middle of heel | Diagnosed by symptoms

Tests may be performed if conservative treatment does not relieve symptoms | Massage is locally contraindicated until the symptoms subside. Massage peripheral to the heel may be supportive. |
| Ankylosing spondylitis | Pain often begins in the low back unilaterally and progresses bilaterally to the upper back, throughout the thorax, and possibly into the joints of the extremities

Fatigue and anemia may develop | MRI

Blood tests | Massage is indicated to reduce pain, maintain mobility, and slow the progress of joint distortion. |
| Reiter's syndrome (reactive arthritis) | Often preceded by infection, low-grade fever, or conjunctivitis

Calcaneal tendon pain

Heel pain

Joint pain

Skin lesions in palms or soles

Redness, burning, or discharge from eyes

Urinary urgency or burning | Physical exam

Joint X-ray

Urinalysis

HLA-B27 antigen test | Massage is contraindicated until the infection is resolved and during active flare-ups of arthritis.

Work with the health care provider to tailor the treatment plan to meet the individual's needs. Avoid skin lesions. |

Table 11-1	Differentiating Conditions Commonly Confused with or Contributing to Plantar Fasciitis (Continued)		
Condition	**Typical Signs and Symptoms**	**Testing**	**Massage Therapy**
Bone spur	Pain in heel, particularly with weight-bearing activity Local skin lesion may be present Reduced ROM	X-ray MRI CT scan	Massage will not reduce a bone spur but may be effective in reducing further damage due to tension in soft tissue. Be cautious with techniques that may fragment the spur.
Bursitis (retrocalcaneal)	Heel pain, particularly with activity or palpation Heat, redness, swelling, or tenderness at the back of the heel	Physical exam ROM tests X-ray or MRI if conservative treatment is not successful	Massage is systemically contraindicated if bursitis is due to infection, and locally contraindicated in the acute stage to avoid increased swelling. In the subacute stage, massage of the structures surrounding the joint is indicated.
Morton's neuroma	Burning and pain in the ball of the foot that radiates into the toes Numbness or tingling in the toes Symptoms most common between third and fourth toes	Palpation assessment for tender mass X-ray	Massage is indicated to reduce adhesions or scar tissue that may contribute to nerve irritation and to increase the space between the third and fourth metatarsals. Take care not to reproduce symptoms.
Gout	Redness, heat, and swelling Sudden, intense pain, often at night, that diminishes gradually over a couple of weeks	Physical exam Blood and urine uric acid concentration tests Synovial fluid test	Local massage is contraindicated during acute attacks. Gout may indicate other systemic conditions. Work with health care team.
Rheumatoid arthritis	Periods of flare-ups and remission Pain, swelling Aching and stiffness, particularly after rest or inactivity Reduced ROM Distortion of joint Rheumatic nodules Occasional low-grade fever and malaise	Physical exam Blood tests Synovial fluid tests Radiography	Massage is indicated in nonacute stages. Work with the health care team.

consult a pathology text for massage therapists before proceeding. These are a few general cautions:

- **Underlying pathologies.** Arthritis, bone fractures, or symptoms common to systemic conditions like diabetes may be contributing factors. If you suspect an underlying condition (consult Table 11-1 and your pathology book for signs and symptoms), refer the client to his or her health care provider for medical assessment before initiating treatment. If the client is diagnosed with an underlying pathology that is not a contraindication for massage, work with the health care team to develop a treatment plan that is appropriate for that individual.
- **Endangerment sites.** Be cautious with pressure around the dorsalis pedis artery where you feel its pulse.

- **Producing symptoms.** Symptoms may occur during treatment. If treatment produces symptoms, adjust the client to a more neutral posture. Reducing dorsiflexion may help. If this does not relieve the symptoms, reduce your pressure or move away from the area. You may be able to treat around the site that reproduced the symptoms, but proceed with caution.
- **Treatment duration and pressure.** If the client is elderly, has degenerative disease, or has been diagnosed with a condition that diminishes activities of daily living, you may need to adjust your pressure as well as the treatment duration. Frequent half-hour sessions may suit the client better. Take care when applying pressure or friction around the calcaneal attachment of the plantar fascia, particularly if there is any risk of tearing or rupture. If the client's symptoms are severe or his or her activities of daily living have been significantly reduced due to pain, recommend medical assessment to determine the degree of degeneration of tissue. If bone spurs are present, do not apply pressure directly, and avoid any techniques that might chip or detach the spur.
- **Friction.** Do not use deep frictions if the client has a systemic inflammatory condition such as rheumatoid arthritis, if the health of the underlying tissues is at risk for rupture, or if the client is taking anti-inflammatory medication. Friction creates an inflammatory process, which may interfere with the intended action of anti-inflammatory medication. Recommend that the client refrain from taking such medication for several hours before treatment if his or her health care provider agrees.
- **Injections.** If the client has had a steroid or analgesic injection within the previous 2 weeks, avoid the area. These injections reduce sensation, which may prevent the client from assessing your pressure adequately. Steroid injections may also alter the physiology of the tissues, increasing the risk of injury from deep massage techniques.
- **Tissue length.** It is important when treating myofascial tissues that you do not lengthen those that are already stretched. Assess for myofascial restrictions first and treat only those that are clearly present. Likewise, overstretched muscles should not be stretched from origin to insertion. If you treat trigger points in overstretched tissue, use heat or a localized pin and stretch technique instead of full ROM stretches.
- **Hypermobile joints and unstable ligaments.** Be cautious with mobilizations if the client has hypermobile joints or if ligaments are unstable due to injury, pregnancy or a systemic condition.

Massage Therapy Research

A thorough review of the literature revealed no research, case studies, or peer-reviewed articles specifically about the benefits of massage therapy for plantar fasciitis or heel pain. Many of the research studies of effective treatment for plantar fasciitis include stretching, although little attention is given to lengthening the muscles manually. In "A Combined Treatment Approach Emphasizing Impairment-Based Manual Physical Therapy for Plantar Heel Pain: A Case Series," Young et al. (2004) report the benefits of physical therapy techniques to mobilize the joints of the ankle and foot using manual therapy. Although this study involved treatment goals similar to those of massage therapy, the methods used to achieve them followed an impairment-based physical therapy approach, focused largely on mobilization, and did not include methods more common in massage therapy such as reducing adhesions, increasing local circulation, and releasing trigger points.

Several studies of treatment options including the use of orthotics, Botox, shock wave therapy, and splinting the ankle into dorsiflexion during sleep included "deep tissue massage" as part of the treatment, although none of these specified a procedure. Several articles reviewing recent literature regarding effective treatments suggest that while stretching increases ROM, it has not proven to be an effective, long-term solution for plantar fasciitis without other interventions. These results suggest a need for detailed studies of the specific benefits of massage therapy for treating not only the muscles but also the noncontractile tissues affected in plantar fasciitis. It may be possible that focused stretching of the muscles without attention to fascia may not be sufficient for positive, long-term results.

The January 2001 issue of *The Journal of Bodywork and Movement Therapies* presented an interesting interdisciplinary look at plantar fasciitis. The survey begins with a case study of a single client with heel pain, followed by individual articles that consider the case from the perspectives of Chinese medicine, body-mind healing, neuromuscular therapy, physical therapy, and chiropractic care. While it provides no conclusive evidence of the benefits of these treatments, this series offers a rare and comprehensive examination into the variety of possible factors contributing to chronic pain.

WORKING WITH THE CLIENT

Client Assessment

While the symptoms of plantar fasciitis are fairly consistent, the biomechanical factors can vary. For this reason, each case should be considered individually. For example, pes planus often presents with eversion of the ankle; short and tight peroneal muscles, gastrocnemius, and soleus; and weakened tibialis muscles. With pes cavus, you may find the ankle inverted with a short and tight tibialis anterior, tibialis posterior, and the muscles that flex the toes. The impact on the knees, hips, and low back may also vary. Common presentations of plantar fasciitis are described here, but it is essential to assess every joint involved to put together an accurate picture for each individual client.

Assessment begins during your first contact with a client. In some cases, this may be on the telephone when an appointment is requested. Ask in advance if the client is seeking treatment for a specific area of pain so that you can prepare yourself.

Table 11-2 lists questions to ask the client when taking a health history.

POSTURAL ASSESSMENT

Allow the client to walk and enter the room ahead of you while you assess his or her posture and movements. Look for imbalances or patterns of compensation for deviations common with plantar fasciitis. Watch as the client climbs steps, looking for reduced mobility or favoring one side. Assess for joint instability, limping, rotation of the femur or tibia, or hyper- or hypolordosis. Have the client sit to fill out the assessment form, watching to see if he or she plantar flexes the ankle or flexes the toes to avoid stretching the calcaneal tendon and plantar fascia. Watch also as the client stands up to see if he or she can stand without assistance or if he or she avoids bearing weight on the affected foot.

When assessing the standing posture, be sure that the client stands comfortably. If he or she deliberately attempts to stand in the anatomic position, you may not get an accurate assessment of his or her posture in daily life. Excessive eversion of the ankle is noted when the inferior aspect of the calcaneal tendon bends laterally. The medial malleolus may also protrude more prominently (Fig. 11-3). With excessive inversion, the inferior aspect of the calcaneal tendon may bend medially, although this may not be as visible as the lateral curve of an everted ankle. With inversion, the lateral malleolus may protrude more prominently (Fig. 11-4). You can also inspect the soles of the client's shoes for wearing of the inside or outside edges, indicating an atypical position of the foot. The calcaneal tendon and fascia of the plantar flexors may appear thick or dimpled. Assess the arches of the feet for pes cavus or pes planus. Pes planus is more common with plantar fasciitis, particularly if the ankle is everted. Some extension of the metatarsophalangeal joint is normal but may be exaggerated with plantar fasciitis. Hyperextension of the metatarsophalangeal joint may force hyperflexion of the interphalangeal joints.

Table 11-2	Health History

Questions for the Client	Importance for the Treatment Plan
Was there a precipitating event, or can you remember a specific moment when the pain began?	The details of the activity or posture that initiated the pain may help you to determine contributing factors such as tendon injuries or stress fractures. A new regimen of running, a new activity that requires weight-bearing movement, or a newly developed sedentary posture may contribute to the symptoms of plantar fasciitis.
Where do you feel symptoms?	The location of symptoms gives clues to the location of trigger points, injury, or other contributing factors. Plantar fasciitis generally causes pain near the anterior, inferior calcaneus. Pain elsewhere in the foot, ankle, or calf is not uncommon and may suggest a coexisting condition.
Describe what your symptoms feel like.	Differentiate between possible origins of symptoms, and determine the involvement of bones, nerves, and soft tissues. See Chapter 1 for descriptions of pain sensations and possible contributing factors.
Do any movements make your symptoms worse or better?	Locate tension, weakness, or compression in structures producing such movements. Dorsiflexion, toe extension, and weight bearing often exacerbate symptoms of plantar fasciitis.
Have you seen a health care provider for this condition? What was the diagnosis? What tests were performed?	Medical tests may reveal stress fractures, bone spurs, nerve involvement, or other conditions. If no tests were performed to make a diagnosis of plantar fasciitis, use the tests described in this chapter for your assessment. If your assessment is inconsistent with the diagnosis, ask the client to discuss your findings with his or her health care provider or ask for permission to contact the provider directly.
Have you been diagnosed with a condition such as arthritis or diabetes? Are you pregnant?	Arthritis, diabetes, and other systemic conditions may contribute to signs and symptoms, may require adjustments to treatment, and may impact treatment outcomes. Pregnancy leads to weight gain and affects hormones that may contribute to symptoms.
Have you had a previous injury or surgery?	Injury or surgery and resulting scar tissue may cause adhesions, hyper- or hypotonicity, and atypical ROM.
What type of work, hobbies, or other regular activities do you do?	A new physical training program, repetitive motions that stress the ankle and foot, and static postures that shorten the plantar fascia may contribute to the client's condition.
Are you taking any prescribed medications or herbal or other supplements?	Medications of all types may contribute to symptoms or involve contraindications or cautions.
Have you had a corticosteroid or analgesic injection in the past 2 weeks? Where?	Local massage is contraindicated. A history of repeated corticosteroid injections may affect the integrity of the plantar fascia and calcaneal tendon, thus increasing the risk of tearing or rupture. Use caution when applying pressure or cross-fiber strokes.
Have you taken a pain reliever or muscle relaxant within the past 4 hours?	The client may not be able to judge your pressure.
Have you taken anti-inflammatory medication within the past 4 hours?	Deep friction initiates an inflammatory process and should not be performed if the client has recently taken anti-inflammatory medication.

Improper alignment of the knee, hip, and pelvis, as well as calcaneal tendinitis, may coexist with plantar fasciitis. Review Chapters 8 (hyperlordosis), 9 (piriformis syndrome), 10 (patellofemoral syndrome), and 14 (tendinopathies) to assess for possible coexisting conditions.

Figure 11-5 compares a healthy posture to a posture affected by plantar fasciitis with pes planus and ankle eversion.

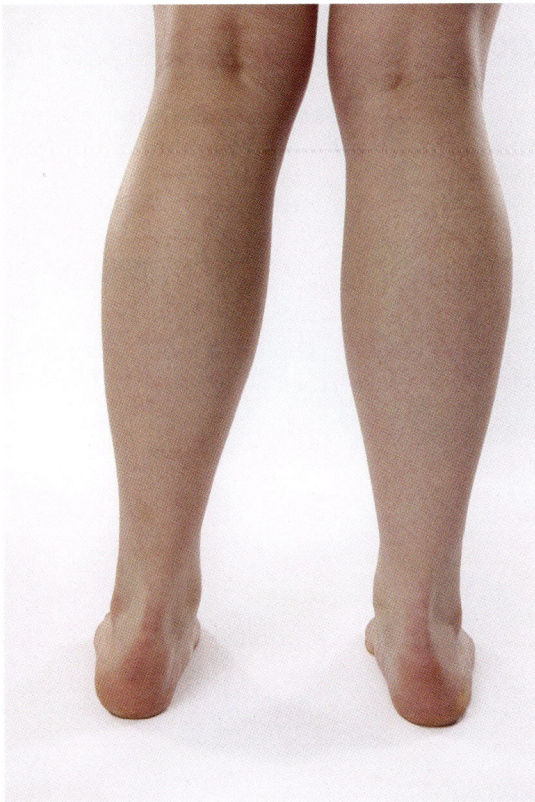

Figure 11-3 **Everted ankles.** Note the lateral bend of the inferior aspect of the calcaneal tendons and the prominence of the medial malleoli.

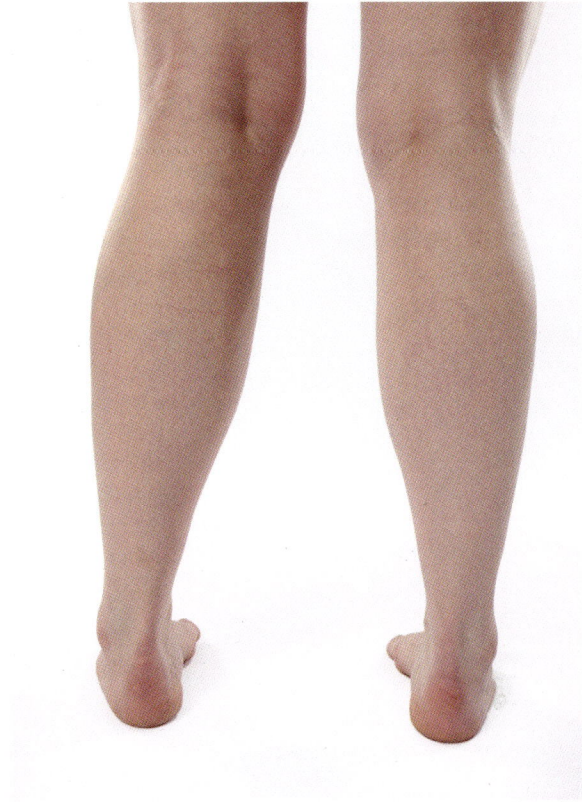

Figure 11-4 **Inverted ankles.** Note the medial bend of the inferior aspect of the calcaneal tendons and the prominence of the lateral malleoli.

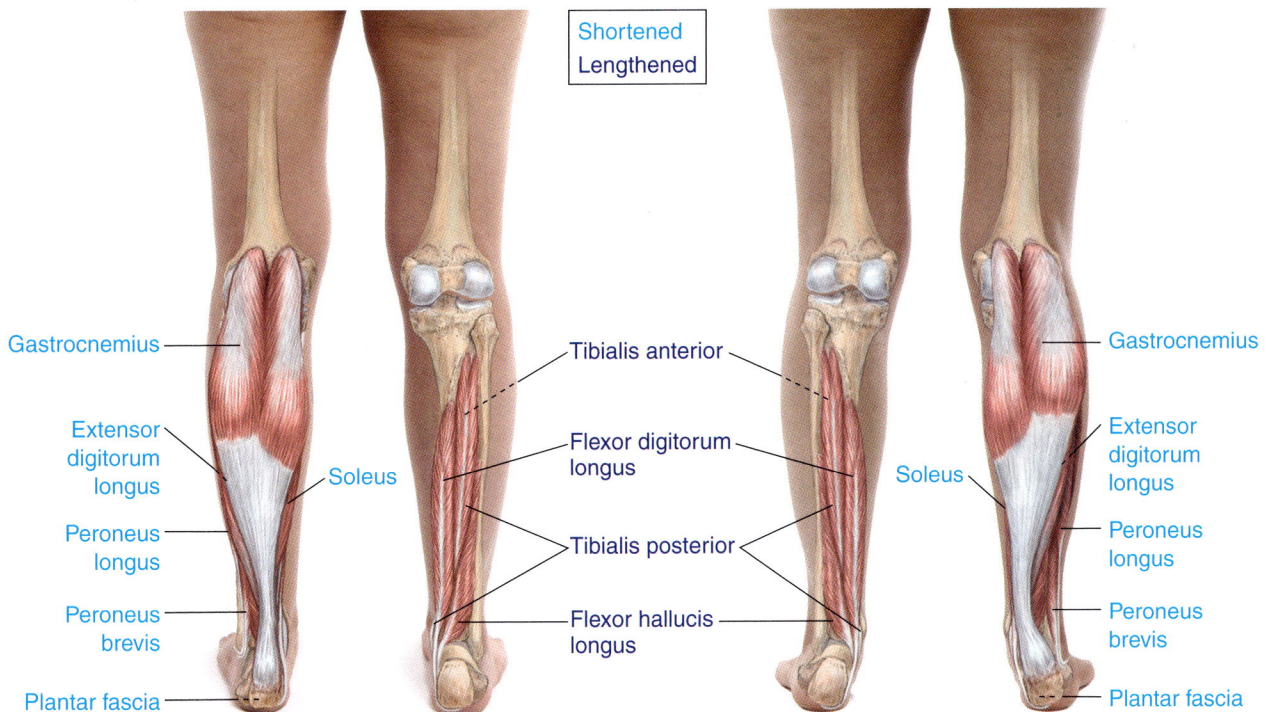

Shortened
Lengthened

Gastrocnemius

Extensor digitorum longus

Peroneus longus

Peroneus brevis

Plantar fascia

Tibialis anterior

Flexor digitorum longus

Soleus

Tibialis posterior

Flexor hallucis longus

Gastrocnemius

Extensor digitorum longus

Soleus

Peroneus longus

Peroneus brevis

Plantar fascia

Figure 11-5 **Postural assessment comparison.** Compare the healthy posture in the image on the left to the deviated posture in the image on the right. Note the flat arch, curved calcaneal tendon, and prominent medial malleolus in the figure on the right.

Box 11-1 **AVERAGE ACTIVE ROM FOR JOINTS INVOLVED IN PLANTAR FASCIITIS**

Ankle
Dorsiflexion 20°
   Tibialis anterior
   Extensor digitorum longus
   Extensor hallucis longus

Plantar Flexion 50°
   Gastrocnemius
   Soleus
   Tibialis posterior
   Peroneus longus
   Peroneus brevis
   Flexor digitorum longus
   Flexor hallucis longus
   Plantaris

Inversion 45–60°
   Tibialis anterior
   Tibialis posterior

   Flexor digitorum longus
   Flexor hallucis longus
   Extensor hallucis longus

Eversion 15–30°
   Peroneus longus
   Peroneus brevis
   Extensor digitorum longus
   First toe

Flexion 45°
   Flexor hallucis longus
   Flexor hallucis brevis
   Abductor hallucis

Extension 70°
   Extensor hallucis longus
   Extensor hallucis brevis

Second to Fifth Toes
Flexion 40°
   Flexor digitorum longus
   Flexor digitorum brevis
   Lumbricals
   Dorsal and plantar interossei
   Abductor digiti minimi
   Flexor digiti minimi
   Quadratus plantae

Extension 40°
   Extensor digitorum longus
   Extensor digitorum brevis
   Lumbricals

ROM ASSESSMENT

Test the ROMs of the ankle and toes involving muscles as both agonists and antagonists. Since it allows the client to control the amount of movement and stay within a pain-free range, only active ROM should be used in the acute stage of injury to prevent undue pain or re-injury. Box 11-1 presents the average active ROM results for the joints involved in plantar fasciitis.

Active ROM

Compare your assessment of the client's active ROM to the values in Box 11-1. Pain and other symptoms may not be reproduced during active ROM assessment because the client may limit movement to a symptom-free range.

- **Active dorsiflexion of the ankle** may be restricted when tight plantar flexors limit movement.
- **Active extension of the toes** may be limited and cause pain when this action stretches the plantar fascia. In addition, because the flexor digitorum brevis, abductor digiti minimi, and abductor hallucis attach to the plantar surface of the calcaneus, extension of the toes may add tension to the attachment site they share with the plantar fascia.

Passive ROM

Compare the client's P ROM on one side to the other when applicable. Note and compare the end feel for each range (see Chapter 1 for an explanation of end feel).

- **Passive dorsiflexion of the ankle** may produce a painful stretch to the plantar flexors and plantar fascia.
- **Passive extension of the toes** may cause pain as the plantar fascia and toe flexors are stretched.

Resisted ROM

Use resisted tests to assess the strength of the muscles that cross the ankle. Compare the strength of the affected side to the unaffected side.

- **Resisted dorsiflexion of the ankle** may reveal weakness.

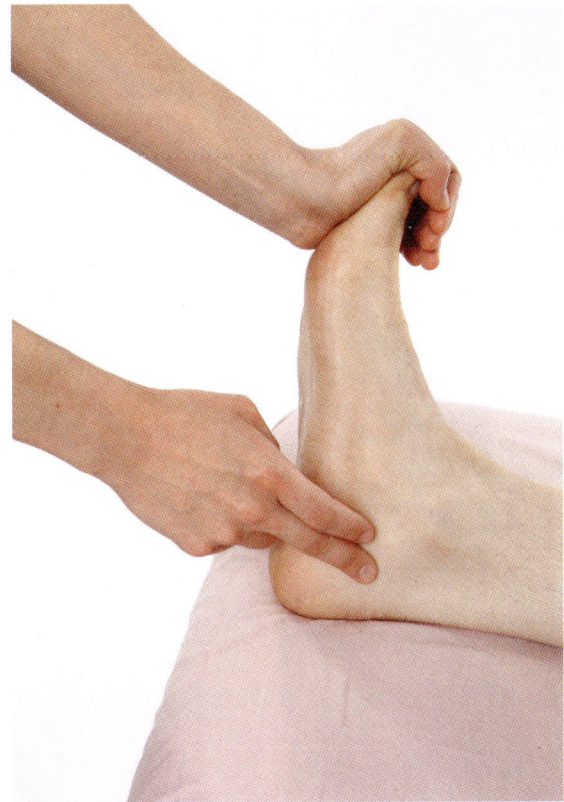

Figure 11-6 **Dorsiflexion eversion test with Tinel's sign.** This test is performed to assess for compression of the tibial nerve in the tarsal tunnel.

SPECIAL TESTS

The following special tests will help you to determine which structures are contributing to pain and when a client should be evaluated by a medical professional using X-ray or other tools, which may reveal conditions that contraindicate massage or require special considerations when planning treatment.

The **dorsiflexion eversion test** is used to assess compression of the tibial nerve within the tarsal tunnel—the space formed by the medial malleolus, calcaneus, and the flexor retinaculum through which the tendons of the tibialis posterior, flexor digitorum longus, and flexor hallucis longus along with the tibial artery, tibial vein, and tibial nerve pass (Fig. 11-6). **Tinel's sign**—a test that can be used to assess nerve conduction anywhere in the body—is often added when simple dorsiflexion and eversion alone do not reproduce symptoms. Use these tests together to assess for the possibility of tarsal tunnel syndrome in clients with heel pain:

1. Begin with the dorsiflexion eversion test. With the client supine, maximally dorsiflex the ankle and toes, and evert the ankle. This position pushes soft tissues deeper into the tarsal tunnel to assess their involvement in compressing the tibial nerve.
2. Hold the position for up to 15 seconds or until symptoms of numbness or tingling are produced.
3. Reproducing symptoms of numbness and tingling along the distribution of the nerve into the foot suggests compression of the nerve.
4. If no symptoms are produced, add Tinel's sign by tapping the tibial nerve between the medial malleolus and the medial aspect of the calcaneus.
5. Reproducing symptoms of numbness and tingling along the distribution of the nerve into the foot suggests nerve involvement.

The windlass test is used to assess whether the windlass mechanism of the plantar fascia produces pain (Fig. 11-7). The test is performed in non-weight-bearing and weight-bearing postures.

1. Begin with the non-weight-bearing test by asking the client to sit with the legs hanging off the edge of the table.

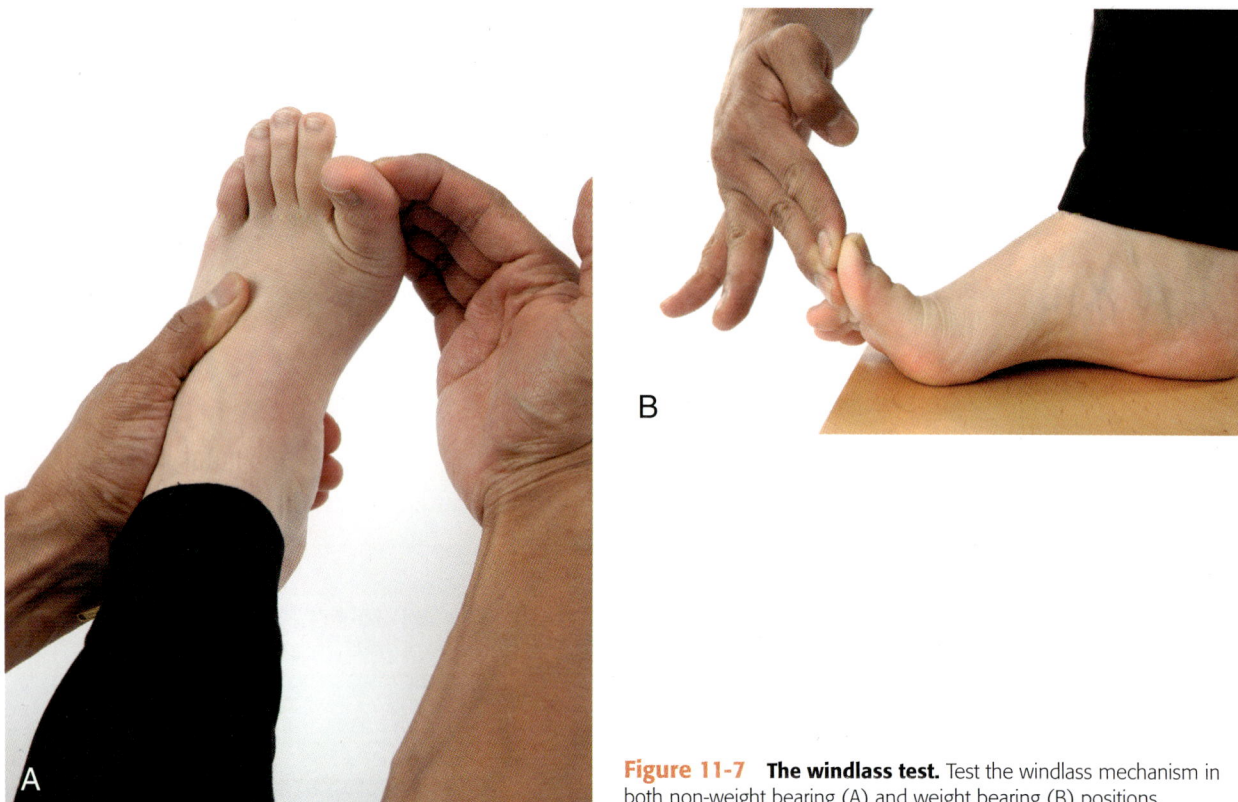

Figure 11-7 **The windlass test.** Test the windlass mechanism in both non-weight bearing (A) and weight bearing (B) positions.

2. With one hand, gently stabilize the ankle in a neutral position, free from plantar flexion and dorsiflexion.
3. With the other hand, fully extend the first toe passively at the metatarsophalangeal joint until you reach the end point or pain is reproduced.
4. Pain in the arch indicates a positive test for dysfunction of the plantar fascia when the windlass mechanism is activated. If no pain is produced, perform the test during weight bearing.
5. Ask the client to stand on a chair, stair, or other stable surface that allows a secure stance with the metatarsal heads at the edge, so the toes are uninhibited.
6. Passively extend the metatarsophalangeal joint of the first toe until you reach the end range or pain is reproduced.
7. Pain in the arch indicates a positive test for dysfunction of the plantar fascia when the windlass mechanism is activated.

PALPATION ASSESSMENT

Dysfunction in any joint from the sacroiliac to the metatarsals may cause or result from plantar fasciitis. Because contributing factors may vary widely, it is essential to assess the tissues of each individual client from the hips to the toes. It should not be surprising to find minor or even major differences in the ways the tissues respond to this dysfunction.

Assess the ankle and foot for atypical temperature, color, and texture. You may find inflammation, adhesions, fibrotic tissue, or tenderness around the malleoli or calcaneus or in the intrinsic muscles of the foot. The tenderest spot may be felt at the anterior calcaneus, where the plantar fascia attaches to the calcaneal tubercle. The gastrocnemius and soleus may be tight and the calcaneal tendon may be thick and dense. If eversion of the ankle is a factor, the peroneus longus and brevis and the extensor digitorum longus may be short and tight.

Trigger points that refer pain into the heel and plantar surface of the foot may be found in the gastrocnemius, soleus, flexor digitorum longus, tibialis posterior, abductor hallucis, and quadratus plantae. See Figure 11-8 for common trigger points with referrals into the heel and plantar surface of the foot.

Condition-Specific Massage

Because the causes of heel pain vary widely, the exact cause can be difficult to pinpoint and more than one condition may coexist. Systemic conditions that involve cautions or contraindications for massage may be the underlying cause of heel pain. If you feel uncertain that the client's symptoms are caused by irritation or inflammation of the plantar fascia or by any of the soft tissue dysfunctions listed earlier, refer the client to his or her health care provider for medical assessment prior to treatment with massage.

It is essential for the treatment to be relaxing. You are not likely to eliminate the symptoms associated with plantar fasciitis or any coexisting conditions in a single treatment. Do not attempt to do so by treating aggressively. Be sure to ask your client to let you know if the amount of pressure you are applying keeps him or her from relaxing. If the client responds by tensing muscles or has a facial expression that looks distressed, reduce your pressure. Remember that you are working on tissue that is compromised. Ask the client to let you know if any part of your treatment reproduces symptoms, and always work within his or her tolerance. Deep palpation of a trigger point may cause pain at the upper end of the client's tolerance. Explain this to your client, describe a pain scale and what level of pain should not be exceeded, and ask him or her to breathe deeply during the application of the technique. As the trigger point is deactivated, the referral pain will also diminish.

The following suggestions are for treating heel pain caused by irritation or inflammation of the plantar fascia with weak dorsiflexion and increased eversion of the ankle. This is the most common presentation, although each client should be assessed for individual needs. If the client has an acute injury, the protocol is PRICE. You may work conservatively proximal or distal to the site, but avoid the area of injury until the subacute or chronic stage.

- Begin in the prone position with the ankles bolstered to reduce passive plantar flexion of the ankle.

- If you notice any swelling, apply superficial draining strokes toward the nearest lymph nodes.

- If swelling is minor or absent, apply moist heat to the plantar flexors and calcaneal tendon.

- Use your initial warming strokes to increase superficial circulation, soften tissues, and assess the tissues from the low back down to the feet. You should be able to minimally assess the tissues of the low back, hips, and leg, which may help you to determine where to focus the time remaining after treating the lower leg.

Treatment icons: Increase circulation; Reduce adhesions; Reduce tension; Lengthen tissue; Treat trigger points; Passive stretch; Clear area

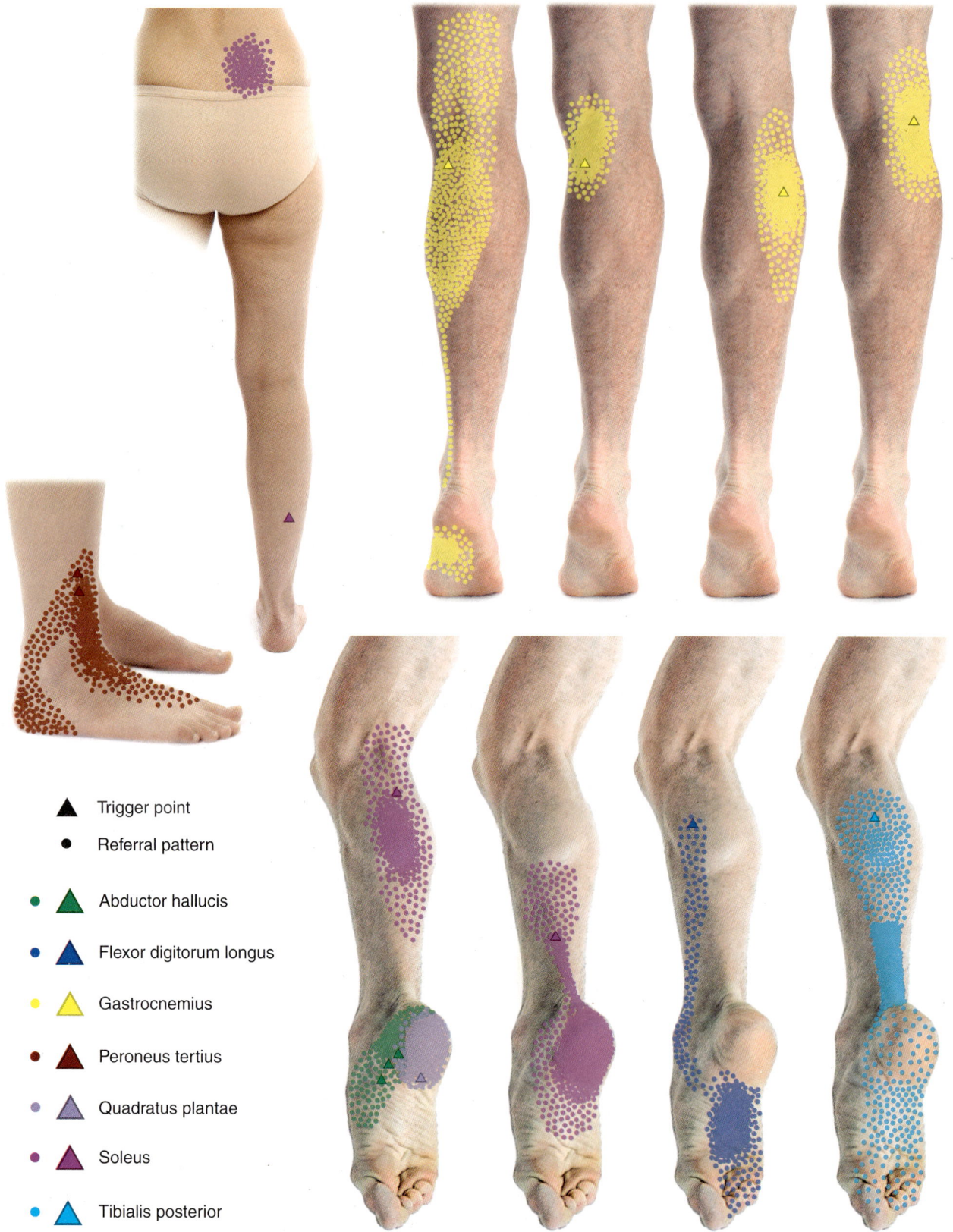

Trigger point ▲

Referral pattern ●

● ▲ Abductor hallucis

● ▲ Flexor digitorum longus

● ▲ Gastrocnemius

● ▲ Peroneus tertius

● ▲ Quadratus plantae

● ▲ Soleus

● ▲ Tibialis posterior

Figure 11-8 **Common trigger points associated with plantar fasciitis and their referral patterns.**

- Before applying emollient, assess for and treat fascial restrictions in the lower leg. You may find restrictions along the gastrocnemius and soleus (Fig. 11-9).

- Once the superficial tissues are pliable enough to allow for deeper work, apply lengthening strokes to tissues that are short and tight. Plantar flexors and evertors of the ankle include the gastrocnemius, soleus (Fig. 11-9), peroneus longus and brevis, extensor digitorum longus (Fig. 11-10), tibialis posterior, flexor digitorum longus, and flexor hallucis longus (Fig. 11-11), although all of the muscles of the lower leg should be assessed. These muscles should be treated along their full length with special attention to the sections that cross the ankle.

- Treat any trigger points that are found.

- Apply moderate traction to the ankle to increase mobility between the talus and the tibia and fibula, which may improve dorsiflexion.

- Assess and treat the muscles of the foot if they are tight or adhered or contain trigger points. Gently knead the tissues between the metatarsals within the client's tolerance (Fig. 11-12).

- Soften the plantar fascia with kneading strokes. Begin superficially and progress into the deeper tissues (see Fig. 11-1).

- Once you feel pliability in the fascia, use cross-fiber strokes to reduce any adhesions. Treating the tissues near the calcaneal attachment may provide the greatest relief, but it is essential to take great care around this attachment, particularly in the first treatments, to avoid rupture of the tissue or encouraging bone spurs.

- Treat the flexor digitorum brevis, abductor digiti minimi, and abductor hallucis for hypertonicity, taking care with pressure at the calcaneal attachments.

- Apply lengthening strokes to the plantar fascia, beginning superficially and progressing to deeper tissues. Unless you are certain that there are no bone spurs or risk of rupture, apply strokes from the metatarsal heads toward the calcaneus to avoid pulling the plantar fascia away from the calcaneal attachment.

- Clear the leg from the foot toward the hips.

- Turn the client supine, and with the knee extended, stretch the plantar flexors, calcaneal tendon, and plantar fascia by performing passive dorsiflexion of the ankle and toes.

- Use PIR if you feel resistance to lengthening the plantar flexors.

- If time permits, assess and treat the muscles involved in any coexisting conditions.

The treatment overview diagram summarizes the flow of treatment (Fig. 11-13).

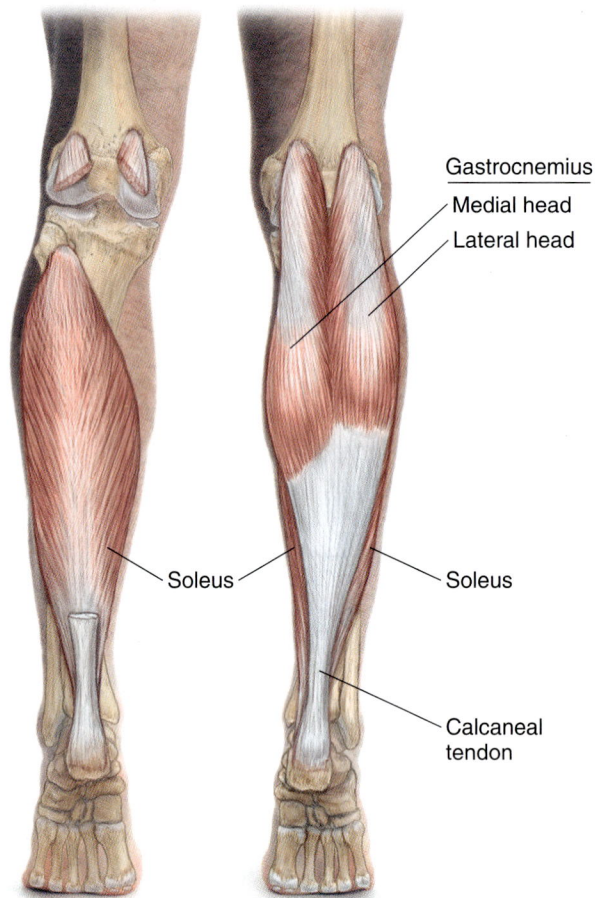

GASTROCNEMIUS

Origin	Condyles of the femur, posterior surface of fibula and tibia.
Insertion	Calcaneus via calcaneal tendon.
Action	Flex knee, plantar flex ankle.
Nerve	Tibial.

SOLEUS

Origin	Soleal line, posterior surface of fibula and tibia.
Insertion	Calcaneus via calcaneal tendon.
Action	Plantar flex ankle.
Nerve	Tibial.

Figure 11-9   Gastrocnemius and soleus. Adapted from Clay JH, Pounds DM. *Basic Clinical Massage Therapy: Integrating Anatomy and Treatment,* 2nd ed. Philadelphia: Lippincott Williams & Wilkins, 2008.

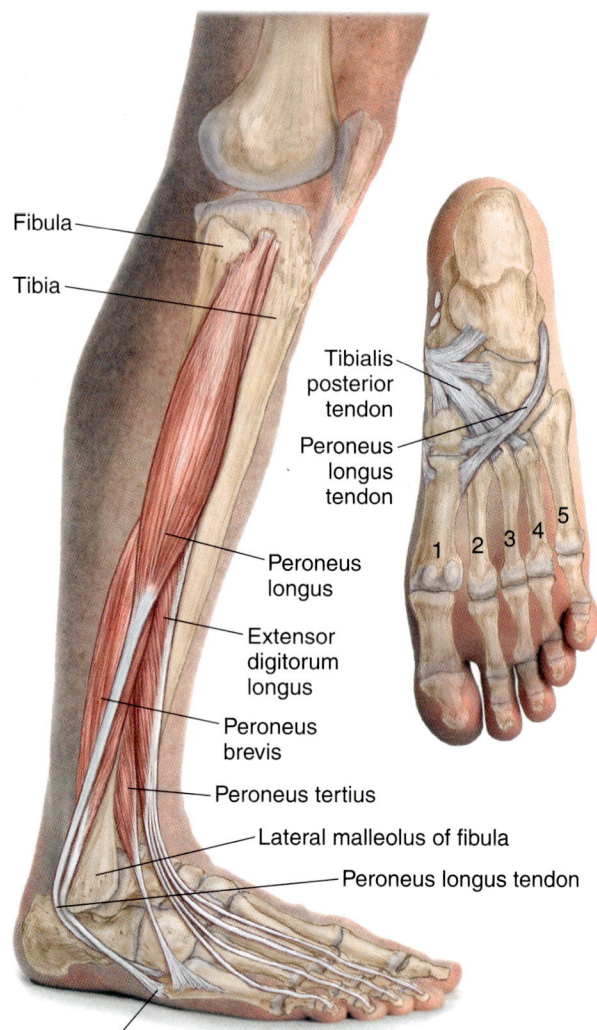

PERONEUS LONGUS

Origin	Proximal, lateral fibula.
Insertion	Base of 1st metatarsal and medial cuneiform.
Action	Evert ankle, assist in plantar flexion of ankle.
Nerve	Superior peroneal.

PERONEUS BREVIS

Origin	Distal lateral fibula.
Insertion	Tuberosity of 5th metatarsal.
Action	Evert ankle, assist in plantar flexion of ankle.
Nerve	Superior peroneal.

EXTENSOR DIGITORUM LONGUS

Origin	Proximal anterior fibula, interosseus membrane.
Insertion	Middle and distal phalanges of toes 2–5.
Action	Extend toes 2–5, dorsiflex ankle, evert ankle.
Nerve	Deep peroneal.

Figure 11-10   Muscles that evert the ankle. Adapted from Clay JH, Pounds DM. *Basic Clinical Massage Therapy: Integrating Anatomy and Treatment,* 2nd ed. Philadelphia: Lippincott Williams & Wilkins, 2008.

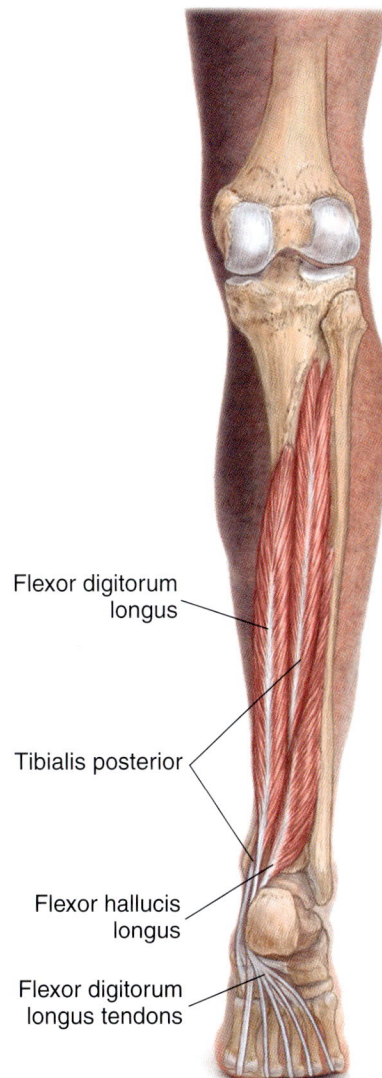

Flexor digitorum
longus

Tibialis posterior

Flexor hallucis
longus

Flexor digitorum
longus tendons

TIBIALIS POSTERIOR

Origin	Proximal tibia, fibula and interosseus membrane.
Insertion	Navicular, cuneiforms, cuboid, base of metatarsals 2–4.
Action	Invert ankle, plantar flexion.
Nerve	Tibial.

FLEXOR DIGITORUM LONGUS

Origin	Middle, posterior tibia.
Insertion	Distal phalanges of toes 2–5.
Action	Flex toes 2–5, plantar flexion, invert ankle.
Nerve	Tibial.

FLEXOR HALLUCIS LONGUS

Origin	Middle posterior fibula.
Insertion	Distal phalanx of 1st toe.
Action	Flex 1st toe, plantar flexion, invert ankle.
Nerve	Tibial.

Figure 11-11 **Deep muscles that plantar flex and invert the ankle.** Adapted from Clay JH, Pounds DM. *Basic Clinical Massage Therapy: Integrating Anatomy and Treatment,* 2nd ed. Philadelphia: Lippincott Williams & Wilkins, 2008.

Dorsal view

- Quadratus plantae
- Flexor digiti minimi brevis
- Extensor hallucis brevis
- Extensor digitorum brevis
- Dorsal interossei
- Flexor hallucis longus tendon
- Flexor digitorum longus tendon
- Lumbricals
- Flexor hallucis longus tendon

Plantar view

- Abductor hallucis
- Flexor digitorum brevis
- Abductor digiti minimi

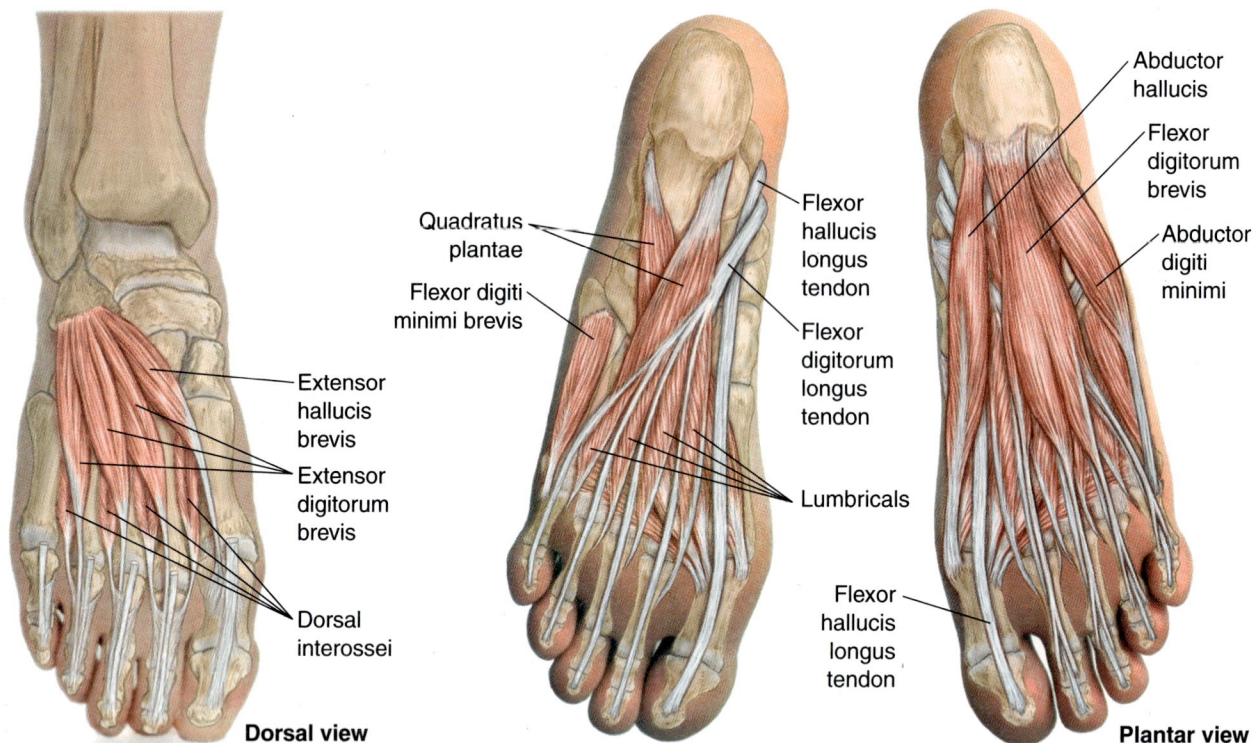

EXTENSOR DIGITORUM BREVIS

Origin	Calcaneus.
Insertion	Toes 2–5 via extensor digitorum longus tendons.
Action	Extend toes 2–4.
Nerve	Deep peroneal.

EXTENSOR HALLUCIS BREVIS

Origin	Calcaneus.
Insertion	Proximal phalanx of 1st toe.
Action	Extend 1st toe.
Nerve	Peroneal.

FLEXOR HALLUCIS BREVIS

Origin	Plantar surfaces of cuboid and lateral cuneiform.
Insertion	Proximal phalanx of 1st toe.
Action	Flex first toe.
Nerve	Medial plantar.

DORSAL INTEROSSEI

Origin	Metatarsals 1–5.
Insertion	Proximal phalanges of toes 2–4.
Action	Abduct toes 2–4.
Nerve	Lateral plantar.

PLANTAR INTEROSSEI

Origin	Base of metatarsals 3–5.
Insertion	Proximal phalanx of toes 3–5.
Action	Adduct and flex toes 3–5.
Nerve	Lateral plantar.

QUADRATUS PLANTAE

Origin	Plantar surface of calcaneus.
Insertion	Flexor digitorum tendons.
Action	Flex toes 2–5.
Nerve	Lateral plantar.

ABDUCTOR HALLUCIS

Origin	Calcaneus.
Insertion	Proximal phalanx of 1st toe.
Action	Abduct and flex 1st toe.
Nerve	Medial plantar.

ABDUCTOR DIGITI MINIMI

Origin	Calcaneus.
Insertion	Proximal phalanx of 5th toe.
Action	Flex and abduct 5th toe.
Nerve	Lateral plantar.

ADDUCTOR HALLUCIS

Origin	Base of metatarsals 2–4.
Insertion	Proximal phalanx of 1st toe.
Action	Adduct 1st toe, assist in maintaining arch.
Nerve	Lateral plantar.

FLEXOR DIGITORUM BREVIS

Origin	Calcaneus.
Insertion	Middle phalanges of toes 2–5.
Action	Flex middle phalanges of toes 2–5.
Nerve	Medial plantar.

FLEXOR DIGITI MINIMI

Origin	Base of 5th metatarsal.
Insertion	Base of proximal phalanx of 5th toe.
Action	Flex 5th toe.
Nerve	Lateral plantar.

LUMBRICALS

Origin	Tendons of flexor digitorum longus.
Insertion	Base of proximal phalanges 2–5.
Action	Flex proximal phalanges of toes 2–5, extend middle and distal phalanges 2–5.
Nerve	Medial and lateral plantar.

Figure 11-12 Muscles of the foot. Adapted from Clay JH, Pounds DM. *Basic Clinical Massage Therapy: Integrating Anatomy and Treatment,* 2nd ed. Philadelphia: Lippincott Williams & Wilkins, 2008.

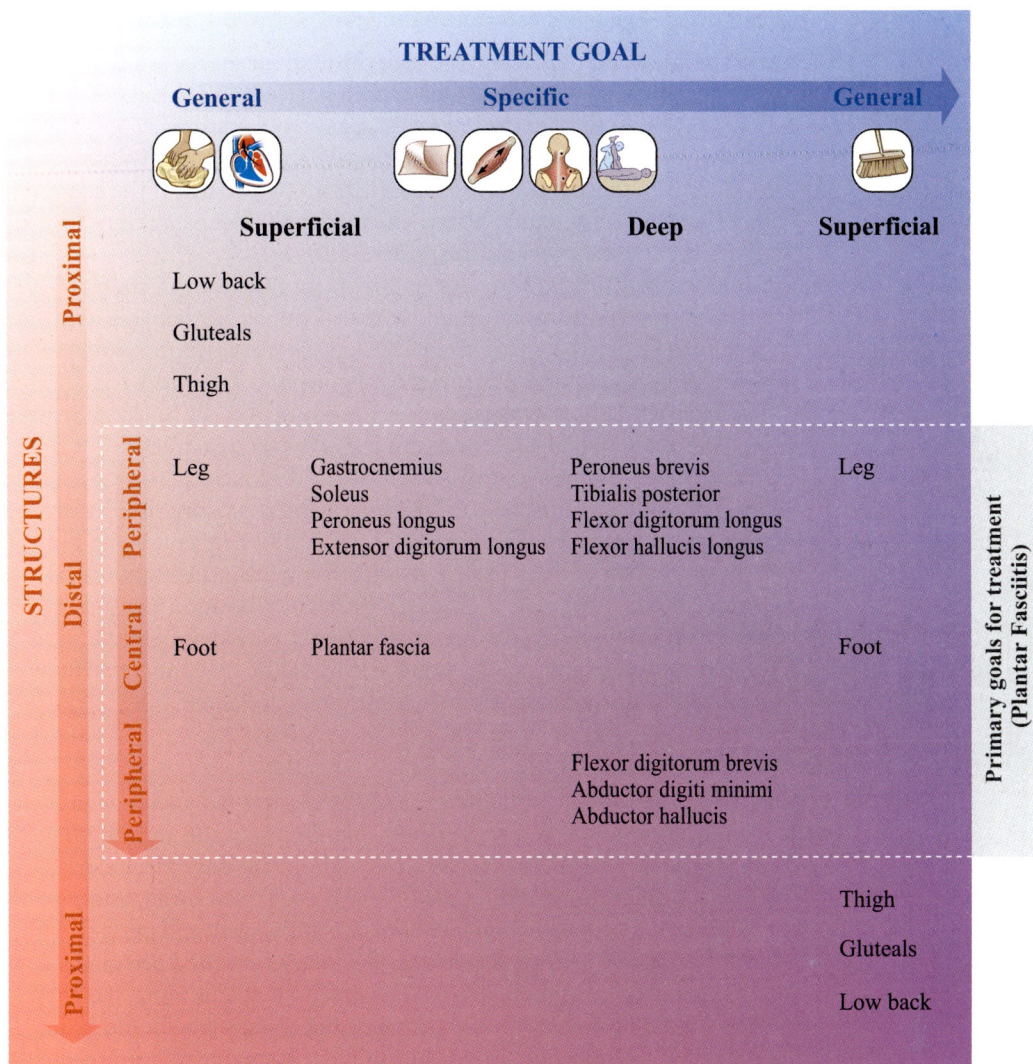

TREATMENT GOAL

General   Specific   General

STRUCTURES		Superficial		Deep	Superficial
Proximal		Low back			
		Gluteals			
		Thigh			
Distal — Peripheral	Leg	Gastrocnemius	Peroneus brevis		Leg
		Soleus	Tibialis posterior		
		Peroneus longus	Flexor digitorum longus		
		Extensor digitorum longus	Flexor hallucis longus		
Central	Foot	Plantar fascia			Foot
Peripheral			Flexor digitorum brevis		
			Abductor digiti minimi		
			Abductor hallucis		
Proximal					Thigh
					Gluteals
					Low back

Primary goals for treatment (Plantar Fasciitis)

Figure 11-13 **Plantar fasciitis treatment overview diagram.** Follow the general principles from left to right or top to bottom when treating plantar fasciitis.

CLIENT SELF-CARE

When plantar fasciitis significantly reduces the client's activities of daily living, the individual should rest or at least minimize weight-bearing activity as much as possible to give the tissue time to initiate healing. Elevating the leg and applying ice to the plantar fascia are indicated to reduce inflammation. A client with chronic plantar fasciitis should also minimize weight-bearing activities that may re-injure tissues and prolong the healing process, reintroducing these activities as gradually as healing allows. That said, moderate activity to keep the tissues mobile and prevent chronic adhesions is an important part of the healing process. The client should be diligent in stretching the plantar flexors before activity. The client will likely benefit from wearing shoes with good arch support or tailored orthotic inserts to support pes cavus, slow the progression of pes planus, or to reduce eversion. Heel cups are used to cushion the heel of a client with fat pad atrophy. These should be used in all shoes and worn regularly, not just when participating in sports or other intensive activities. For chronic cases, the client may wear a night splint that prevents plantar flexion.

The following are intended as general recommendations for stretching and strengthening muscles involved in the client's condition. The objective is to create distance between the attachment sites of muscles that have shortened and to perform repetitions of movements that decrease the distance between the attachments of muscles that have weakened. If you have had no training in remedial exercises and do not feel that you have a functional understanding of stretching and strengthening, refer the client to a professional with training in this area.

Clients often neglect self-care due to time constraints. Encourage them to follow these guidelines:

- Instruct the client to perform self-care throughout the day, such as while talking on the phone, reading e-mail, washing dishes, or watching television instead of setting aside extra time.
- Encourage the client to take regular breaks from stationary postures or repetitive actions. If the client's daily activities include hours of sitting, suggest walking for at least a few minutes every hour to prevent the plantar fascia from tightening. If the client's daily activities require standing for long periods or repetitive actions that contribute to plantar fasciitis, suggest sitting for at least a few minutes every hour.
- Demonstrate gentle self-massage of the plantar fascia and the tissues surrounding the plantar fascia to keep adhesions and hypertonicity at bay between treatments. If no swelling is present, instruct the client to gently roll the foot over a tennis ball, can, or other sturdy round object, from the calcaneus to the metatarsals and back, to keep the tissues pliable. Soaking the feet in warm water prior to rolling over the object may soften the superficial tissues. If bone spurs are present, avoid the affected area or leave out this exercise.
- Demonstrate all strengthening exercises and stretches to your client and have him or her perform these in your presence before leaving to ensure that he or she is performing them properly and will not harm himself or herself when practicing alone. Stretches should be held for 15–30 seconds and performed frequently throughout the day within the client's limits. The client should not force the stretch or bounce. The stretch should be slow, gentle, and steady, trying to keep every other joint as relaxed as possible.
- Stretching and strengthening exercises should be recommended according to your findings in ROM testing and palpation.

Stretching

Maintaining the proper length and tone of the plantar flexors is essential to reduce hyperflexion and eversion of the ankle and to reduce the flattening of the arch that may contribute to plantar fasciitis. Stretches should be performed throughout the day, particularly before and after activity.

Instruct the client to stand at an arm's length away from a wall, leaning against it. Bring the toes of the unaffected foot forward close to the edge of the wall, and bend that knee. This will place the opposite, affected ankle into passive dorsiflexion. When the knee of the affected leg is extended, the gastrocnemius gets the best stretch. To stretch the soleus more, flex the knee of the affected leg. Both heels should be on the floor at all times, and the stretch should be held for 15–30 seconds or as long as is comfortable (Fig. 11-14). If the client is unable to keep the heel on the floor, instruct him or her to reduce the distance between the feet. Stretch the opposite ankle as needed.

To stretch the plantar flexors while seated, instruct the client to sit comfortably with the back supported, and then extend the knees, dorsiflex the ankles, and hold for 15–30 seconds (Fig. 11-15). This action also helps to strengthen the dorsiflexors. Suggest that the client repeat this action a few times, and then get up and walk around to mobilize the ankle and the foot.

If eversion is a contributing factor, instruct the client to simultaneously stretch the evertors and strengthen the invertors by actively inverting the ankle fully and holding for as long as it is comfortable. Repeat this action a few times, and then get up and walk around to mobilize the ankle.

Strengthening

Strengthening the dorsiflexors may prime them to better oppose plantar flexion. The seated calf stretch described above also strengthens the dorsiflexors. In addition, strengthening the intrinsic muscles of the foot may increase their ability to absorb shock and maintain both flexibility and structural support. Instruct the client to perform exercises in which he or she grasps items with the toes. Begin with bigger, flexible items, like a towel. As the foot becomes stronger, gradually progress to smaller items, such as a pen or marbles, picking them up between the toes as well (Fig. 11-16). Drawing the alphabet in the air with the foot is a simple exercise for strengthening the ankle and improving ROM. Instruct the client to make the movements only as big as is comfortable and to draw only as many letters as possible until he or she feels fatigue.

SUGGESTIONS FOR FURTHER TREATMENT

Ideally, a client with plantar fasciitis will have treatments twice a week until he or she can perform activities of daily living with minimal or no pain for at least 4 days. Once this is achieved, reduce

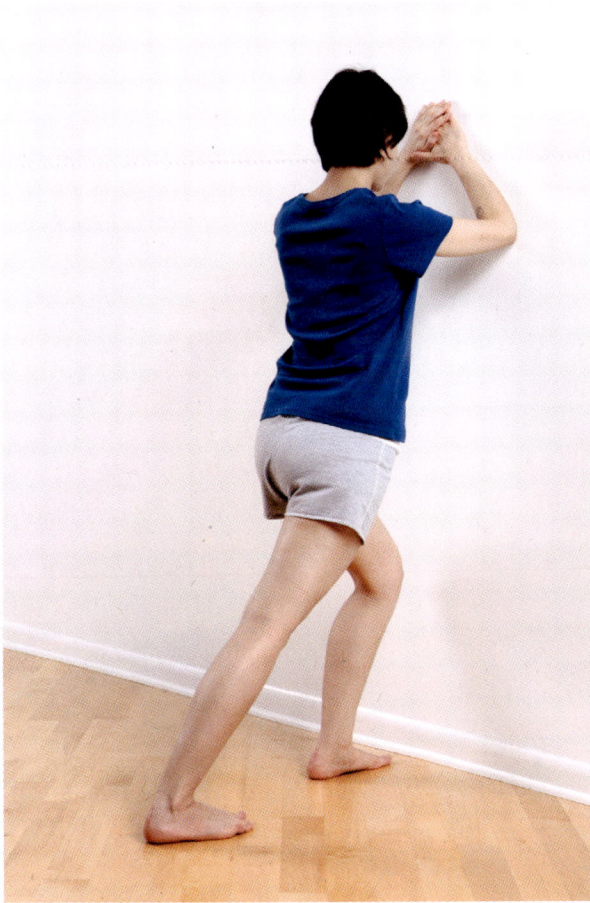

Figure 11-14   **Stretch the plantar flexors.**

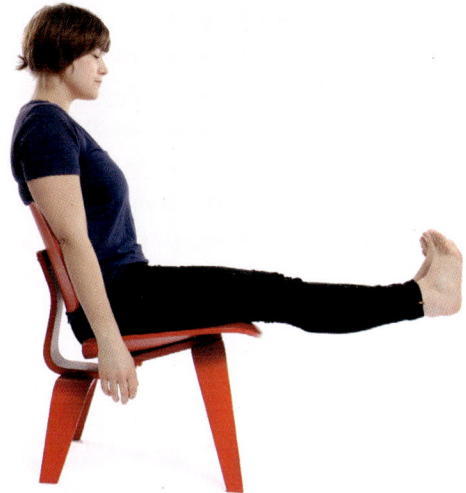

Figure 11-15   **Stretch the hamstrings and plantar flexors while strengthening the quadriceps.** Sit comfortably with the back supported, and then extend the knees and dorsiflex the ankles.

frequency to once per week until symptoms are absent for at least 7 days. When the client reports that he or she has been pain-free for more than 7 days, treatment can be reduced to twice per month. If the client is pain-free for 3 or more consecutive weeks, he or she can then schedule once per month or as necessary. If the client's symptoms are localized and other postural deviations are minimal, half-hour treatments may be sufficient to effect a change in plantar fasciitis. When treating plantar fasciitis caused by soft tissue dysfunction, there should be some improvement with each session. If this is not happening, consider the following possibilities:

- There is too much time between treatments. It is always best to give newly treated tissues 24–48 hours to adapt, but if too much time passes between treatments in the beginning, the client's activities of daily living may reverse any progress.
- The client is not adjusting activities of daily living or is not keeping up with self-care. As much as we want to fix the problem, we cannot force a client to make the adjustments we suggest. Explain the importance of his or her participation in the healing process, and encourage the client to follow your recommendations, but be careful not to judge or reprimand a client who does not.
- The condition is advanced or has other musculoskeletal complications that are beyond your basic training. Refer this client to a massage therapist with advanced clinical massage training. Continuing to treat a client whose case is beyond your training could turn the client away from massage therapy altogether and hinder healing.
- The client has an undiagnosed, underlying condition. Discontinue treatment until the client sees a health care provider for medical assessment.

If you are not treating the client in a clinical setting or private practice, you may not be able to take this client through the full program of healing. Still, if you can bring some relief in just one

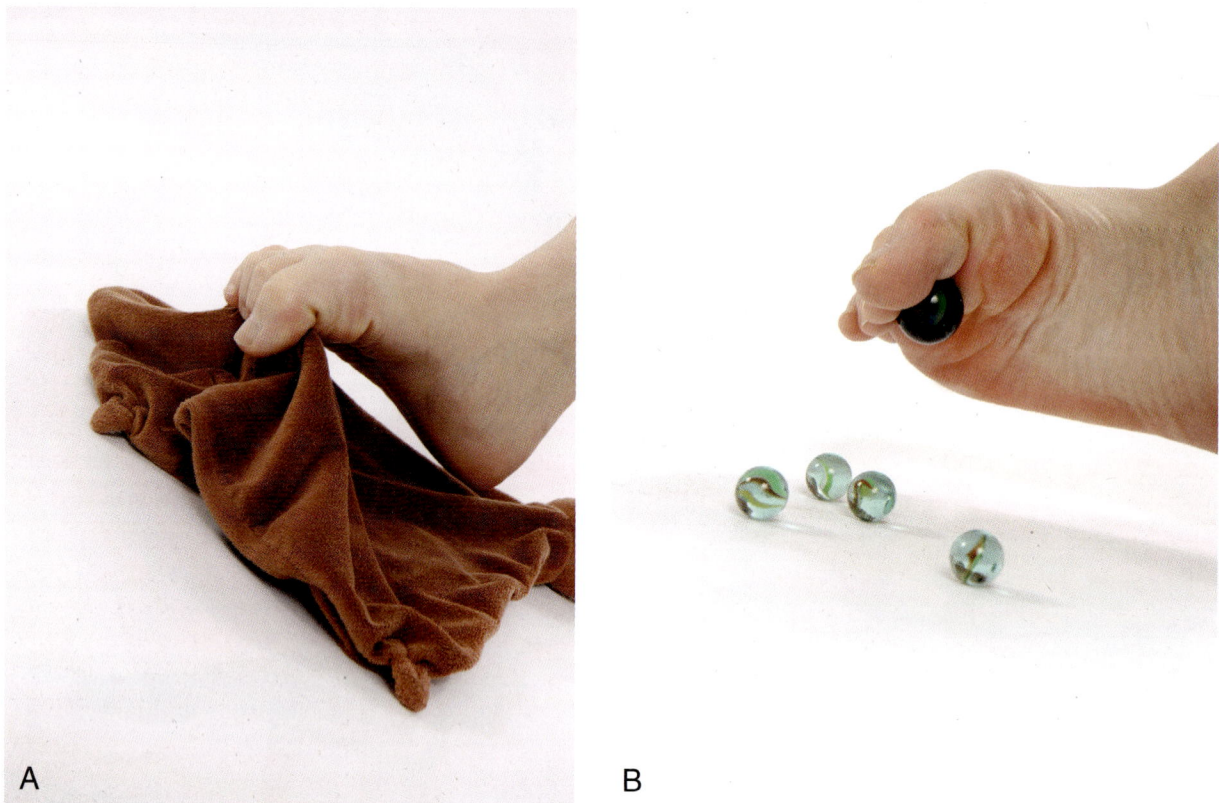

Figure 11-16   **Strengthen the muscles of the foot.** Begin with items that are easy to grasp (A) and progress to items that require more fine motor skill (B).

treatment, it may encourage the client to discuss this change with his or her health care provider and seek manual therapy rather than more aggressive treatment options. If the client agrees to return for regular treatments, the symptoms are likely to change each time, so it is important to perform an assessment before each session. Once you have released superficial tissues in general areas, you may be able to focus more of your treatment on deeper tissues in a specific area. Likewise, once you have treated the structures specific to plantar fasciitis, you may be able to pay closer attention to compensating structures and coexisting conditions.

PROFESSIONAL GROWTH

CASE STUDY

Dewan is a 45-year-old married male. Four years ago, he moved from a small Caribbean island, where he was a professional soccer player and coach, to the United States to attend university. He began feeling pain in his right foot approximately 1 month ago, which has gradually gotten worse.

Subjective

Dewan complained of pain in his right foot, which began approximately 1 month ago and has gotten progressively worse. Prior to moving to the United States to attend school, Dewan was a professional soccer player and soccer coach. He played soccer nearly every day. After moving to the United States, his life has become more sedentary. Between his studies and work, he had little time for physical fitness. Now that he has completed his degree and secured a job, he has returned to coaching his son's high school soccer team. The pain in his right foot began within the first week of coaching soccer 3 days a week. When it first began, he felt the pain during practice and in the mornings after. When he had more than 48 hours between practices, he felt no pain. Over the past month, the pain has become more regular. He stated that he feels it most often in the morning, at the beginning of a practice, and in the evenings after practice. He stated that icing the foot brings temporary relief, but that his first steps in the morning and his first run of a practice are very painful. Because he goes to practice right after work, he has not made time to properly stretch before practice, and he stated that stretching after practice is painful.

Dewan described a healthy diet. He had several minor injuries to his legs and ankles while playing soccer that he stated never kept him from playing for more than a day or two with the exception of a kick to the posterior right leg that resulted in myositis ossificans. This required 1 week of rest followed by a few weeks of manual therapy to encourage reabsorption of calcium and to restore normal tone. He has not consulted his health care provider about his foot pain. His soccer team in the Caribbean had a full-time massage therapist on staff, and he thought massage might help his foot pain. His goal is to be able to continue coaching soccer without pain.

Objective

Dewan appears very healthy and vibrant, lean and muscular. He showed no signs of pain or dysfunction when climbing the stairs, walking, or standing from a seated position. He sat with his feet flat on the floor.

Postural assessment revealed a slight increase in the kyphotic curve with internally rotated shoulders. His knees remain slightly flexed when standing, and his ankles are slightly everted bilaterally. The four lateral toes of the right foot are hyperextended at the metatarsophalangeal joint, and flexed at the interphalangeal joint. The arches are within normal height, very slightly flatter on the right.

The passive dorsiflexion-eversion test reproduced a level 3 pain, on a scale of 1–10, near the calcaneus with no referral, numbness, or tingling. Tinel's sign was negative for tarsal tunnel syndrome. Weight-bearing plantar flexion with passive extension of the toes, performed by asking the client to stand on his tip-toes, reproduced pain that the client suggested was closest to what he feels during activity. The non-weight-bearing windlass test was positive and produced pain at level 8. I did not perform the weight-bearing test. There is no visible or palpable swelling in the foot or ankle. The calcaneal tendon and superficial fascia into the mid calf are dense and adhered. There is an area of dimpled, dense tissue in the right leg just below the musculotendinous junction of the gastrocnemius. When asked, Dewan answered that this was the area of his past myositis ossificans. The right calcaneal tendon is less flexible than the left. The skin of the plantar surface of both feet is thick, dry, and cracked superficially around the edges of the heel. There was no local or specific pain with palpation of the calcaneus, and there is no indication of a bone spur. The tenderest spot on the sole of the foot is approximately 1 cm distal to the medial calcaneal tubercle. Still, only deep cross-fiber strokes reproduced pain at a level 3.

Action

Treatment today focused on lengthening shortened plantar flexors, reducing adhesions in the intrinsic muscles of the feet, reducing adhesions and lengthening the plantar fascia. I treated both legs, with more aggressive treatment on the right. I began with general massage to the low back, gluteal area, and thighs bilaterally. Nothing remarkable was noted.

I used myofascial release on the posterior leg with special attention paid to the distal tendinous area. I used kneading followed by longitudinal gliding and deeper muscle stripping to the plantar flexors and evertors, namely the gastrocnemius, soleus, tibialis posterior, peroneus longus and brevis, and the extensor digitorum longus. I applied specific, localized cross-fiber strokes followed by superficial and deep muscle stripping to the area affected by myositis ossificans. A trigger point was found in the soleus, approximately 2 inches superior and slightly posterior to the lateral malleolus, and it referred into the heel. Ischemic compression followed by muscle stripping reduced pain from level 7 to level 3. I used cross-fiber strokes followed by longitudinal strokes to the calcaneal tendons bilaterally. There was no change in texture. I applied gentle kneading to the intrinsic muscles of the foot followed by longitudinal stripping between the metatarsals. I used gliding and kneading to warm and soften the plantar fascia until the tissue felt pliable enough to apply deeper pressure. I applied cross-fiber strokes to the plantar fascia, beginning superficially and slowly working deeper, avoiding the medial calcaneal tubercle until pain with the extension of the first toe reduced to a level 3. I also applied deep muscle stripping to the plantar fascia from distal to proximal. Finally, I used clearing strokes on the full leg.

Turning the client supine with no bolster, I stretched the plantar flexors and plantar fascia with a passive dorsiflexion of the ankle. This produced pain at the medial calcaneal tubercle at a level 2. Adding passive extension of the toes increased pain to level 6. Decreasing the extension of the toes reduced pain to a level 3. I held the stretch for 15 seconds. At the end of the stretch, the pain remained at level 3. I applied general Swedish techniques to the anterior leg. I found that the iliotibial bands were dense and adhered bilaterally. I cleared the whole leg, and then attempted to stretch the plantar flexors and plantar fascia again. Dorsiflexion alone produced no pain. Adding extension of the toes increased pain to a level 3. After holding the stretch for 15 seconds, the client's pain reduced to a level 2.

Plan

As a life-long athlete, Dewan is familiar with stretching and strengthening exercises, so simple demonstrations were sufficient. His symptoms are not debilitating and do not severely hinder his activities of daily living. For this reason, I think it is unnecessary for him to stop coaching but suggested that he take it slowly and be gentle on the feet until symptoms become less frequent. It is essential that he make time to thoroughly stretch the plantar flexors and plantar fascia before each practice. I suggested making this the first activity for the whole team at each practice. I recommended applying ice to the sole of the foot for approximately 3 minutes after practice. Icing for too long could stiffen the tissues and increase the risk of tearing. I also suggested stretching the plantar flexors and plantar fascia and strengthening the dorsiflexors by extending the knees and dorsi-flexing the ankles while seated during the workday. I suggested avoiding extending the toes during this exercise until this action no longer produced pain greater than level 3.

Dewan will return for treatment 3 days from today and twice next week. As symptoms decrease and the risk of tearing is minimized, treatment can be reduced to once weekly.

I will plan to focus more intently on lengthening the flexor hallucis during the next treatment.

CRITICAL THINKING EXERCISES

1. Excessive eversion of the ankles is commonly seen with plantar fasciitis and is described in the treatment guidelines above. Create a SOAP chart with history, assessment, and a treatment plan that describes a case of plantar fasciitis due to excessive inversion of the ankle. How might inversion of the ankle affect posture at the knees, hips, or low back? Treatment goals should include lengthening shortened tissues, strengthening weak muscles, and restoring proper neuromuscular function.

2. A client calls to schedule a massage for foot pain. She states that she sprained the ankle of the affected leg a few times. She was also diagnosed with calcaneal tendonitis in the affected leg for which she received no treatment. A month or so after the diagnosis, the daily pain was gone, but the tendon continued to hurt when she stretched her calves deeply in yoga. Discuss the possible relationship between the injuries and plantar fasciitis. What questions would you ask this client? Are there questions that you need to ask her health care provider?

3. Develop a 10-minute stretching and strengthening routine for a client that covers all of the muscles involved in plantar fasciitis. Use Box 11-1 and Figure 11-5 as a guide. Remember that a stretch increases the distance between the origin and insertion of a muscle and is important for those muscles that are shortened while strengthening is performed by actively bringing the origin and insertion closer together and is important for the antagonists of shortened muscles. Describe each step of the routine in enough detail that the client can refer to these descriptions in your absence and perform them without harm.

4. Conduct a short literature review to learn about the relationship between symptoms resembling plantar fasciitis and the following:
   - Diabetes
   - Rheumatoid arthritis
   - Morton's toe
   - Night splinting

BIBLIOGRAPHY AND SUGGESTED READINGS

Alshami AM, Souvlis T, Coppieters MW. A review of plantar heel pain of neural origin: Differential diagnosis and management. Manual Therapy. 2008;13(2):103–111.

American College of Foot and Ankle Surgeons. Tarsal Tunnel Syndrome. Available at http://www.footphysicians.com/footankleinfo/tarsal-tunnel-syndrome.htm#2. Accessed Spring 2009.

Barrett SL. A guide to neurogenic etiologies of heel pain. Podiatry Today. 2005;18(11):36–44. Available at http://www.podiatrytoday.com/article/4735. Accessed Spring 2009.

Biel A. *Trail Guide to the Body: How to Locate Muscles, Bones and More*, 3rd ed. Boulder, CO: Books of Discovery, 2005.

Bolgla LA, Malone TR. Plantar fasciitis and the windlass mechanism: A biomechanical link to clinical practice. Journal of Athletic Training. 2004;39(1):77–82.

Burns J, Crosbie J, Hunt A, et al. The effect of pes cavus on foot pain and plantar pressure. Clinical Biomechanics. 2005;20(9):877–882.

Clarkson HM. *Joint Motion and Function Assessment: A Research-Based Practical Guide*. Baltimore, MD: Lippincott Williams & Wilkins, 2005.

Cornwall MW, McPoil TG. Plantar fasciitis: Etiology and treatment. Journal of Orthopaedic and Sports Physical Therapy. 1999;29(12):756–760.

Hambrick T. Plantar fascitis: A chiropractic perspective. Journal of Bodywork and Movement Therapies. 2001;5:49–55.

Hertling D, Kessler RM. *Management of Common Musculoskeletal Disorders: Physical Therapy Principles and Methods*, 4th ed. Philadelphia, PA: Lippincott Williams & Wilkins, 2006.

Kullman J, Steinbock K. Plantar fascitis: Chinese medicine perspective. Journal of Bodywork and Movement Therapies. 2001;5(1):31–33.

Lowe W. *Orthopedic Massage: Theory and Technique*. St Louis, MO: Mosby-Elsevier, 2003.

Mayo Foundation for Medical Education and Research. Bursitis. Available at http://www.mayoclinic.com/health/bursitis/DS00032. Accessed Spring 2009.

Mayo Foundation for Medical Education and Research. Plantar Fasciitis. Available at http://www.mayoclinic.com/health/plantar-fasciitis/DS00508. Accessed Spring 2009.

Mayo Foundation for Medical Education and Research. Rheumatoid Arthritis. Available at http://www.mayoclinic.com/health/rheumatoid-arthritis/DS00020. Accessed Winter 2009.

McPoil TG, Martin RL, Cornwall MW, et al. Heel pain–plantar fasciitis: Clinical practice guidelines linked to the International Classification of Functioning, Disability, and Health (ICF), presented by the Orthopaedic Section of the American Physical Therapy Association. Journal of Orthopaedic & Sports Physical Therapy. 2008;38(4):A1–A18.

Oatis C. *Kinesiology: The Mechanics and Pathomechanics of Human Movement*, 2nd ed. Baltimore, MD: Lippincott Williams & Wilkins, 2009.

Potts J. Plantar Fascitis: Physical therapy perspective. Journal of Bodywork and Movement Therapies. 2001; 5:45–49.

Rattray F, Ludwig L. *Clinical Massage Therapy: Understanding, Assessing and Treating over 70 Conditions*. Toronto, ON: Talus Incorporated, 2000.

Rosenholz C. Plantar fascitis: Body-mind perspective. Journal of Bodywork and Movement Therapies. 2001;5:33–36.

Rosenholz C. Plantar fascitis: Introduction. Journal of Bodywork and Movement Therapies. 2001;5:29–30.

Simons DG, Travell JG, Simons LS. *Myofascial Pain and Dysfunction: The Trigger Point Manual*, 2nd ed. Philadelphia, PA: Lippincott Williams & Wilkins, 1999.

U.S. National Library of Medicine and the National Institutes of Health. Broken Bone. Available at http://www.nlm.nih.gov/medlineplus/ency/article/000001.htm. Accessed Spring 2009.

U.S. National Library of Medicine and the National Institutes of Health. Gout. Available at http://www.nlm.nih.gov/medlineplus/ency/article/000424.htm#Symptoms. Accessed Winter 2009.

U.S. National Library of Medicine and the National Institutes of Health. Reactive Arthritis. Available at https://www.nlm.nih.gov/medlineplus/ency/article/000440.htm. Accessed Spring 2009.

Werner R. *A Massage Therapist's Guide to Pathology*, 4th ed. Philadelphia, PA: Lippincott Williams and Wilkins, 2009.

Witt P. Plantar Fasciitis: Neuromuscular perspective. Journal of Bodywork and Movement Therapies. 2001; 5:36–45.

Young B, Walker MJ, Strunce J, et al. A combined treatment approach emphasizing impairment-based manual physical therapy for plantar heel pain: A case series. Journal of Orthopaedic & Sports Physical Therapy. 2004;34(11):725–733.

Muscle Strains

UNDERSTANDING MUSCLE STRAINS

Muscle strain, often called a pulled muscle, occurs when muscle fibers are overstretched. Increased tensile stress—force that elongates a muscle—is the primary cause of muscle strains. Overstretching may result in tears to the muscle fibers and tendons at the musculotendinous junction or at the site of attachment to the bone (Fig. 12-1). Overstretching can occur if the muscle is forced to lengthen beyond its normal range when the muscle is activated during a stretch or when a muscle affected by spasm, fatigue, scar tissue, dehydration, or other dysfunction is stressed by quick, intense movement, particularly against resistance, even within the normal ROM. Eccentric contraction of a compromised muscle is a common cause of strains. For example, a person with a sedentary lifestyle may develop shortened hip flexors with a high resting tone. If this person stands too quickly, the poorly conditioned hip flexors may not adapt to the quick, eccentric contraction, and strain may occur.

Strains can occur in any muscle but are most likely in muscles that cross two joints, particularly when the muscle lengthens across both joints simultaneously. Muscles commonly strained include the hamstrings, quadriceps, gastrocnemius, the muscles of the rotator cuff, pectoralis major, biceps brachialis, and the muscles of the neck (particularly with whiplash). An acute strain occurs when a muscle is recruited to perform a contraction quickly and intensely, particularly against resistance. Muscles with a high concentration of fast-twitch fibers that are frequently recruited to contract eccentrically are most susceptible to acute strain. A chronic strain occurs when a muscle is regularly recruited to perform repetitive actions or when an acute strain is not fully treated and continues to contribute to dysfunctional patterns. Postural muscles such as the erector spinae, which contract against gravity for long periods throughout the day, are most susceptible to chronic strain. Strain can occur in any part of a muscle and may involve just a few or all of its fibers (Fig. 12-2). The most common site of strain is at or near the musculotendinous junction, where the very elastic muscle fibers meet the less malleable tendon. The risk of acute strain increases when the health of the muscle is compromised.

The more a muscle is lengthened, the less able it is to absorb stress. As a muscle approaches its maximum length, muscle spindles initiate a reflex response to resist further stretching by activating or tensing the stretched fibers. This activation of the muscle increases its ability to absorb stress, protecting the muscle from injury. The velocity of contraction and reflex response, resistance against the action, muscle fatigue, weakness, tension, temperature, and prior injuries all affect whether the contraction is smooth and healthy or results in an injury.

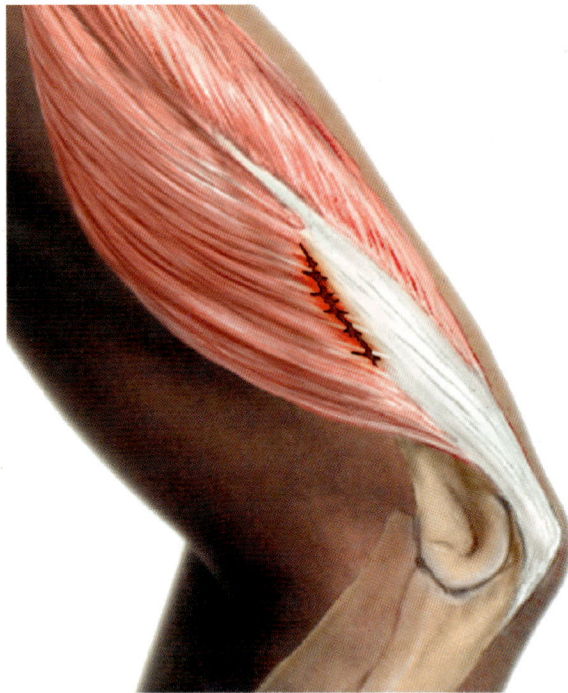

Figure 12-1 **Muscle strain.** Fibers in the muscle, tendon, or musculotendinous junction or at the attachment site tear due to overstretching.

Common Signs and Symptoms

The signs and symptoms of muscle strains differ depending on the grade (severity of the injury) and stage (duration of symptoms) of the injury. Table 12-1 outlines the common signs and symptoms for each grade and stage of muscle strain.

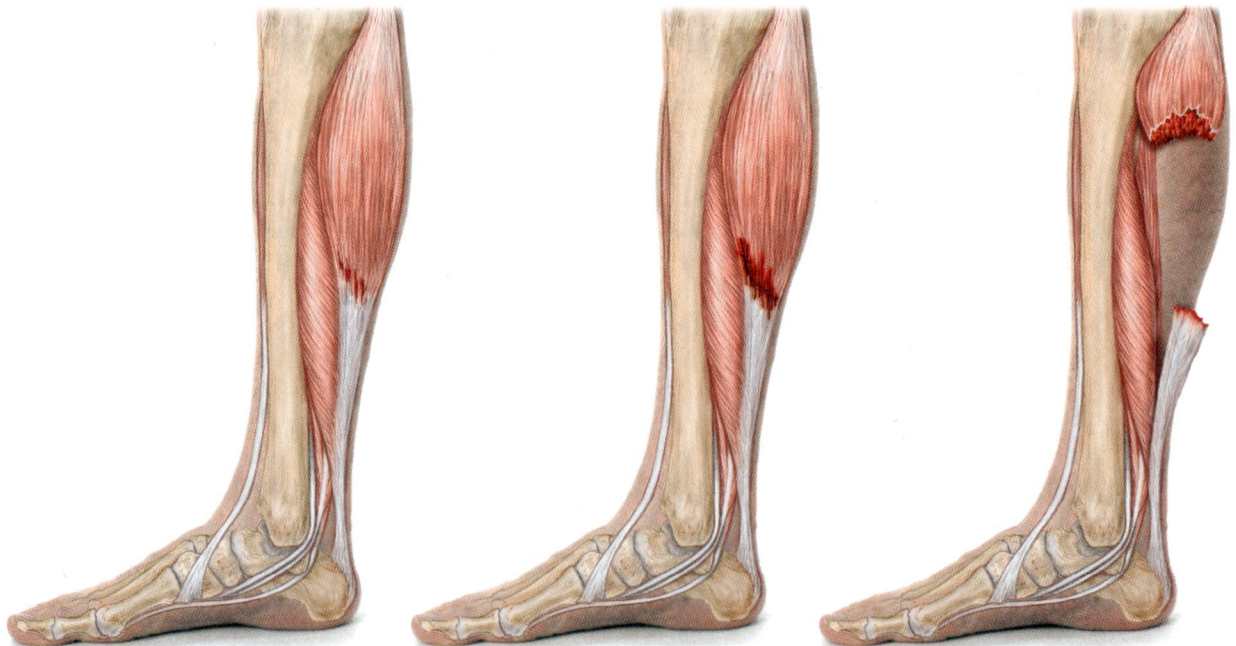

Figure 12-2 **Degrees of strain.** Few fibers are torn in a first-degree strain (left). Several fibers are torn in a second-degree strain (middle). All fibers are torn in a third-degree strain (right). The muscle and tendons may shorten and bunch up near the attachment site. Adapted from Clay JH, Pounds DM. *Basic Clinical Massage Therapy: Integrating Anatomy and Treatment,* 2nd ed. Philadelphia: Lippincott Williams & Wilkins, 2008.

Table 12-1	Grades and Stages of Muscle Strain		
	Grade 1	**Grade 2**	**Grade 3**
	Mild strain	Moderate strain	Severe strain
	Minor stretch or tear	Tearing of several to the majority of fibers	Complete rupture of muscle belly, separation of muscle from tendon, or tendon from bone.
	Client can continue activity with mild pain	Pain and weakness may make continued activity difficult	Pain and weakness halt continued activity.
Acute stage (symptoms typically last 3–4 days following injury)	Minimal loss of strength Mild discomfort with activity Minimal or no local edema Minimal or no bruising Mild local tenderness	Snapping sound or sensation at moment of injury Moderate local edema Moderate bruising, red or purple Possible hematoma Possible palpable gap at site of injury Moderate local tenderness Moderate pain with activity Moderate weakness with activity Moderate decrease in ROM Protective muscle spasm crossing affected joint(s)	Snapping sound or sensation at moment of injury Severe pain Immediate loss of strength Immediate loss of ROM Inability to perform activity involving the affected muscle Considerable local edema Considerable bruising, red or purple Possible hematoma Palpable gap at site of injury Ruptured muscle may contract and gather into a palpable mass Protective muscle spasm crossing affected joint(s)
Subacute stage (symptoms typically remain from 3 days to 3 weeks following acute stage)	Minimal to no pain Minimal to no reduction of strength Scar developing at site of injury Adhesions developing at site of injury and between surrounding muscles and other soft tissues Trigger points in affected muscle, synergists, and antagonists	Moderate to minimal pain improved since the acute stage Moderate to minimal reduction of strength improved since the acute stage Bruising remains and may be changing color to yellow or green Possible hematoma Palpable inconsistency in muscle shape at the site of injury Injury may be splinted or casted Scar at the site of injury Adhesions developing at the site of injury and between the surrounding muscles and other soft tissues Protective muscle spasm may diminish and may be replaced by hypertonicity Trigger points in affected muscle, synergists, and antagonists	Significant pain Significantly reduced strength, particularly against resistance Bruising remains, may be changing color to yellow or green Possible hematoma Palpable gap at the site of injury if muscle was not surgically repaired Significant scarring if muscle was surgically repaired. Injury may be splinted or casted Protective muscle spasm may continue, or may diminish and may be replaced by hypertonicity Trigger points developing in affected muscle, synergists, and antagonists

(continued)

Table 12-1	Grades and Stages of Muscle Strain (Continued)		
	Grade 1	**Grade 2**	**Grade 3**
Chronic stage (symptoms continue beyond the subacute stage)	Bruising has cleared	Bruising has cleared	Bruising has cleared
	Trigger points, scars, adhesions, and hypertonicity may still affect injured muscle and compensating structures and may cause ischemia	Trigger points, scars, adhesions, and hypertonicity affect the injured muscle and compensating structures and may cause ischemia	Trigger points, scars, adhesions, and hypertonicity affect the injured muscle and compensating structures and may cause ischemia
	Discomfort when affected muscle is stretched	Discomfort or pain when the affected muscle is stretched	Reduce ROM in joint(s) crossed by the affected muscle
	Increased risk of re-injury if not properly treated	ROM in joint(s) crossed by the affected muscle has improved but is still restricted	Reduced strength if the affected muscle was not surgically repaired
	Chronic inflammation if not properly treated	Increased risk of re-injury if not properly treated	Increased risk of re-injury if not properly treated
		Chronic inflammation if not properly treated	Increased risk of overuse injury to synergists if the affected muscle was not surgically repaired
		Possible atrophy if not properly treated	Chronic inflammation if not properly treated
			Possible atrophy if not properly treated

In general, strains produce local pain, stiffness, pain on resisted movement or passive stretch, reduced strength, and impaired ROM.

Possible Causes and Contributing Factors

The cause of strain is overstretching with too much tensile stress. The affected muscle lengthens beyond its capability when the joint it crosses is forced beyond its maximum range, particularly when the movement occurs quickly and passively. Strain can also occur when an unhealthy muscle is unable to lengthen within the average normal range. Previous injury, even if the injury was minor and caused no reduction in activities of daily living, may result in scar tissue, weakness, hypertonicity, spasm, or trigger points, which if left untreated, increases the risk of strain. When scar tissue forms, it alters the shape and impedes the function of the affected fibers. Collagenous scar tissue does not have the flexibility or contractile strength of healthy muscle tissue, putting the torn fibers at risk for re-injury if the muscle is overstretched (Fig. 12-3). This dysfunction also increases the load that the healthy fibers must bear, putting them at risk for tearing and the muscle as a whole at risk for more serious injury including rupture. Previous strains, sprains, contusions, and dislocations often alter biomechanics and increase the risk of chronic strain if they are not properly treated.

When the antagonists of an action are much weaker than the agonists, an intense concentric contraction may overpower the eccentric contraction, forcing the joint beyond the antagonist's capability. This can also occur when the antagonist is fatigued and unable to adequately regulate motion at the joint. When a muscle is hypertonic, in spasm, or contains trigger points, it may be less capable of lengthening to accommodate an eccentric contraction. In this case, a strong or quick concentric contraction of an opposing muscle intensifies the tensile stress in the antagonist and may lead to tearing of its fibers. In addition, when the health of a muscle is compromised, the reflex response may be insufficient to inhibit overstretching.

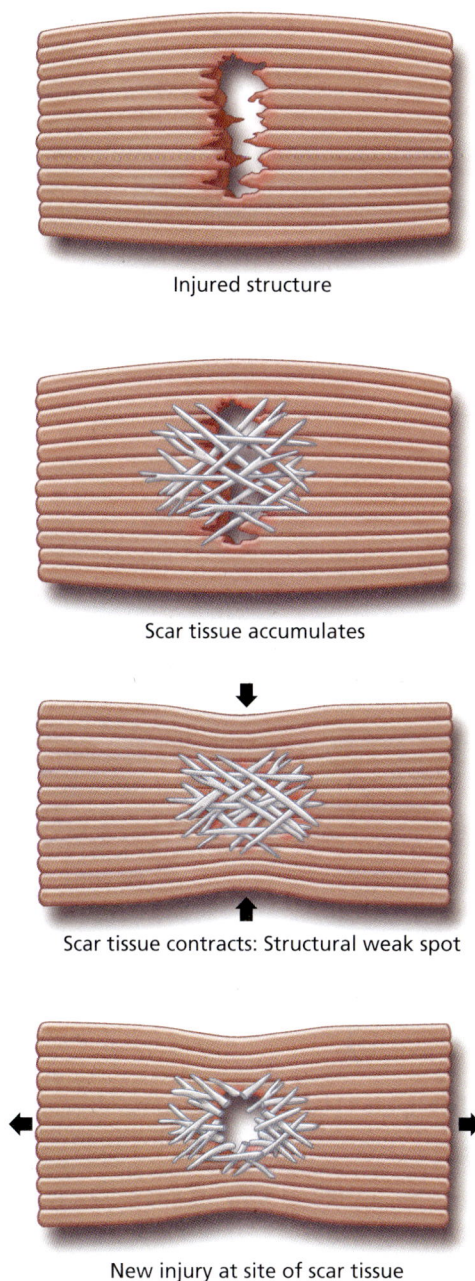

Injured structure

Scar tissue accumulates

Scar tissue contracts: Structural weak spot

Figure 12-3 **Injury–re-injury cycle.** Scar tissue alters the shape and function of the affected fibers, leaving the muscle at risk for re-injury. From the top, overstretch tears muscle fibers; new scar tissue forms to restore integrity of fibers; scar tissue contracts and becomes dense, altering the shape of the muscle and leaving a weak spot; fibers with remaining dense scar tissue are at risk for re-injury. From Werner R. *A Massage Therapist's Guide to Pathology*, 4th ed. Philadelphia, PA: Lippincott Williams & Wilkins, 2009.

New injury at site of scar tissue

Athletes are particularly prone to strains, particularly in sports involving quick, intense movements using maximum strength. Athletes are also more prone to other injuries, which, if they do not properly heal, increase the risk of strains. Athlete or not, the muscles of a person participating in an intense activity following a period of relative inactivity may not be well conditioned and may suffer from strains. In general, using improper techniques when participating in sports, dancing, or other intense activity increases the risk of muscle strains.

Age may also play a role in the increased risk for muscle strains. In adolescents, growth spurts sometimes increase the length of the bones more quickly than the muscle can adapt. This increases tensile stress and the risk of strain until the muscles grow to fit the joint. In older adults, the tone, strength, and general health of tissues begins to deteriorate, putting muscle fibers at risk for tearing. Temperature may also play a role in the risk of strain injuries. In cold temperatures, superficial vessels contract to prevent substantial heat loss. This cooling affects elasticity and may increase the risk of muscle fiber rupture. Simple contractions performed before intense activity can increase muscle temperature by a full degree or two.

Because strains can occur anywhere in the body, they can be confused with many other conditions throughout the body. For example, pain in the back of the calf may be a muscle strain, but it may also be a Baker's cyst or blood clot. Low back pain may involve strains, a herniated disc, or both. Pain in the chest could indicate a strain to the pectorals but can also be a symptom of a cardiac event. Muscle strain is usually associated with a precipitating event, whether a single, acutely painful injury or the introduction of new activity after a period of inactivity. Palpation of the area usually produces more intense pain at the specific site of the injury. Table 12-2 lists some general conditions commonly confused with or contributing to muscle strains. Because the pattern of pain from strains can present so differently, it is particularly important to understand the client's health history, precipitating events, and other possible causes of pain in the area before treatment. Consult your pathology book for more detailed information. If you are unsure and the client's symptoms resemble a more serious condition, particularly if the client has other risk factors, refer him or her to a health care provider for medical assessment.

Contraindications and Special Considerations

First, it is essential to understand the cause of the client's pain. If the client is unable to move the joint, heard a popping sound, or has significant weakness or if you suspect the client has a fractured bone or significant tearing to the tissues, work with the client's health care provider, and consult a pathology text for massage therapists before proceeding. These are a few general cautions:

- **Protective muscle splinting.** When a muscle is injured, its synergists and antagonists may spasm reflexively in an attempt to keep the joint's movement within a range that prevents further injury. Do not reduce protective muscle splinting in the acute stage of injury. Wait until the subacute or chronic stage, when sufficient scarring and muscle fiber regeneration reduces the need for protective splinting.
- **Bruises.** A bruise indicates damage to blood vessels allowing blood to accumulate in surrounding tissue. Avoid direct pressure to a bruise that is still healing. As the vessels heal and blood is reabsorbed, the color changes from red or purple to green or yellow. Severe bruising may result in a hematoma—a localized pooling of blood outside the vessels. In some cases, a sac-like enclosure forms around the pool of blood to minimize internal bleeding. A hematoma often resolves on its own, like a simple bruise, but if it grows or hardens it may require medical attention. Avoid direct pressure to a hematoma, and refer the client to a health care professional if the area becomes hard, if the client reports feeling pressure from the hematoma, or if it does not show signs of resolving over the course of a week or two.
- **Muscle testing.** Use only active ROM testing in the acute stage of a grade 2 or 3 strain. The client usually limits active movement to the pain-free range. P ROM and R ROM testing in the acute stage may cause further injury.
- **Hydrotherapy.** Do not apply heat near the edges of a cast to prevent the accumulation of fluid under the cast.
- **Reproducing symptoms.** Symptoms may occur during treatment. If treatment reproduces symptoms, adjust the client to a more neutral posture. Shortening or adding slack to the muscle may help. If this does not relieve the symptoms, reduce your pressure or move away from the area. You may be able to treat around the site that reproduced the symptoms, but proceed with caution.
- **Treatment duration and pressure.** If the client is older, has degenerative disease, or has been diagnosed with a condition that diminishes activities of daily living, you may need to adjust your pressure as well as the treatment duration. Frequent half-hour sessions may suit the client better.
- **Friction.** Do not use deep frictions if the health of the underlying tissues is at risk for rupture or if the client is taking anti-inflammatory medication or anticoagulants. Allow time for scarring and tissue regeneration to avoid re-injury. Friction creates an inflammatory process, which may interfere with the intended action of anti-inflammatory medication.

Table 12-2	Differentiating Conditions Commonly Confused with or Contributing to Muscle Strains		
Condition	**Typical Signs and Symptoms**	**Testing**	**Massage Therapy**
Sprain	Inflammation, heat, redness, and pain in acute stage Remaining inflammation and weakness reduce ROM in subacute and chronic stages	Often self-assessed	Massage is indicated. See Chapter 13.
Tendinitis	Often has gradual onset Pain, tenderness, and swelling at affected tendon	Physical exam Localized pain on full passive stretch X-ray may be performed to rule out other conditions	Massage is indicated. See Chapter 14.
Spasm/cramp (contracture)	Sudden, often sharp pain in affected voluntary muscle Palpable and often visible mass of hypertonic muscle tissue	Most often self-assessed X-ray or MRI may be used to assess extent of damage	Massage is indicated. Discuss with health care provider if repeated spasm is related to an underlying condition or medication.
Myofascial pain syndrome	Persistent muscle aches or pain Muscle or joint stiffness Muscle tension Trigger points Pain interrupts sleep	Physical exam Palpate for trigger points Referred pain or twitch response Other tests may be performed to rule out other sources of pain	Massage is indicated. Myofascial pain syndrome is associated with trigger points. See Chapter 3.
Delayed onset muscle soreness (DOMS)	Stiffness and discomfort 24–72 hours after activity Common when new activity is initiated after a period of inactivity Risk increases with activities involving eccentric contractions Temporary reduction in strength Temporary reduction in ROM Continuing activity and increasing the frequency and intensity may improve symptoms	By signs and symptoms	Treatment is not necessary, although massage may improve symptoms and prevent further injury
Avulsion fracture	Bone fragments at the attachment site of a tendon or ligament Often accompanies strains and sprains Moderate local pain Bruising and inflammation	X-ray	Local massage is contraindicated in the acute stage. Caution is used when treating the surrounding tissues to avoid further injury. Massage may help to prevent further injury when muscle tension is a contributing factor.

(continued)

Table 12-2	Differentiating Conditions Commonly Confused with or Contributing to Muscle Strains (Continued)		
Condition	**Typical Signs and Symptoms**	**Testing**	**Massage Therapy**
Bursitis	Pain, particularly with activity or palpation Heat, redness, swelling, or tenderness	Physical exam ROM tests X-ray or MRI if conservative treatment is not successful	Massage is systemically contraindicated if bursitis is due to infection, and locally contraindicated in the acute stage to avoid increased swelling. In the subacute stage, massage to the structures surrounding the joint is indicated.
Hernia	Bulge in the area Pain or discomfort, particularly when bending, coughing, sneezing, or lifting heavy objects	Physical exam	Massage is locally contraindicated until the hernia is repaired.

Recommend that the client refrain from taking such medication for several hours before treatment if the health care provider agrees. Because anticoagulants reduce clotting, avoid techniques that may cause tearing and bleeding.

Massage Therapy Research

Many articles and research studies describe a healing program for muscle strains including massage, deep friction, and stretching. There are also many articles that include massage as part of a program to prevent muscle strains in athletes. However, a thorough review of the literature resulted in no research, case studies, or peer-reviewed articles testing the benefits of massage therapy alone in the treatment of muscle strains, and none of the studies that include massage in a healing program specifies the treatment used. While massage is cited as an important element in healing strains, no study has tested the specific effect of massage therapy on the healing process, reduction of scar tissue and adhesions, release of protective muscle splinting, regeneration of muscle tissue, restoration of strength and ROM, or reduction in the risk of re-injury.

In "Evaluation of the Effect of Two Massage Techniques on Hamstring Muscle Length in Competitive Female Hockey Players," Hopper et al. (2005) reported that reduced muscle length predisposes the athlete to injury; they studied the benefits of two forms of massage therapy in lengthening the hamstrings of 35 subjects treated over 3 consecutive days. Treatment was performed by experienced physiotherapists. One group received what the authors refer to as "standardized classic massage intervention," which included proximal to distal effleurage, circular kneading, proximal to distal picking up, and shaking. Each massage lasted 8 minutes. The second group received what the authors refer to as "dynamic soft tissue mobilisation (DSTM)," which involved the classic massage described above for a shorter duration, followed by longitudinal and cross-fiber strokes to the specific tissues identified as tight. The technique was applied during passive then active extension of the knee. DSTM treatments also lasted 8 minutes. Hamstring length was measured before, directly after, and 24 hours after treatment. Both groups showed a significant increase in hamstring length following treatment, and there was no significant difference between the two groups. While the benefits were not maintained 24 hours after treatment, the authors recommended a study of the two treatments on subjects in the subacute phase of injury and recommended investigating treatment designed to reflect the clinical setting.

Delayed onset muscle soreness (DOMS) results from the breakdown of muscle fibers following exercise, seen more often following resisted eccentric contractions than following concentric contractions. Several sources refer to DOMS as mild muscle strain, although DOMS is differentiated as a random pattern of injury to muscle belly fibers that do not require rest for recovery while strain refers to an identifiable pattern of tearing—frequently involving the tendon or musculotendinous junction—which requires a period of rest for proper healing. In "The Effects of Therapeutic Massage on Delayed Onset Muscle Soreness and Muscle Function Following Downhill Walking," Farr et al. (2002) described performing a 30-minute massage to one leg of each of eight male subjects 2 hours after each performed a 40-minute, downhill treadmill walk. Massage included only effleurage and petrissage to all major muscles of the leg and did not include deep tissue massage. Participants experienced reduced pain in the leg massaged, but there was no significant improvement in the strength or function of the affected muscles. While treatment did not focus on a single strained muscle, the study did show the benefit of massage for reducing the pain associated with muscle damage due to repeated eccentric contraction by increasing local circulation, reducing edema and the accumulation of metabolites, and decreasing nerve sensitization and pain. Further study of the effects of massage on the healing process of muscle strains is needed.

WORKING WITH THE CLIENT

Client Assessment

Muscle strain is a common cause of musculoskeletal pain, experienced in some degree by most people. Strain is often one element of musculoskeletal injuries or chronic pain conditions. For example, when short plantar flexors contribute to plantar fasciitis, lengthening those muscles against resistance, such as when walking, can cause tearing of the fibers. When mild, first-degree strains contribute to the symptoms of other conditions, the following treatment recommendations can aid healing and reduce the risk of re-injury. Reducing adhesions and scar tissue, reorienting muscle fibers, lengthening shortened muscles, and strengthening weak muscles are the basic goals for treating muscle strains.

More serious second- and third-degree strains require more focused attention. An acute third-degree strain requires medical attention. You are not likely to see a client in the acute stage of a third-degree strain. When surgical repair presents more risk than benefit, the muscle may be left detached. In most cases, the muscle is surgically repaired, and the client is prescribed physical therapy. You are most likely to see a client in this condition as part of a program to reduce pain, limitations in ROM, or compensating patterns that may have developed. Swelling and bruising in the acute stage of a second-degree strain can be significant enough to contraindicate treatment locally or to a broad area surrounding the injury. Significant swelling that occurred within 20 minutes of injury may indicate bleeding that poses a greater risk for the development of a hematoma or injury to structures other than muscle and requires medical attention.

Because any muscle can be strained, the following descriptions do not identify specific muscles to be treated, as previous chapters have. Use the resources in the previous chapters as needed to determine fiber direction, joints crossed, superficial versus deep muscles, common trigger points and referral areas, and so on.

Assessment begins during your first contact with a client. In some cases, this may be on the telephone when an appointment is requested. Ask in advance if the client is seeking treatment for a specific area of pain so that you can prepare yourself.

Table 12-3 lists questions to ask the client when taking a health history.

Table 12-3	Health History

Questions for the Client	Importance for the Treatment Plan
Where do you feel symptoms?	Location of the symptoms helps to identify the precise location of stretched or torn fibers and contributing factors.
Describe what your symptoms feel like.	A description of symptoms including weakness, heat, or fullness in the area may help you to determine the stage and degree of strain. See Chapter 1 for descriptions of pain sensations and possible contributing factors.
What activity were you performing when you first felt the pain? Did you hear or feel a snap in the area at the time of injury?	The details of the activity or posture that initiated the pain may help you to determine its cause. A new regimen of exercise, weight-bearing activity, or repetitive action, particularly following a period of inactivity, may contribute to a strain.
When did the symptoms begin?	The date of the injury may help you to determine the stage of the injury and the health of the tissue.
To what degree were you able to continue activity following the injury?	The activity level after the injury may help you determine the degree of strain. An inability to continue activity suggests a third-degree strain and should be referred for medical assessment.
Do you have a history of injury or surgery to this area?	An explanation of prior injury to the area may help you to locate the strain and determine contributing factors. Surgery and resulting scar tissue may increase the risk of strain.
Do any movements make your symptoms worse or better?	Locate weakness in the structures producing such movements. Resisted activity of the affected muscle is likely to increase symptoms. Adding slack or reducing tension in the muscle may decrease symptoms.
Have you seen a health care provider for this condition? What was the diagnosis? What tests were performed?	Medical tests may reveal the degree of strain, fractures, or coinciding injuries. If no tests were performed to make a diagnosis, use the tests described in this chapter for your assessment. If your assessment is inconsistent with a diagnosis, ask the client to discuss your findings with a health care provider or ask for permission to contact the provider directly.
Are you taking any prescribed medications or herbal or other supplements?	Medication of all types may contribute to symptoms or have contraindications or cautions.
Have you had a corticosteroid or analgesic injection in the past 2 weeks? Where?	Local massage is contraindicated. A history of repeated corticosteroid injections may affect the integrity of the muscle and tendons, increasing the risk of tearing or rupture. Use caution when applying pressure or cross-fiber strokes even after the period of contraindication has passed. Analgesics reduce sensation and may cause the client to allow you to work too aggressively.
Have you taken a pain reliever or muscle relaxant within the past 4 hours?	The client may not be able to judge your pressure and may allow you to work too aggressively.
Have you taken anti-inflammatory medication within the past 4 hours?	Deep friction initiates an inflammatory process and should not be performed if the client has recently taken anti-inflammatory medication.

POSTURAL ASSESSMENT

Allow the client to walk and enter the room ahead of you while you assess his or her posture and movement. Look for imbalances in movement of the joint(s) crossed by the affected muscle or muscle group or patterns of compensation that may develop to protect the injured structures. If the lower body is affected, watch as the client walks or climbs steps. If the upper body is affected, watch as the client opens the door, takes off his or her coat or lifts a pen. If the thorax is affected, notice how the client moves the spine. Look for reduced mobility or favoring of one side. Watch as the client sits, stands from sitting, lifts or sets down objects, turns to talk to you, and so on to see if he or she can perform these activities without assistance or if he or she avoids bearing weight on the affected joint. The grade and stage of the strain will influence the level of imbalance and compensation.

When assessing the client's standing posture, be sure that the client stands comfortably. If he or she deliberately attempts to stand in the anatomic position, you may not get an accurate assessment of his or her posture in daily life. When strain affects the lower body, the client may stand in a position that keeps weight off the affected joint(s). When the upper body is affected, the client may hold the joint in a position that keeps the injured muscle from stretching. If the client has a removable device bracing the injured area, ask him or her to remove it if it is possible to bear the weight without it so that you can get an accurate picture of the strength of the injured muscles.

ROM ASSESSMENT

Test the ROM of the joint(s) crossed by the strained muscle. Only active ROM testing should be performed with a second- or third-degree strain in the acute stage to avoid further injury.

Active ROM

Compare your assessment of the client's active ROM in the affected joint(s) to the values listed for the joint's average ROM in Chapters 4–11. Pain and other symptoms may not be reproduced during active ROM assessment because the client may limit movement to a symptom-free range.

- **Active ROM of the affected joint** will be limited. Limitations are more significant with more severe grades of strain and diminish as the stage of injury progresses from acute to chronic. A first-degree strain in the acute stage may be limited by discomfort caused by stretching the affected muscle; second-degree strains may be limited by pain with concentric and eccentric contraction; third-degree strains produce severe pain and allow little or no movement of the affected joint.

Passive ROM

P ROM should not be performed in the acute stage of a second- or third-degree strain to avoid further injury. Compare the client's P ROM on one side to that on the other when applicable. Note and compare the end feel for each range (see Chapter 1 for an explanation of end feel).

- **P ROM of the affected joint** in the acute stage of a first-degree strain may be slightly limited, may cause pain due to reflexive muscle spasm, and may cause pain when ROM lengthens the affected muscle. Results may be similar in the subacute and chronic stages for all grades of strain with varying degrees of limitation and pain according to grade. Note that ROM testing following a third-degree strain that was not surgically repaired is intended to assess the synergists and antagonists of the ruptured muscle.

Resisted ROM

R ROM should not be performed in the acute stage of a second- or third-degree strain to avoid further injury. Use resisted tests to assess the strength of the muscles that cross the affected joint for a first-degree strain and in the subacute or chronic stages of second- and third-degree strains. Compare the strength of the affected side to that of the unaffected side when possible.

- **R ROM of the affected joint** in the acute stage of a first-degree strain in all stages may be slightly limited or painful. R ROM with a second- or third-degree strain in the subacute and chronic stages should be performed with a gradual increase in resistance to avoid further injury when assessing muscle strength. R ROM is limited by reduced strength and pain at the injury site. The structure being tested may tremble as the client reaches his or her limit of strength. Note that ROM testing following a third-degree strain that was not surgically repaired tests the synergists and antagonists of the ruptured muscle.

SPECIAL TESTS

Because strains can occur in any muscle, there is no single special test. Length and strength assessment of the affected muscle, its synergists, and antagonists along with locating the specific site of injury are the primary assessment strategies for strains. Use ROM testing as described above to assess strength and length. When appropriate for the grade and stage of strain, test the strength of the muscle(s) you suspect to be injured with active and resisted concentric contraction. Test the length of the muscle(s) you suspect to be injured with passive or active eccentric contractions. Refer to Chapters 4–11 for special tests of the muscles affected by the conditions covered in those chapters.

PALPATION ASSESSMENT

Bruises may be present in the acute and early subacute stages (Fig. 12-4). Avoid direct pressure on a fresh bruise. Minor bruising may occur with a first-degree strain or with the second-degree strain of a small muscle or of relatively few fibers in a larger muscle. A larger bruise may be evident with a second-degree strain to a larger muscle or more than one muscle or with a third-degree strain. As the injury heals, bruising changes colors and then disappears. In the chronic stage, the bruise is usually gone unless repeated tearing continues to occur. Edema may also be present in all stages. Avoid direct pressure on an edematous area in the acute stage. In the acute stage, when the inflammatory process is active, the area may be red and hot, and the texture of the edematous area may be dense or hard as if the area is too full and stretching the skin. When the inflammatory process diminishes, the edematous area may feel softer and less dense. In the chronic stage, the edematous area may feel boggy or gelatinous. Swelling that persists and continues to feel dense or hard may indicate a hematoma. Refer the client to his or her health care provider for medical assessment.

On palpation, the site of injury may be tender in all stages. Tenderness diminishes as the injury heals. Tenderness on palpation may radiate to the surrounding tissue, and the area of radiating

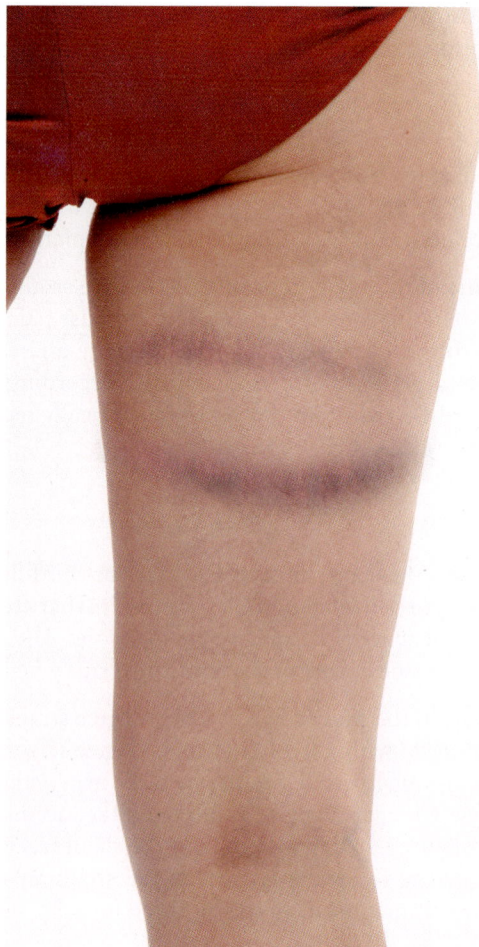

Figure 12-4 **Bruise following muscle strain.** The darkest area of bruising suggests the precise location of torn fibers.

pain also diminishes as the injury heals. You may feel a gap in the affected fibers, particularly with a second- or third-degree strain. The gap will fill in with scar tissue as the injury heals. If a third-degree strain is not surgically repaired, the gap remains and can often be seen and palpated. You may feel the remaining muscle bunched up near one of the attachment sites if it ruptured at the opposite musculotendinous junction or detached from the bone, or more rarely, at both attachment sites if the muscle belly ruptured.

As time passes, scar tissue becomes thicker, denser, and possibly fibrous. Adhesions may develop, reducing mobility between the skin and affected muscle or between the affected muscle and those surrounding it. If not properly treated, scarring, adhesions, and remaining edema may reduce local circulation, resulting in ischemia. The ischemic area may feel cool to the touch. When assessing muscle tone, you may find protective spasms in the affected muscle, its synergists, or its antagonists in the acute and early subacute stages. This protective spasm serves to keep the joint from moving through a range that may cause further injury. Do not attempt to reduce protective spasms in the early stages. As healing progresses and the risk of re-injury diminishes, the spasm may cease naturally or can be treated manually. In the late subacute and chronic stages, the affected muscle and synergists may remain hypertonic. Holding the injured muscle in a shortened position to reduce the risk of pain or re-injury is a natural impulse and may cause the antagonists to remain overstretched and stressed. Trigger points may develop in any of the muscles involved in the movement of the joint crossed by the strained muscle. If the severity of the injury prevents movement of the joint or if the injury was not treated well enough to restore ROM, you may find atrophy in the affected muscle(s) or synergists.

To effectively treat a strain, it is essential to locate the precise site of injury and to know the direction of fibers of the affected muscle. Refer to the images of specific muscles throughout this text for fiber direction. Take your time palpating the location. Once you have identified the affected muscle(s) with ROM testing, palpate them slowly, covering approximately 1 inch of tissue in 5–10 seconds. Stay focused and allow the receptors in your fingers to transmit important information. Feel for gaps, scars, or other anomalies in texture, tone, temperature, and tenderness.

Condition-Specific Massage

This section focuses on first-degree strains in all stages and second- or third-degree strains in the late subacute or chronic stage. While massage therapy may be beneficial for second-degree strains in an earlier stage, the potential contraindications and complications require more advanced training. An acute third-degree strain requires medical attention. Healing in the subacute stage of a third-degree strain is best supervised by a professional experienced in treating severe muscle strains.

The treatment goals and techniques are the same for first-degree strains in all stages and second- or third-degree strains in the subacute or chronic stage, but the intensity of treatment should be adjusted according to the severity of injury. For example, a first-degree chronic strain that has developed minor scarring and dysfunction does not present as significant a risk of re-injury during a stretch as a second-degree strain with moderate scarring or a third-degree stain with severe scarring. A third-degree strain is likely to have developed much more extensive protective muscle spasms, adhesions, and scars, and requires more warming of superficial tissues and a slower pace approaching the deeper tissues. You are more likely to be able to focus directly on the injured muscle with a first-degree strain while a second-degree strain requires more attention to the compensating and surrounding structures before addressing the torn fibers directly.

It is essential for the treatment to be relaxing. You may not be able to eliminate the symptoms associated with muscle strain or any coexisting conditions in a single treatment. Do not attempt to do so by treating aggressively. Be sure to ask your client to let you know if the amount of pressure you are applying keeps him or her from relaxing. If the client responds by tensing muscles or his or her facial expression looks distressed, reduce your pressure. Remember that you are working on tissue that is compromised. Ask the client to let you know if any part of your treatment reproduces symptoms, and always work within his or her tolerance. Deep palpation of a trigger point may cause pain at the upper end of the client's tolerance. Explain this to your client, describe a pain scale and what level of pain should not be exceeded, and ask him or her to breathe deeply during the application of the technique. As the trigger point is deactivated, the referral pain will also diminish.

The following suggestions are for treating pain, weakness, and limited ROM caused by over-stretching or tearing of muscle fibers. The following are general principles for any muscle affected by strain. Refer to Chapters 4-11 for resources pertaining to specific muscles.

■ Positioning and bolstering depends on which muscles are to be treated. In the early stages following injury, the affected muscles should rest comfortably in a position that prevents stretching. Full lengthening of the affected muscle may cause pain and increase the risk of re-injury.

■ If you find edema, apply superficial draining strokes toward the nearest lymph nodes and, when possible, bolster the area to allow gravity to draw fluid toward the thorax.

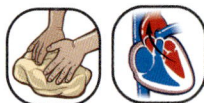

■ If swelling is minor or absent and bruises have sufficiently faded, apply moist heat to the affected area to soften scars and adhesions and increase local circulation.

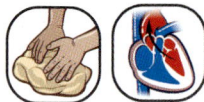

■ Use your initial warming strokes to increase superficial circulation, soften tissues, and assess the tissues broadly surrounding the site of injury or compensating for the injured muscle. If time permits, apply initial warming strokes to the whole body. You should be able to minimally assess tissues surrounding the injury for adhesions, hypertonicity, protective muscle spasm, and tensile stress, which will help you to determine how to focus your time.

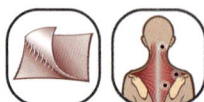

■ Based on your findings, treat muscles proximal to the site of injury for adhesions, shortening, hypertonicity, and trigger points.

■ Before applying emollient, assess for and treat fascial restrictions around the injured area. Tissues that have shortened to prevent re-injury, particularly those closest to the injury are most likely to develop fascial restrictions.

■ Reduce tension in the tissues that surround the site of injury. Pay special attention to the synergists of the muscle's primary actions. If the antagonists are accessible, treat these now, or perform this after the client changes position.

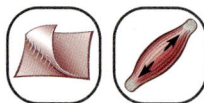

■ Once the superficial tissues are pliable enough to allow for deeper work, apply friction strokes to reduce the remaining adhesions and lengthening strokes to tissues that are short and tight. Muscles with fiber direction and actions in common with the injured muscle are likely to have shortened, possibly in spasm, to protect the injured muscle from overstretch and re-injury.

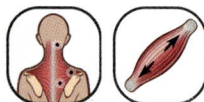

■ Treat any trigger points found in the synergists of the affected muscle or in muscles compensating for the injury. Treat trigger points in antagonists if they are accessible now, or treat them later after the client changes position. Follow trigger point treatment with lengthening strokes, but do not stretch the muscles until you have treated the precise site of injury.

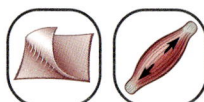

■ Locate the precise site of the strain, and assess the direction of the tear. Using short, slow strokes within the client's pain tolerance, apply cross-fiber strokes to reduce scar tissue at the site of injury. Follow this with longitudinal strokes to redirect the fibers. Alternate rounds of cross-fiber and longitudinal strokes until you feel a change in texture. If the area gets hot or begins to swell, discontinue this step, and briefly ice the area.

Treatment icons: Increase circulation; Reduce adhesions; Reduce tension; Lengthen tissue; Treat trigger points; Passive stretch; Clear area

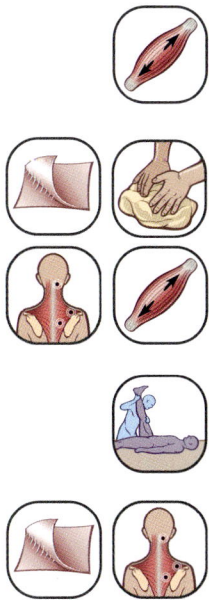

- Apply longitudinal strokes to the full length of the injured muscle.

- Treat tissues distal to the injury for compensating patterns if needed.

- Passively stretch the affected muscle or perform PIR within the client's tolerance to lengthen the affected muscle and its synergists. This may require repositioning the client.

- If you were earlier unable to address the antagonists of the injured muscle, reposition the client and address them now.

The treatment overview diagram summarizes the flow of treatment (Fig. 12-5).

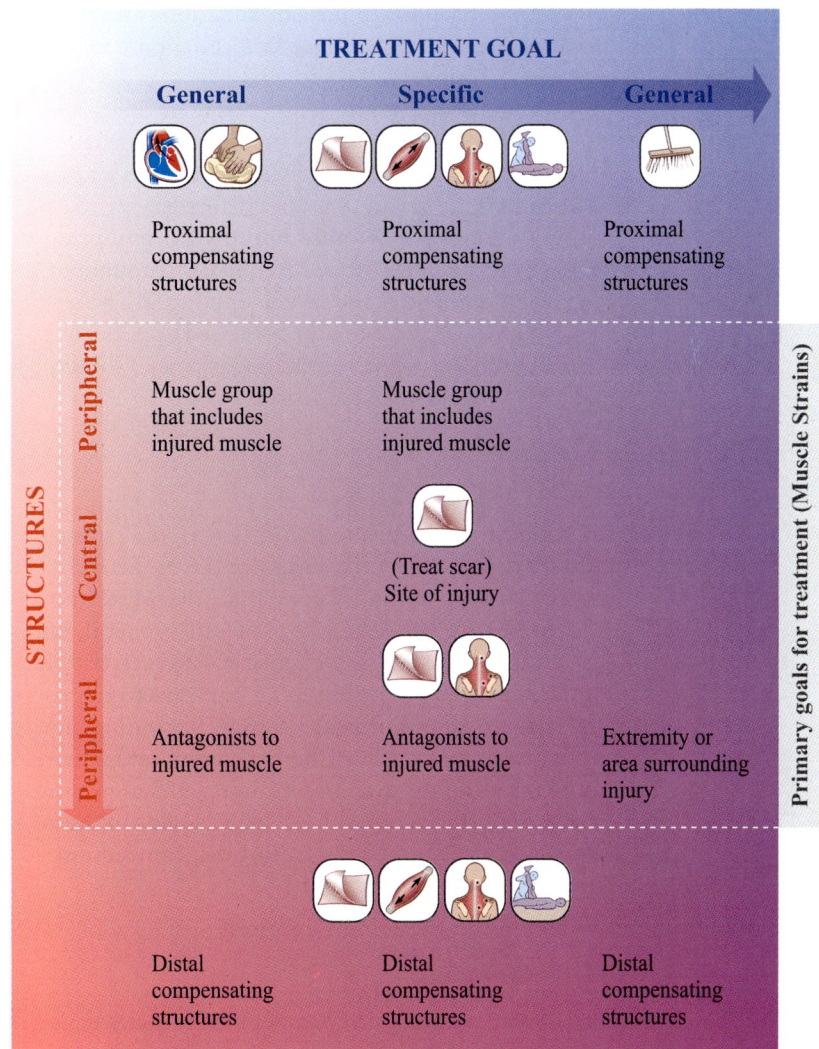

Figure 12-5 **Muscle strains overview diagram.** Follow the general principles from left to right or top to bottom when treating muscle strains.

CLIENT SELF-CARE

Avoiding re-injury is a primary concern when recommending self-care. Clients with an acute or subacute second- or third-degree strain should be prescribed self-care by a professional with advanced training and experience in treating severe musculoskeletal injuries. For clients with first-degree strains, or those in the chronic stage of a second- or third-degree strain, the following suggestions may encourage proper healing.

These suggestions are intended as general recommendations for stretching and strengthening the muscles involved in the client's condition. The objective is to create distance between the attachment sites of muscles that have shortened and to perform repetitions of movements that decrease the distance between the attachments of muscles that have weakened. If you have had no training in remedial exercises and do not feel that you have a functional understanding of stretching and strengthening, refer the client to a professional with training in this area.

Clients often neglect self-care due to time constraints. Encourage them to follow these guidelines:

- Instruct the client to perform self-care throughout the day, such as while talking on the phone, reading e-mail, washing dishes, or watching television instead of setting aside extra time.
- Encourage the client to take regular breaks from stationary postures or repetitive actions. If the client's daily activities include hours of inactivity, suggest moving for at least a few minutes every hour to prevent adhesions and reduced circulation. If the client's daily activities require repetitive actions that contribute to strains, suggest resting for at least a few minutes every hour.
- Demonstrate gentle self-massage of the tissues surrounding the injury to keep adhesions and hypertonicity at bay between treatments.
- Demonstrate all strengthening exercises and stretches to the client and have him or her perform these in your presence before leaving to ensure that he or she is performing them properly and will not cause harm when practicing alone. Stretches should be held for 15–30 seconds and performed frequently throughout the day within the client's limits. The client should not force the stretch or bounce. The stretch should be slow, gentle, and steady, trying to keep every other joint as relaxed as possible.
- Stretching and strengthening exercises should be recommended based on your findings in ROM testing and palpation.

Stretching

Maintaining proper length and tone of the strained muscle, its synergists, and its antagonists is essential to reduce the risk of re-injury. Stretches should be performed throughout the day, particularly before and after activity. ROM testing and palpation identify which muscles have shortened and need to be stretched. In general, stretching occurs when the distance between the attachment sites of the muscle is increased. Refer to Chapters 4–11 for stretches to specific muscles or groups of muscles. Take care to instruct the client to stretch slowly and to limit stretches to the comfortable range, beginning slowly and gradually increasing the stretch as symptoms diminish and the risk of re-injury is reduced. Stretching an injured muscle too quickly or too deeply may initiate a reflex response that may result in spasm. In addition, when the affected muscle is lengthened, its antagonists are shortened. If the antagonists are involved in protective splinting, contracting them too quickly or too deeply may also result in spasm.

Strengthening

Strengthening weakened or atrophied muscles is also important for restoring proper function of the affected joint. ROM testing and palpation identify which muscles have weakened and need to be strengthened. In general, active or resisted concentric contractions strengthen muscles. As with stretching, a strengthening program should progress gradually. Pain-free, active ROM is effective for gradually restoring strength to weakened muscles. As healing progresses and the risk of re-injury diminishes, add resistance to active ROM. Refer to Chapters 4–11 for exercises to strengthen specific muscles or muscle groups.

SUGGESTIONS FOR FURTHER TREATMENT

Ideally, a client with a strained muscle will have treatments twice a week until the client can perform activities of daily living with minimal or no pain for at least 4 days. Once this has been achieved, reduce frequency to once per week until symptoms are absent for at least 7 days. When the client reports that he or she has been pain-free for more than 7 days, treatment can be reduced to twice per month. If the client is pain-free for 3 or more consecutive weeks, he or she can then schedule once per month or as necessary. There should be some improvement with each session. If this is not happening, consider the following possibilities:

- There is too much time between treatments. It is always best to give the newly treated tissues 24–48 hours to adapt, but if too much time passes between treatments in the beginning, the client's activities of daily living may reverse any progress.
- The client is not adjusting activities of daily living or is not keeping up with self-care. As much as we want to fix the problem, we cannot force a client to make the adjustments we suggest. Explain the importance of his or her participation in the healing process, and encourage the client to follow your recommendations, but be careful not to judge or reprimand a client who does not.
- The condition is advanced or has other musculoskeletal complications that are beyond your basic training. Refer this client to a massage therapist with advanced training. Continuing to treat a client whose case is beyond your training could turn the client away from massage therapy altogether and hinder healing.
- The client has an undiagnosed, underlying condition. Discontinue treatment until the client sees a health care provider for medical assessment.

If you are not treating the client in a clinical setting or private practice, you may not be able to take this client through the full program of healing. Still, if you can bring some relief in just one treatment, it may encourage the client to discuss this change with a health care provider and seek manual therapy rather than more aggressive treatment options. If the client receives regular treatments, the signs and symptoms are likely to change each time, so it is important to perform an assessment before each session. Once you have released superficial tissues in general areas, you may be able to focus more of your treatment on deeper tissues in a specific area. Likewise, once you have treated the specific symptoms of the strain, you may be able to pay closer attention to compensating structures and coexisting conditions.

PROFESSIONAL GROWTH

CASE STUDY

Andy is a 32-year-old male. Two weeks ago while playing basketball, he heard and felt a snap at the back of his thigh, immediately followed by pain. He could walk using the leg but felt pain and limped. Within half an hour after injury, only minimal swelling at the site of injury was present. Within 24 hours the back of his thigh was covered with bruises. He called this office, and PRICE plus a visit to his health care provider was recommended before scheduling a massage. He iced the area immediately after returning home and intermittently for 1 week following injury. He also elevated the injured thigh and wrapped the injury. He felt the worst pain when seated due to pressure on the thigh against the chair, so he sat at the edge of the chair, which led to low back pain.

Andy's health care provider diagnosed a second-degree strain to the right semimembranosus. No MRI was performed. Diagnosis was made by palpation and the pattern of bruising and swelling, which followed the long, proximal musculotendinous junction of the semimembranosus. Andy stated that his provider agreed with the recommendation to rest, ice, and compress the area and to allow healing to start before beginning massage treatment. His first massage treatment was 1 week after the injury. At that time, Andy stated that the pain on walking had diminished somewhat but that he still felt sharp pain when the seat of a chair compressed the area of injury. He had been sitting on the edge of his seat at work to avoid contact with the injury, which he stated was causing some low back pain. He stated that he felt moderate pain when extending the knee upon lying down but noticed that if he extended the knee slowly, pain was minimal. Upon visual assessment, a spiral pattern of accumulated blood was evident, suggesting that the injury had been wrapped with a narrow ACE bandage, possibly too tightly. A solid compressive bandage without elastic edges contacting the bruised area was recommended to minimize this accumulation.

At the time of his first appointment, bruising was still too significant to work directly on the site of injury. Treatment focused on reducing compensatory low back pain and treating the uninjured leg to prevent hypertonicity and trigger points. Treatment to the injured leg focused on reducing edema at the site of injury, increasing local circulation, and reducing adhesions and hypertonicity in the synergists and antagonists. The injury is now 2 weeks old, and Andy has returned for a second treatment.

Subjective

Today, Andy states that he has been more mobile since his massage last week. He still feels some discomfort with activity but feels significant pain only at the end of the day when he is fatigued. He is still unable to fully extend the knee without pain, although the pain has decreased. Andy followed my recommendation to rest the foot of the injured leg on a box or stack of books while sitting to prevent his thigh from contacting his chair while at work, as an alternative to sitting at the edge of the chair. He has not experienced low back pain since the last session.

Objective

Andy is still limping slightly but can bear more weight on the injured leg. When standing still, Andy still bears weight on the left leg. The left hip is elevated slightly. The right hip and knee are flexed, and the right femur is slightly rotated medially. The bruise is now green and fading. Inflammation that followed the proximal musculotendinous junction of the semimembranosus is now gone, and the gap at the middle third of the proximal semimembranosus tendon has filled with scar tissue. It is still tender to the touch, but he can tolerate moderate pressure. ROM has improved, although he was unable to fully extend the knee and flex the hip due to pain.

Andy felt no tenderness on palpation of the proximal and distal ends of the hamstrings, minimal tenderness surrounding the injury, and pain upon palpation of the site of strain that radiated to the area immediately surrounding the strain. The local and radiating pain have diminished somewhat since last week. The texture of the surrounding muscles is dense and adhered.

The left gluteus maximus and the posterior fibers of the gluteus medius remain hypertonic, although they have improved since the last treatment. The hypertonicity of the right gastrocnemius has improved. Andy is able to rest the right foot flat when standing.

Action

I began in a prone position with the ankles bolstered to reduce hamstring stretch. I applied general Swedish and deep tissue strokes to the low back and glutes to assess the remaining compensatory patterns. I applied kneading, cross-fiber, and longitudinal strokes to continue reducing adhesions and hypertonicity in synergists and compensating limb. I applied slow muscle stripping to assess for trigger points. The client felt pain and referral upon crossing the site of injury. It is still unclear if this is due to a trigger point in the semitendinosus or scar tissue and referred pain from the semimembranosus strain. As healing continues and referred pain from the injury ceases, I will revisit this area to determine if compression produces trigger point referral. A trigger point in the adductor magnus referred into the pelvis, and I treated it with compression and muscle stripping, reducing the referral from level 5 pain to level 3.

I applied cross-fiber strokes to the precise site of injury. The client's pain tolerance continues to prevent deep, direct access to the semimembranosus, but I was able to mobilize tissues through the semitendinosus and by working toward the injury from its periphery. I followed this with longitudinal strokes. The area was warm to the touch following treatment. I applied ice to prevent possible swelling, but removed the ice within 2 minutes to avoid chilling the muscle before the stretches. I used general kneading and gliding strokes to the distal limb to increase circulation and reduce remaining compensatory hypertonicity. I treated the unaffected leg with general Swedish techniques to keep hypertonicity and adhesions at bay.

Turning the client supine, I applied a slow and minimal passive stretch to the hamstrings and adductors but was unable to stretch either to full ROM because of the client's discomfort. I applied kneading and longitudinal strokes to the quadriceps of the affected leg and found minimal tension in the rectus femoris. I used general Swedish techniques on the unaffected leg and clearing strokes bilaterally toward the thorax.

Plan

Because the bruising is resolving and the protective muscle splinting is no longer needed, I suggested that warm hydrotherapy to the synergists and antagonists followed by gentle stretches may be effective to maintain pliability if he feels stiffness. I recommended continuing mild, pain-free exercises including gentle flexion and extension of the hip and knee and walking to maintain circulation and prevent adhesions and shortening of the muscles. I suggested increasing activity as tolerance permits but cautioned against stretching the hamstrings quickly or fully until the scar is strong enough to withstand tension. I suggested avoiding resisted activity for at least another week. I will reassess at the next appointment. Andy rescheduled for one week from today. If symptoms continue to improve, I will attempt to access the semimembranosus directly and continue to treat the scar. If this is possible, we will increase visits to twice per week for 1 or 2 weeks while realigning the scar tissue. Goals include softening and redirecting scar tissue, continuing to reduce hypertonicity, treating trigger points if found, and continuing to gradually increase ROM and strength. I explained that second-degree strains can take 1–2 months to heal completely.

CRITICAL THINKING EXERCISES

1. Your client states that she feels pain in her left shoulder and points to the medial border and superior angle of the scapula up to the neck. Her neck is laterally flexed and rotated to the right. Which muscle(s) might be strained? Which muscle(s) may be contributing to the strain because they are stronger, shortened, or hypertonic, causing the strained muscle(s) to lengthen? Write a SOAP note for this client. Create a scenario that describes how this pattern may have developed, signs and symptoms, possible coinciding conditions, a postural assessment, testing, precautions or contraindications, and specific treatment. Use a reference book that describes the actions of the affected muscles to help you associate signs and symptoms. There is no single, correct SOAP note for this exercise. Be creative as the possibilities are virtually endless.

2. This chapter contains references to the coincidence of strains with the individual conditions described in Chapters 4–11. Choose one of the conditions described in those chapters and identify which muscles could be strained or are at risk for strain based on the client's posture or activities. Strains may occur when impaired muscles are forced to stretch beyond their capacity or to contract quickly and intensely. How would you add treatment of the strain into the treatment described for the other condition?

3. Conduct a short literature review to learn about the relationship between chronic strains and the following:
   - Age
   - Insufficient hydration
   - Lactic acid accumulation

BIBLIOGRAPHY AND SUGGESTED READINGS

Biel A. *Trail Guide to the Body: How to Locate Muscles, Bones and More*, 3rd ed. Boulder, CO: Books of Discovery, 2005.

Connolly DAJ, Sayers SP, McHugh MP. Treatment and prevention of delayed onset muscle soreness. Journal of Strength and Conditioning Research. 2003;17(1):197–208.

Farr T, Nottle C, Nosaka K, et al. The effects of therapeutic massage on delayed onset muscle soreness and muscle function following downhill walking. Journal of Science and Medicine in Sport. 2002;5(4):297–306.

Garrett WE. Muscle strain injury: Clinical and basic aspects. Medicine and Science in Sports and Exercise. 1990;22(4):436–443.

Hertling D, Kessler R. *Management of Common Musculoskeletal Disorders: Physical Therapy Principles and Methods*, 4th ed. Philadelphia, PA: Lippincott Williams & Wilkins, 2006.

Hopper D, Conneely M, Chromiak F, et al. Evaluation of the effect of two massage techniques on hamstring muscle length in competitive female hockey players. Physical Therapy in Sport. 2005;6(3):137–145.

Lowe W. *Orthopedic Massage: Theory and Technique*. St Louis, MO: Mosby-Elsevier, 2003.

Mayo Foundation for Medical Education and Research. Avulsion Fracture: How is it Treated? Available at http://www.mayoclinic.com/health/avulsion-fracture/AN00200. Accessed Spring 2009.

Mayo Foundation for Medical Education and Research. Bursitis. Available at http://www.mayoclinic.com/health/bursitis/DS00032. Accessed Spring 2009.

Mayo Foundation for Medical Education and Research. Inguinal Hernia. Available at http://www.mayoclinic.com/health/inguinal-hernia/DS00364. Accessed Spring 2009.

Mayo Foundation for Medical Education and Research. Myofascial Pain Syndrome. Available at http://www.mayoclinic.com/health/myofascial-pain-syndrome/DS01042. Accessed Spring 2009.

Mayo Foundation for Medical Education and Research. Sprains and Strains. Available at http://mayoclinic.com/health/sprains-and-strains/DS00343. Accessed Spring 2009.

Orchard J. Biomechanics of muscle strain injury. New Zealand Journal of Sports Medicine. 2002;30:92–98.

Rattray F, Ludwig L. *Clinical Massage Therapy: Understanding, Assessing and Treating over 70 Conditions*. Toronto, ON: Talus Incorporated, 2000.

Werner R. A *Massage Therapist's Guide to Pathology*, 4th ed. Philadelphia, PA: Lippincott Williams and Wilkins, 2009.

Ligament Sprains

UNDERSTANDING LIGAMENT SPRAINS

A sprain is an overstretch injury to a ligament. Ligaments are tough but flexible fibrous bands composed mainly of collagen. They function to stabilize joints, restrict excessive movement, and prevent the movement of a joint in a direction that may cause injury. Some ligaments, such as the flexor retinaculum of the wrist, also form structures like the carpal tunnel that contain tendons, nerves, and vessels that cross a joint. Ligaments vary in shape, allowing specific bundles of fibers to be recruited for a specific movement within the full ROM of the joint. They are functional only under tensile stress. During a contraction that moves a joint, the ligament that lengthens functions to keep the joint from moving out of its normal range. A ligament that is compressed during the movement of a joint has no real function.

In order to manage the complex, multidirectional forces associated with joint movement, ligaments are formed from dense regular connective tissue with fibers arranged in a slightly less parallel manner than tendon fibers (Fig. 13-1). Like tendons, the collagen fibers in ligaments are crimped to allow lengthening without causing damage (Fig. 13-2). When the tensile load increases, the collagen fibers begin to uncrimp, and the ligament lengthens. As tension increases due to additional load or when the load continues for an extended period, more fibers uncrimp, the ligament stiffens to resist the stretch, and energy is absorbed. This is referred to as creep. When this lengthening occurs slowly and the load does not exceed the ligament's ability, the ligament adapts to manage the load. On the other hand, swift and high-impact movements, as well as constant or repetitive tensile stress, reduces the ligament's ability to adapt to the load. If the tensile load exceeds the ligament's ability to resist, it can stretch to the point of failure—termed a sprain. In many cases, ligaments that are severely or repeatedly sprained never recover their full structural or functional strength; however, the joints they cross can recover full function if other structures affecting the joint are healthy.

If the tensile load that lengthens a ligament is constant or repetitive, the ligament may deform into a shape that is less effective for preventing movements that may cause injury. Likewise, if the position of a joint is repeatedly altered due to poor body mechanics or is constantly altered when tight muscles prevent the joint from maintaining an ideal posture, the ligament may deform to adapt to the postural deviation. As collagen regenerates, tension can be restored in the ligament if it is given enough time to recover. The greater the deformation, the longer it takes to recover. Constant or repetitive distortion can lead to ligament laxity, which puts the ligament at greater risk for sprain and increases the risk of injury to other structures crossing the joint.

Injury to a ligament often initiates an inflammatory response. Acute inflammation accompanies the healing process, and with rest, aids in restoring strength and proper functioning. Without sufficient rest and healing, however, inflammation can become chronic. Chronic inflammation can lead to atrophy, potentially weakening the ligament permanently. Scar tissue also forms during the healing process of a ligament injury. However, scar tissue has inferior

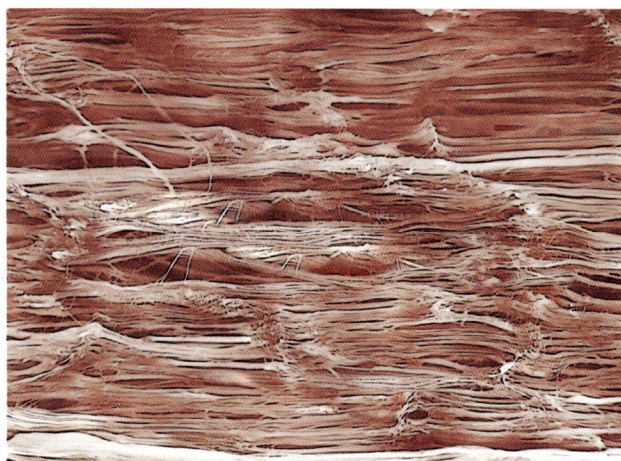

Figure 13-1 **Ligament structure.** Ligaments are made of dense collagen fibers arranged to manage multidirectional forces.

biomechanical function and stability compared to healthy ligaments. It deforms more easily under tensile stress and can bear only a fraction of the load that a healthy ligament can.

When a ligament is injured, neurological signals activate reflexive muscle activity to stabilize the joint. A reflexive contraction may develop on one side of the joint to compensate for the lost stability resulting from the ligament injury while reflexive inhibition may develop to keep opposing muscles from contracting intensely enough to pull the weakened joint out of place and further damage the ligament. For example, the radial collateral ligament of the wrist limits ulnar deviation. If it is sprained, the muscles that produce radial deviation (extensor carpi radialis longus and brevis and flexor carpi radialis) may contract while the muscles that produce ulnar deviation (extensor carpi ulnaris and flexor carpi ulnaris) may be inhibited to limit movements previously controlled by the now-injured ligament. In addition, muscles that do not cross the affected joint may also be activated or inhibited to improve stability indirectly.

Damage to a ligament also affects its mechanoreceptors and nerve endings, affecting proprioception, altering the client's perception of the normal position and function of the joint. During

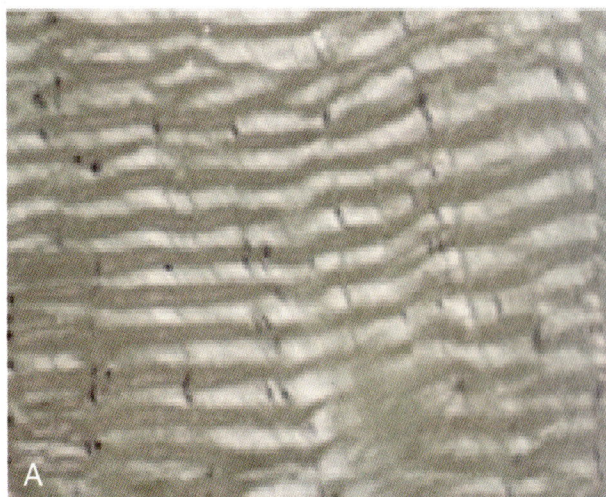

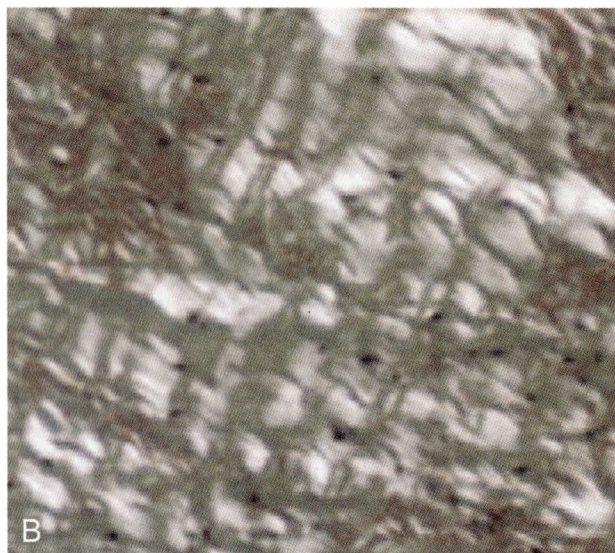

Figure 13-2 **Crimped ligament fibers. (A)** The collagen fibers in a healthy anterior cruciate ligament are crimped to allow lengthening without causing damage. **(B)** Once damaged, fibers with unhealthy crimps become more susceptible to tearing. From Murray MM. Effect of the intra-articular environment on healing of the ruptured anterior cruciate ligament. Journal of Bone & Joint Surgery. 2000;82-A:1390. Available at http://www.jbjs.org/Comments/c_p_murray.shtml.

the healing process, this compensation is essential to minimize the risk of re-injury. Once scar tissue has formed, collagen is regenerated, and the relative strength of the ligament is restored, rehabilitation must include restoring the normal resting tone of the muscles crossing the joint as well as normalizing proprioception.

Common Signs and Symptoms

Sprains can occur in any joint but occur most often in the ankles, knees, wrists, and fingers (Fig. 13-3). Overstretching may result in injury ranging from minor tears to a complete rupture of the ligament. Signs and symptoms differ depending on the grade (severity of the injury) and stage (duration of symptoms) of the sprain. In general, sprains produce local pain, stiffness, pain on passive stretch, and impaired ROM. Bruises and inflammation may be present in the acute and early subacute stages (Fig. 13-4). Table 13-1 outlines the common signs and symptoms for each grade and stage of ligament sprain.

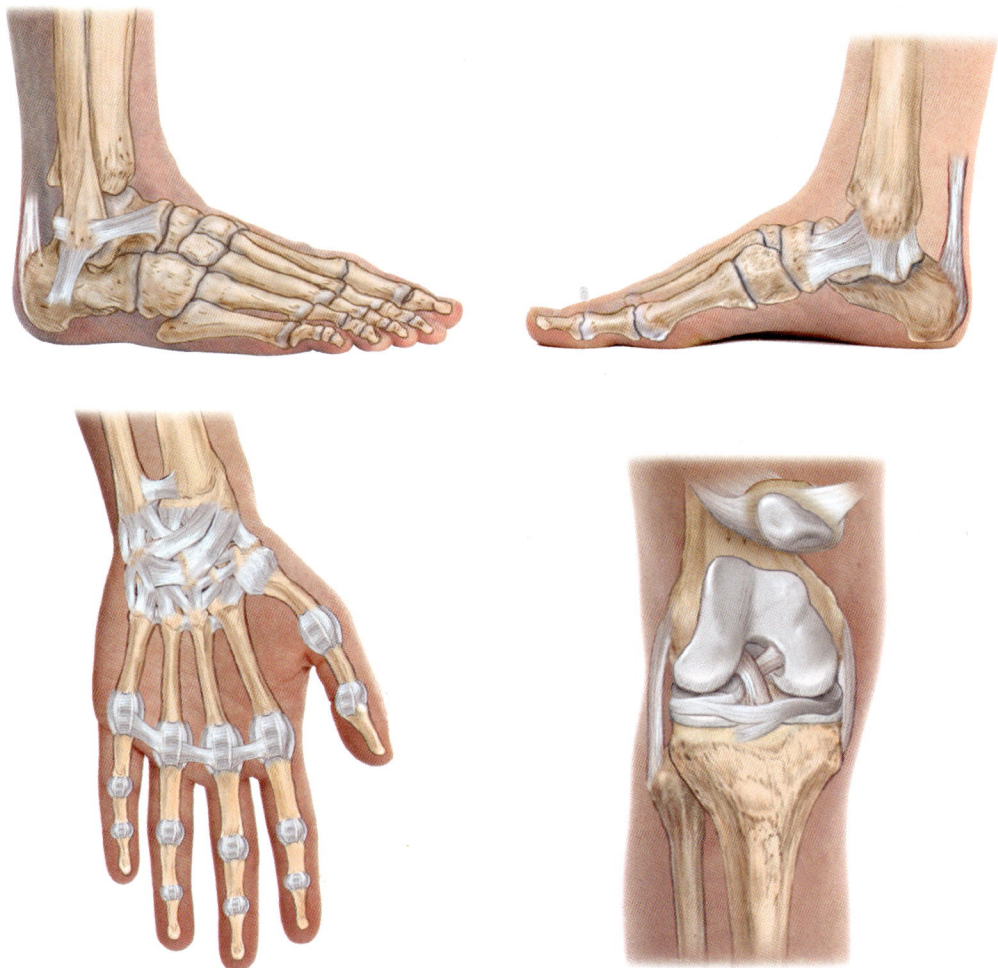

Figure 13-3 **Ligaments that cross the joints most commonly injured.** It is essential to know the fiber direction of each of the ligaments that cross an injured joint in order to properly assess and treat the sprained ligament(s). Adapted from Clay JH, Pounds DM. *Basic Clinical Massage Therapy: Integrating Anatomy and Treatment,* 2nd ed. Philadelphia: Lippincott Williams & Wilkins, 2008.

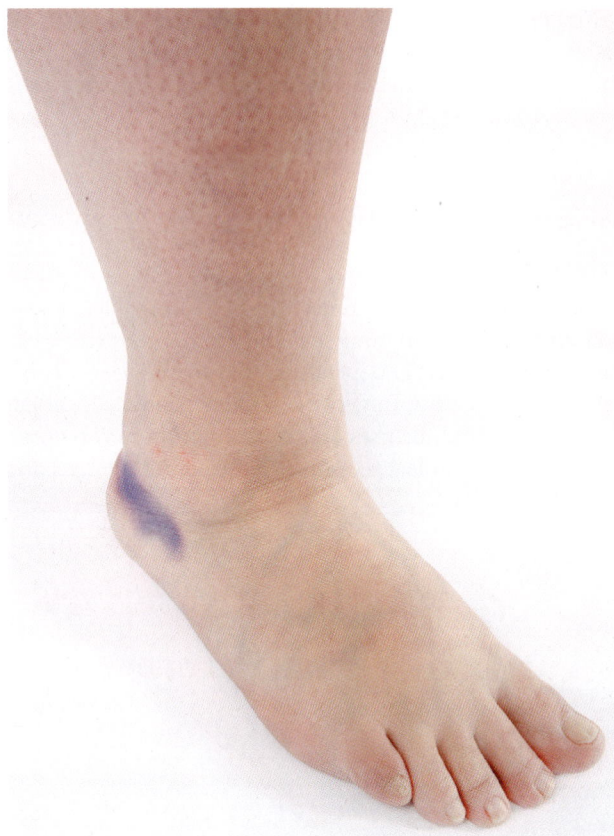

Figure 13-4 Acute ankle sprain.
Common signs of an acute sprain include inflammation and bruising.

Possible Causes and Contributing Factors

The most common cause of sprain is a swift, high-impact movement that stretches the ligament beyond its capacity. This often occurs in sports and other high-impact activities but may also occur when factors including systemic disorders, deconditioning, or repetitive actions weaken the ligament and destabilize the joint; in this situation, the ligament may sprain during common activities of daily living. Beginning a new activity following a period of inactivity without gradual reconditioning increases the risk of sprain. Similarly, sufficient warm-up prior to vigorous activity increases ROM and may help prevent sprain. Poor technique during new, intense, or repetitive activities increases the risk of sprain. Structures that are fatigued due to prolonged activity, improper warm-up, or poor technique may not be able to support the joint properly, thus, increasing the risk of sprain.

Once a sprain occurs, failing to allow sufficient time for healing in the early stages can slow or halt the natural healing process. When overstretching or small tears in the ligament results in scar tissue that is not strong enough to resist further tearing, the inflammatory process will continue, compromising the structure's integrity, and the risk of repeated injury increases. Similarly, continuing activity that encourages the inflammatory process may weaken the structure and cause compensating patterns to become habitual. Continuing aggravating activities once degeneration has begun may inhibit regeneration of collagen and continue to weaken the ligament.

However, immobility can also cause the ligament to degenerate and weaken, increasing the risk of injury with activity. Reduced loading can lead to rapid tissue degeneration. Sensible activity followed by rest strengthens the ligament, aids in collagen regeneration, and over time increases stability during more taxing activities. For this reason, it is important to ease into new activities after periods of inactivity to prevent injury and to ease into moderate activity as soon as possible following an injury to aid healing. While some rest or at least limiting of the aggravating activity is necessary to allow healing to begin, movement also keeps adhesions at bay and reduces ischemia.

Table 13-1	**Grades and Stages of Ligament Sprains**		
	Grade		
Stage	**Grade 1 or First Degree**	**Grade 2 or Second Degree**	**Grade 3 or Third Degree**
	Mild sprain	Moderate sprain	Severe sprain
	Minor stretch or tear	Tearing of several to most fibers	Complete rupture of ligament or separation of ligament from bone
Acute (symptoms typically last 2-3 days following injury)	Joint remains stable	Joint becomes slightly unstable	Joint is unstable
	Mild, localized discomfort with activity and at rest	Snapping sound or feeling when injured	Snapping sound or feeling when injured
	Minimal or no local edema	Moderate local edema	Severe pain at time of injury
	Minimal or no bruising	Moderate bruising	Difficulty or inability to continue activity
		Moderate local tenderness	ROM is impaired
		Moderate pain with activity and at rest	Considerable local edema
		Moderate decrease in ROM	Considerable red or purple bruising
		Possible strain to muscles crossing the injured joint	Possible hematoma, particularly if joint capsule is injured
		Possible protective muscle spasm crossing affected joint(s)	Possible strain to muscles crossing the injured joint
			Possible protective spasm in muscles crossing affected joint(s)
Subacute (symptoms typically remain from 2-4 weeks following the acute stage)	Joint is stable	Joint is stable but may be hypermobile in the direction normally restricted by the injured ligament	Joint remains unstable and hypermobile in the direction normally restricted by the injured ligament
	Minimal to no pain	Pain improved since acute stage	Pain may have improved since the acute stage
	Scar developing at site of injury if tearing occurred	Bruising remains and may be changing color to yellow or green	Bruising remains and may be changing color to yellow or green
	Adhesions developing at and around site of injury	Scar developing at site of injury	Adhesions developing at and around the site of injury
	Reduced ROM	Reduced ROM	Significant scarring if ligament was surgically repaired
	Possible trigger points in muscles crossing the affected joint	Adhesions developing at and around the site of injury	Reduced ROM
		Protective muscle spasm may diminish and may be replaced by hypertonicity	Protective muscle spasm may continue or may diminish and may be replaced by hypertonicity
		Possible trigger points in muscles crossing affected joint	Possible trigger points in muscles crossing the affected joint
		Impaired proprioception at the joint	Impaired proprioception at the joint

(continued)

Table 13-1	Grades and Stages of Ligament Sprains (Continued)

	Grade		
Stage	**Grade 1 or First Degree**	**Grade 2 or Second Degree**	**Grade 3 or Third Degree**
Chronic (symptoms continue beyond the subacute stage)	Joint is stable	Joint is stable	Joint may remain unstable if the ligament was not surgically repaired
	Trigger points, scars, adhesions, and hypertonicity may still be present in compensating structures and surrounding tissues	Bruising has cleared	Bruising has cleared
		Trigger points, scars, adhesions, and hypertonicity affect compensating structures and surrounding tissues	Atrophy may result if a joint has been immobilized
	Discomfort when affected ligament is stretched	Discomfort or pain when affected ligament is stretched	Trigger points, scars, adhesions, and hypertonicity affect compensating structures and surrounding tissues
	Increased risk of re-injury if not properly treated	Reduced ROM in affected joint	Reduced ROM in affected joint
	Chronic edema if not properly treated	Increased risk of re-injury if not properly treated	Increased risk of overuse injury to compensating structures if affected ligament was not surgically repaired
	Loss of proprioception at joint if not properly treated	Chronic edema if not properly treated	Chronic edema if not properly treated
		Possible atrophy if not properly treated	Loss of proprioception at joint if not properly treated
		Loss of proprioception at joint if not properly treated	

Insufficient rehabilitation following a sprain, as well as repeated sprain to the same ligament, reduces tension in the ligament and often leaves a joint unstable. Joint instability significantly increases the risk of injury. As the body ages, regeneration of collagen and elastin fibers slows. Once this occurs, ligaments are at greater risk for sprain, and it becomes increasingly less likely that full function of an injured ligament will be restored. Maintaining strong, healthy muscles increases joint stability and may reduce the risk of injury.

Being overweight as a result of pregnancy or weight gain increases demand on the musculoskeletal system during all activities and may increase the risk of spraining a ligament, particularly in weight-bearing joints. During pregnancy, women also produce higher levels of the hormone relaxin, which softens collagen and loosens the ligaments to allow the uterus and surrounding structures to adapt to the growing fetus and prepare for childbirth. This can cause systemic ligament laxity, increasing the risk for sprain. Similarly, fluctuations of estrogen and progesterone during the menstrual cycle may also affect the integrity of ligaments. Ligament laxity can also be a genetic condition, often associated with Marfan Syndrome, Stickler's Syndrome, and Ehlers-Danlos Syndrome. With these conditions, other organs and connective tissues may be affected. Consult your pathology book for contraindications and special considerations for clients with these conditions. Rheumatoid arthritis and osteoarthritis may also predispose a client to ligament injuries.

Sprains have fairly distinct signs and symptoms but can be confused with other conditions or may contribute to pain associated with another condition. For example, pain and swelling with minimally reduced ROM may result from a grade 1 sprain but can also be a symptom of tendinosis. Sprains can be confused with or can contribute to many of the conditions common to specific joints, such as carpal tunnel syndrome and patellofemoral syndrome. Neck pain, back pain, and low back pain can involve sprains to the ligaments that stabilize the vertebrae, which should be considered in treatment. A swift, high-impact movement that causes a sprain may also fracture a bone. If you suspect a fractured bone, refer the client for medical assessment before initiating treatment.

Table 13-2	Differentiating Conditions Commonly Confused with or Contributing to Ligament Sprains		
Condition	**Typical Signs and Symptoms**	**Testing**	**Massage Therapy**
Muscle strain	Swelling, bruising, and local pain Reduced ROM Pain on active contraction or stretching of the affected muscle Weakness	Often self-assessed Physical exam	Massage is indicated. See Chapter 12.
Tendinopathy	Often has gradual onset Pain, tenderness, and swelling at affected tendon	Physical exam Localized pain on full passive stretch X-ray may be performed to rule out other conditions	Massage is indicated. See Chapter 14.
Avulsion fracture	Bone fragments at the attachment site of a tendon or ligament often accompany strains and sprains Moderate local pain Bruising and inflammation	X-ray	Local massage is contraindicated in the acute stage. Caution is used when treating surrounding tissues to avoid further injury. Massage may help to prevent further injury when muscle tension is a contributing factor.
Bursitis	Pain, particularly with activity or palpation Heat, redness, swelling, or tenderness local to the affected bursa	Physical exam ROM tests X-ray or MRI if conservative treatment is not successful	Massage is systemically contraindicated if bursitis is due to infection. Massage is locally contraindicated in the acute stage to avoid increased swelling. In the subacute stage, massage to the structures surrounding the joint is indicated.

It is important to understand the client's health history, precipitating events, and other possible causes of pain in the area before proceeding with treatment. Table 13-2 lists some general conditions commonly confused with or contributing to sprains. Consult your pathology book for more detailed information. If you are unsure and the client's symptoms resemble those of a more serious condition, particularly if the client has other risk factors, refer him or her to a health care provider for medical assessment.

Contraindications and Special Considerations

First, it is essential to understand the cause of pain. If the client is unable to move the joint, heard a popping sound, or has significant weakness, or if you suspect the client has a fractured bone or experienced significant tearing to the tissues, work with the client's health care provider, and consult a pathology text for massage therapists before proceeding. These are a few general cautions:

- **Hemarthrosis.** Significant swelling that occurs within the first 20 minutes of injury to a joint may indicate hemarthrosis—bleeding in the joint capsule (Fig. 13-5). Other signs may include burning or tingling in the joint and a feeling of fullness that may prevent movement

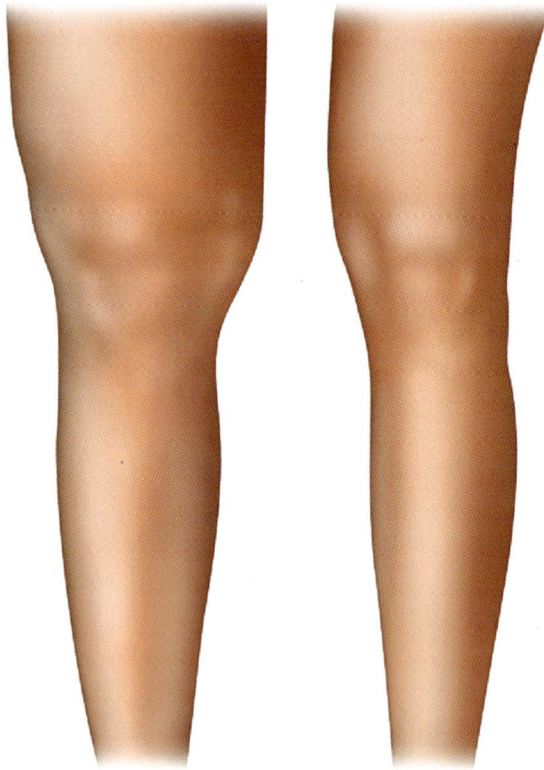

Figure 13-5 **Acute hemarthrosis.** Rapid, significant swelling following an injury may indicate hemarthrosis.

of the joint. The client should be referred to a medical professional for assessment and possible aspiration of the joint.

- **Bruises.** A bruise indicates damage to capillaries allowing blood to accumulate in surrounding tissue. Avoid direct pressure on a bruise that is still healing. As the capillaries heal and blood is resorbed, the color changes from red or purple to green or yellow. In some cases, severe bruising may result in a hematoma—a localized pooling of blood outside the vessels. In some cases, a sac-like enclosure forms around the pool of blood to minimize internal bleeding. A hematoma often resolves on its own, similarly to a simple bruise, but if it grows or hardens, it may require medical attention. Avoid direct pressure to a hematoma, and refer the client to a health care professional if the area becomes hard, if the client reports feeling pressure from the hematoma, or if it does not show signs of resolving over the course of a week or two.

- **Muscle testing.** Use only active ROM testing in the acute stage of a grade 2 or 3 sprain. The client usually limits active movements to the pain-free range. P ROM and R ROM testing may cause further injury.

- **Protective muscle splinting.** When a ligament is injured, the muscles that cross the affected joint may spasm reflexively in an attempt to limit the joint's movement to prevent further injury. Do not reduce protective muscle splinting in the acute stage of injury. Wait until the late subacute or chronic stage, when sufficient scarring and fiber regeneration reduce the need for protective splinting.

- **Re-injury.** Avoid ROM and traction techniques that stretch the injured ligament until the integrity of the structure is restored.

- **Treatment duration and pressure.** If the client is elderly, has degenerative disease, or has been diagnosed with a condition that diminishes activities of daily living, you may need to adjust your pressure as well as the treatment duration. Frequent half-hour sessions may suit the client better.

- **Friction.** Do not use deep frictions if the health of the underlying tissues is at risk for rupture. Allow time for scarring and fiber regeneration to avoid re-injury. Do not use friction if the client is taking anti-inflammatory medication or anticoagulants. Friction creates an inflammatory process, which may interfere with the intended action of anti-inflammatory medication. Recommend that the client refrain from taking such medication for several hours prior to treatment if the health care provider is in agreement. Because anticoagulants reduce clotting, it is best to avoid techniques that may cause tearing and bleeding.

Massage Therapy Research

Several reports on the use of massage in the treatment of sprains were written in the late nineteenth and early twentieth century. While we have learned much more about the structure and function of ligaments since then, as well as about the benefits of massage, few studies investigating the specific effects of massage therapy on the healing of sprains have been conducted more recently. Several studies do report significant improvement of sprains treated with a combination of therapies including ultrasound, acupuncture, chiropractic manipulation, and massage techniques such as transverse friction. Because it is impossible to distinguish the specific value of massage techniques when combined therapies are used, these studies are not cited here.

In "A Theoretical Model for Treatment of Soft Tissue Injuries: Treatment of an Ankle Sprain in a College Tennis Player," Gemmell et al. (2005) present a case study exemplifying the potential benefits of manual therapy for the healing of sprains. The subject was a 21-year-old male tennis player with ankle pain for 6 weeks following an inversion sprain. Although the subject was able to walk pain-free after 6 weeks of cryotherapy, electrotherapy, and anti-inflammatory medication prescribed by the team physician, he was unable to perform activities such as running or jumping and could not return to tennis, reporting a pain level of 8 out of 10. When asked to indicate the area of pain, he pointed to the anterior aspect of the ankle and the lateral, distal lower leg. At the time of his initial visit with the study's authors, 6 weeks after the injury, the subject presented with mild swelling, no bruising or crepitus, limited dorsiflexion, and tenderness on palpation of the anterior talofibular and tibiofibular ligaments. The study's authors diagnosed a mild sprain with dysfunction of the anterior ankle ligaments and myofascial distortions in the peroneal muscles. Manual therapy consisted of firm stroking of the peroneal attachment sites and muscle stripping to the peroneal muscles to repair myofascial distortions. The subject played tennis for 2 days following treatment and returned with mild discomfort when jumping. The peroneals were treated once more, and 1 week later, the subject returned to competitive tennis. Nine months after treatment, the client reported no pain or dysfunction of the ankle.

WORKING WITH THE CLIENT

Client Assessment

While swift, high-impact movements often cause obvious, and often self-diagnosed, sprains, less obvious sprains can result from poor body mechanics and repetitive actions. For example, improper lifting, twisting, and obesity can affect the spinal ligaments and those that connect the spine to the pelvis and may contribute to low back pain. Consistently standing with the weight on one leg forces changes in the alignment of the leg, pelvis, and spine, increasing the risk of spraining ligaments that cross those joints. Assessing sprains with less obvious signs may require advanced training, although some clues may be present. Pain upon palpation along the length of a ligament or its attachment sites that is greater than tenderness in muscles around it may suggest a sprain. Localized pockets of inflammation may also suggest a sprain. In addition, unexplained spasm of muscles that cross a joint may be a protective mechanism for a sprained ligament. The good news is that with these sorts of sprains, reducing muscle spasm and hypertonicity, releasing fascial restrictions and adhesions, and adjusting body mechanics can greatly encourage the ligament's natural healing process.

With readily recognizable sprains, assessment and treatment of the surrounding soft tissues is essential. When mild, grade 1 sprains contribute to the symptoms of another condition, the following treatment recommendations are meant to aid healing and reduce the risk of re-injury. Reducing adhesions and scar tissue, reorienting ligament fibers, lengthening shortened muscles, and strengthening weak muscles are the basic goals of treating sprains.

More serious grade 2 and 3 sprains require more focused attention. If you do not have the advanced training necessary to treat a complicated case or if symptoms in the subacute stage continue to significantly reduce activities of daily living, the client should be assessed by a health care provider and cleared for massage therapy prior to treatment. Swelling and bruising in the acute stage of a grade 2 sprain can be significant enough to contraindicate local treatment. Significant swelling that occurred within 20 minutes of the injury may indicate bleeding that poses a greater risk for hemarthrosis, hematoma, or injury to structures other than a ligament; this requires medical attention. An acute, grade 3 sprain requires medical attention. If surgical repair poses more risk than benefit, the ligament may be left severed, although in most cases the ligament is surgically repaired, and the client is prescribed physical therapy. Regardless of whether the ligament has been surgically repaired, you are most likely to see a client in subacute or chronic stage of a grade 3 sprain as part of a program to reduce pain, limitations in ROM, or compensating patterns that may have developed.

Because sprain can occur in any ligament, the following descriptions do not specify structures as in previous chapters. Refer to the previous chapters as needed to determine fiber direction, joints crossed, superficial versus deep structures, and so on.

Assessment begins during your first contact with a client. In some cases, this may be on the telephone when an appointment is requested. Ask in advance if the client is seeking treatment for specific area of pain so that you can prepare yourself.

Table 13-3 lists questions to ask the client when taking a health history.

POSTURAL ASSESSMENT

Allow the client to enter the room ahead of you while you assess his or her posture and movement. Look for imbalances in movement of the joint crossed by the affected ligament or patterns of compensation that may develop to protect the injured structures. If the lower body is affected, watch as the client walks or climbs steps. If the upper body is affected, watch as the client opens the door, takes off his or her coat or lifts a pen. If the thorax is affected, notice how the client moves the spine. Look for reduced mobility or a favoring of one side. Watch as the client sits, stands from sitting, lifts or sets down objects, turns to talk to you, and so on to see if he or she performs these activities without assistance or if he or she avoids bearing weight with the affected joint. The grade and stage of the sprain influence the level of imbalance and compensation.

When assessing standing posture, be sure that the client stands comfortably. If he or she deliberately attempts to stand in the anatomic position, you may not get an accurate assessment of his or her posture in daily life. When sprain affects the lower body, the client may stand in a position that keeps weight off the affected joint. When the upper body is affected, the client may hold the joint in a position that keeps the injured ligament from stretching. If the client has braced the injury with a removable device, ask him or her to remove it if it is possible to bear the weight without it so that you can get an accurate picture of the strength of the injured joint.

ROM ASSESSMENT

Test the ROM of the joint crossed by the sprained ligament. Only active ROM testing should be performed with a grade 2 or 3 sprain in the acute and early subacute stages to avoid further injury. In the chronic stage, the client may have developed compensating patterns, causing pain in other joints that should also be tested. Advanced training that includes more detailed instruction and precautions for ROM testing in the acute and early subacute stages is necessary.

Table 13-3	Health History

Questions for the Client	Importance for the Treatment Plan
Where do you feel symptoms?	The location of symptoms helps to identify the precise location of stretched or torn fibers and contributing factors.
Describe what your symptoms feel like.	A description of symptoms including weakness, heat, or fullness in the area may help you to determine the stage and degree of sprain and whether there may be more significant damage. See Chapter 1 for descriptions of pain sensations and possible contributing factors.
When did the symptoms begin?	The date of injury may help you to determine the stage of the injury and the health of the tissue.
What were you doing when you first felt the pain? Did you hear a snap or feel a twinge in the area at the time of injury?	In the absence of a clear incident of swift, forceful stretching of a ligament, the details of the activity or posture that initiated the pain may help you to determine its cause.
To what degree were you able to continue activity following the injury?	The level of activity following injury may help you to determine the degree of the sprain. Inability to continue activity suggests a grade 3 sprain and should be referred for medical assessment.
Did significant swelling occur within the first 20 minutes of injury?	Rapid swelling at the time of injury may indicate hemarthrosis or hematoma. The client should be referred for medical assessment.
Do you have a history of injury or surgery to this area?	An explanation of a prior injury to the area may help you to locate the sprain and determine contributing factors. Surgery and resulting scar tissue may increase the risk of sprain.
Do any movements make your symptoms worse or better?	Locate weakness in structures producing such movements. Lengthening of the affected ligament is likely to increase symptoms. Adding slack or reducing tension in the ligament may decrease symptoms.
Have you seen a health care provider for this condition? What was the diagnosis? What tests were performed?	Medical tests may reveal the degree of sprain, fractures, or coexisting injuries. If no tests were performed to make a diagnosis, use the tests described in this chapter for your assessment. If your assessment is inconsistent with a diagnosis, ask the client to discuss your findings with a health care provider or ask for permission to contact the provider directly.
Are you taking any prescribed or over-the-counter medications or herbal or other supplements?	Medication of all types may contribute to symptoms or involve contraindications or cautions.
Have you had a corticosteroid or analgesic injection in the past 2 weeks? Where?	Local massage is contraindicated. A history of repeated corticosteroid injections may affect the integrity of soft tissues increasing the risk of tearing or rupture. Use caution when applying pressure or cross-fiber strokes. Analgesics reduce sensation and may cause the client to allow you to work too aggressively.
Have you taken a pain reliever or muscle relaxant within the past 4 hours?	The client may not be able to judge your pressure and may allow you to work too aggressively.
Have you taken anti-inflammatory medication within the past 4 hours?	Deep friction initiates an inflammatory process and should not be performed if the client has recently taken anti-inflammatory medication.

Active ROM

Compare your assessment of the client's active ROM in the affected joints to the values listed in the Average ROM boxes in Chapters 4-11. Pain and other symptoms may not be reproduced during active ROM assessment because the client may limit movement to a symptom-free range. Protective muscle spasm may reduce ROM in the direction that would stretch the ligament.

■ **Active ROM of the affected joint** will be limited, particularly in the direction that stretches the injured ligament. Limitations are more significant with more severe grades of sprain and diminish as the stages of injury progress from acute to chronic. A grade 1 or 2 sprain in the acute stage may be limited by discomfort upon stretching of the affected ligament; grade 3 sprains produce severe pain and little to no movement of the affected joint(s), due in part to swelling and protective muscle spasm.

Passive ROM

P ROM should not be performed in the acute or early subacute stages of a grade 2 or 3 sprain to avoid further injury. In the late subacute or chronic stage, perform P ROM slowly to pinpoint which ligament is injured. Note and compare the end feel for each range (see Chapter 1 for an explanation of end feel). Compare the client's P ROM on one side to the other when applicable.

■ **P ROM of the affected joint** in the acute stage of a grade 1 sprain may be slightly limited and may cause pain when movement lengthens the affected ligament. Results may be similar in the subacute and chronic stages for all grades of sprain with varying degrees of limitation and pain depending on the stage of healing. ROM testing following a grade 3 sprain that was not surgically repaired is intended to assess whether the muscles crossing the joint are strong enough to stabilize it and whether persistent muscle spasm restricts mobility.

Resisted ROM

R ROM should not be performed in the acute or early subacute stages of a grade 2 or 3 sprain to avoid further injury. Use resisted tests to determine if muscles crossing the affected joint were also strained and to assess the strength of the muscles that cross the affected joint for a grade 1 sprain, and in the late subacute or chronic stages of grade 2 or 3 sprains. Compare the strength of the affected side to the unaffected side when possible.

■ **R ROM of the affected joint(s)** with a grade 1 sprain in all stages and with a grade 2 or 3 sprain in the subacute and chronic stages may be limited because of pain if the muscles were also injured. R ROM should be applied with a gradual increase in resistance to avoid further injury while assessing muscle strength. ROM is limited by reduced strength and pain at the site(s) of injury to the muscle. If protective muscle spasm persists into the subacute and chronic stages of sprain, ROM may be limited because of pain on contraction of the muscle(s) in spasm or of their weakened antagonists.

SPECIAL TESTS

A swift, high-impact movement causing a ligament sprain may also injure the muscles crossing the affected joint. In the subacute and chronic stage of the sprain, use ROM testing to assess the strength and length of muscles that may have been strained. In addition, protective muscle spasm may occur to help stabilize the injured joint. Once protective muscle spasm is no longer necessary, treating muscles that cross the injured joint and those that compensate for joint instability is essential for recovery. Refer to Chapter 12 for a more detailed description of testing and treating muscle strains and to Chapter 1 for a more detailed description of end feel.

A ligamentous stress test is used in the late subacute and chronic stages of sprains to determine which ligament crossing the injured joint is sprained and the grade of the sprain. Because the ligamentous stress test involves applying overpressure at the end of the ROM that stretches the ligament, it is not used in the acute stage to avoid further injury before natural healing has begun to strengthen the affected structures.

Ligamentous stress test (Fig. 13-6):

1. Passively move the joint in the direction that stretches the ligament. To determine which ligament(s) is sprained, it is necessary to know the attachment sites of each ligament crossing the joint in order to move the joint in the precise direction that stretches each ligament.

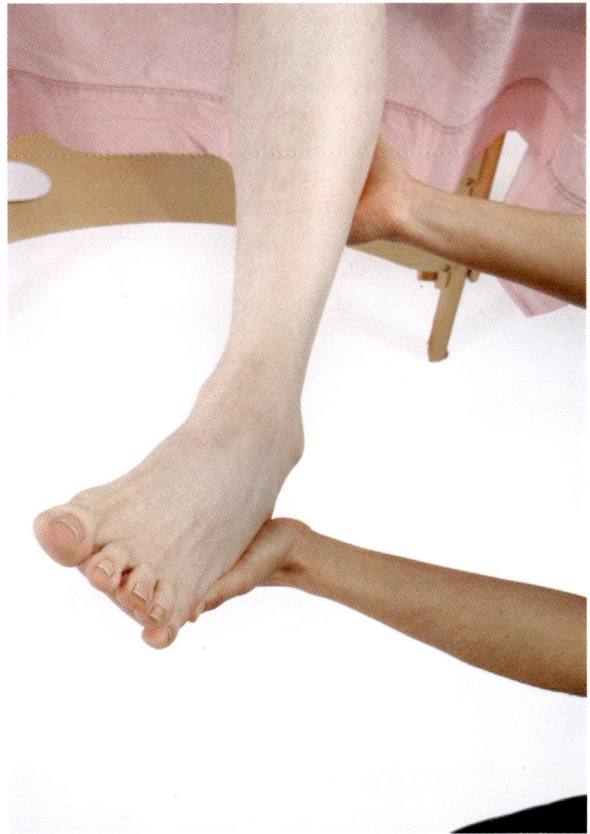

Figure 13-6 **Ligamentous stress test.**
Determine which ligament crossing an injured joint may be sprained.

2. In the late subacute or chronic stage of sprain, carefully apply slight overpressure at the end of the ROM to minimally stress the ligament without causing further injury or undue pain.

3. A grade 1 sprain will produce local pain specific to the injured ligament with overpressure. There is a soft capsular end feel with no joint laxity. A grade 2 sprain will produce significant local pain specific to the injured ligament with overpressure. There is a loose ligamentous end feel with possible joint laxity. Because a grade 3 sprain is the complete rupture of a ligament, ROM will not stretch the injured ligament, and any pain produced with overpressure is not specific to the injured ligament. Pain produced with ROM of a known grade 3 sprain may indicate a lesser grade sprain to another ligament, a muscle strain, or a tendinopathy, or it may occur if the client contracts opposing muscles to prevent further ROM. The end feel is empty with joint laxity.

PALPATION ASSESSMENT

Avoid direct pressure on a fresh bruise or an edematous area in the acute stage. In the acute stage, when the inflammatory process is active, the area may be red and hot, and the texture of the edematous area may be dense or hard as if the area is too full and stretching the skin. When the inflammatory process diminishes, the edematous area may feel softer and less dense. In the chronic stage, the edematous area may feel boggy or gelatinous, and the area may feel cool due to ischemia. Swelling that persists and continues to feel dense or hard beyond the acute stage may indicate a hematoma. Refer the client to a health care provider for medical assessment.

The site of injury may be tender to the touch in all stages, although the amount of pressure needed to elicit a response differs according to the grade of sprain and increases as the injury progresses into later stages. Tenderness diminishes as the injury heals. Although most ligaments are very deep, you may be able to feel a gap in the affected fibers, particularly with a grade 2 or 3 sprain. The gap will fill in as scar tissue forms and collagen regenerates. If a grade 3 sprain was not surgically repaired, the gap will remain. As time passes, scar tissue that forms to stabilize the affected structures will become thicker, denser, and possibly fibrous. Adhesions may develop, reducing mobility between the ligament and surrounding tissues. If not properly treated, scarring, adhesions, and remaining edema may reduce local circulation, resulting in ischemia, which may feel cool to the touch. When assessing muscle tone, you may find protective spasms in the muscles crossing the affected joint in the acute and early subacute stages. This protective spasm occurs to keep the joint from moving to a point that may cause further injury. Do not reduce protective spasms in the early stages. As healing progresses, the spasm may cease naturally, but the muscles may remain hypertonic. Trigger points may develop in any of the compensating soft tissues. If the severity of the injury prevents movement of the joint or if the injury was not treated well enough to restore ROM, you may find atrophy in the affected muscles.

To effectively treat a sprain, you must locate the precise site of injury and know the direction of the fibers of the affected ligament. Take your time palpating the location. Once you have identified the affected ligament(s) with ROM testing, palpate them slowly, covering approximately 1 inch of tissue over 5-10 seconds. Stay focused, and allow the receptors in your fingers to transmit important information. Feel for gaps, scars, or other anomalies in texture, tone, temperature, and tenderness.

Condition-Specific Massage

The remainder of this chapter focuses on grade 1 sprains in all stages and grade 2 and 3 sprains in the late subacute and chronic stages. While massage therapy may be beneficial for grade 2 sprains in earlier stages, because of the potential for contraindications and complications, advanced training is needed. An acute grade 3 sprain requires medical attention. In the later stages of healing following a grade 3 sprain that was not surgically repaired, focus on releasing restrictive adhesions, hypertonicity, and trigger points to compensating structures, and restoring ROM and strength in the affected joint(s). If the ligament was surgically repaired and is accessible, releasing restrictive adhesions and realigning scar tissue are an integral part of restoring ROM and strength. For sprains to ligaments that are inaccessible manually, such as the cruciate ligaments of the knee, focus on the surrounding structures with the goal of restoring ROM, strength, and stability.

The treatment goals and techniques are the same for grade 1 sprains in all stages and grade 2 or 3 sprains in the late subacute and chronic stages, but the intensity of treatment should be adjusted according to the severity of injury. For example, a grade 1 chronic sprain resulting in minor scarring and dysfunction does not present as significant a risk of re-injury during a stretch as a grade 2 sprain with moderate scarring or a surgically repaired grade 3 sprain with severe scarring. A grade 3 sprain is likely to have developed much more extensive protective muscle spasms and adhesions than lower grade sprains, and it will require more warming of superficial tissues and a slower pace when approaching the deeper tissues than lower grade sprains require. You are more likely to be able to focus directly on the injured ligament in the earlier stages of a grade 1 sprain, while a grade 2 sprain requires more attention to the compensating and surrounding structures before addressing the torn fibers directly.

In general, it is best to wait at least 24–48 hours after a grade 1 or 2 sprain before beginning treatment to allow the natural healing process to set in. Following this period, the extent of treatment depends on the severity of the sprain. A grade 1 sprain can be treated with manual therapy directly following the waiting period. For a grade 2 sprain, the focus for the initial treatment is short sessions focused on gentle mobilization, particularly if swelling persists and the tissues are tender to the touch. As the ligament heals and the client is better able to tolerate pressure, longer and more focused treatment including friction is indicated. Massage for a grade 3 sprain is best applied in the subacute stage under the supervision of a health care provider, or in the chronic stage when the joint has stabilized, and can be of a longer duration.

It is essential for treatment to be relaxing. You may not be able to eliminate the symptoms associated with a ligament sprain or any coexisting conditions in a single treatment. Do not attempt to do so by treating aggressively. Be sure to ask your client to let you know if the amount of pressure that you are applying keeps him or her from relaxing. If the client responds by tensing muscles or has a facial expression that looks distressed, reduce your pressure. Remember that you are working on tissue that is compromised. Ask the client to let you know if any part of your treatment reproduces symptoms, and always work within his or her tolerance.

The following are suggestions for treating pain, weakness, and limited ROM caused by the overstretching or tearing of a ligament. These suggestions are generalized for any ligament affected by sprain. Refer to Chapters 4–11 for resources pertaining to specific muscles crossing the affected joint.

- Positioning and bolstering depends on the structures being treated. The affected joint should rest comfortably in a position that prevents overstretching of the injured ligament.

- If you find local inflammation, bolster the area when possible to allow gravity to draw fluid toward the nearest lymph nodes, and apply superficial draining strokes. If necessary, apply ice to the area for just a few minutes to reduce swelling, taking care not to chill the surrounding tissues that are hypertonic or in spasm.

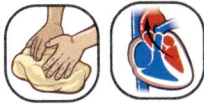

- If local swelling is minor or absent and bruises have sufficiently faded, apply brief, moist heat to the affected ligament to soften scar tissue and adhesions and to increase circulation. If protective muscle spasm is no longer beneficial to prevent re-injury, apply moist heat to hypertonic, compensating muscles.

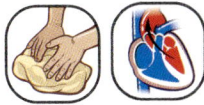

- Use your initial warming strokes to increase superficial circulation, soften tissues, and assess the tissues broadly surrounding the site of injury and compensating for the injured joint. You should be able to initially assess for adhesions, hypertonicity, protective muscle spasm, and tensile stress, which will help you to determine how to focus your time.

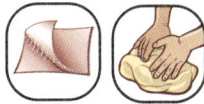

- Based on your findings, treat compensating muscles proximal to the site of injury for myofascial restrictions, adhesions, shortening, and hypertonicity.

- Assess for and treat trigger points that may have developed in compensating structures during the protective phase of healing and those that refer to the general area of injury.

- Assess and treat fascial restrictions surrounding the injured ligament.

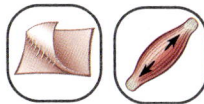

- Using focused palpation, locate the precise site of the sprain and, if possible, the direction of tearing. Using short, slow strokes within the client's pain tolerance, apply cross-fiber friction to reduce adhesions and scar tissue at the site of injury. Follow this with longitudinal strokes to realign the developing scar tissue in the functional direction. Alternate rounds of cross-fiber and longitudinal strokes until you feel a change in texture.
- Apply pain-free ROM techniques that gently stretch the ligament to further encourage re-alignment of the fibers. While it is important to use techniques that gently stress the ligament by increasing the distance between its attachments, take care not to overstretch the ligament to avoid re-injury.
- If the area became hot or began to swell while applying friction, apply ice for just a few minutes to reduce heat and swelling without overly chilling the area.

Treatment icons: Increase circulation; Reduce adhesions; Reduce tension; Lengthen tissue; Treat trigger points; Passive stretch; Clear area

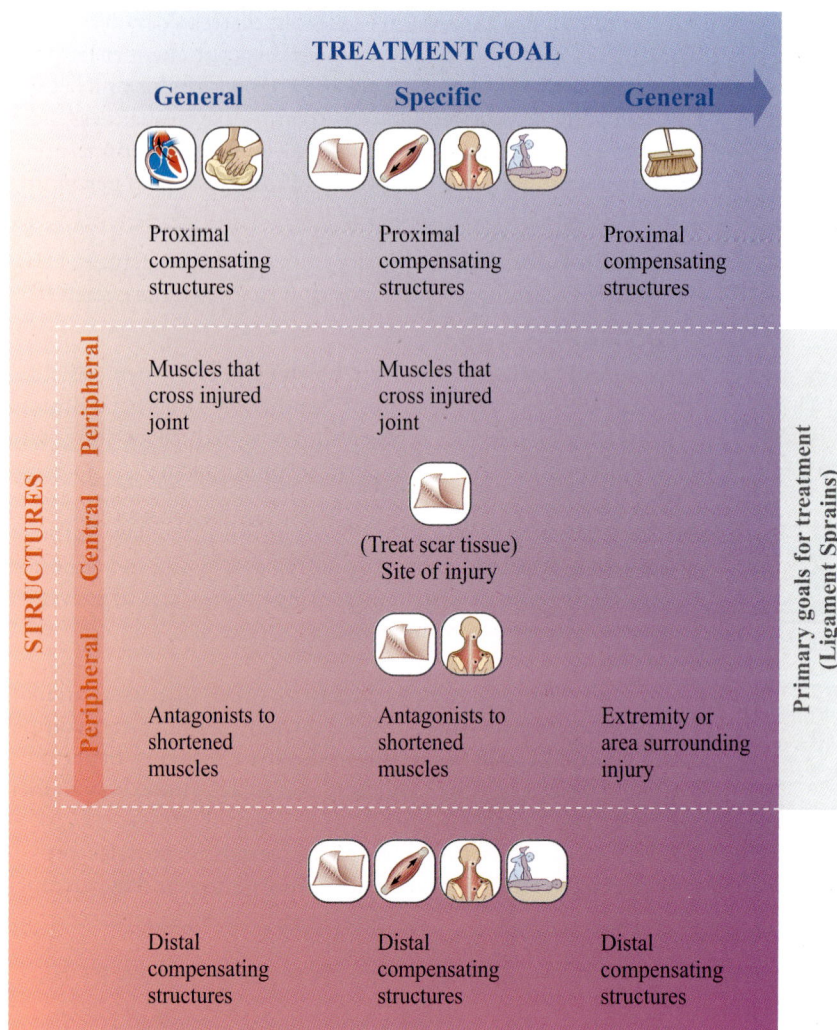

Figure 13-7 **Ligament sprains overview diagram.** Follow the general principles from left to right or top to bottom when treating ligament sprains.

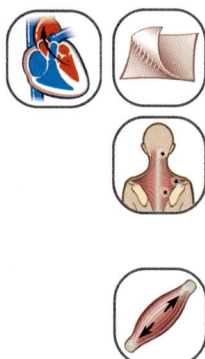

■ Treat tissues distal to the injury for compensating patterns, if needed, and to increase circulation.

■ Passively stretch or perform PIR to local, compensating muscles within the client's tolerance as necessary. This may require repositioning the client.

The treatment overview diagram summarizes the flow of treatment (Fig. 13-7).

CLIENT SELF-CARE

Avoiding re-injury is a primary concern when recommending self-care. For clients with a grade 1 sprain in any stage, or a grade 2 or 3 sprain in the late subacute or chronic stage, the following suggestions may encourage proper healing.

These suggestions are intended as general recommendations for stretching and strengthening structures involved in the client's condition. The objective is to create distance between the attachment sites of muscles that have shortened and to perform repetitions of movements that decrease the distance between the attachments of muscles that have weakened. If you have had no training in remedial exercises and do not feel that you have a functional understanding of stretching and strengthening, refer the client to a professional with training in this area.

- Instruct the client to perform self-care throughout the day, such as while talking on the phone, reading e-mail, washing dishes, or watching television if this can be accomplished without stressing the injured ligament or compensating structures. This minimizes the need to set aside extra time.
- Encourage the client to take regular breaks from stationary postures or repetitive actions that may affect the health of a ligament or the joint it crosses. If the client's daily activities include hours of inactivity, suggest moving for a few minutes every hour to prevent adhesions and reduced circulation. If the client's daily activities require repetitive actions that contribute to sprains or compensating patterns resulting from sprains, suggest resting for a few minutes every hour.
- Demonstrate gentle self-massage of the tissues surrounding the injury to keep adhesions and hypertonicity at bay between treatments.
- Demonstrate all strengthening exercises and stretches to your client and have him or her perform these in your presence before leaving to ensure that he or she is performing them properly and will not cause harm when practicing alone. In all stages of a sprain in any degree, it is essential not to stretch the joint to the extent that the injured ligament is over-stretched or re-injured. In the chronic stage or when appropriate for a healing sprain, stretches should be held for 15–30 seconds and performed frequently throughout the day within the client's limits. The client should not force the stretch or bounce. Stretching should be slow, gentle, and steady, trying to keep every other joint as relaxed as possible.
- Stretching and strengthening exercises should be recommended according to your findings in ROM testing and palpation.

Stretching

Depending on the severity of the injury, early mobilization and moderate, controlled stress to an injured ligament may aid the healing process. Mobilization increases circulation to the area, reduces adhesions, and helps to restore normal proprioception when performed within the client's tolerance. When possible, moving the injured joint to produce the shapes of the letters of the alphabet may help to restore and maintain mobility. Instruct the client to draw small letters, and to draw only as many letters as possible without feeling pain or excessive fatigue, taking care not to fully stretch the injured ligament. In the later stages of healing, recommend increasing the ROM by drawing bigger letters so that controlled but pain-free stress is placed on the joint.

Because muscles crossing the injured joint may also have been injured or may have responded to protect the joint, it is important to recommend self-care to aid in healing. For strained muscles, refer to Chapter 12. Muscles that have shortened to maintain stability in the joint may need stretching once their protective splinting is no longer necessary. The results of ROM testing and palpation will help you to determine which muscles have shortened and need to be stretched. Refer to Chapters 4–11 for stretches to specific muscles or groups of muscles. Take care to instruct the client to stretch slowly and to limit stretches to the comfortable range, gradually increasing the stretch as symptoms diminish and the risk of re-injury is reduced.

Strengthening

Strengthening weakened or atrophied muscles is equally important for restoring proper function of the affected joint. The results of ROM testing and palpation determine which muscles have weakened and need to be strengthened. In general, active or resisted concentric contractions strengthen muscles. As with stretching, a strengthening program should progress gradually. Pain-free, active ROM is effective for gradually restoring strength to weakened muscles. As healing progresses and the risk of re-injury diminishes, add resistance to active ROM by including weight-bearing activities. Refer to Chapters 4–11 for exercises to strengthen specific muscles or muscle groups.

SUGGESTIONS FOR FURTHER TREATMENT

In the acute stage, shorter treatments focused on reducing inflammation and increasing mobility are recommended until inflammation is minimal and the client can tolerate manual pressure to the tissues. A grade 1 sprain often heals in approximately 1 week, and treatments can be scheduled twice per week until symptoms subside. Grade 2 sprains can heal in as little as 2 weeks, but could take up to 6 weeks to heal well enough to return to activity without symptoms. Treatments can be scheduled twice per week until mobility and strength are restored, and weekly after that until compensating patterns are resolved. Grade 3 sprains, depending on whether the ligament is surgically repaired, may take up to 2 months to heal sufficiently to perform normal activities of daily living without symptoms. Depending on the progress of healing and complications, you may want to discuss the injury with the client's health care provider before initiating treatment. With proper clearance, treatments can be scheduled twice per week until mobility and strength are restored, and weekly after that until compensating patterns resolve.

There should be some improvement with each session. If this is not happening, consider the following possibilities:

- There is too much time between treatments. It is always best to give the newly treated tissues 24–48 hours to adapt, but if too much time passes between treatments in the beginning, the client's activities of daily living may reverse any progress.
- The client is not adjusting activities of daily living or is not keeping up with self-care. As much as we want to fix the problem, we cannot force a client to make the adjustments we suggest. Explain the importance of his or her participation in the healing process, and encourage the client to follow your recommendations, but be careful not to judge or reprimand a client who does not.
- The condition is advanced or has other musculoskeletal complications that are beyond your basic training. Refer this client to a massage therapist with advanced training. Continuing to treat a client whose case is beyond your training could turn the client away from massage therapy altogether and hinder healing.
- The client has an undiagnosed, underlying condition. Discontinue treatment until the client sees a health care provider for medical assessment.

If you are not treating the client in a clinical setting or private practice, you may not be able to take this client through the full program of healing. Still, if you can bring some relief in just one treatment, it may encourage the client to discuss this change with a health care provider and seek manual therapy rather than more aggressive treatment options. If the client agrees to return for regular treatments, the symptoms are likely to change each time, so it is important to perform an assessment before each session. Once you have released the superficial tissues in general areas, you may be able to focus more of your treatment on deeper tissues in a specific area. Likewise, once you have treated symptoms specific to sprains, you may be able to pay closer attention to compensating structures and coexisting conditions.

PROFESSIONAL GROWTH

CASE STUDY

Adila is a 39-year-old mother of three. She has sprained her left ankle three times, each time toward the end of the second trimester of her three pregnancies. The last sprain was about 1 year ago. Since the first sprain, she has always been very protective of the ankle because she is worried that it is weak. After each of the three sprains, she was able to use the ankle without symptoms within a few days of twisting it, and until recently, she has had no limitations in mobility and no pain. Approximately 1 month ago, she began to feel pain in the ankle and lower leg when she walks long distances and when she climbs stairs, particularly when carrying a child, laundry, or other heavy load. Fearing the ankle would sprain again, she has been using a brace for stability. This decreases the level of pain in the ankle, but she continues feeling pain in the leg, creeping up toward the knee. She has also been feeling some discomfort in her lower back recently.

Subjective

When asked, Adila explained that there was minimal swelling and bruising each time she sprained the ankle. She used ice each time, and after resting for a day, she continued activity with the ankle braced. She did not seek medical attention because she read on the Internet that if she was able to bear weight, had minimal swelling, and noticed improvement 48 hours after injury, there was little chance of a broken bone, and the sprain would probably heal on its own. She explained that she had gained more weight with her last pregnancy and has been unable to lose it as easily as with the first two. She described herself as being 20 pounds heavier than her normal weight. When asked, she described the pain she feels as a tightness that begins to fatigue after walking for about 5–10 minutes and when climbing up the stairs.

Objective

Adila is not limping. When standing still, she carries her body weight on the right leg. The left hip is slightly more laterally rotated compared to the right. The right hip is slightly elevated. She has slight hyperlordosis. The ankle is slightly everted and dorsiflexed when not bearing weight. There is no hypermobility in the ankle. Active inversion and plantar flexion are reduced compared to the right ankle. Passive inversion is restricted without pain, and passive inversion and plantar flexion produced an "uncomfortable stretching feeling" along the anterior leg. Resisted inversion is weak. There is a small pocket of edema just anterior to the left lateral malleolus with minor, superficial adhesions along the inferior extensor retinaculum and significant adhesions with dense scar tissue along the anterior talofibular ligament. This area is tender to the touch. I found nothing remarkable along the calcaneofibular ligament. Tissues of the left anterior and lateral leg are dense and adhered. The iliotibial band is dense and adhered.

Action

The primary treatment goals include reducing adhesions along the anterior talofibular ligament and anterior lateral leg and reducing adhesions and lengthening the peroneus longus, peroneus brevis, and extensor digitorum longus. Future goals include reducing adhesions and density in the iliotibial band, reducing hyperlordosis, and leveling the pelvis.

I elevated the left leg to initiate drainage of the edema. I applied superficial strokes toward the lymph nodes at the ankle and knee to continue draining. I used general Swedish massage on the thighs and right leg while drainage continued. The pocket of edema reduced sufficiently to allow more specific palpation and treatment of the area. I applied myofascial release to the left anterior lateral leg and ankle. I used superficial and deep kneading to the full left leg with a focus on reducing adhesions along the anterior lateral leg. I used muscle stripping to the peroneus longus, peroneus brevis, and extensor digitorum longus. I applied deep transverse friction to the anterior talofibular ligament followed by longitudinal strokes to reduce adhesions and scar tissue and to realign ligament fibers. I applied gentle mobilization of the left ankle with a focus on placing tensile stress on the anterior talofibular ligament. Each mobilization ended with inversion and plantar flexion of the ankle. Very localized heat and minor swelling developed along the ligament. I applied ice for approximately 5 minutes, followed by a minimal, general mobilization of the ankle.

I began releasing the superficial tissues of the left thigh, bilateral gluteals, and low back. The thoracolumbar fascia is dense and adhered. The right sacroiliac joint is less mobile than the left. The right quadratus lumborum is dense with a possible trigger point. I will return to these areas as time permits in subsequent visits. I will also assess the iliopsoas.

Plan

I recommended self-care beginning with drawing the alphabet with her ankle. I instructed Adila to begin slowly, within her pain tolerance, and to only draw as many letters as she can before the leg feels weak or fatigued. After drawing the alphabet, I instructed her to walk around for approximately 1 minute, and then stretch the lateral leg by inverting the ankle within her tolerance, using external surfaces if necessary to feel a stretch along the lateral leg and ankle. As symptoms improve, I suggested she consider adding jumping exercises and activities that include criss-cross steps to continue strengthening the ankle and to restore proper proprioception. Adila rescheduled 4 days out to reassess the leg and continue with treatment if necessary and to assess the hips and low back and treat as necessary.

CRITICAL THINKING EXERCISES

1. Choose two joints and describe which muscles may be reflexively activated or inhibited if a ligament providing stability to that joint is injured. Remember that muscles that cross the joint may have a direct effect while muscles that do not cross the joint may have an indirect effect. Describe how reflexive activity in these muscles may protect the affected joint.

2. Your client started feeling pain in her wrist, particularly when she works at her computer. She believes she has carpal tunnel syndrome, but she has no tingling in her fingers and your tests are negative for carpal tunnel. She mentions that she fell off her bicycle about a year ago and hurt her wrist, but she did not have it evaluated at the time. Discuss the possible injuries that may have occurred when she fell that may mimic symptoms of carpal tunnel syndrome a year later. In what direction may the impact have bent the wrist? Which soft tissue structures may have been stressed? Is there a ligament sprain in the wrist that, if untreated, may produce symptoms in the chronic stage that resembles carpal tunnel syndrome? How will you treat this client?

3. Your client had a grade 3 complete rupture of the anterior cruciate ligament during a skiing accident 6 months ago. He opted not to have the ligament surgically repaired but had six sessions of physical therapy following the injury to restore ROM. He is able to walk without limping and has no pain in the knee but has been experiencing low back pain and pain along the spine. Describe how the injury may contribute to his current dysfunctions. Would compensating patterns contribute to back pain? Which muscles or other structures may have been affected during the healing process? There are many possibilities here, so take your time thinking about it, and be creative.

4. Discuss which ligaments might be affected in clients with the following chronic conditions:
   - Hyperkyphosis
   - Hyperlordosis
   - Plantar fasciitis
   - Piriformis syndrome
   - Patellofemoral syndrome
   - Tension headaches

5. Conduct a short literature review to learn about the relationship between chronic sprains and the following:
   - Age
   - Rheumatoid arthritis
   - Osteoarthritis
   - Generalized ligament laxity
   - Thyroid dysfunction
   - Down or Asperger Syndrome

BIBLIOGRAPHY AND SUGGESTED READINGS

Biel A. *Trail Guide to the Body: How to Locate Muscles, Bones and More*, 3rd ed. Boulder, CO: Books of Discovery, 2005.

Culav EM, Clark CH, Merrilees MJ. Connective tissues: Matrix composition and its relevance to physical therapy. Physical Therapy. 1999;79(3):308–319.

Frank CB. Ligament structure, physiology and function. Journal of Musculoskeletal and Neuronal Interactions. 2004;4(2):199–201.

Gemmell H, Hayes B, Conway M. A theoretical model for treatment of soft tissue injuries: treatment of an ankle sprain in a college tennis player. Journal of Manipulative and Physiological Therapeutics. 2005;28(4):285–288.

Lowe W. *Orthopedic Massage: Theory and Technique*. St Louis, MO: Mosby-Elsevier, 2003.

Mayo Foundation for Medical Education and Research. Avulsion Fracture: How is it Treated? Available at http://www.mayoclinic.com/health/avulsion-fracture/AN00200. Accessed Spring 2009.

Mayo Foundation for Medical Education and Research. Bursitis. Available at http://www.mayoclinic.com/health/bursitis/DS00032. Accessed Spring 2009.

Mayo Foundation for Medical Education and Research. Sprains and Strains. Available at http://mayoclinic.com/health/sprains-and-strains/DS00343. Accessed Spring 2009.

Rattray F, Ludwig L. *Clinical Massage Therapy: Understanding, Assessing and Treating over 70 Conditions*. Toronto, ON: Talus Incorporated, 2000.

Solomonow M. Ligaments: A source of musculoskeletal disorders. Journal of Bodywork and Movement Therapies. 2009;13(2):136–154.

Werner R. *A Massage Therapist's Guide to Pathology*, 4th ed. Philadelphia, PA: Lippincott Williams & Wilkins, 2009.

Tendinopathy

UNDERSTANDING TENDINOPATHY

In the past, research into musculoskeletal pain and injury often considered the muscle and tendon as one mechanism. In recent years, the tendon itself has been studied in more clinical detail, revealing remarkable details about its composition, function, and role in injury. Because of this, many previously held beliefs about tendon injuries have been revised, and new research continues to reevaluate our understanding of tendons. Knowledge of the mechanisms of tendon failure and the pain originating from injured tendons continues to become more specific and refined. The term "tendinopathy" refers generally to pathology that affects a tendon. This chapter covers three common tendinopathies: tendinosis, tendinitis, and tenosynovitis. These tendinopathies have several similar qualities. The treatments for each are also similar. They vary in underlying causes, however, so while the treatment for each may be similar, the treatment goal for each differs. In all three cases, an untreated tendinopathy increases the risk for rupture of the tendon. Understanding the form and function of tendons helps one differentiate these conditions and their treatment.

Muscle fibers contract to produce the force that moves a joint. That force is transmitted to the bones by tendons. Tendons are tough structures made largely of collagen and protein that are less flexible and less elastic than muscles but have tensile strength comparable to that of bones. The structure and composition of the body's many tendons differ slightly according to their particular function. These differences also play a role in the risk of injury and the process of repair. Tendons under high functional demand, such as the superior tendon of the long head of the biceps brachii, have a higher level of collagen remodeling than those that are under lower demand, such as the inferior tendon of the biceps brachii.

In general, collagen fibers in tendons are densely packed and arranged longitudinally, parallel to each other and parallel to the forces commonly applied to them. This arrangement reinforces their resistance to tensile stress. These collagen fibers are bundled into fascicles (Fig. 14-1). Each fascicle is wrapped in connective tissue called the endotenon, which also wraps around groups of fascicles forming the tendon. Vessels and nerves that supply the tendon are found mainly in the endotenon. Endotenons are wrapped in a layer of continuous, loose connective tissue called the peritenon. Tendons that work together, such as the wrist flexors, may be wrapped in an additional layer called the epitenon. Tendons that bend around joints or pass beneath a retinaculum are subject to greater amounts of friction. These tendons are each encased in a sleeve-like synovial sheath called the tenosynovium (Fig. 14-2). These sheaths contain synovial fluid that lubricates the tendons, allowing them to glide freely and protecting the tendon itself from friction. Between the tendon and its synovial sheath is a fatty connective tissue matrix called the paratenon.

In a relaxed tendon, the parallel collagen fibers are slightly crimped (Fig. 14-3). This structure, like a spring, provides shock absorption during activity. When a muscle contracts, its tendon lengthens before shortening. As tensile stress is applied, these crimps flatten, allowing the tendon

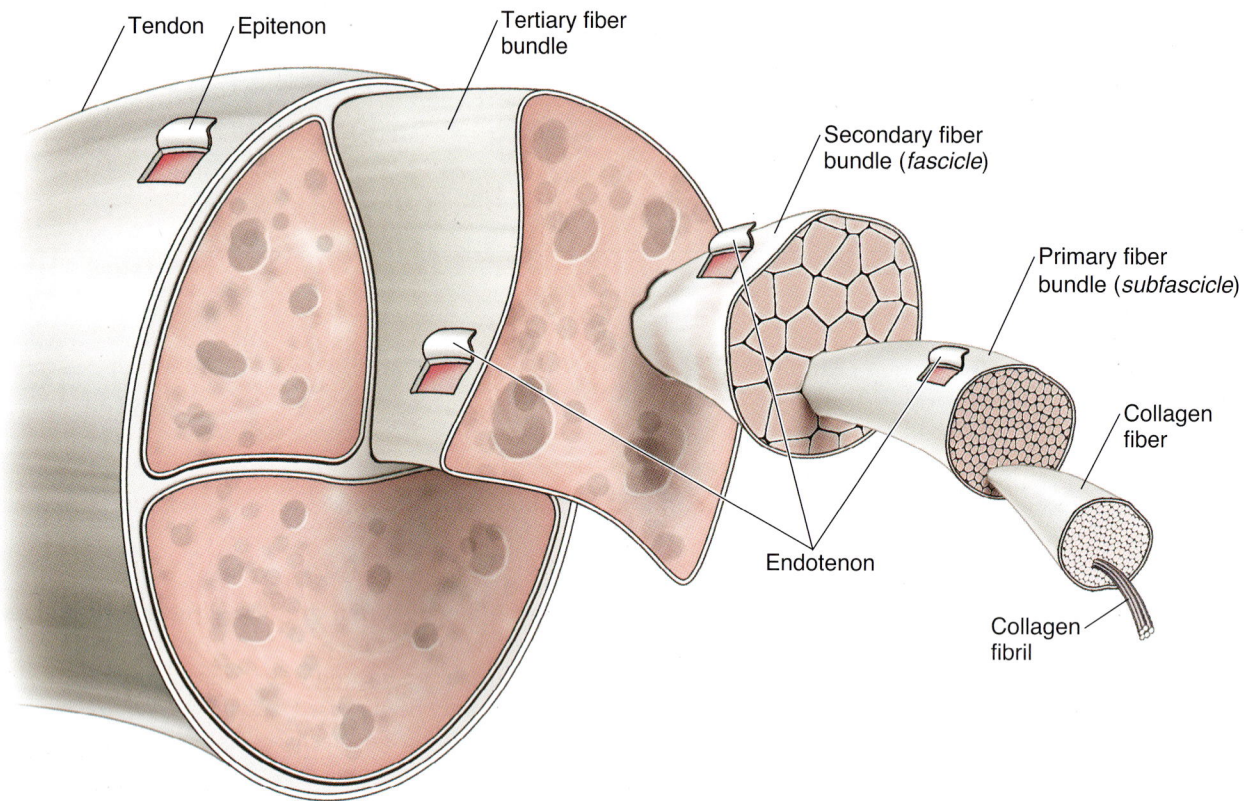

Figure 14-1   Tendon structure. Tendons are made of dense, parallel collagen fibers wrapped in layers of connective tissue.

to lengthen slightly while making it stiffer and resistant to further lengthening. This protects both the tendon and its muscle from overstretching and strain. The breaking point (when fibers tear under tensile stress) is reached when tension increases the length of a tendon by approximately 8%. Golgi tendon organs—proprioceptors found at the musculotendinous junction—detect muscle tension during a contraction. When healthy muscles contract in a controlled manner, a reflex response initiated by the Golgi tendon organs relaxes the muscle when the

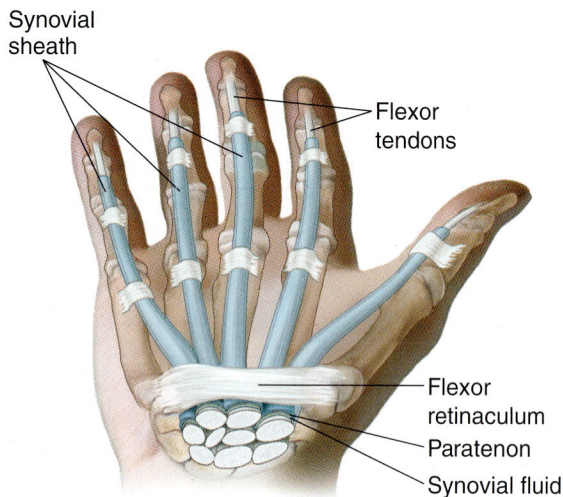

Figure 14-2   Tenosynovium. Tendons subject to great amounts of friction are encased in sleeve-like synovial sheaths called tenosynovium.

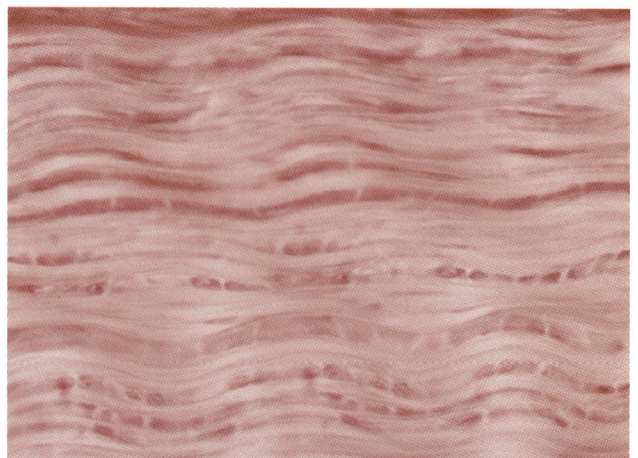

Figure 14-3   Crimped tendon fibers. The parallel collagen fibers of tendons are slightly crimped when relaxed, providing shock absorption during activity. Adapted from http://www.sacs.ucsf.edu/home/cooper/Anat118/ConnTiss/conntiss2.htm

amount of tension approaches the point of failure. When the muscle, tendon, or proprioceptors that detect tension are not healthy, or when a contraction occurs too quickly or forcefully for the reflex response to protect the musculotendinous unit, overloading can occur. Because the tendon is so much stronger than muscle, when tearing does occur, it usually occurs in the muscle belly or the musculotendinous junction or the tendon detaches from the bone. Although rare, tearing of the tendon fibers does occur. These tears, the underlying cause of tendinitis, are also called strains, as described in Chapter 12.

Like a spring, as the tendon lengthens and stiffens, it also stores energy. At the end of a ROM, the tendon recoils, releasing energy and generating a greater force for movement, which reduces the energy expenditure required by the muscle. Similar to a rubber band, the size and shape of a tendon influences the amount of stretch and the amount of energy released in recoil. A long, thin tendon stretches further, requires less force from its muscle to stiffen, and accumulates more energy for release on recoil to produce broad movement. This is ideal for muscles that primarily propel the body and that fatigue quickly as well as those that control fine motor skills. A short, flat tendon stretches less, requires more force by the muscle to stiffen, and accumulates less energy to be released on recoil, producing strong but more subtle movement. This is ideal for muscles that maintain posture and that fatigue slowly and for tendons that assist in stabilizing joints.

Painful conditions involving a tendon are often referred to as tendinitis. Tendinitis is the inflammation of a tendon, usually resulting from acute injury or chronic overuse that results in small tears in tendon fibers and interrupts the already limited blood supply (Fig. 14-4, *A*). The treatment goal for tendinitis is to reduce inflammation, reduce adhesions and scar tissue, and realign fibers. Rest is often recommended in the early stage to allow the fibers to begin healing naturally. Treatment involves transverse strokes to reduce adhesions and scar tissue and to increase circulation that supplies nutrients as well as longitudinal strokes and stretching to realign the torn fibers and encourage collagen repair. However, current studies assessing cellular changes to injured tendons have shown that inflammation—the response to tearing and repair—is not as frequently involved in tendon injuries as previously believed and that tendinitis is actually quite rare. The suffix "-itis," which denotes inflammation, has been incorrectly applied for common tendon injuries. Instead, new research has demonstrated that tendon injuries are more often the result of chronic collagen degeneration, disorganized fiber arrangement, and increased vascularization. Inflammation seems mainly to be an issue when fibers have torn.

The suffix "-osis" denotes degeneration, and the term "tendinosis" has since become more widely used in describing chronic tendon injuries (Fig. 14-4, *B*). The treatment goals for tendinosis are to reduce adhesions, encourage collagen regeneration, and realign the collagen fibers. Mechanical loading, characteristic of friction, firm pressure, and stretching or eccentric exercise encourages collagen remodeling. Tendinitis and tendinosis can affect any tendon, but most commonly affected are the tendons of the rotator cuff, the long head of the biceps brachii, the common flexor and extensor tendons at the elbow, the patellar tendon, the tendons of popliteus and tibialis posterior, and the Achilles tendon.

Tenosynovitis, an inflammation of the tenosynovium, can occur in any tendon wrapped in a synovial sheath (Fig. 14-4, *C*). Inflammation of the synovium is often the result of injury or overuse that causes a roughening of the otherwise smooth tendon, hindering efficient movement through the sheath, creating friction and inflammation and impeding the restoration of synovial fluid. Tenosynovitis can also result from infection in the synovium, usually as a result of an injection, bite, or other injury that pierces the tendon or from complications of gonorrhea. These cases are often accompanied by rash and fever, and the client should be referred to his or her health care provider for medical treatment. Gout may also contribute to tenosynovitis, particularly in the lower extremities. If the client is at risk for gout, refer him or her to a health care provider for uric acid testing. In this case, massage is contraindicated in the acute stage. Refer to a pathology book for detailed suggestions for treating a client with gout. The treatment goal for tenosynovitis that is not infectious in origin is to reduce the adhesions between the tendon and synovial sheath, smooth the roughened surface of the tendon within the sheath, and encourage the restoration of synovial fluid. Again, transverse friction and lengthening the tendon are preferred techniques for these goals. Common areas of tenosynovitis include the abductor and extensor pollicis tendons

A

Tear in tendon

B

Collagen fiber

C

Cross section of sheath
surrounding tendon

Inflammation

Tendon   Tenosynovium

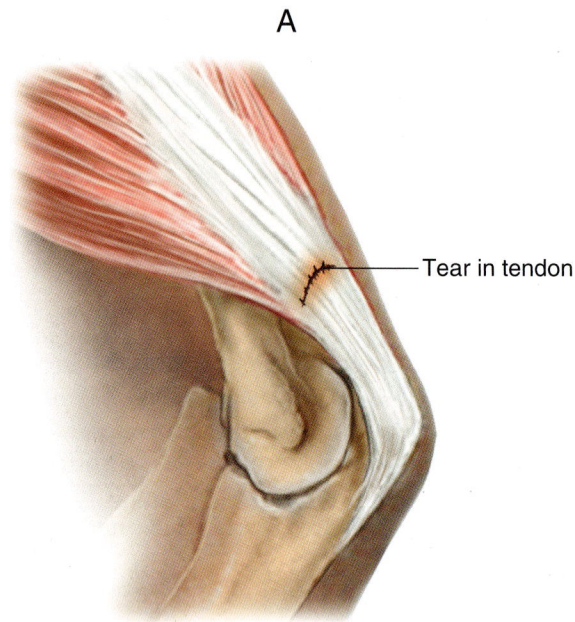

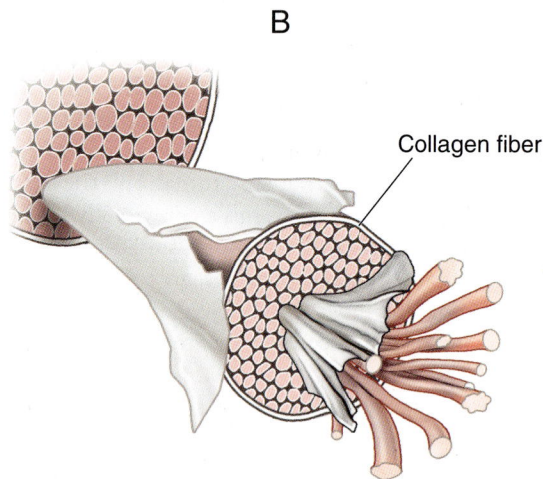

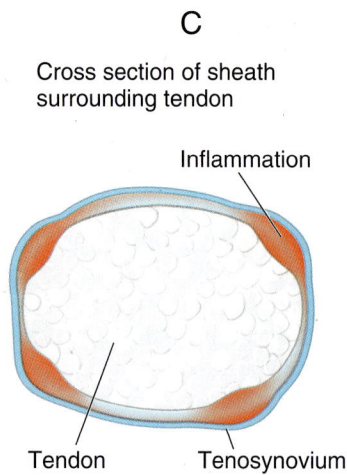

Figure 14-4 **Tendinopathies. (A)** Tendinitis is inflammation of the tendon due to tearing of tendon fibers. **(B)** Tendinosis is degeneration of collagen fibers. **(C)** Tenosynovitis is inflammation of the tenosynovium due to increased friction or trauma.

(called DeQuervain's tenosynovitis), finger flexors (called trigger finger), and the tendons of the ankle dorsiflexors.

Common Signs and Symptoms

The signs and symptoms of tendinopathies often develop gradually as a result of overuse, improper biomechanics, or the degenerative process that results from illness or aging. Acute injuries including grade 2 or 3 strains to a musculotendinous unit do occur and are sometimes the first sign that a tendinopathy was developing. Tendinopathy, the general condition of tendon injury, is marked by pain or tenderness local to the tendon, decreased strength of the musculotendinous unit, and crepitus, stiffness, and reduced ROM in the joint it crosses. These symptoms often increase with use, particularly during repetitive and resisted activities, and especially when the tendon is stretched or recoils. Symptoms may wake one from sleep, and pain and stiffness are often worse in the morning or after immobility. Gentle movement often improves symptoms that result from immobility, although intense activity may aggravate the condition. A full passive stretch of the affected tendon may elicit pain at the tendon. Local pain at the site of a tendon helps to differentiate tendinopathy from injury to a muscle belly. The muscle of the affected tendon may be hypertonic, hypotonic, or adhered and may contain trigger points. The synergists and antagonists of the affected muscles may develop compensating patterns including hypertonicity, adhesions, and trigger points. When the client compensates by avoiding lengthening the tendon, the joint may begin to lock into the shortened position.

It may be difficult to differentiate tendinitis, tendinosis, and tenosynovitis without medical testing. However, a few distinguishing characteristics may give you some clues. Tendinitis is an inflammatory condition and is often accompanied by swelling, redness, and heat at the site of the tendon. Because tendinitis involves torn fibers, eliminating the aggravating activity and allowing the tendon to rest and form scar tissue supports the healing process. Additionally, inflammation characteristic of tendinitis is interrupted by anti-inflammatories and corticosteroids, minimizing pain and other symptoms while supporting the healing process. If your client has rested, iced the injury, and used anti-inflammatory medication for a few weeks with only short-term relief that returns when the medication is not used, this may indicate that inflammation is not a primary contributing factor and that the condition is not tendinitis. With rest, improvement often begins shortly after the acute stage. With treatment, tendinitis usually resolves completely in a few weeks. Without proper treatment, the tendon may continue to degenerate, putting the client at greater risk for rupture or tendinosis.

Tendinosis is not an inflammatory condition. Therefore, while anti-inflammatories may temporarily reduce pain, they are not likely to improve symptoms over the long term. In fact, studies have shown that anti-inflammatories may inhibit collagen regeneration, and thus, healing. Corticosteroids have also been shown to reduce collagen regeneration, and while they may offer temporary relief of pain, they can ultimately hinder healing and increase the risk of further injury. Ice, which is often used to reduce inflammation, also initiates vasoconstriction. Since increased vascularity is a sign of tendinosis, ice may reduce symptoms and encourage healing. Because tendinosis is the result a degenerative process, and regeneration of collagen occurs more slowly than repair of torn tissues, improvement may take several weeks to months. The presence of heat and swelling, the duration of symptoms, and the effect of medication may help you differentiate between tendinitis and tendinosis.

Signs and symptoms of tenosynovitis include pain, swelling, and heat at the joint crossed by the tendon, reduced mobility of the affected joint, and pain with movement of the joint. Crepitus may also be present. When infection is the underlying cause of tenosynovitis, fever and redness may also be present. If you suspect infection, refer the client to a health care provider for medical assessment. Palpable nodules may also be found in the affected tendon. Nodules may be recognized before the client experiences other symptoms. ROM is limited, particularly when attempting to lengthen the tendon, sometimes requiring passive force to release the tendon from adhesion to its sheath. While movement may be painful, immobility reduces the production of synovial fluid and may lead to adhesions and locking of the joint in the shortened position. Movement is essential to prevent adhesions and immobility.

Possible Causes and Contributing Factors

Repetitive activity is a common contributing factor in tendinopathies. Tailors and seamstresses, computer and cash register operators, and musicians are at risk for tendinopathies, particularly in the upper extremities. Poor biomechanics and postural or muscle imbalances may cause overloading of a tendon during sport or recreational activities, work, or general activities of daily living and may contribute to a tendinopathy. Improper warming prior to activity, improper technique during activity, and unsuitable accessories such as shoes can also contribute to overloading a tendon. Athletes and assembly line employees are particularly affected by tendinopathies due to overloading. Golfers and tennis players are at risk for tendinopathies in the elbows, while runners are more likely to develop tendinopathies in the knees or ankles. Assembly line work that involves lifting puts the employee at greater risk of tendinopathies in the shoulder.

Once a tendinopathy arises, failing to allow sufficient time for healing in the early stages can slow or halt the natural healing process. With tendinitis, if small tears in the tendon do not form scars that are strong enough to resist further tearing, the inflammatory process will continue, compromising the structure's integrity, and the risk of further injury increases. Similarly, continuing activity that encourages the inflammatory process characteristic of tenosynovitis may weaken the structure and cause compensating patterns to become habitual. With tendinosis, continuing aggravating activities once degeneration has begun may inhibit the regeneration of collagen and continue to weaken the tendon.

However, recent studies have begun to reveal that inactivity or underuse may also play a role in chronic tendinopathy. Movement encourages collagen regeneration and the production of synovial fluid. Immobility discourages collagen regeneration, encourages adhesions, and can lead to atrophy. While some rest or at least limiting the aggravating activity is necessary to allow healing to begin, movement is an important element of the natural healing process.

Being overweight increases demand on the musculoskeletal system during all activities and may contribute to tendinopathies. Diabetes—often associated with obesity—as well as drugs used to control diabetes may cause metabolic changes that increase fibrosis and may alter the structure of tendons. Statins—the drugs used to reduce cholesterol—and some antibiotics include risk factors for both muscle and tendon pathologies. Rheumatoid arthritis—a systemic inflammatory pathology—increases the risk of tendinitis and tenosynovitis and may exacerbate symptoms. Gout—an accumulation of uric acid in the joints—may also contribute to inflammatory tendinopathies. Most commonly, the process of aging, which reduces elasticity and increases intolerance to tensile stress in both muscles and tendons, is a contributing factor. Infectious tenosynovitis can be caused by injuries that expose the tendon to bacteria, improper injection technique, IV drug use, and injuries that require medical attention. Individuals with a compromised immune system may be at greater risk for infectious tenosynovitis.

Because tendinopathies can occur anywhere in the body, they can be confused with many other conditions throughout the body. For example, pain in the toe may be a tendinopathy, but it can also be the result of gout. Wrist pain may be the result of tendinopathy, carpal tunnel syndrome, or both. Table 14-1 lists some general conditions commonly confused with or contributing to tendinopathies. Because tendinopathies may be difficult to distinguish, it is particularly important to understand the client's health history, precipitating events, and other possible causes of pain in the area before treatment. Consult your pathology book for more detailed information. If you are unsure and the client's symptoms resemble those of a more serious condition, particularly if the client has other risk factors, refer him or her to a health care provider for medical assessment.

Contraindications and Special Considerations

First, it is essential to understand the cause of pain. If the client cannot move the joint, heard a popping sound, or has significant weakness or if you suspect the client has a fractured bone or significant tearing to the tissues, work with the client's health care provider and consult a pathology text for massage therapists before proceeding. These are a few general cautions:

Table 14-1	Differentiating Conditions Commonly Confused with or Contributing to Tendinopathy		
Condition	**Typical Signs and Symptoms**	**Testing**	**Massage Therapy**
Calcific tendinitis (inflammation of tendon due to calcium deposits)	Can affect any tendon, most common in the shoulder Pain, inflammation, stiffness, weakness, crepitus Aggravated by activity Symptoms worsen during periods of calcium shedding and reabsorption	X-ray	Massage is indicated within the client's pain tolerance. Client should be made aware that shedding of calcium deposits may temporarily intensify symptoms. ROM techniques may prevent frozen shoulder.
Osteoarthritis	Tenderness with pressure on joint Stiffness, particularly after rest or inactivity Inflexibility Swelling Grating sensation or sound	Physical exam X-rays Blood tests Synovial fluid tests Arthroscopy	Massage is contraindicated during an acute flare-up, indicated otherwise.
Rheumatoid arthritis	Periods of flare-ups and remission Pain, swelling Aching and stiffness, particularly after rest or inactivity Reduced ROM Distortion of joint Rheumatic nodules Occasional low-grade fever and malaise	Physical exam Blood tests Synovial fluid tests Radiography	Massage is indicated in nonacute stages. Work with the health care team.
Reiter's syndrome (reactive arthritis)	Often preceded by infection, low-grade fever, or conjunctivitis Tendon pain Joint pain Skin lesions in palms or soles Redness, burning, or discharge from eyes Urinary urgency or burning	Physical exam Joint x-ray Urinalysis HLA-B27 antigen	Massage is contraindicated until infection is resolved, and during active flare-ups of arthritis. Work with the health care provider to tailor the treatment plan to meet the individual's needs. Avoid skin lesions.
Carpal tunnel syndrome	Pain, numbness, and tingling in thumb, index, and middle fingers, and lateral half of ring finger Gradual atrophy and reduced fine motor skills	Phalen's test Tinel's sign EMG Nerve conduction test	Massage is indicated. See Chapter 7

(continued)

Table 14-1	Differentiating Conditions Commonly Confused with or Contributing to Tendinopathy (Continued)		
Condition	**Typical Signs and Symptoms**	**Testing**	**Massage Therapy**
Plantar fasciitis	Often develops gradually but can be acute Sharp, burning, or aching pain in arch of foot Swelling in arch Symptoms worse at push-off phase of gait, particularly after periods of inactivity Possible tearing of fibers and bone spur in calcaneus	X-ray, MRI to rule out other causes of pain Dorsiflexion-eversion test Windlass test	Massage is indicated. See Chapter 11
Sprain	Usually acute Inflammation, heat, redness, and pain in acute stage Remaining inflammation, weakness, reduced ROM in chronic stage	Often self-assessed Physical exam MRI	Massage is indicated. See Chapter 13.
Spasm/cramp (contracture)	Sudden, often sharp pain in the affected voluntary muscle Palpable and often visible mass of hypertonic muscle tissue	Often self-assessed X-ray or MRI may be used to assess extent of damage	Massage is indicated. Discuss with health care provider if repeated spasm is related to an underlying condition or side effects from medication.
Myofascial pain syndrome	Persistent muscle aches or pain Muscle or joint stiffness Muscle tension Trigger points Pain interrupts sleep	Physical exam Palpate for trigger points Referred pain or twitch response Other tests may be performed to rule out other sources of pain	Massage is indicated. Myofascial pain syndrome is associated with trigger points. See Chapter 3.
Bursitis	Pain, particularly with activity or palpation Heat, redness, swelling, or tenderness	Physical exam ROM tests X-ray or MRI if conservative treatment is not successful	Massage is systemically contraindicated if bursitis is due to infection, and locally contraindicated in the acute stage to avoid increased swelling. In the subacute stage, massage to the structures surrounding the joint is indicated.
Diabetes	Frequent urination, frequent thirst, increased appetite, fatigue, nausea	Physical exam Fasting blood sugar test	Indicated when tissues and circulation are not compromised.
Gout	Redness, heat, and swelling Sudden, intense pain, often at night, which diminishes gradually over a couple of weeks	Physical exam Blood and urine uric acid concentration tests Synovial fluid test	Massage is contraindicated during acute attacks. Gout may indicate other systemic conditions. Work with health care team.

- **Infection.** When tenosynovitis is infectious, massage is contraindicated until the infection has resolved and the client receives clearance from his or her health care provider.
- **Reproducing symptoms.** Symptoms may occur during treatment. If treatment reproduces symptoms beyond the client's pain tolerance, adjust the client to a more neutral posture. Shortening or adding slack to the tendon may help. If this does not relieve the symptoms, reduce your pressure or move away from the area. You may be able to treat around the site that reproduced the symptoms and return to it after treating superficial and peripheral tissues, but proceed with caution.
- **Treatment duration and pressure.** If the client is elderly, has degenerative disease, or has been diagnosed with a condition that diminishes activities of daily living, you may need to adjust your pressure as well as the treatment duration. Frequent half-hour sessions may suit the client better.
- **Friction.** Do not use deep frictions if the health of the underlying tissues is at risk for rupture. Allow time for scarring and tissue regeneration to avoid re-injury. Do not use friction if the client is taking anti-inflammatory medication or anticoagulants. Friction initiates an inflammatory process, which may interfere with the intended action of anti-inflammatory medication. Recommend that the client refrain from taking such medication for several hours prior to treatment if the health care provider agrees. Because anticoagulants reduce clotting, avoid techniques that may cause tearing and bleeding.

Massage Therapy Research

Tendinopathy is being studied intensely. New research continues to revise our understanding of the structure and function of tendons, the causes of pathology, and treatment options. Because of this, there are as many new questions as there are answers.

In 1999, Gehlsen et al. conducted a study titled "Fibroblast Responses to Variation in Soft Tissue Mobilization Pressure" that assessed morphologic changes in the Achilles tendon of rats after applications of augmented soft tissue mobilization therapy (ASTM). The study supports the premise that microtrauma, such as pressure or friction, facilitates the healing process in tendons and asks what magnitude of microtrauma is necessary to induce change. Thirty rats were randomly assigned to one of five groups: tendinitis, tendinitis plus light ASTM, tendinitis plus medium ASTM, tendinitis plus extreme ASTM, and a control group (healthy tendon). Tendinitis was induced using an injection of collagenase. The three ASTM groups received a massage every 4 days, totaling six treatments. Fibroblasts were assessed by microscope 1 week after the final ASTM treatment. The control group showed parallel collagen fibers, as in healthy tendons. The tendinitis group showed fiber misalignment. The ASTM groups also exhibited fiber misalignment with an increased number of tendon fibroblasts indicating the healing process, with the extreme ASTM group exhibiting the greatest number of fibroblasts. The authors concluded that ASTM stimulates fibroblast proliferation and that the amount of pressure used affects the level of cellular response. ASTM involves the use of instruments other than the hands to apply pressure to the soft tissues. This is generally performed to spare the practitioner from developing overuse injuries. It is unclear whether applying the same amount of pressure with the hands instead of instruments would significantly alter the outcomes.

In a 2008 study titled "The Effect of Mechanical Load on Degenerated Soft Tissue," Warren Hammer presents three case studies in which he assesses the Graston Technique of soft tissue mobilization for the treatment of supraspinatus tendinosis, Achilles tendinosis, and plantar fasciosis (degeneration of the plantar fascia). Like ASTM, the Graston Technique is a form of mechanical loading of soft tissues that uses stainless steel instruments with curved edges contoured to fit shapes of the body. The client with supraspinatus tendinosis was treated twice a week for 5 weeks. The client with Achilles tendinosis was treated twice a week for 6 weeks and performed eccentric exercises at home. Both of these clients were asymptomatic following this regimen. The client with plantar fasciosis was treated 12 times over the course of 6 weeks and advised to use orthotics. She reported 95% improvement but had to discontinue treatment due to insurance conflicts. Hammer's conclusions support previous studies suggesting that mechanical loading of soft tissues facilitates fibroblast production and collagen remodeling and is thus effective in treating conditions in which collagen degeneration is a primary contributing factor. He also suggests the need for further study to examine how Graston Technique compares to other manual techniques, how mechanical loading differs in the case of acute versus chronic injuries, and how the magnitude of load relates to anti-inflammatory versus pro-inflammatory processes of healing. It is important to note that the conclusions of this study are based solely on the clients' reports of symptom relief, ROM and strength testing, and comparative palpation following treatment. No histological studies were performed to measure fibroblast proliferation.

Pedrelli et al. (2009) concentrated their inquiry on the role of fascial restrictions in tendinopathies. In their study titled "Treating Patellar Tendinopathy with Fascial Manipulation," 18 patients with a history of unilateral patellar tendon pain were treated with the fascial manipulation technique described by physiotherapist Luigi Stecco, with the goal of restoring gliding between intrafascial fibers. Pain with movement was evaluated before treatment, immediately after treatment, and one month after treatment. A single therapist performed all treatments, which included applying pressure mid thigh between the vastus lateralis and rectus femoris with force toward the vastus intermedius. Deep friction or mobilization of the fascia was subsequently applied. Participants were asked not to perform sports for 4 days following treatment to avoid stressing the structures. All participants reported reduced pain immediately following treatment. Two participants reported complete relief that was maintained 1 month after treatment. Nine participants reported a relief following treatment that continued to improve between treatment and the 1-month follow-up. Three participants reported feeling pain relief immediately following treatment, with a recurrence of some pain between treatment and the 1-month follow-up, but the level of pain was still less than before treatment.

While these studies are encouraging, it is important to note that while pain is reduced and strength is regained, it is still somewhat unclear how or why this occurs. Without fully understanding the mechanism of tendon pathologies, treatments are more frequently geared toward symptom relief. While valuable, symptom relief does not necessarily result in long-term recovery or reducing the risk of re-injury. Further studies are needed to determine the exact effect that massage techniques have on repairing or regenerating the collagen fibers in tendons or in reducing inflammation.

WORKING WITH THE CLIENT

Client Assessment

Assessment begins during your first contact with a client. In some cases, this may be on the telephone when an appointment is requested. Ask in advance if the client is seeking treatment for specific area of pain so that you can prepare yourself.

Table 14-2 lists questions to ask the client when taking a health history.

POSTURAL ASSESSMENT

Allow the client to enter the room ahead of you while you assess his or her posture and movement. Look for imbalances in the movement of the joint crossed by the affected tendon or patterns of compensation that may develop to protect the injured structures. Watch as the client walks and climbs steps if the lower body is affected. Watch as the client opens the door, takes off his or her coat, or picks up a pen if the upper body is affected. Watch as the client sits, stands from sitting, lifts or sets down objects, turns to talk to you, and so on to see if he or she can perform these activities without assistance or if he or she avoids resistance against the affected tendon. Look for reduced mobility or the favoring of one side.

Table 14-2	Health History

Questions for the Client	Importance for the Treatment Plan
Where do you feel symptoms?	The location of symptoms helps to locate the injured tendon or to differentiate tendinopathy from other soft tissue injuries.
Describe what your symptoms feel like.	A description of symptoms including weakness, heat, or fullness in the area may help you to differentiate tendinosis, tendinitis, and tenosynovitis. See Chapter 1 for descriptions of pain sensations and possible contributing factors.
What activity were you performing when you first felt the pain?	The details of the activity or posture that initiated the pain may help you to determine its cause. A new regimen of exercise, weight-bearing activity, or repetitive action, particularly following a period of inactivity may contribute to tendinopathies.
When did the symptoms begin?	Onset of symptoms may help you to determine the stage of the injury and the health of the tissue.
Do you have a history of injury or surgery to this area?	An explanation of prior injury to the area may help you to determine contributing factors. Surgery and resulting scar tissue may increase the risk of tendinopathy.
Do any movements make your symptoms worse or better?	Locate weakness in structures producing such movements. Resisted activity or activities that stretch the tendon are likely to increase symptoms. Adding slack or reducing tension in the tendon may decrease symptoms.
Have you seen a health care provider for this condition? What was the diagnosis? What tests were performed?	Medical tests may reveal the location and stage of tendinopathy or coinciding injuries. If no tests were performed to make a diagnosis, use the tests described in this chapter for your assessment. If your assessment is inconsistent with a diagnosis, ask the client to discuss your findings with a health care provider or ask for permission to contact the provider directly.
Are you taking any prescribed or over-the-counter medications or herbal or other supplements?	Medication of all types may contribute to symptoms or have contraindications or cautions.
Have you had a corticosteroid or analgesic injection in the past 2 weeks? Where?	Local massage is contraindicated. A history of repeated corticosteroid injections may affect the integrity of muscle and tendons, increasing the risk of injury. Use caution when applying pressure or cross-fiber strokes. Analgesics reduce sensation and may cause the client to allow you to work too aggressively.
Have you taken a pain reliever or muscle relaxant within the past 4 hours?	The client may not be able to judge your pressure and may allow you to work too aggressively.
Have you taken anti-inflammatory medication within the past 4 hours?	Deep friction initiates an inflammatory process and should not be performed if the client has recently taken anti-inflammatory medication. Regular use of anti-inflammatories may also contribute to collage degeneration.

When assessing the standing posture, be sure that the client stands comfortably. If he or she deliberately attempts to stand in the anatomic position, you may not get an accurate assessment of his or her posture in daily life. If the client has the joint braced with a removable device, ask him or her to remove it if it is possible to bear weight without it so that you can get an accurate picture of the strength of the injured structures. When tendinopathy affects the lower body, the client may stand in a position that keeps the weight off the affected joint. This, in turn, may initiate imbalances in posture from the feet up to the spine. Check for irregularities in the ankles, knees, hips, and low back. When the upper body is affected, the client may hold the joint in a position that keeps the injured tendon from stretching. This may initiate compensating patterns that protect the affected tendon. Look for imbalance in the shoulders, rotations in the arm, forearm, and cervical or thoracic spine. You may not be able to attend to all of the compensating patterns in the early treatments but may be able to return to them once the aggravating injury begins to heal.

ROM ASSESSMENT

Test the ROM of both the agonists and antagonists that cross the joint also crossed by the injured tendon. Since it allows the client to control the amount of movement and stay within a pain-free range, only active ROM testing should be performed in the acute stage to avoid further injury. In the chronic stage, the client may have developed compensating patterns causing pain in other joints that should also be tested.

Active ROM

Compare your assessment of the client's active ROM in the affected joints to the values listed in the Average ROM boxes in Chapters 4–11.

- **Active ROM of the affected joint** may be limited but will not likely produce localized pain when tendinosis or tendinitis is present. The client may limit movement to the pain-free range. More likely, an active contraction without resistance may not stress the tendon to the point of discomfort, but may cause discomfort in the affected muscle or compensating structures. With tenosynovitis, pain will likely result with any activity that involves the tendon gliding within its sheath. If the joint is already stuck in a flexed position, the value of active ROM testing is limited.

Passive ROM

Compare the client's P ROM on one side to the other when applicable. Note and compare the end feel for each range (see Chapter 1 for an explanation of end feel). P ROM should not be used in the acute stage of injury.

- **P ROM of the affected joint** may produce no symptoms or demonstrate restriction when shortening the muscle, but often produces pain on a full passive stretch. The location of pain during a full passive stretch of the affected joint may help to determine if the injury is in the muscle belly or the tendon. Pain local to the tendon suggests tendinopathy. With tenosynovitis, passive movement that requires the tendon to move through its sheath may be painful. A full passive stretch may require more force than usual, and clicking, grating, or crepitus may be present as the tendon detaches from its sheath. Apply the passive stretch slowly, and limit it to a range within the client's pain tolerance.

Resisted ROM

Use resisted tests to assess the strength of the affected musculotendinous unit. Compare the strength of the affected side to the unaffected side when possible. R ROM should not be used in the acute stage of injury.

- **R ROM of the affected joint** may produce pain at the tendon that may refer into the muscle. It may be necessary to perform the test in a variety of positions to elicit symptoms and to assess synergists to the affected musculotendinous unit. Weakness is not likely in the early stages of tendinitis or tendinosis but may develop if the condition is not treated. With tenosynovitis, if the joint is stuck in the shortened position there is no benefit to performing R ROM of the affected joints.

SPECIAL TESTS

There are numerous orthopedic tests for tendinopathies that are specific to the affected tendon. These specific, named tests are largely comprised of combinations of passive lengthening and resisted contractions of the affected muscles. It will be important to learn these orthopedic tests if you choose to focus your advanced training on clinically oriented treatments or research. At a beginner's level, length and strength assessment, a full passive stretch of the affected tendon, and palpation are sufficient assessment tools for distinguishing tendinopathies from other potential causes of pain. Use ROM testing as described above, and refer to Chapters 4-11 for special tests of the muscles affected by those conditions.

PALPATION ASSESSMENT

If the affected tendon passes directly over a bone, the bursa beneath it may be inflamed. Treating bursitis requires advanced training. If you suspect bursitis as a coexisting condition, avoid deep pressure and friction locally in all stages. In the subacute stage of bursitis, massage to the surrounding structures is indicated, but direct pressure is avoided. Additionally, if you suspect bursitis that may be infectious in nature, refer the client to his or her health care provider for assessment before providing massage therapy.

The area around the affected tendon may be warm or swollen due to inflammation, particularly if the affected tendon is superficial and if tendinitis or tenosynovitis is the condition to be treated. The site of injury may be tender on palpation. Tenderness diminishes as the injury heals. Tenderness on palpation may radiate to surrounding tissue, and the area of radiating pain will also diminish as the injury heals. The tendon itself may feel thick and dense. Adhesions may be present around the affected tendon and among the synergists and antagonists of the affected musculotendinous unit. Crepitus may be notable around the affected tendon and with movement of the affected joint. With tenosynovitis, grating may be evident when making the tendon glide within its sheath by lengthening the affected musculotendinous unit. If the tendon is pulled taut over the bones of the joint it crosses, it may strum over the bone with movement of the joint or with manual manipulation. Hypertonicity and trigger points may be found in the affected musculotendinous unit, its synergists, and its antagonists. If the joint has been immobilized for an extended period, if the client has developed protective patterns, or if the injury involves serious strain or compression or lesions to the nerves, the affected muscles may begin to atrophy. In addition, if the injury coincides with a strain, which is often the case with tendinitis, scar tissue may form to heal tears. If not properly treated, scarring and adhesions may reduce local circulation, resulting in ischemia. The ischemic area may feel cool to the touch.

To effectively treat a tendinopathy, it is essential to locate the precise tendon and to know the direction of fibers of the affected tendon and muscle. Refer to the illustrations of specific muscles throughout this text to determine fiber direction. Take your time palpating the location, and be very precise. Once you have identified the affected tendon, palpate slowly, covering approximately 1 inch of tissue in 5–10 seconds. Stay focused, and allow the receptors in your fingers to transmit important information. Feel for adhesions, scars, or other anomalies in texture, tone, temperature, and tenderness.

Condition-Specific Massage

Tendinopathy may be one element of a musculoskeletal injury or chronic pain condition. For example, carpal tunnel syndrome may involve a tendinopathy of a flexor tendon; strains that occur at the musculotendinous junction may be the cause or result of a tendinopathy; and the pain associated with patellofemoral syndrome may involve or be confused with patellar tendinopathy. These are just a few examples. Always consider the health of the tendon when assessing musculoskeletal conditions. When tendinopathy contributes to the symptoms of another condition, the following recommendations are incorporated into the treatment and meant to aid healing and reduce the risk of re-injury of the tendon. Reducing adhesions, reducing scar tissue if present, encouraging collagen regeneration and reorienting collagen fibers, reducing hypertonicity and tensile stress, and strengthening weak muscles are the basic goals of treating tendinopathies. When tendinopathy is the primary condition, the following suggestions can be used alone.

Because tendinopathy can occur in any tendon, the following descriptions do not specify particular muscles as in earlier chapters. Use the resources in Chapters 4–11 when needed to determine fiber direction, joints crossed, superficial versus deep tissues, and so on. Although the treatment goals for tendinitis, tendinosis, and tenosynovitis differ, transverse friction, pressure, and controlled tensile stress applied to the tendon, along with treating the affected muscle and its synergists and antagonists, are common to all treatments. In some cases, tendinopathies are complicated by other conditions such as infection, entrapment, or a compartment syndrome. A complicated case of tendinopathy is best supervised by a professional with advanced training.

It is essential for the treatment to be as relaxing as possible. Deep friction of a tendon can be somewhat painful and requires the client to allow you to reach the upper limit of his or her tolerance. Explain this to your client, and ask him or her to let you know when the amount of pressure you are applying causes him or her to tense up. In addition, because treatment to the affected tendon can be uncomfortable, it is best to alternate 30-60 seconds of treatment directly to the tendon with more general treatment to the muscles, stretches, and joint mobilizations. You are not likely to eliminate the symptoms associated with tendinopathies or any coexisting conditions in a single treatment. Do not attempt to do so by treating overly aggressively. Remember that you are working on tissue that is compromised. Ask the client to let you know if any part of your treatment reproduces symptoms, and always work within his or her tolerance. Deep palpation of a trigger point may cause pain at the upper end of the client's tolerance. Explain this to your client, describe a pain scale and what level of pain should not be exceeded, and ask him or her to breathe deeply during the application of the technique. As the trigger point is deactivated, the referral pain will also diminish.

The following suggestions are for treating pain, weakness, and limited ROM caused by a tendinopathy. This is generalized for any affected tendon. Refer to Chapters 4–11 for treatment suggestions pertaining to specific muscles.

- Positioning and bolstering depend on which tendon is to be treated.

- If you find swelling, apply superficial draining strokes toward the nearest lymph nodes, and when possible, bolster the area to allow gravity to draw fluid toward the thorax.

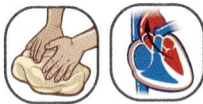

- If swelling is minor or absent, apply brief moist heat to the affected area to soften adhesions and to increase circulation. Just a few minutes of moist heat is sufficient. If inflammation is present, do not use heat.

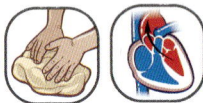

- Use your initial warming strokes to increase superficial circulation, soften tissues, and to assess the tissues broadly surrounding the site of injury and those that may be compensating for the injured musculotendinous unit. You should be able to initially assess tissues for adhesions, hypertonicity, protective muscle spasm, and tensile stress, which will help you determine how to focus your time.

- Before applying emollient, assess for and treat fascial restrictions around the injured area and compensating structures. Tissues that have shortened to prevent re-injury, particularly those closest to the joint, are most likely to develop fascial restrictions.

- Soften the tissues peripheral to the site of injury, beginning proximal. Pay special attention to the muscle of the affected tendon and its synergists. If the antagonists are accessible, treat these now, or return to this step when the client changes position.

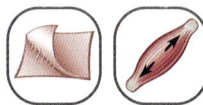

- Once the superficial tissues are pliable enough to allow for deeper work, apply transverse strokes to reduce the remaining adhesions and apply lengthening strokes to the peripheral tissues that are short and tight, beginning proximal. Muscles with fiber direction and actions in common with the muscle of the injured tendon are likely to have shortened, possibly in spasm, to protect the injured tendon and muscle from further injury.

Treatment icons: Increase circulation; Reduce adhesions; Reduce tension; Lengthen tissue; Treat trigger points; Passive stretch; Clear area

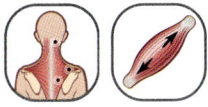

- Treat any trigger points found in the synergists of the affected muscle or in muscles compensating for the injury. Treat trigger points in antagonists if they are accessible, or return to this step when the client changes position. Follow trigger point treatment with lengthening strokes, but do not stretch the muscles until you have treated the injured tendon to avoid reflexive contractions.

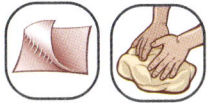

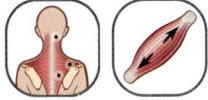

- Assess and treat the muscle belly of the affected tendon for adhesions, tension, and trigger points. Follow trigger point treatment with lengthening strokes, but do not stretch the muscles until you have treated the injured tendon to avoid reflexive contractions.

- Locate the injured tendon. With tendinosis and tendinitis, passively position the affected joint so that the tendon is lengthened but not overstretched. Reproducing symptoms may indicate overstretching. With tenosynovitis, the tendon should be fully lengthened and taut, within the client's tolerance.

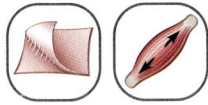

- Working slowly within the client's pain tolerance, apply short, deep transverse strokes to the full length of the injured tendon. Begin with strokes in one transverse direction, and continue with strokes in the opposite transverse direction. Transverse strokes both reduce adhesions and scar tissue, and encourage collagen repair. Follow this with longitudinal strokes to redirect tendon fibers, and mobilizations that lengthen the tendon. Alternate rounds of transverse strokes, longitudinal strokes, and mobilizations until you feel a change in texture. If the area gets hot or begins to swell, discontinue this step, and apply ice to the area for a few minutes to slow down the inflammatory process and cool the area.

- Apply longitudinal strokes to the full length of the injured tendon and muscle.

- Passively stretch the affected musculotendinous unit as fully as possible within the client's tolerance. This may require repositioning the client. Hold the stretch for 10-15 seconds. This step is essential for realigning the fibers and increasing the load on the tendon, which facilitates collagen remodeling.

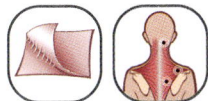

- If you were unable to address the antagonists of the muscle with an injured tendon, reposition the client and address them now.

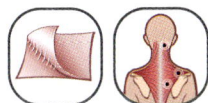

- If time permits, assess and treat any compensating patterns found.

The treatment overview diagram summarizes the flow of treatment (Fig. 14-5).

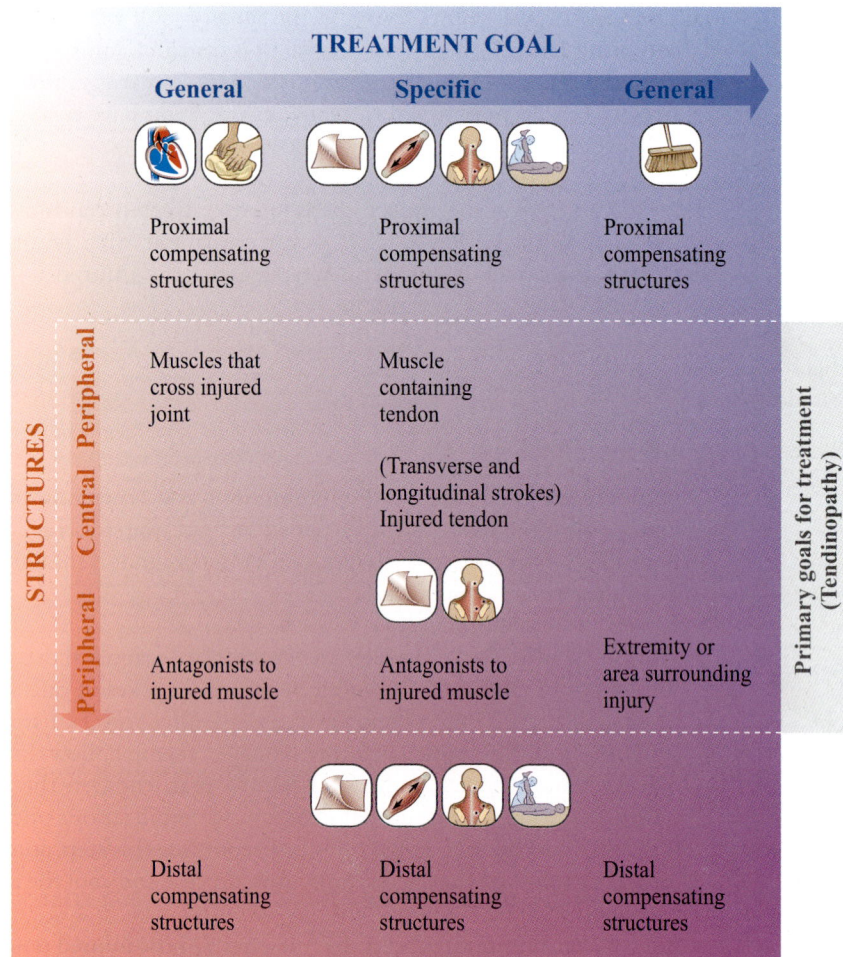

Figure 14-5 **Tendinopathy treatment overview diagram.** Follow the general principles from left to right or top to bottom when treating tendinopathies.

CLIENT SELF-CARE

Avoiding further injury is a primary concern when recommending self-care. While reducing aggravating activities and decreasing loads will help reduce friction, inflammation, and strain, activity is essential for collagen regeneration and to reduce adhesions. During the healing process, the client may choose to wear a brace or other protective device while performing activities that aggravate symptoms. It is best to wear these only when participating in aggravating activities and to allow the joint to be mobile otherwise. Arch supports may be helpful with tendinopathies of the lower extremity and if prescribed, should always be worn. Proper biomechanics are crucial to avoid re-injury. Ask your client to show you the repetitive activity that he or she performs or the action that initiated pain, and suggest ways of moving that will minimize aggravating factors.

The following are intended as general recommendations for stretching and strengthening muscles involved in the client's condition. The objective is to create distance between the attachment sites of musculotendinous units that have shortened and to perform repetitions of movements that decrease the distance between the attachments of units that have weakened. If you have had no training in remedial exercises and do not feel that you have a functional understanding of stretching and strengthening, refer the client to a professional with training in this area.

Clients often neglect self-care due to time constraints. Encourage them to follow these guidelines:

- Instruct the client to perform self-care throughout the day, such as while talking on the phone, reading e-mail, washing dishes, or watching television instead of setting aside extra time.
- Encourage the client to take regular breaks from stationary postures or repetitive actions. If the client's daily activities include hours of inactivity, suggest moving for at least a few

minutes every hour to prevent adhesions and reduced circulation. If the client's daily activities require repetitive actions that contribute to a tendinopathy, suggest resting for at least a few minutes every hour or reducing the aggravating activity as much as possible.

- Demonstrate gentle self-massage of the tissues surrounding the injury to keep adhesions and hypertonicity at bay between treatments.
- Demonstrate all strengthening exercises and stretches to your client and have him or her perform these in your presence before leaving to ensure that he or she is performing them properly and will not cause harm when practicing alone. Stretches should be held for 15–30 seconds and performed frequently throughout the day within the client's limits. The client should not force the stretch or bounce. The stretch should be slow, gentle, and steady, trying to keep every other joint as relaxed as possible.
- Stretching and strengthening exercises should be recommended according to your findings in ROM testing and palpation.

Stretching

Maintaining proper length and tone of the musculotendinous unit, its synergists, and its antagonists is essential to reduce the risk of re-injury. Stretches should be performed throughout the day, particularly before and after activity. The results of ROM testing and palpation will determine which muscles have shortened and need to be stretched. In general, stretching occurs when the distance between the attachment sites of the muscle is increased. Refer to Chapters 4–11 for stretches to specific muscles or groups of muscles. Take care to instruct the client to stretch slowly and to limit stretches to the comfortable range, beginning slowly, and gradually increasing the stretch as symptoms diminish and the risk of re-injury is reduced. Stretching an injured muscle too quickly or too deeply may initiate a reflex response, which may result in spasm. In addition, when the affected muscle is lengthened, its antagonists are shortened. If the antagonists are involved in protective splinting, contracting them too quickly or too deeply may also result in spasm.

Strengthening

Eccentric exercise has been shown to improve recovery from tendinopathies since increasing the load on the tendon encourages collagen proliferation. Eccentric exercises are those that lengthen the injured muscle. For example, if the long head of the biceps brachii is affected by tendinosis, extension of the shoulder increases eccentric loading to the biceps tendon and encourages healing. Eccentric exercise also strengthens the antagonists of the injured muscle, which helps to balance strength on either side of the joint. These exercises should be introduced slowly and increased in intensity only within the client's tolerance.

Strengthening weakened or atrophied muscles is equally important for restoring proper function of the affected joint. The results of ROM testing and palpation will determine which muscles have weakened and need to be strengthened. In general, active or resisted concentric contractions strengthen muscles. As with stretching, a strengthening program should progress gradually. Pain-free, active ROM is effective for gradually restoring strength to weakened muscles. As healing progresses and the risk of re-injury diminishes, add resistance to active ROM. Refer to Chapters 4–11 for exercises to strengthen specific muscles or muscle groups.

SUGGESTIONS FOR FURTHER TREATMENT

Ideally, a client with a tendinopathy will have treatments two or three times a week until the client can perform activities of daily living with minimal or no pain for at least 4 days. Once this has been achieved, reduce frequency to once per week until symptoms are absent for at least 7 days. When the client reports that he or she has been pain-free for more than 7 days, treatment can be reduced to twice per month. If the client is pain-free for 3 or more consecutive weeks, he or she can then schedule appointments once per month or as necessary.

There should be some improvement with each session. If this is not happening, consider the following possibilities:

- There is too much time between treatments. It is always best to give the newly treated tissues 24–48 hours to adapt, but if too much time passes between treatments in the beginning, the client's activities of daily living may reverse any progress.

- The client is not adjusting activities of daily living or is not keeping up with self-care. As much as we want to fix the problem, we cannot force a client to make the adjustments we suggest. Explain the importance of his or her participation in the healing process, and encourage the client to follow your recommendations, but be careful not to judge or reprimand a client who does not.
- The condition is advanced or has other musculoskeletal complications that are beyond your basic training. Refer this client to a massage therapist with advanced training. Continuing to treat a client whose case is beyond your training could hinder healing and turn the client away from massage therapy altogether.
- The client has an undiagnosed, underlying condition. Discontinue treatment until the client sees a health care provider for medical assessment.

If you are not treating the client in a clinical setting or private practice, you may not be able to take this client through the full program of healing. Still, if you can bring some relief in just one treatment, it may encourage the client to discuss this change with a health care provider and seek manual therapy rather than more aggressive treatment options. If the client agrees to return for regular treatments, the symptoms are likely to change each time, so it is important to perform an assessment before each session. Once you have addressed symptoms specific to the tendinopathy, you may be able to pay closer attention to compensating structures and coexisting conditions.

PROFESSIONAL GROWTH

CASE STUDY

Elisa is a 25-year-old student studying fashion design. She has pain in her thumb and palm that began while sewing a piece for her final project. She uses her computer daily, draws sketches of fashion designs with fine detail, and frequently sends text messages and plays games on her cell phone.

Subjective

Elisa stated that she has had episodes of pain in her right hand for the past year, particularly when sewing and sending text messages. She also feels some pain when carrying groceries or other heavy items in bags with handles instead of in a backpack. The worst of the pain is between her thumb and index finger. She does not feel pain in the left hand regularly but has noted that lately it seems weaker than usual. She explained that in the past year, the aching in her right hand has become more frequent and more intense and that, at least a couple of times per week, her thumb and index finger lock and she feels pain in her forearm. She also started feeling general aching in her shoulders. She bought a brace to support her hand but has a hard time performing tasks while wearing it, so she has not used it much. She has tried ibuprofen and felt some relief, but only when she was not using her hands. When she used ibuprofen and continued to work, the pain persisted. When she first felt the symptoms, she had a manicure that included a forearm and hand massage. She said that for that day and the next she had some relief. She hopes that focused massage will have even better, long-term results. She has no known underlying conditions. Her mother, who was a seamstress before retiring, had received a diagnosis of DeQuervain's tenosynovitis. Elisa wants to avoid developing the same condition. When asked, she stated that she has felt no unusual fatigue or malaise and has had no fever, sharp pain, or other unusual symptoms other than the pain in her hand. When asked, she stated that the pain does not wake her from her sleep but that she occasionally feels weakness in the morning when picking up her coffee cup.

Objective

Elisa appears healthy and vibrant. Her handshake was firm with no signs of pain. She had no difficulty turning the doorknob and seemed comfortable using a pen to fill out her intake forms. The right hand is slightly swollen compared to the left. Swelling is general, not specific to any finger. The skin is slightly dry and chapped bilaterally. There is no difference in temperature between the hands. When asked to fully extend the thumb and fingers of both hands, extension on the right side was visibly reduced compared to the left, and Elisa felt aching in her thumb and along the anterior forearm. Passive extension of each individual finger revealed reduced ROM in the thumb and forefingers of both hands with pain on full passive extension of the right thumb. Palpation of the flexor tendons resulted in a level 5 pain on the right flexor pollicis longus, level 2 pain on the right first digit tendon of the flexor digitorum, level 2 pain on the left flexor pollicis. No remarkable results were seen from the passive stretch or palpation of other fingers. Palpation revealed tenderness and hypertonicity in the adductor pollicis and opponens pollicis. Palpation of the forearms revealed adhesions and hypertonicity in the flexors, particularly on the right, and taut bands in the extensors, which were also more pronounced on the right. Palpation of the common flexor tendon produced no pain, and Elisa stated that it felt good. No trigger points were found. Signs and symptoms suggest right flexor pollicis longus tendinosis with short, tight wrist flexors and taut wrist extensors. Shoulder aches may be the result of compensation.

Action

I began in the supine position, bolstering the right arm and applying drainage strokes to reduce minor fluid accumulation in the right hand. I applied general Swedish massage to the pectorals, shoulders, neck, and arms. I proceeded with treatment to the bilateral forearms and hands, beginning on the right with myofascial release using wringing to the forearms and deep fascial techniques to reduce adhesions among flexors and extensors. Adhesions were most significant in the right distal flexors. I applied kneading and stripping to the adductor and opponens pollicis and transverse friction to the forearm muscles, followed by lengthening the flexors and applying broad pressure and circular strokes to the extensors. No trigger points were found. With the forearm supinated, the wrist slightly extended with a bolster, and the fingers held in extension with one hand, I applied transverse friction to the tendons of the flexor pollicis longus and the flexor digitorum. I applied stripping to the same tendons followed by deep effleurage to the same muscles. I performed four rounds of treatment, alternating between friction and the lengthening of tendons with the lengthening of muscles. I applied a full deep stretch to the thumb and fingers, followed by clearing strokes toward the axilla, and 3 minutes of icing to frictioned tendons.

Plan

Following treatment, Elisa stated that she felt much less discomfort in her hands. She continued to feel discomfort on passive extension of the R. thumb and first finger, though less than before treatment. Elisa rescheduled for another treatment in 3 days. I recommended full stretches to the fingers and wrist several times throughout the day. I suggested that she ask her roommate to apply wringing to her forearms occasionally to keep adhesions at bay and demonstrated self-massage to continue reducing adhesions and hypertonicity in the forearms and between the thumb and first digit. I also suggested reducing activities that are least necessary (e.g., texting less during times when she is sewing a lot). I explained that her simple tendinosis could develop into a more serious case. I explained DeQuervain's tenosynovitis, so she can monitor for symptoms. Currently, there is no tenderness in the extensor pollicis, no pain or crepitus with passive flexion of the thumb, and no heat or swelling in the radial aspect of the wrist.

CRITICAL THINKING EXERCISES

1. Your client mentions feeling pain in the left shoulder and points to the anterior aspect, near the head of the humerus. Active extension of the left shoulder is limited compared to extension of the right shoulder, but causes little pain. Full passive extension of the left shoulder causes pain at the very spot the client originally pointed to. Write a SOAP note for this client. Is tendinopathy a possibility? Which tendon might be affected? How will you determine if it is tendinosis, tendinitis, or tenosynovitis? Which muscles may be compensating? Create a scenario that describes how this pattern developed, the signs and symptoms, possible coexisting conditions, a postural assessment, testing, precautions or contraindications, and specific treatment. Use a reference that describes the actions of the muscles to help you correlate the signs and symptoms. There is no single, correct SOAP note for this exercise. Be creative, as the possibilities are virtually endless.

2. This chapter contains references to the coinciding of tendinopathy with one of the conditions described in Chapters 4–11. Choose one of the conditions described in those chapters and discern which tendon could be injured or at risk for tendinopathy based on the client's posture or activities. How will you incorporate tendinopathy into the treatment description for that condition?

3. Conduct a short literature review to learn about the relationship between tendinopathies and the following:
   - Statin medication
   - Fluoroquinolone antibiotics
   - Mesenchymal syndrome
   - Genetic collagen variations

BIBLIOGRAPHY AND SELECTED READINGS

Anderson O. RunnersWeb.com. Science of Sport: Do You Really Have Tendonitis–Or is it Tendinosis? Available at http://www.runnersweb.com/running/news/rw_news_20050513_RRN_Tendons.html. Accessed Spring 2009.

Biel A. *Trail Guide to the Body: How to Locate Muscles, Bones and More*, 3rd ed. Boulder, CO: Books of Discovery, 2005.

Franchi M, Fini M, Quaranta M, et al. Crimp morphology in relaxed and stretched rat Achilles tendon. Journal of Anatomy. 2007;210(1):1–7.

Gehlsen GM, Ganion LR, Helfst R. Fibroblast responses to variation in soft tissue mobilization pressure. Medicine & Science in Sports & Exercise. 1999;31(4):531–535.

Hammer W. The effect of mechanical load on degenerated soft tissue. Journal of Bodywork and Movement Therapies. 2008;12(3):246–256.

Hertling D, Kessler R. *Management of Common Musculoskeletal Disorders: Physical Therapy Principles and Methods*, 4th ed. Philadelphia, PA: Lippincott Williams & Wilkins, 2006.

James R, Kesturu G, Balian G, et al. Tendon: Biology, biomechanics, repair, growth factors, and evolving treatment options. Journal of Hand Surgery. 2008;33(1):102–112.

Khan KM, Cook JL. Overuse tendon injuries: Where does the pain come from? Sports Medicine and Arthroscopic Review. 2000;8(1):17–31.

Khan KM, Cook JL, Taunton JE, et al. Overuse tendinosis, not tendinitis. The Physician and Sports Medicine. 2000;28(5):5.

Lowe W. *Orthopedic Massage: Theory and Technique*. St Louis, MO: Mosby-Elsevier, 2003.

Mayo Foundation for Medical Education and Research. Bursitis. Available at http://www.mayoclinic.com/health/bursitis/DS00032. Accessed Spring 2009.

Mayo Foundation for Medical Education and Research. Myofascial Pain Syndrome. Available at http://www.mayoclinic.com/health/myofascial-pain-syndrome/DS01042. Accessed Spring 2009.

Mayo Foundation for Medical Education and Research. Sprains and Strains. Available at http://mayoclinic.com/health/sprains-and-strains/DS00343. Accessed Spring 2009.

Oatis C. *Kinesiology: The Mechanics and Pathomechanics of Human Movement*, 2nd ed. Baltimore, MD: Lippincott Williams & Wilkins, 2009.

Pedrelli A, Stecco C, Day JA. Treating patellar tendinopathy with fascial manipulation. Journal of Bodywork and Movement Therapies. 2009;13(1):73–80.

Rattray F, Ludwig L. *Clinical Massage Therapy: Understanding, Assessing and Treating over 70 Conditions*. Toronto, ON: Talus Incorporated, 2000.

Riley G. Tendinopathy—From basic science to treatment. Nature Clinical Practice Rheumatology. 2008;4 (2):82–89. Available at http://www.nature.com/nrrheum/journal/v4/n2/full/ncprheum0700.html. Accessed Spring 2009.

Shoulder-Pain-Management. Calcific tendonitis. Available at http://www.shoulder-pain-management.com/CalcificTendonitis.html. Accessed Spring 2009.

Vogel KG. Tendon structure and response to changing mechanical load. Journal of Musculoskeletal Neuron Interaction. 2003;3(4):323–325.

Werner R. *A Massage Therapist's Guide to Pathology*, 4th ed. Baltimore, MD: Lippincott Williams and Wilkins, 2009.

Zatsiorsky VM. *Biomechanics in Sport: Performance Enhancement and Injury Prevention*. Malden, MA: Blackwell Science, 2000.

Index

Note: Page locators followed by b, f and t indicates box, figure and table respectively.